Practical FDG Imaging

Springer Science+Business Media, LLC

Dominique Delbeke, MD, PhD
William H. Martin, MD
James A. Patton, PhD
Martin P. Sandler, MD
Department of Radiology and Radiological Sciences,
Vanderbilt University Medical Center, Nashville, Tennessee

Editors

Practical FDG Imaging

A Teaching File

With a Foreword by R. Edward Coleman, MD

With 146 Illustrations in 316 Parts

Springer

Dominique Delbeke, MD, PhD
William H. Martin, MD
James A. Patton, PhD
Martin P. Sandler, MD
Department of Radiology and Radiological Sciences
Vanderbilt University Medical Center
Nashville, TN 37232
USA

Library of Congress Cataloging-in-Publication Data
Practical FDG imaging : a teaching file / Dominique Delbeke . . . [et al.].
p. ; cm.
Includes bibliographical references and index.
ISBN 978-1-4757-7688-1 ISBN 978-0-387-22453-4 (eBook)
DOI 10.1007/978-0-387-22453-4

1. Tomography, Emission. I. Delbeke, Dominique.
[DNLM: 1. Tomography, Emission-Computed—methods. 2. Fludeoxyglucose F 18—diagnostic use. 3. Fluorine Radioisotopes—diagnostic use. WN 206 P895 2001]
RC78.7.T62 P733 2001
616.07'575—dc21 2001032004

Printed on acid-free paper.

Production coordinated by Chernow Editorial Services, Inc., and managed by MaryAnn Brickner; manufacturing supervised by Jerome Basma.
Typeset by SNP Best-set Typesetter Ltd., Hong Kong.

9 8 7 6 5 4 3 2

ISBN 978-1-4757-7688-1 SPIN 10956618

To our families

Philippe, Cerine, and Cedric Jeanty
Cynthia, Lauren, and David Martin
Beverly, Jimmy, and David Patton
Glynis, Kim, and Carla Sandler

Foreword

FDG imaging is one of the most rapidly growing techniques in radiology. Even though the technology that has led to modern day PET scanning was developed in the early 1970s, PET scanning was only used clinically in any significant numbers starting in the late 1990s. It took so long for PET to be used clinically simply because of the absence of policy for reimbursement until 1998. One limitation for reimbursement was related to absence of approval of FDG by the Food and Drug Administration (FDA). In 1997, Congress passed the Food and Drug Administration Modernization Act that gave PET radiopharmaceuticals the equivalence of FDA approval. In January 1998, following the approval of FDG, the Health Care Financing Administration (HCFA) developed a policy to cover PET scans for evaluation of solitary pulmonary nodules and the initial staging of lung cancer. This policy was followed by an expansion of the policy in July 1999, when the following indications were covered: detection of recurrent colorectal cancer with rising CEA, detection of recurrent malignant melanoma and initial staging and restaging of lymphoma. Other third parties developed coverage policies similar to those of the HCFA, and many third-party payers covered more than the indications approved by the HCFA.

As the number of indications covered by third-party payers increased, the use of PET scanning increased. This increase in usage resulted in more investment going into PET imaging, and the instrumentation industry made major efforts to improve PET instrumentation. These improvements have been in both camera-based and dedicated systems. Marked improvements have occurred in the camera-based systems with thicker crystals which result in studies that have more counts in the images, better methods of attenuation correction including CT-based attenuation correction, and fusion imaging of the PET scan with the CT scan. The dedicated systems have improvements consisting of being able to acquire the studies in a shorter time period because of the use of iterative reconstruction algorithms and segmented attenuation correction. There are combined CT-dedicated PET scanners, and the images are dramatically improved because of the noise-free attenuation correction. Furthermore, the ability to have fusion imaging of the PET and CT scans makes these studies more useful diagnostically.

The rapid increase in the availability of PET imaging has resulted in the need for more training in FDG imaging. This training is being performed at regional and national meetings and at a few academic medical centers that provide CME courses on PET imaging. Books devoted to current techniques for performing and interpreting FDG PET studies are now being widely sought.

This book provides information necessary for performing FDG imaging and interpreting the studies. The book is unique for several reasons: It is current; it has both camera-based and dedicated PET scans; it is authored by individuals with extensive experience in clinical PET imaging; it covers both the technical and clinical aspects of FDG imaging; and it presents cases of all the malignancies that one is likely to see in a clinical PET practice.

The authors provide examples of normal variants and frequently found imaging artifacts. The characteristic findings in disorders of the central nervous system, cardiac disease, and oncology are included.

Dr. Delbeke and her colleagues are to be congratulated for providing this important information in a timely fashion. Individuals who are starting to do PET imaging will find the information in this book helpful in their practice and will find it worthwhile to have this as a reference book.

R. Edward Coleman, MD
Professor of Radiology
Vice-Chairman of Department of Radiology
Duke University Medical Center
Durham, North Carolina

Preface

Practical FDG Imaging: A Teaching File is intended to provide a reference source of cases with FDG images obtained both on dedicated PET tomographs and hybrid scintillation gamma cameras. The cases are presented in depth so that they will be of value to both the specialist physician and resident in training who need to learn the indications and interpretation of FDG images and the advantages and limitations of hybrid scintillation gamma cameras compared to dedicated PET tomographs. The book is designed to be used by residents training in nuclear medicine and radiology, by nuclear medicine physicians and radiologists in private or academic practice who need to become familiar with this technology, and those whose specialties carry over to FDG imaging. The first three chapters cover the technical aspects of FDG imaging, including the history of PET development, physics of positron imaging, and FDG production and distribution. Chapters 4, 5, and 6 are devoted to clinical applications in the fields of neurology, cardiology, and oncology. Each chapter begins with an introduction summarizing the literature, principles for interpretation of FDG images and clinical indications. Chapter 6 begins with a section describing the normal and physiologic variations of FDG distribution, as well as the related pitfalls in image interpretation. The following sections of Chapter 6 are devoted to the role of FDG imaging in different types of body tumors. After the introduction, each of the clinical chapters includes a series of cases presentations ranging from the simple to the more complex. In an attempt to simulate normal clinical practice, cases have been organized without any order of priority.

We sincerely hope this text will provide nuclear physicians, radiologists, trainees, and those with an interest in FDG imaging with a reference text of teaching files that will enhance their practice of clinical PET and help those preparing for board examinations.

Dominique Delbeke, MD, PhD
William H. Martin, MD
James A. Patton, PhD
Martin P. Sandler, MD

Acknowledgments

We wish to acknowledge the work of our Vanderbilt PET technologists, Janine E. Belote, M. Dawn Shone, and Sarah A. Washburn, for their outstanding technical assistance in acquiring and processing the images shown in this book. We are particularly indebted to Ronald C. Arildsen and Thomas A. Powers from body CT and Dr. Robert M. Kessler from neuroradiology in the Department of Radiology and Radiological Sciences at Vanderbilt University Medical Center for their invaluable help in interpreting the correlative studies. We would like to thank all contributors, including the authors and publishers, who have granted us permission to reproduce their illustrations.

Dominique Delbeke, MD, PhD
William H. Martin, MD
James A. Patton, PhD
Martin P. Sandler, MD

Contents

Contributors

Jeroen J. Bax, MD, PhD
Faculty, Department of Cardiology, Leiden University Medical Center, 2333 AA Leiden, The Netherlands

Eric Boersma, PhD
Faculty, Division of Cardiology, Thorax Center, Erasmus Medical Center, 3015 GD Rotterdam, The Netherlands

Jeff Clanton, MS, PhD, BCNP
Associate in Radiology and Radiological Sciences, Chief of Radiopharmacy, PET Center, Department of Radiology and Radiological Sciences, Vanderbilt University Medical Center, Nashville, TN 37232-2675, USA

Dominique Delbeke, MD, PhD
Director and Professor, Division of Nuclear Medicine/PET Center, Department of Radiology and Radiological Sciences, Vanderbilt University Medical Center Nashville, TN 37232-2675, USA

Abdou Elhendy, MD, PhD
Faculty, Division of Cardiology, Thorax Center, Erasmus Medical Center, 3015 GD Rotterdam, The Netherlands

Amy B. Gibson, MD
Clinical Instructor, Department of Radiology and Radiological Sciences, Vanderbilt University Medical Center, Nashville, TN 37232-2675, USA

Marcus V. Grigolon, MD
Clinical Fellow, Division of Nuclear Medicine, Department of Radiology, School of Medical Sciences, Campinas State University, Campinas 13024, Brazil

Orlin Woodie Hopper, MD
Clinical Instructor, Department of Radiology and Radiological Sciences, Vanderbilt University Medical Center, Nashville, TN 37232-2675, USA

Darrin L. Johnson, MD
Clinical Instructor, Department of Radiology and Radiological Sciences, Vanderbilt University Medical Center, Nashville, TN 37232-2675, USA

Chris Y. Kim, MD
Clinical Fellow, Division of Cardiology, Department of Internal Medicine, Vanderbilt University Medical Center, Nashville, TN 37232, USA

Tsuyoshi Komori, MD, PhD
Instructor, Department of Radiology, Osaka Medical College, Osaka, Japan

Mark Kuzucu, MD
Clinical Instructor, Department of Radiology and Radiological Sciences, Vanderbilt University Medical Center, Nashville, TN 37232-2675, USA

William H. Martin, MD
Associate Professor of Radiology and Medicine, Division of Nuclear Medicine/PET, Co-Director of Nuclear Cardiology, Department of Radiology and Radiological Sciences, Vanderbilt University Medical Center, Nashville, TN 37232-2675, USA

James A. Patton, PhD
Professor of Radiology and Physics, Department of Radiology and Radiological Sciences, Vanderbilt University Medical Center, Nashville, TN 37232-2675, USA

Michael E. Phelps, PhD
Chair, Department of Molecular and Medical Pharmacology, Director, Crump Institute for Biological Imaging, Associate Director, Laboratory of Structural Biology and Molecular Medicine, Chief, Division of Nuclear Medicine, University of California, Los Angeles, Los Angeles, CA 90024, USA

Don Poldermans, MD, PhD
Faculty, Division of Cardiology, Thorax Center, Erasmus Medical Center, 3015 GD Rotterdam, The Netherlands

Stanley L. Pope, MD
Clinical Instructor, Department of Radiology and Radiological Sciences, Vanderbilt University Medical Center, Nashville, TN 37232-2675, USA

Martin P. Sandler, MD
Professor of Radiology and Medicine, Chairman of Radiology, Department of Radiology and Radiological Sciences, Vanderbilt University Medical Center, Nashville, TN 37232-2675, USA

A.F.L. Schinkel, MD
Faculty, Division of Cardiology, Thorax Center, Erasmus Medical Center, 3015 GD Rotterdam, The Netherlands

Gerrit W. Sloof, MD, PhD
Faculty, Division of Cardiology, Thorax Center, Erasmus Medical Center, 3015 GD Rotterdam, The Netherlands

LeAnn Simmons-Stokes, MD
Clinical Instructor, Department of Radiology and Radiological Sciences, Vanderbilt University Medical Center, Nashville, TN 37232-2675, USA

1
History of PET

Michael E. Phelps

There are three major technical components of positron emission tomography (PET): PET scanner, cyclotron production of radiopharmaceuticals, and biological assays of normal and disease processes. A historical perspective from the early development stages through today is given for each of these technology areas, as well as some predictions for the future. Details of the technologies are given on PET scanners and cameras in Chapter 2 and for cyclotron production of radiopharmaceuticals in Chapter 3.

Molecular Imaging with PET

The overall process for performing a molecular imaging examination of the biological nature of disease with PET is shown in Figure 1.1. This figure illustrates the imaging of glucose metabolism within organ systems of the body using the labeled molecule 2-[F-18]-2-deoxy-2-fluoro-D-glucose (FDG). FDG represents a molecular imaging probe labeled with a positron emitting radionuclide, fluorine-18. The action of FDG as a glucose analog is shown in Figure 1.2, along with another molecular imaging probe, 3′-deoxy-3′-[F-18]fluorothymidine (FLT) for imaging DNA replication.[1]

Glucose metabolism is imaged by injecting FDG intravenously, after which FDG is delivered to the organ systems of the body via the bloodstream. FDG is transported from plasma into cells via the glucose facilitated carrier system and trapped in cells by phosphorylation to provide a record of glucose metabolism. The PET scanner is a camera that records the location and tissue concentration of positron emission by the unique coincidence detection of the 180° emission of the two 511 keV photons from positron annihilation (Figure 1.1). A reconstruction algorithm is used to convert the data collected at various angles around the subject into three-dimensional tomographic images in any desired planes, that is, transverse, coronal, or sagittal.

Why Was PET Developed?

As discussed later in this chapter and more extensively in Chapter 2, the unique simultaneous emission of two 511 keV photons 180° apart and the use of electronic coincidence detection provide high spatial resolution that is nearly depth independent, high detection efficiency, and an accurate way to correct for tissue attenuation of 511 keV photons.[2–4] As a result, PET scanners accurately satisfy the mathematical requirements of the image reconstruction algorithm and provide high image quality and quantitative measurements of biological processes for research and clinical practice.[5,6]

Further, the only radioactive forms of the major natural elements of the body—oxygen, nitrogen, and carbon—that can be detected externally are positron emitters. There is no positron emitting form of hydrogen, and therefore, fluorine-18 is used as a hydrogen substitute. Fluorine is, in its own right, a common molecule used in biochemistry and the pharmaceutical industry as a modifier of the

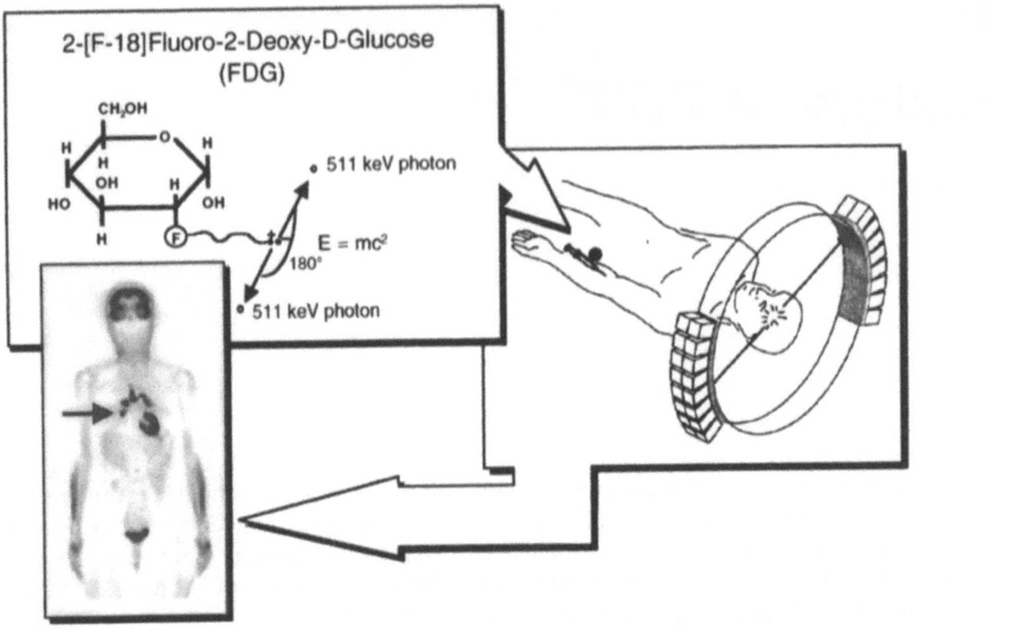

FIGURE 1.1. Principles of PET. A biologically active molecule is labeled with positron-emitting radioisotope. The example shown is of FDG, for imaging glucose metabolism. Two 511-keV photons produced from positron annihilation ($E = mc^2$) are detected when these two photons strike opposing detectors, providing a unique form of electronic collimation. One line of coincidence detection is shown, but in modern tomographs, approximately 1 to 70 million detector pair combinations or more can record events simultaneously. Detectors are arranged either in the dual-head configuration shown or around the entire circumference. Modern dual-head and circumferential PET scanners collect sufficient data to form more than 60 tomographic image planes simultaneously. Tomographic images are collected for the selected organ or for the entire body. The figure shows a single 6mm thick coronal image in a woman with bilateral metastasis to lung (arrow) from previous ovarian cancer that was surgically resected. Black is the highest metabolic rate in the image. (Reprinted with permission from the Journal of Nuclear Medicine.[5])

properties of molecules. For example, fluorine is a small element that forms strong carbon-fluorine bonds (110 kilo calories), and so, it is often used to limit unwanted properties while retaining desired ones. FDG is a good example of this. Fluorine is substituted for an OH in the 2 position of glucose. The result is that FDG remains a substrate for glucose facilitated transport carriers across capillary and cell membranes and competes with glucose as a substrate for hexokinase to be phosphorylated to FDG-6-PO_4. The fluorine in the 2 position, however, inhibits metabolism of FDG-6-PO_4 to continue down the glycolytic pathway as well as its dephosphorylation (Figure 1.2). While the small size and properties of fluorine maintain FDG as a substrate for transport and phosphorylation, going to any of the next halogens, Cl, Br, or I, removes these properties.

FDG originated from the development of [C-14]-2-deoxyglucose (DG) imaging with autoradiography in animals by Sokoloff et al.[7] DG is formed by substituting H for OH in the 2 position in the glucose molecule. FDG is formed by substituting F for H in the 2 position of DG. FDG was first synthesized by Ido et al.[8] and tracer kinetic models were developed for PET and FDG by Phelps et al.,[9] Reivich et al.,[10] and Huang et al.[11] to provide the means to calculate the rate of glucose metabolism in units of micromoles/min/g tissue. Interestingly, DG and FDG were originally developed as drugs to

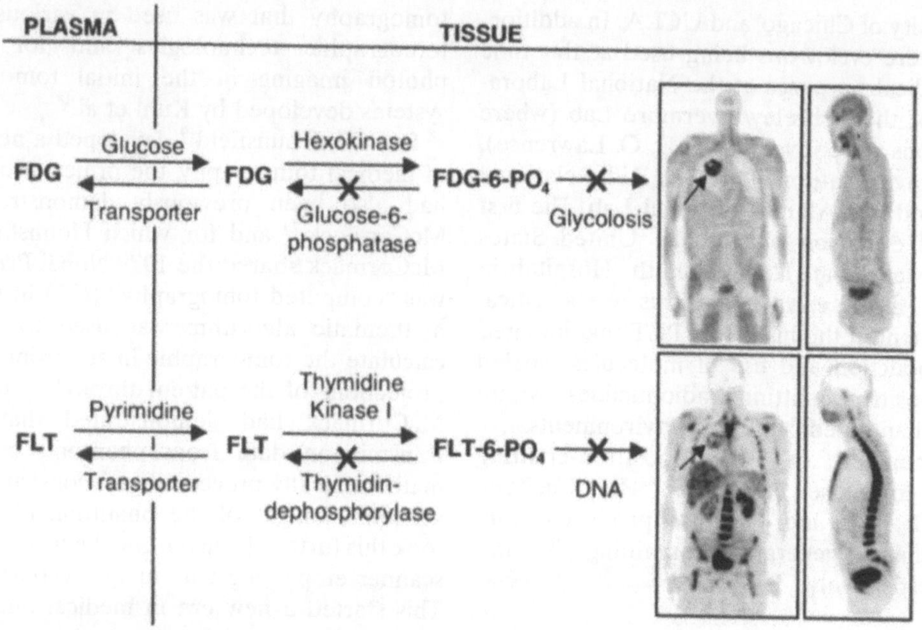

FIGURE 1.2. Tracer kinetic models for FDG and FLT. The arrows show forward and reverse carrier mediated transport between plasma and tissue phosphorylation. Both FDG and FLT phosphates are not significant substrates for dephosphorylation or further metabolism at normal imaging times of 40 to 60 minutes after injection. Models taking dephosphorylation reaction into account at much later image times have been developed.[9,11] Images are 6 mm thick longitudinal tomographic sections of a patient with a non–small-cell lung cancer (arrows), with high glucose metabolism and DNA replication. The rest of the images show normal distribution of glucose utilization and DNA replication, exceptions being clearance of both tracers to bladder (arrowhead) and, in the case of FLT, the glucuronidation by hepatocytes in liver. (Courtesy of Anthony Shields.)

block accelerated rates of glycolysis in tumors[12] because at pharmacologic doses, FDG (DG)-6-PO_4 builds up in cells and shuts down further phosphorylation of glucose by binding to hexokinase. Although FDG (DG) was successful in shutting down glycolysis in tumors at pharmacologic doses, it was not successful as a drug because in these high mass amounts it also shut down glycolysis of the brain that cannot switch to other substrates, at least not in adults.

The example with FDG illustrates that PET is a quantitative molecular imaging technique for examining the biological properties of normal cellular function, as well as those of disease. Over 500 different molecular imaging probes[13] have been developed to examine various biological and biochemical processes, ranging from blood flow, metabolism, synthesis, receptor modulated signal transduction, and hormone functions to the expression of genes.[5,6]

Production of PET Imaging Probes

The positron emitting radionuclides of O-15, N-13, C-11, and F-18 are produced with particle accelerators, typically cyclotrons. Cyclotrons were originally developed for research in nuclear physics. Michel Ter Pogossian in the United States lead the way in introducing cyclotrons into hospitals for research using positron-emitting radionuclides. The Department of Energy (DOE) under Ter Pogossian's urging, installed cyclotrons in a number of hospitals throughout the United States in the mid-1960s to early 1970s. These initial sites were Washington University, Sloan-Kettering,

University of Chicago, and UCLA. In addition, there were cyclotrons being used at this time for medical purposes at the National Laboratories of the Berkeley/Livermore Lab (where cyclotrons were invented by E. O. Lawrence), Brookhaven National Lab, Oak Ridge National Labs, and Los Alamos National Lab. The first medical cyclotron outside the United States was installed at Hammersmith Hospital in London in the early 1960s. This was a critical experiment in the history of PET that initiated the production and use of molecules labeled with positron-emitting radionuclides within hospital and medical school environments.

A number of other positron-emitting radioisotopes used in PET are ^{82}Rb, ^{64}Cu, ^{68}Ga, and ^{124}I. ^{82}Rb and ^{68}Ga are produced from ion-exchange generators containing ^{82}Sr and ^{68}Ge, respectively.

PET Imaging Systems

Studies of positron labeled compounds in animals and patients began with detector systems that were used to record the kinetics of positron labeled compounds in vivo, but not to image them. Two major developments changed this: the development of positron imaging cameras and, subsequently, the development of PET. Positron imaging began with Brownell and colleagues'[14,15] development of a dual-head camera made up of discrete NaI (Tl) detectors and coincidence detection to form two-dimensional images of positron labeled components in animals and patients. Muehllehner et al.[16] modified a NaI (Tl) gamma camera to have dual opposing detector heads and coincidence detection. Robertson et al.[17] developed a circular array of NaI (Tl) using coincidence detection. Brownell et al.[14,15] also developed a method to sort data into focal planes at various depths between the detector heads. Robertson et al. used a circular design to collect data at various angles around the subject and formed tomographic images by projecting the data from each detector pair across the space between the detector pair and then adding all the detector pair data from all angles collected to form an image. These approaches were a class of imaging approaches called "blurring" tomography that was used in various X-ray tomographic technologies and for single-photon imaging in the initial tomographic systems developed by Kuhl et al.[18]

In 1973, Hounsfield[19] developed a new form of medical tomography, the principle of which had also been previously demonstrated by McCormack,[20] and for which Hounsfield and McCormack shared the 1979 Nobel Prize. This was "computed tomography" (CT) in which a mathematic algorithm was used to actually calculate the tomographic image from angular projections of the patient through a 180° arc. McCormack had demonstrated that X-ray transmission data from phantoms could be mathematically processed to reconstruct cross-sectional images of the phantom. Hounsfield took this further by inventing the first X-ray CT scanner employing true image reconstruction. This started a new era in medical imaging of computed tomography.

PET began in 1973 and 1974, with the development of a circumferential array of NaI (Tl) detectors arranged in a hexagonal geometry (Figure 1.3) by Phelps et al.[2,21,22] This system employed coincidence detection, proper linear and angular sampling, attenuation correction for 511 keV photons in tissue, and near spatially invarient resolution to meet mathematical criteria of the computed tomography algorithm. Images were then reconstructed with a proper convolution based image reconstruction algorithm. This system was called a positron emission transaxial tomograph (PETT). The first scanner was called PETT II and was used for phantom and animal studies to define the physical and mathematical requirements of PET.[2] The first human system was called PETT III.[21,22] PETT I was a system of the same geometric design but used conventional lead collimators and was quickly converted to coincidence detection because of its favorable properties to meet the mathematical criteria of the image reconstruction algorithm.

This initiated a time when many labs and companies would contribute to the evolution of PET scanner technology as it is today[3,4] (Chapter 2). Subsequently, Phelps changed the name from PETT to PET by dropping the word "transaxial" because tomographic images could

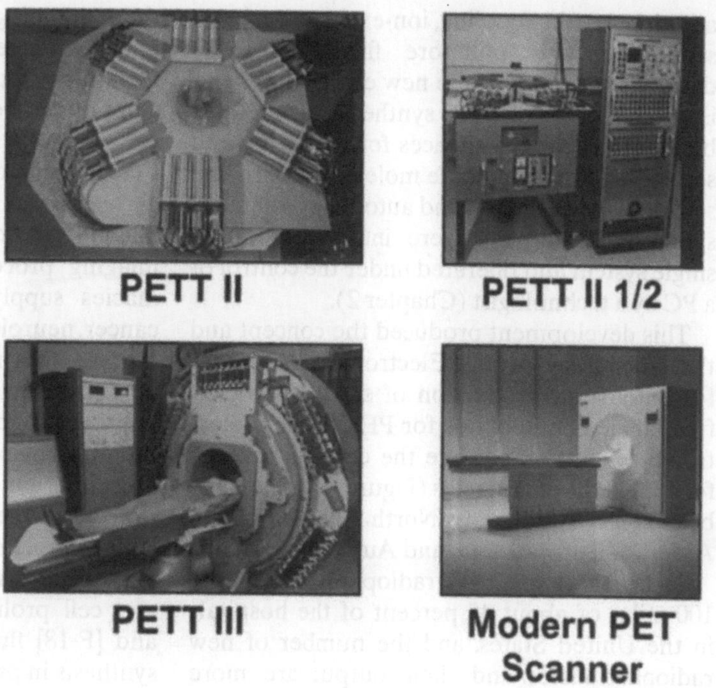

FIGURE 1.3. Photographs of the PETT II, PETT II 1/2, PETT III, and a modern commercial PET scanner. In the PETT II photograph, a phantom can be seen in the field of view of the 24 NaI (Tl) detectors. PETT II was developed in November 1973. By February 1974, PETT II had been converted to PETT II 1/2, having a hole in the center with a computer controlled turntable that automatically rotated phantoms and animals 60 degrees. The computer of the system was used to collect, attenuation correct, reconstruct, and display tomographic images. PETT III had a transparent cover so the 48 Na(Tl) detectors arranged in a hexagonal array could be seen. An example of a typical commercial scanner of today is also shown.

be reconstructed and displayed in many planes other than transaxial.

Purpose of PET in Medicine

PET grew out of a need to merge imaging with biochemistry and biology. PET was also used to take the lead in defining a new field of molecular imaging. In a similar way, biochemistry and biology were also being merged with medicine to form molecular medicine. Molecular medicine is focused on identifying the original molecular errors of disease and developing molecular corrections for them, including gene therapy. Molecular imaging with PET is part of this new molecular medicine with a role of examining the biological nature of disease, for its proper characterization and to guide the selection and evaluation of treatments based on these biological criteria, and eventually developing a new biological classification of disease. Molecular imaging is part of the new approaches to molecular diagnostics, from molecular imaging to chip technologies, that are coming together with the new molecular therapeutics.

Preparation of Molecular Imaging Probes

PET radioisotopes are produced by particle accelerators, typically cyclotrons. The early cyclotrons used in PET were relatively large cyclotrons from a nuclear physics origin that had to be placed in "vaults" with four feet thick (or greater) concrete walls, had complicated control systems and required sophisticated chemistry labs for labeling biological molecules with a high level of professional staffing for the cyclotron and chemistry. This was costly and impractical for clinical medicine. A solution had to be invented.

What began as a severe handicap for PET was turned into an advantage through innovation. In the mid-1980s, cyclotron technology was developed to specifically meet the needs of PET. First, small, self-shield, single-particle cyclotrons were developed. Second, automated chemical synthesis technology was developed for the production of routinely used positron labeled compounds. These devices consisted of a series of unit operations, such as solvent and reagent addition, heating/cooling, ion-exchange column separation, and millipore filtration. These devices are similar to the new electronic chemistry technology of DNA synthesizers and combinatorial chemistry devices for preparing and separating drug candidate molecules. Third, the self-shielded cyclotron and automated chemical synthesis technology were integrated into a single system and operated under the control of a PC by a technologist (Chapter 2).

This development produced the concept and the technology of an "Electronic Generator" for automated production of sterile, pyrogen-free labeled compounds for PET.[23] These electronic generators became the core technology for PET radiopharmacies (Figure 1.4) that have been constructed across North America, South America, Europe, Asia, and Australia.

Today, there is a PET radiopharmacy within 100 miles of about 45 percent of the hospitals in the United States, and the number of new radiopharmacies and their output are more than doubling each year. These PET radiopharmacies removed the burden of cyclotron technology and synthesis of positron labeled compounds from clinics that provide PET clinical service. PET radiopharmacies provide the delivery of PET labeled compounds, just as occurs for conventional nuclear medicine, allowing the clinical practices to focus on the imaging procedures. Today, these radiopharmacies supply FDG for clinical studies in cancer, neurological disorders, and cardiovascular disease. This will, however, be the source of new positron labeled imaging probes as they are approved for clinical use. A number of new PET radiopharmaceuticals for clinical service are presently under review or entering the review process of the Food and Drug Administration (FDA). Examples include [F-18]FDOPA for movement disorders, FLT for DNA replication and cell proliferation in cancer (Figure 1.2), and [F-18] fluorocholine for accelerated lipid synthesis in prostate cancer.

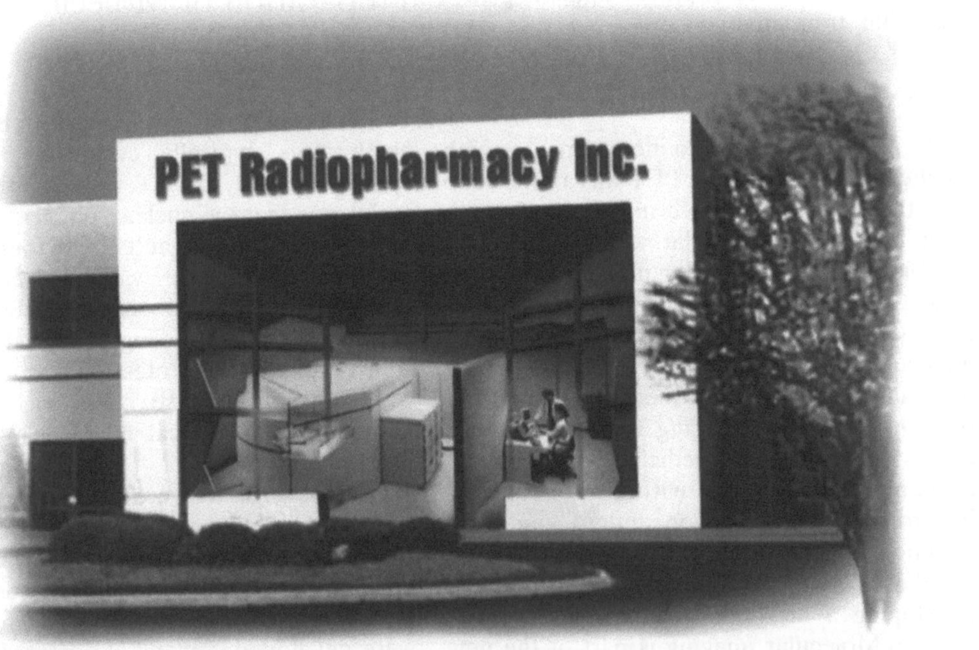

FIGURE 1.4. PET radiopharmacy using "electronic generators." The electronic generator is a miniaturized self-shielded cyclotron integrated with automated chemical synthesizers into a single system operated by personal computer. (PET Radiopharmacy Inc. is generic name.) (Reprinted with permission from the Journal of Nuclear Medicine.[5])

Biological Basis of FDG

The value of FDG is based on the importance of glucose metabolism in normal cellular function and as an indicator of disease that has been well established in biochemistry and biology. This is exemplified by the fact that glucose metabolism is:

- Critical to proper cell function.
- Provides greater than 95 percent of ATP for cerebral function.
- Protective and increased in ischemic tissue.
- Increased 19- to 25-fold in malignant cancers.

The utility of FDG resulting from the preceding is that FDG:

- Measures glucose metabolism.
- Differentiates malignant from benign lesions.
- Differentiates malignant tissue from edemous, necrotic, and scar tissues.
- Differentiates reversible from irreversible ischemic tissue.
- Detects early, even asymptomatic disease[5,6] that has no detectable anatomical abnormality on CT and magnetic resonance imaging (MRI).

Merger of PET and Pharmaceutical Discovery Processes

An interesting development is now occurring in the merger of the development of PET molecular imaging probes and the drug discovery process. This is occurring for several reasons. One reason is that molecular imaging probes and drugs share a number of common properties and provide benefits to each other's discovery process. PET molecular imaging molecules are used in low mass amounts to image and measure the function of the molecular disease target. Drugs are used in high mass amounts to modify the function of the molecular disease target. They use, however, the same molecule or analogs of the same molecule to achieve these purposes. Most of the desired properties for both applications are the same, although there are some differences that are desired or allowable for each as shown in Table 1.1.

TABLE 1.1. Desired properties of biological imaging probes and drugs.

Property	Imaging probe	Drug
Small molecule	Yes	Yes
High affinity for target	Yes	Yes
Low affinity for nontargets	Yes	Yes
Require target to background ratio to be >1	Yes	No
Sufficient lipophilicity or carrier system for crossing cell membranes rapidly	Yes	Yes
Clearance from plasma with a halftime of minute to hours	Yes	No*
Is not rapidly metabolized systematically	Yes	Yes

* Prefer halftimes of hours to days.

The development of the microPET scanner by Cherry et al.[24,25] for mice and the development of genetically engineered and human disease cell transplant models of disease in mice have provided a common in vivo mammalian platform to study the biological nature of disease and develop new molecular therapies. The drug discovery process needed a technology to study the pharmacokinetics, pharmacodynamics, titration of the drug to the molecular disease target, and methods for accessing the biological outcome in living mouse models of disease. MicroPET provides this.

In addition, the field of PET research needed access to the proprietary molecular libraries and combinatorial chemistry and high throughput chemical screening technologies within the drug industry. Many partnerships have been developed that have brought together the PET molecular probe and drug discovery processes. These include technology transfer agreements between academic PET programs and pharmaceutical companies, as well as the establishment of molecular imaging programs with PET, MRI, and optical imaging technologies within pharmaceutical companies, focused on biological selection and screening of drugs in the living animal, particularly the mouse.[5,6] This brings the enormous intellectual, technical, and financial resources of the pharmaceutical companies to the PET molecular imaging probe discovery process. PET also provides the pharmaceutical companies with a pathway from microPET in mice to clinical PET in patients based on a commonality of methods used.

PET Scanners and Cameras

Principles of a PET Scanner

In positron decay, the positron is emitted from the nucleus and travels a short distance colliding with electrons until coming to rest bound to an electron. Since the positron is an antielectron, the positron/electron combination annihilates, releasing two 511 keV photons 180° apart. The unique form of emission allows for an "electronic collimation" to define the origin of the emission, as shown in Figure 1.1. This is called "coincidence detection" because of the requirement that the two photons strike opposing detectors within a short time of typically 5 to 15 nanoseconds. Electronic circuits record the coincidence event, determining that the original positron emission occurred along a line between the two opposing detectors.

Coincidence detection also allows one detector element to register events with many detectors on the opposing side of the detector array. This can be in a fan beam geometry, or if there are multiple planes of detectors, a cone beam of events can be collected. This provides for an efficient mode of detection. In comparison, one resolution element in the use of lead collimators can only have one line of response at a time to detect gamma rays, and the resolution worsens with distance from the collimator. This is contrasted to PET in which each resolution element can have hundreds of lines of response detecting the 511 keV photons simultaneously, with nearly depth independent resolution.

Sufficient data are collected in a linear direction across the object and sufficient angles through an 180° arc around the subject to quantitatively reconstruct tomographic images of the tissue concentration of the positron-emitting radionuclides. This quantitative feature of the PET scanner is used with tracer kinetic models to calculate the concentrations and reaction rates of biochemical and biological processes.[5,6]

Early PET Scanners

Figure 1.3 shows the evolution from the first prototype PET scanners (PETT II, PETT II 1/2)[2] to the first human PET scanner (PETT III)[21,22] and an example of a modern commercial PET scanner. PETT II and PETT II 1/2 were used to develop the physical and mathematical principles and design approaches of PET using phantom studies and physical measures of performance. They were also used to perform animal studies of the brain, heart, and other organ systems of the body. The results from PETT II and PETT II 1/2 led to the design and construction of PETT III, the results of which led to the first commercial PET scanner through a technology transfer to industry, Emission Computed Axial Tomography (ECAT)[26,27] by ORTEC/EG & G. The rights to ECAT were later acquired by CTI who partnered with Siemens. The early commercial supply of ECAT scanners allowed PET research programs to be established worldwide. Today there are numerous commercial sources of PET scanners such as CTI/Siemens, GE, ADAC/Philips, Marconi, and Positron Corporation. In addition, there are a number of mobile PET companies, such as Radiology Corporation of America, Mobile PET and Alliance.

The PETT II and PETT III scanners employed a hexagonal array of NaI (Tl) detectors. Brownell et al.[28] also adopted a proper image reconstruction algorithm to his dual-head camera of discrete NaI (Tl) detectors to provide both two-dimensional camera images and tomographic images after rotation through an 180° arc.

In 1976, two other major events occurred, the introduction of bismuth oxygerminate (BGO) as a high-efficiency detector for PET and the circular geometry of PET scanners by Cho et al.[29,30] and Derenzo et al.[31–33] BGO and circular geometry became the standard for PET scanners until today.

During the late 1970s and early 1980s, the complexity of PET scanners increased substantially to provide higher resolution and higher efficiency. The initial PETT II was composed of 24 NaI (Tl) detectors, each with a diameter of 5 cm. There were only 12 coincidence lines of response (LOR) between detectors, although additional LORs were collected by rotating the object under study by 60 degrees to collect the necessary angular data to reconstruct tomographic images. An external source of a positron emitter was used with and without the object in the scanner to provide corrections for attenuation. Tomographic images were reconstructed with a convolution based image reconstruction algorithm.

The PETT III was composed of 48 NaI (Tl) detectors with 192 coincidence lines of response and employed a fan beam configuration of LOR. Each detector was 3.8 cm in diameter. In the PETT III, the detectors were moved laterally over the distance of a detector diameter (3.8 cm) and the gantry rotated 60 degrees to collect the necessary linear and angular data. After attenuation corrections, images were reconstructed. Some of the performance and design characteristics from PETT II to modern PET scanners are shown in Table 1.2, and image comparisons are shown in Figures 1.5 and 1.6.

Since the spatial resolution of PET scanners is improved as the size of the detector element is reduced (Chapter 2), the size of PET detector elements started decreasing, and with this, the number of detector elements and the number of coincidence lines of response was increasing rapidly. This complexity was further expanded by using multiple rings of detectors. Up to this point, PET systems used circumferential arrays of individual detectors and photomultiplier tubes to meet the high count requirements of PET. Cost factors were beginning to limit the resolution that could be obtained with PET due to the large numbers of individual small detectors. In addition, photo multiplier tube technology was not being miniaturized to meet the requirements of decreasing detector size.

Transition to Today's PET Scanners

Once again, a solution had to be invented for progress to occur in improving spatial resolution by getting around limitations in photo multiplier tubes and issues of cost. This invention is called the "block detector."[34] The block detector is similar to a small gamma camera for PET. A block detector is formed by cutting a block of detector material into a matrix of small detector elements, typically 16 to 64 per block. A small number of photomultiplier tubes, typically 4, were used on each block to provide a position logic that could identify which of the 16 to 64 individual detector elements in the block had been struck by a 511 keV photon. These blocks were then assembled into a circumferential array or assembled into planar arrays for dual-head PET cameras. An array of discrete block detectors can be seen in Figure 1.1.

Block detectors of BGO became the standard of PET scanners with the circular geometry employed by CTI/Siemens, GE, and Positron Corporation, as well as in the dual-head planar array of CTI/Siemens ART scanner. These systems provided the

TABLE 1.2. Evolution of clinical PET scanner performance with typical values.

	1974	1984	2000
Spatial resolution (mm)	25 × 25	8 × 10	4 × 4
Typical volume resolution (cm³)	117	1.44	0.064
Efficiency (kcps/μCi/cc) 2-D	0.5	40	200
3-D			1,000
Axial field of view (cm)	2.5	8	15
Number of detector elements	24	264	≥20,000
Coincidence lines of response 2-D	12	15,000	$\geq 6 \times 10^6$
3-D			$\geq 75 \times 10^6$
Number of simultaneous image planes recorded			≥60

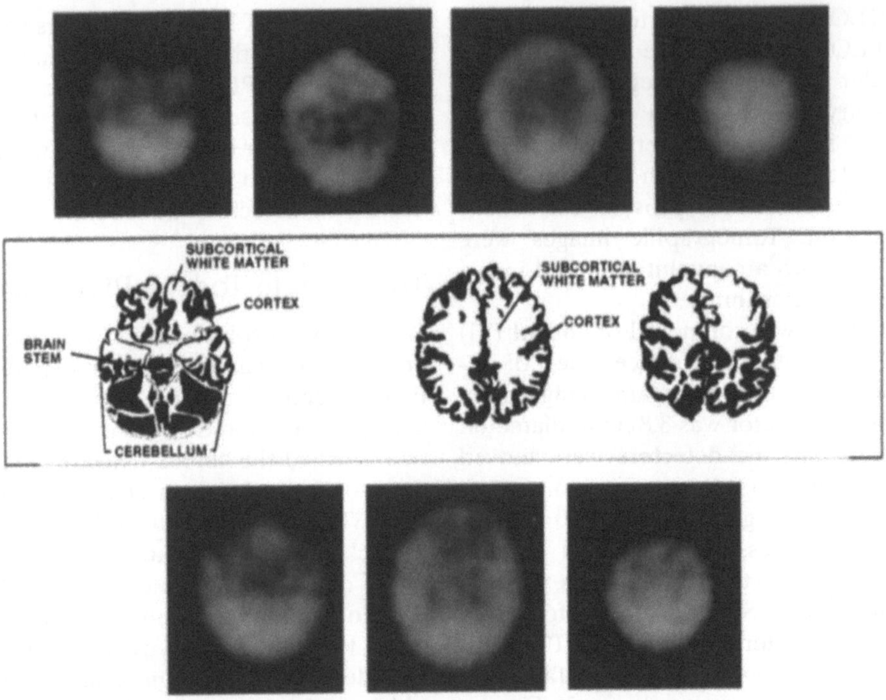

FIGURE 1.5. Images taken with PETT III after injection of [C-11] glucose. The images from left to right are from the cerebellum up to the top of the brain. The bottom images are sections in between those at the top. White is the highest level of activity.

performance standard of PET, while maintaining control of cost in the face of rapidly increasing performance (Table 1.2).

Another event that changed the course of PET was the development of whole-body imaging. This development actually occurred by an unusual circumstance. In the early 1990s, efforts were increasing to incorporate PET into the healthcare system. At the time, there were no FDA approved radiopharmaceuticals and no reimbursement for PET. One way to introduce PET into clinical medicine was to develop a whole-body scanning capability using ^{18}F ion for bone scanning, since it had been previously approved by the FDA. ^{18}F had been the standard for nuclear medicine bone scanning throughout the world in the 1960s and early 1970s until the arrival of the ^{99m}Tc phosphate compounds. Thus, I initiated a project to develop whole-body PET with the goal of providing an FDA approved indication of bone scanning with F-18 ion.

Once the whole-body scanning approach was developed by Guerro et al.[35] and Dahlbom et al.,[36] we began to consider where whole-body scanning would be most valuable to medicine. The answer became obvious when a friend was diagnosed with breast cancer. The oncologist said, "Everything about cancer is determined by metastases." We shifted the focus of the whole-body scanning with PET to FDG and cancer (Figure 1.7). Many programs throughout the world went on to demonstrate and validate the value of whole-body PET in cancer.[37]

NaI (Tl) Coincidence Cameras

NaI (Tl) gamma cameras have a long history in PET, beginning with the first attempts by Muehllehner et al.[16] at imaging positron labeled compounds with two-dimensional imaging, until today. Muehllehner, Karp, and colleagues have refined the gamma camera approach to PET by producing a hexagonal array of 2.54 cm thick NaI (Tl) gamma cameras with high-speed

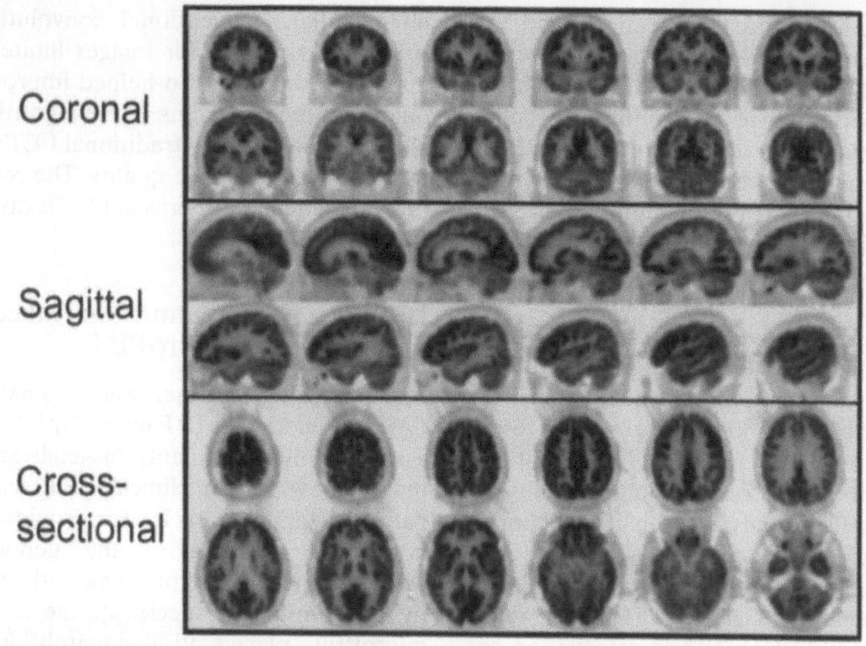

FIGURE 1.6. Images of the cerebral metabolic rate for glucose using a modern PET scanner (Siemens EXACT HR+) and FDG in a normal human subject. The injected dose was 10 mCi, and the imaging time was 30 minutes. Black indicates the highest level of activity.

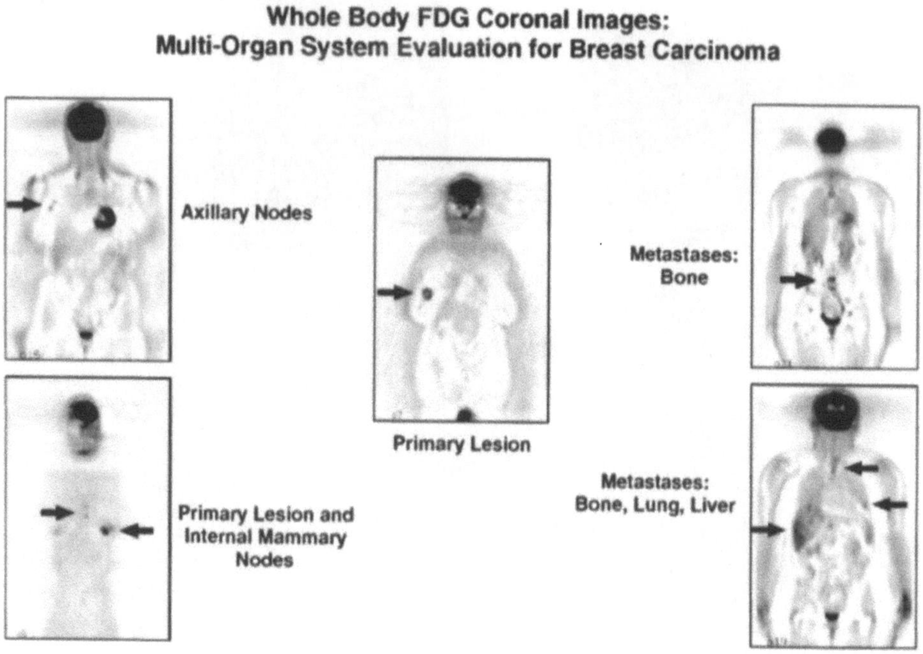

FIGURE 1.7. Whole-body PET with FDG in a patient with breast cancer. The figure illustrates the use of PET to examine all organs of the body for primary and metastatic disease in a single procedure.

electronics, attenuation corrections, and very good image quality for PET. The initial version was called the PENN-PET.[38] Although this system's performance is significantly behind BGO full-ring PET scanners due to its lower efficiency and lower count rate capability, it sets the standard for NaI (Tl) gamma camera technology in PET (Chapter 2). The refined commercial version of the PENN-PET is called the C-PET and is sold by ADAC/Philips.

The use of conventional dual-head NaI (Tl) gamma cameras in PET began in the late 1990s by adding coincidence detection to existing systems that had good intrinsic spatial resolution but very low efficiency and count rate capability and, therefore, low image quality and long acquisition times. The desire to improve PET coincidence camera performance produced systems with thicker NaI (Tl) crystals with thickness from 1.3 to 2.54 cm, as well as higher speed electronics and attenuation correction. The use of algebraic image reconstruction algorithms that produce higher quality images than conventional convolution algorithms, particularly for images limited by the number of counts, also helped improve image quality of these systems. These algorithms have also been adopted by traditional PET scanners, improving their image quality. The role of NaI (Tl) coincidence cameras in PET is discussed in Chapter 2.

Bringing Biology and Pharmaceuticals Together with microPET

The microPET scanner was originally developed by Cherry et al. (Figure 1.8)[24,25] to provide a similar imaging quality in small animals, as that achieved with clinical PET scanners in patients (Figure 1.9). It also provided a technology to help move the genome-based research from genes, proteins, and cells to the living mammalian species of the mouse. The microPET placed PET squarely into basic research in biology, genetics, molecular basis of disease, and molecular therapies. This new

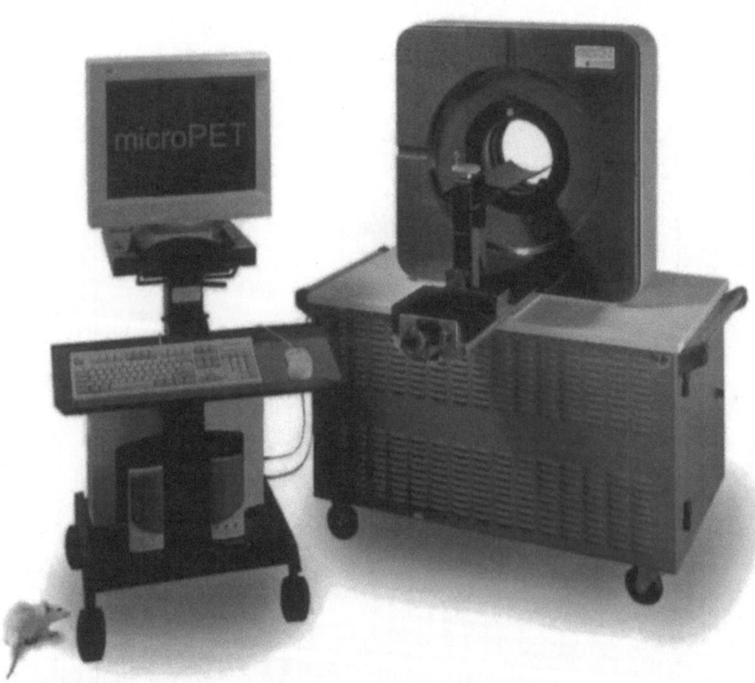

FIGURE 1.8. Photo of the Concorde Microsystems microPET scanner. The scanner can either be placed on a bench top or on the cabinet containing the system electronics as shown below the scanner.

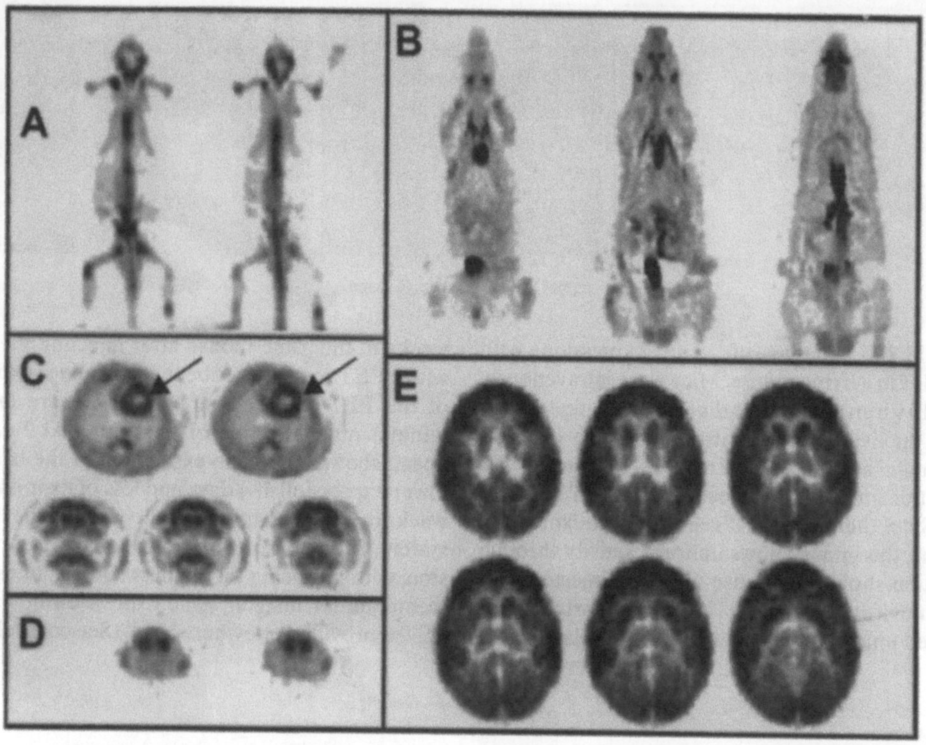

FIGURE 1.9. Image quality of microPET I. (A) Two 1.5 mm thick longitudinal whole body sections of a 25 g mouse using [F-18] fluoride ion to image the skeletal system of a prostate cancer mouse model with bone metastases. (B) Longitudinal whole body FDG images of glucose metabolism in normal 250 g rate. (C Upper) Cross sections through the chest of a rat showing glucose metabolism in left (arrow) and right ventricles. Left ventricle is 9 mm in diameter, with 1 mm wall thickness. Right ventricle is thinner, and metabolic rate is 1/3 left. (C Lower) Coronal sections of glucose metabolism in a rat brain weighing 1 g, showing cortex well-separated from internal structure of striatum. (D) Images of a mouse brain with [C-11] WIN 35,428 that binds to dopamine reuptake transporters showing clear separation of left and right striatum that each weigh about 12 mg. (E) FDG brain images of a two-month-old Vervet monkey with good delineation of cortical and subcortical structures. The dimension across the brain is 2 cm. Cortical convolutions of the brain are not seen because the young monkey has few of them. (Reprinted with permission from the Journal of Nuclear Medicine.[5])

direction in research led to the development of new molecular imaging assays, from metabolism to gene expression (Figure 1.10, see color plate). In addition, the 2,000-fold reduction in size from man to mouse has required the evolution of new detector technology, image reconstruction algorithms, and tomograph design concepts. Thus, microPET will also serve as a platform for providing technologies that will improve clinical PET scanners in the physical performance and in new molecular assays.

FDA and HCFA

FDA

In 1997, Congress passed an FDA Reform Bill that contained special provisions for PET, in a bill sponsored by Senator Stevens (R-AK). This bill required the FDA to streamline the approval process for PET. Further, it required the FDA to create new "Good Manufacturing Processes" that recognized the requirements

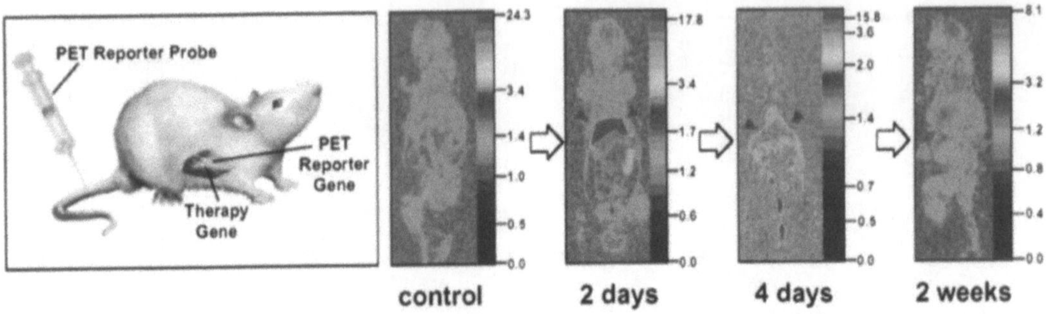

FIGURE 1.10. Images of gene expression with microPET in a living mouse. Mice were intravenously injected with an adenovirus that localizes greater than 90% to the liver. In the control mouse, the virus did not contain a PET reporter gene. The image was taken after intravenous injection of a PET reporter probe. Since there is no PET reporter gene expression to report, the image shows uniform activity through the section shown. A mouse was then injected with an adenovirus containing a PET reporter gene. Repeated images were taken at 2 days, 4 days, and 2 weeks in the same mouse after injecting the mouse with a PET reporter probe that will image expression of the PET reporter gene. Images were taken 60 minutes after injection of the probe. At 2 days, the image shows high gene expression in the liver, with lower expression at 4 days and loss of expression at 2 weeks due to termination of the virus by the immune system. The color scale is proportional to gene expression, with red being the highest. Descriptions of this technique for imaging gene expression in vivo with PET is provided elsewhere.[5,6,43,44] (See color plate)

imposed by the short half-lives of the common PET radionuclides and the devices used for automated production of PET molecular imaging probes. As an outcome of the bill, FDG was broadly approved in safety and effectiveness for all cancers, myocardial viability, and epilepsy. FDA also approved [N-13]NH_3 for detection of cardiovascular disease. The use of FDG for Alzheimer's disease is presently under review and is likely to be approved, as is [F-18] FluoroDOPA for Parkinson's disease. The positron emitter ^{82}Rb was previously approved for the diagnosis of cardiovascular disease.

HCFA

Although several hundred private insurance companies began covering PET early on, the Health Care Financing Administration (HCFA) that is responsible for Medicare and Medicaid was slow to provide coverage. On January 1, 1998, the HCFA provided a limited coverage of PET/FDG for evaluating solitary pulmonary nodules that was added to their previous coverage of the detection of cardiovascular disease with Rb-82.

On July 1, 1998, the HCFA expanded the coverage to include recurrent colorectal cancer with a rising CEA, staging of melanoma and lymphoma. Up to this point, all of the preceding were being evaluated by HCFA for coverage on an indication by indication basis, even though the FDA had provided broad approval of PET for all cancers and cardiovascular disease, as well as some select indications for neurological disorders. December 15, 2000 marked a time of dramatic change in the HCFA's approach to PET. On this date, the HCFA announced a national coverage decision on PET based on a coverage request submitted to the HCFA by UCLA and Duke. This coverage request contained the summary and analysis of the literature of PET studies in cancer, cardiovascular disease, epilepsy and Alzheimers. An expanded version of this document was subsequently published by Gambhir et al.[37] The HCFA National Coverage Document contained four main features:

- The HCFA would now consider evidence for coverage for PET from biology/biochemistry, clinical research/trials, and clinical judgement.

- Broad coverage (diagnosis, staging, therapy assessment, and recurrence) was provided for lung cancer, colorectal, melanoma, lymphoma, head and neck, and esophageal cancers. Coverage of cardiovascular disease was expanded to include detection and viability. Coverage was also included for evaluating patients with refractory seizure disorders for selecting surgical candidates. Thus, for the first time, the physician would be allowed to decide how best to use PET in patient management.
- For new indications, if evidence from biology/biochemistry exists, then it is sufficient to show the accuracy and value in one aspect of the disease to gain broad approval. For example, if PET is shown to be of value in staging breast cancer, then this would be sufficient to provide broad approval for breast cancer.
- HCFA agreed to evaluate coverage for breast (and possible ovarian, cervical, and uterine) cancer and Alzheimer's disease.

The new coverage approved on December 12, 2000, was implimented on July, 2001.

Future Advances in PET

The future is hard to predict. Alan Kay of Macintosh once said, "The best way to predict the future is to invent it." A lot of the development of PET has occurred by inventions. It is likely that the future of PET will be also invented. A number of inventions are already occurring and more will come. The following list illustrates some things arising from today's research and development, as well as predictions about the future.

PET Imaging Instrumentation

- The PET/CT scanners that were invented in the last few years[39–41] will become commonplace in the future. They provide an efficient display of molecular imaging of the biological nature of disease, along with anatomical information to further improve the diagnosis as well as provide fast and accurate attenuation corrections to improve the speed and image quality of PET. In addition, they will provide efficient approaches to radiation and surgical planning and guided biopsies. Systems being commercially produced today are composed of fusing PET and CT scanners together. In the future, new high performance and cost reduced approaches that truly integrate these technologies into a single scanner concept will occur.
- Lutetium orthosilicate (LSO)[42] will become the high performance detector material of choice and replace BGO. It is already used in commercial microPET scanners, and the first commercial clinical systems are being sold by CTI/Siemens.
- Dedicated PET scanners will evolve to new designs that will be in the price range of \$500,000 to \$1.2 million with performance ranging from the dedicated PET scanners of today to ones exceeding today's state-of-the-art by a considerable margin. High image quality whole-body studies will be performed in 10 minutes or less, and local organ examinations like the brain will be done in 2 minutes or less with high image quality.
- NaI (Tl) camera based systems will improve to some degree and play a decreasing role in the overall clinical delivery of PET services. They will be replaced with new detector materials and system designs for both PET and PET/SPECT systems.
- MicroPET will become a standard technology for biology research and drug discovery.

Molecular Imaging Assays

- All nuclear medicine assays of today will be replaced with PET, and to a lesser degree with new SPECT imaging, employing molecular imaging probes designed to target the biological properties of disease coming from advances in genomics, proteomics, molecular biology, and the new molecular pharmacology of molecular medicine.
- New PET molecular imaging probes will come from collaborations between the PET research community and molecular pharmacology and the pharmaceutical industry. Over the next three to five years, the variety of molecular imaging with PET will grow rapidly.

Clinical Studies

- Clinical PET studies will diversify with the diversity of molecular imaging probes, expanding to infectious and inflammatory processes, greater specificity in cancer diagnosis and management, diabetes, a wide variety of neurological disorders, and other disorders as the number of disease targets for molecular therapeutics expands.
- FDG will continue to grow in its clinical utility. Glucose metabolism is such a common process of cellular function and dysfunction, and FDG is such a good imaging probe, that it will have a long lifetime.
- The HCFA and private insurance will continue to expand coverage for PET because of its important molecular imaging role in managing patients in this new era of molecular medicine.
- Molecular imaging diagnostics and molecular therapeutics will come close together in the molecular characterization of disease and the selection of therapy from those criteria.

References

1. Shields AF, Grierson JR, Dohmen BM, et al.: Imaging proliferation in vivo with [F-18]FLT and positron emission tomography. Nature Medicine 1998;4:1334–1336.
2. Phelps ME, Hoffman E, Mullani N, et al.: Application of annihilation coincidence detection to transaxial reconstruction tomography. J Nucl Med 1975;16:210–224.
3. Phelps ME, Cherry SR: The changing design of positron imaging systems. Clin Pos Imaging 1998;1:31–45.
4. Patton JA: Instrumentation for coincidence imaging with multihead scintillation cameras. J Nucl Med 2000;30:239–254.
5. Phelps ME: PET: The merger of biology and imaging into molecular imaging. J Nucl Med 2000;41:661–681.
6. Phelps ME: Positron emission tomography provides molecular imaging of biological processes. Proc Natl Acad Sci (USA) 2000;97:9226–9233.
7. Sokoloff L, Reivich M, Kennedy C, et al.: The (^{14}C) deoxyglucose method for the measurement of local glucose utilization: Theory, procedure and normal values in the conscious and anesthetized albino rat. J Neurochem 1977;28:897–916.
8. Ido T, Wan C-N, Casella JS, et al.: Labeled 2-deoxy-D-glucose analogs: ^{18}F labeled 2-deoxy-2-fluoro-D-glucose, 2-deoxy-2-fluoro-D-mannose and ^{14}C-2-deoxy-2-fluoro-D-glucose. J Labeled Compds Radiopharmacol 1978;14:175–183.
9. Phelps ME, Huang SC, Hoffman EJ, et al.: Tomographic measurement of local cerebral glucose metabolic rate in humans with (F-18) 2-fluorodeoxy-D-glucose: Validation of method. Ann Neurol 1979;6:371–388.
10. Reivich M, Kuhl D, Wolf A, et al.: The (^{18}F)fluorodeoxyglucose method for the measurement of local cerebral glucose utilization in man. Circ Res 1979;44:117–127.
11. Huang SC, Phelps ME, Hoffman EJ, et al.: Noninvasive determination of local cerebral metabolic rate of glucose in man. Am J Physiol 1980;238:E69–E82.
12. Woodward GE, Hudson MT: The effect of 2-deoxy-D-glucose in glycolysis and respiration of tumor and normal tissues. Cancer Res 1954;14: 599–605.
13. Fowler JS, Wolf AP: Positron emitter-labeled compounds: Priorities and programs, in Phelps ME, Mazziotta JC, Schelbert HR (eds): Positron Emission Tomography and Autoradiography: Principles and Applications. New York: Raven Press, 1986, pp 391–450.
14. Burnham C, Brownell G: A multi-crystal positron camera. IEEE Trans Nucl Sci 1972;19:201–205.
15. Brownell G, Burnham C: MGH positron camera, in Freedman G (ed): Tomographic Imaging in Nuclear Medicine. New York: Society of Nuclear Medicine, 1973, pp 154–164.
16. Muehllehner G, Buchin M, Dudek J: Performance parameters of a positron imaging camera. IEEE Trans Nucl Sci 1976;NS-23:528–537.
17. Robertson J, Marr R, Roseblum B: Thirty-two crystal positron transverse section detector, in Freedman G (ed): Tomographic Imaging in Nuclear Medicine. New York: Society of Nuclear Medicine, 1973, pp 151–153.
18. Kuhl D, Edwards R: Cylindrical and section radioisotope scanning of the liver and brain. Radiology 1964;83:926–935.
19. Hounsfield G, Ambrose J: Computerized transverse axial scanning (tomography). Part I: Description of system. Part II: Clinical applications. Br J Radiol 1973;46:1016–1047.
20. McCormack A: Reconstruction of densities from their projections, with applications to radiological physics. Phys Med Biol 1973;18:195–207.

21. Phelps ME, Hoffman E, Mullani N, et al.: Design considerations for a positron emission transaxial tomograph (PETT III). IEEE 1976;NS–23:516–522.
22. Hoffman E, Phelps ME, Mullani N, et al.: Design and performance characteristics of a whole body transaxial tomograph. J Nucl Med 1976;17:493–503.
23. Satyamurthy N, Barrio J, Phelps ME: Electronic generators for the production of positron-emitted labeled radiopharmaceuticals: Where would PET be without them? Clin Positron Imaging 1999;2:233–253.
24. Cherry SR, Shao Y, Silverman RW, et al.: MicroPET: A high resolution PET scanner for imaging small animals. IEEE Trans Nucl Sci 1997;44:1109–1113.
25. Chatziioannou AF, Cherry SR, Shao Y, et al.: Performance evaluation of microPET: A high resolution lutetium oxyorthosilicate PET scanner for animal imaging. J Nucl Med 1999;40:1164–1175.
26. Phelps ME, Hoffman E, Huang S, et al.: A new computerized tomographic imaging system for positron emitting radiopharmaceuticals. J Nucl Med 1978;19:635–647.
27. Hoffman E, Ricci A, van der Stee LMAM, et al.: ECAT III—Basic design considerations. IEEE Trans Nucl Sci 1983;NS–30:729–733.
28. Brownell G, Burkham C, Chesler D, et al.: Transverse section imaging of radionuclide distributions in heart, lung and brain, in Ter Pogossian M, Phelps M, Brownell G, Cox J, Davis D, Evans R (eds): Reconstruction Tomography in Diagnostic Radiology and Nuclear Medicine. Baltimore: University Park Press, 1977, pp 293–308.
29. Cho Z, Chan J, Eriksson L: Circular ring transverse axial positron camera for 3-dimensional reconstruction of radionuclide distribution. IEEE Trans Nucl Sci 1976;NS–23:613–622.
30. Cho Z, Farukhi M: BGO as a potential scintillation detector in positron cameras. J Nucl Med 1977;18:840–844.
31. Derenzo SE, Budinger T, Cahoon J: High resolution computed tomography of positron emitters. IEEE Nucl Sci 1977;NS–24:544–558.
32. Derenzo SE: Monte Carlo calculations of the detection efficiency of arrays of NaI(Tl), BGO, CsF, Ge, and plastic detectors for 511 keV photons. IEEE Trans Nucl Sci 1981;NS–28:131–136.
33. Derenzo SE, Budinger TF, Huessman RH, et al.: Imaging properties of a positron tomograph with 280 BGO crystals. IEEE Trans Nucl Sci 1981;NS–28:81–89.
34. Casey M, Nutt R: A multislice two-dimensional BGO detector system for PET. IEEE Trans Nucl Sci 1986;NS–33:760–763.
35. Guerrero T, Hoffman E, Dahlbom M, et al.: Characterization of a whole-body imaging technique for PET. IEEE Trans Nucl Sci 1990;37:676–680.
36. Dahlbom M, Hoffman E, Hoh CK, et al.: Evaluation of a positron emission tomography (PET) scanner for whole body imaging. J Nucl Med 1992;33:1191–1199.
37. Gambhir S, Czernin J, Schwimmer J, et al.: A tabulated summary of the 2-[F-18]fluorodeoxyglucose (FDG) positron emission tomography (PET) literature. J Nucl Med 2001;42:15.
38. Karp J, Muehllehner G, Mankoff D, et al.: Continuous-slice PENN-PET: A positron tomography with volume imaging capability. J Nucl Med 1990;31:617–627.
39. Beyer T, Townsend DT, Brun T, et al.: A combined PET/CT scanner for clinical oncology. J Nucl Med 2000;41:1369–1379.
40. Patton JA, Delbeke D, Sandler MP: Image fusion using integrated dual-head coincidence camera with x-ray tube based attenuation maps. J Nucl Med 2000;41:1364–1368.
41. Shreve, P: Adding structure to function. J Nucl Med 2000;41:1380–1381.
42. Casey M, Eriksson L, Schmand M, et al.: Investigation of LSO crystals for high spatial resolution positron emission tomography. IEEE Trans Nucl Sci 1997;44:1109–1113.
43. Gambhir SS, Barrio JR, Phelps ME, et al.: Imaging adenoviral-directed reporter gene expression in living animals with positron emission tomography. Proc Natl Acad Sci USA 1999;96:2333–2338.
44. Tjuvajev JG, Chen SH, Joshi A, et al.: Imaging adenoviral-mediated herpes virus thymidine kinase gene transfer expression in vivo. Cancer Res 1999;59:5186–5193.

2
Physics of PET

James A. Patton

Positron Decay and Annihilation Radiation

Positron Emission Tomography (PET) makes use of radiopharmaceuticals labeled with positron-emitting radionuclides. Positron decay is one of the three isobaric processes, which also includes beta minus decay and electron capture. Positron decay is characterized by the following decay equation using ^{18}F as an example.

$$^{18}F \rightarrow {}^{18}O + \beta^{+} + \nu$$

β^{+} is the positron, and ν is a neutrino, a particle with no mass or charge that always accompanies the positron in the decay process due to conservation of energy requirements. This process is characterized by the loss of a proton and the gain of a neutron in the daughter nucleus (atomic mass number remains constant) and occurs in nuclei that are unstable because of an excess of protons compared to the number of neutrons in the nuclei. Positron decay is more prevalent in nuclei with low atomic numbers and can only occur when the energy states of the parent and daughter differ by more than 1.022 MeV due to conservation of energy requirements. A positron and neutrino pair is emitted in the decay of every nucleus undergoing positron decay. The energies of the positron and neutrino are variable but constrained such that their total energy is equal to the difference in energy states of the parent and daughter minus 1.022 MeV. Thus, the positron energy varies from zero to its maximum value, which occurs when the energy of the neutrino is zero (the mean energy is approximately one-third of maximum energy). The decay scheme for ^{18}F is shown in Figure 2.1.

The positron is a positively charged electron and has all of the physical properties of the electron with the exception of its charge. Because of its small mass and positive charge, the positron is highly interactive and travels only a short distance after emission before losing its energy and coming to rest. For example, the mean range of the positrons from ^{18}F decay is only 0.2 mm (see Table 2.1). After coming to rest, the positron will immediately combine with a negatively charged electron to form positronium. However, almost immediately the masses of the two particles are converted into energy. Since the rest mass energy of the electron is 511 keV, a total of 1.022 MeV of energy is released in the process, and this release is accomplished by the formation of two 511 keV photons. This process is termed *annihilation*, and the photons are termed *annihilation radiation*. The photons leave the site of their production at approximately 180 degrees from each other (not exactly 180 degrees due to the residual energies of the positronium mass at the time of annihilation). The collinear emission of these two photons forms the basis for imaging the positron decay process.

Detection of Annihilation Radiation

Detection of an annihilation event is accomplished as shown in Figure 2.2 using the technique of coincidence detection. Since the two

TABLE 2.1. Characteristics of common positron emitters.

Positron emitter	Half-life (min)	Daughter	%β^+	Maximum energy (MeV)	Mean range (mm)
Carbon-11	20.4	^{11}B	99	0.96	0.3
Nitrogen-13	10.0	^{13}C	100	1.19	1.4
Oxygen-15	2.1	^{15}N	100	1.72	1.5
Fluorine-18	110.0	^{18}O	97	0.64	0.2
Gallium-68	68.0	^{68}Zn	88	1.89	1.9
Rubidium-81	1.3	^{81}Kr	96	3.35	2.6

annihilation photons are traveling in opposite directions, they can be localized by a dual opposed detector system. The key to the process is to simultaneously detect the two photons to ensure that they are both from the same annihilation process. This is accomplished by coupling the two detectors to a coincidence circuit. Using this method, the detection of one photon in one detector opens a timing window in the coincidence circuit. This window remains open for 7 to 15 nanoseconds. The detection of the second photon in the other detector during this time frame completes the process, and an annihilation event has been identified. It is known that the annihilation event occurred somewhere along a line drawn between the two detectors, and thus, there is positional information contained in the detection process. In principle, the uncertainty in the measurement of the location of the event and, therefore, the spatial resolution of the imaging device are determined by the size of the detectors (that is, the smaller the detectors, the lower the uncertainty and the higher the spatial resolution). However, this principle is limited by the distance traveled by the positron before annihilation and the deviation from 180 degrees of the two resulting photons. Taking these factors into consideration, the resolution limit in positron emission tomography is typically quoted to be approximately 2 mm.

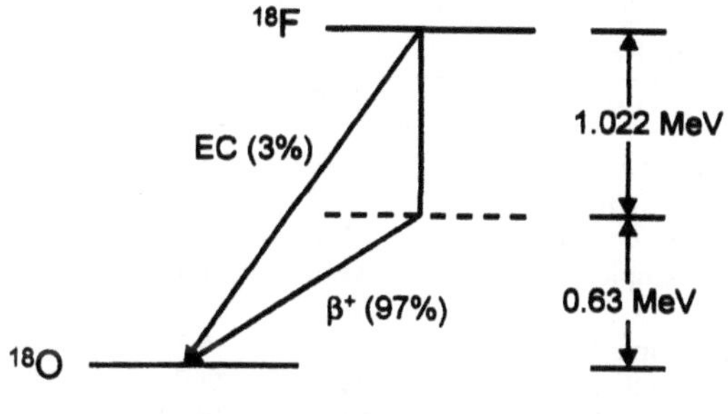

FIGURE 2.1. Decay scheme of ^{18}F.

Detector Materials

For many years, the scintillation detector of choice for PET imaging has been bismuth germanate oxide (BGO) instead of sodium iodide NaI(Tl), which is used in other nuclear medicine imaging devices. BGO is used because of its high density and high effective atomic number, which results in a high intrinsic detection efficiency for 511 keV photons. A 30 mm thick crystal of BGO has an intrinsic detection efficiency of approximately 90% at 511 keV. When two detectors are used in coincidence to simultaneously detect two 511 keV photons, the coincidence detection efficiency is the product of the efficiencies of the two detectors or approximately 81%. Recently a new scintillation material, luthetium oxiorthosilicate (LSO), has been introduced as a possible replacement for BGO.[1] Although currently more expensive than BGO, LSO has the advantage of greater light output (factor of 6) and faster decay time (factor of 7.5), and these improvements can be used to advantage in increasing the count rate capabilities of modern systems. PET systems using LSO are now available from one manufacturer (Siemens-CTI). The properties of BGO, LSO, and NaI(Tl) are shown in Table 2.2.

In practice, imaging is accomplished by surrounding the patient with many small detectors

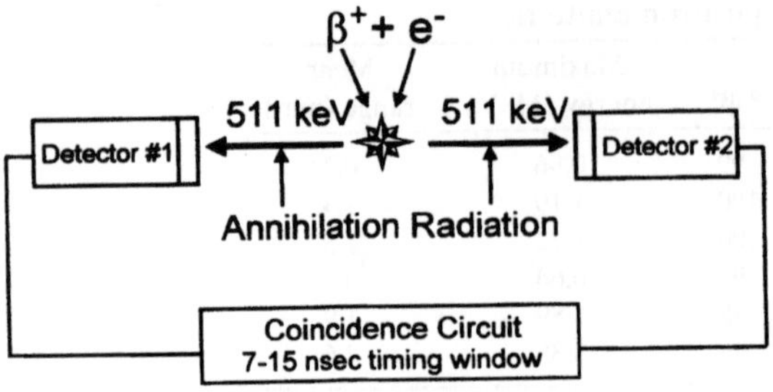

FIGURE 2.2. Block diagram of a two-detector grouping with a coincidence-timing window used to simultaneously detect the two photons resulting from the annihilation of a positron-electron pair using the technique of coincidence counting.

arranged in multiple rings, thus establishing many possible lines of coincidence as shown in Figure 2.3. Current systems have 18 to 32 rings of detectors providing axial fields of view of approximately 15 cm (Figure 2.4). Thus, the imaging of sections of the body greater than 15 cm in the axial direction requires multiple acquisitions obtained by indexing the patient through the system using a movable imaging table under precise computer control. The high spatial resolution of these systems is accomplished using a unique combination of small crystals and photomultipler tubes called detector blocks. An example of this technology is shown in Figure 2.5. A rectangular solid crystal of BGO is modified by the addition of vertical and horizontal grooves partially through its volume to effectively create a block of many small discrete detectors (64 in Figure 2.5). A photon interaction in one of the discrete crystals will result in scintillations localized primarily in that crystal. The crystal in which the interaction occurred is then identified by four photomultiplier tubes using conventional Anger logic and mounted on the base of the crystal. In the detector block shown in Figure 2.5, the discrete crystals are approximately 4 mm × 4.4 mm × 30 mm deep resulting in a transaxial spatial resolution of 4.6 mm. This is the technology that has been used by Siemens-CTI[2,3] in their ECAT EXACT series of systems. A slight modification of this approach is used by General Electric[4] in their Advance system shown in Figure 2.6. Instead of using a group of four photomultiplier tubes and Anger logic, this detector block makes use of two square, position-sensitive photomultiplier tubes to identify the discrete crystal in which the interaction occurred.

Ideally, the only events that are recorded should be those that result from the simultaneous detection of two photons (two *singles* events) from a single annihilation process. These are termed *true coincidences* as shown in Figure 2.7A. However, because of the orientation of the emitted photons or due to attenuation effects, some of the annihilation photons do not reach a detector or are not absorbed in a detector. In addition, as the singles rate increases, the probability increases that two photons from two separate annihilation processes will be detected in two detectors within the coincidence timing window. This results in an invalid event with erroneous positional information, termed a *random coincidence*, being recorded as shown in Figure 2.7B. The rate of random coincidences, R, can be calculated by:

$$R = 2\tau S_1 S_2$$

Where τ is the coincidence timing window, and S_1 and S_2 are the singles rates. There is no way to distinguish between true and random coincidence events. The effect of the random events on image quality is to provide a uniform background to the image that increases as the square of the singles count rate, as shown in the equation. However, since random events are truly random and occur at the same rate regardless of the time difference between the two detected single events, a seperate delayed timing window can be used to measure the

TABLE 2.2. Characteristics at 511 keV of scintillators used in PET.

Characteristic	NaI (Tl)	BGO	LSO
Effective Z	50.00	74.60	66.00
Density (gm/cm^3)	3.67	7.13	7.40
Mean free path (cm)	2.88	1.05	1.16
Hygroscopic	yes	no	no
Fragile	yes	no	no
Decay time (μsec)	0.23	0.30	0.04
Relative light yield	100.00	13.00	65.00
Energy resolution (%)	7.80	10.10	<10.00

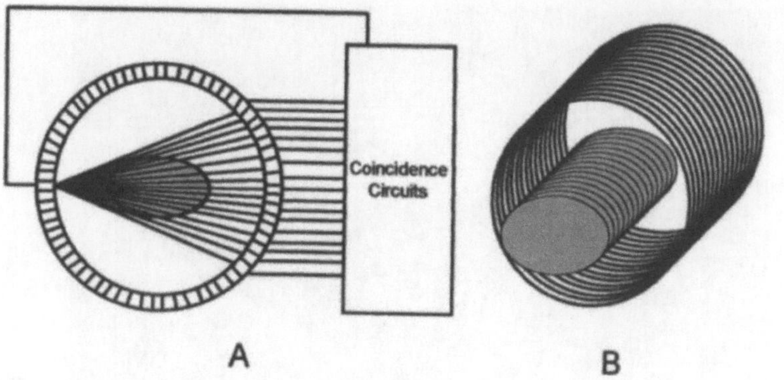

FIGURE 2.3. One ring of detectors from a multiring PET system. Many potential lines of coincidence are possible for each detector in the ring (A). Multiple rings of detectors are used to extend the axial field of view (B).

random coincidence rate, and this value can be used to subtract the random background from the acquired data. The primary disadvantage of this process is the increase in statistical noise in the subtracted image.

Scatter is also of concern in coincidence imaging. If one of the two annihilation photons undergoes Compton scatter in the region being imaged but still reaches the detector as shown in Figure 2.7C, the two photons will still be detected within the coincidence timing window, and an invalid coincidence event with erroneous positional information will be recorded. The performance of pulse height analysis with a lower energy threshold typically set at 300 to 350keV will eliminate the effects of large angle scatter, but the effects of small angle scatter will remain, a problem that also exists in routine single photon imaging. The effect of scatter, as in conventional single photon imaging, is to add an inhomogenous background to the image, which degrades contrast in areas of high scatter from dense organs. However, unlike single photon imaging, recorded coincident events from scattered photons do not necessarily appear to have originated within the body.

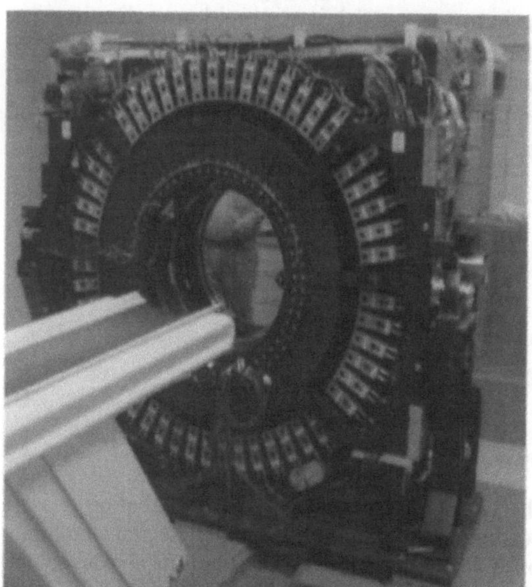

FIGURE 2.4. Photograph of a state-of-the-art multiring PET scanner (General Electric Advance).

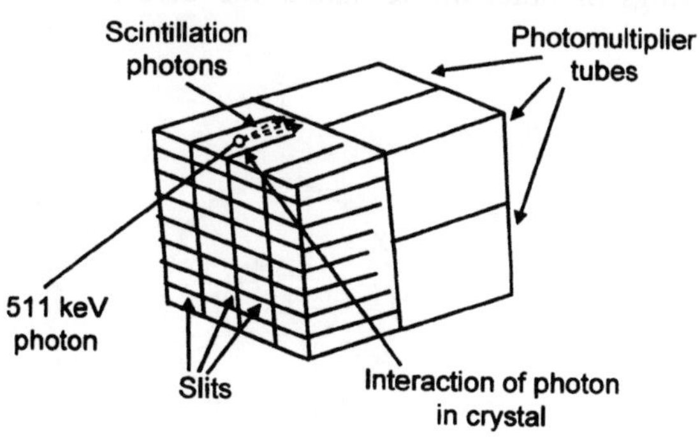

FIGURE 2.5. For high-resolution imaging, a block of bismuth germanate oxide is segmented into many small discrete crystals (64 in this example). The crystal in which an interaction occurs is determined by conventional Anger logic using four photomultiplier tubes positioned at the back of the crystal block.

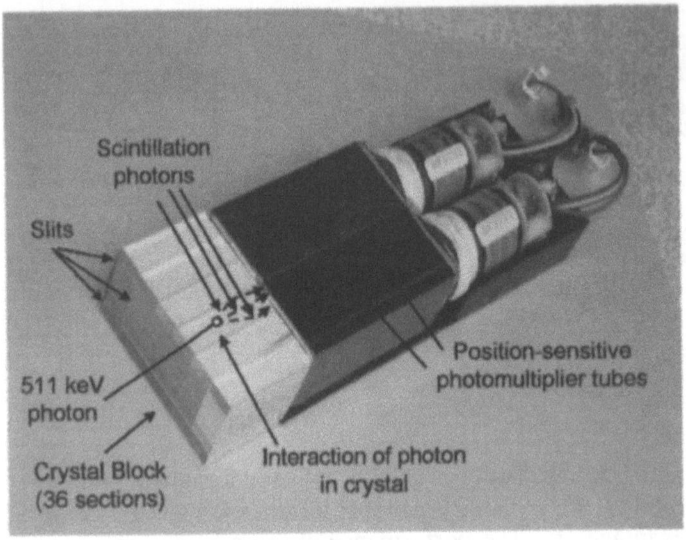

FIGURE 2.6. An alternative approach used in the General Electric Advance for identifying the crystal (one of 32 in this example) is to use position-sensitive photomultiplier tubes.

Based on these possibilities, the *total coincidences* measured in a PET system are actually the sum of true, random, and scatter events.

Two-Dimensional versus Three-Dimensional Imaging

It is possible to reduce the effects of scatter and reduce the singles rate, and therefore, the randoms rate, by adding thin one-dimensional collimators, termed septa, between adjacent rings of detectors to shield the detection of events in the axial direction as shown in Figure 2.8A. These septa are typically constructed from tungsten with a thickness of 1 mm and a spacing to match the axial width of each discrete BGO crystal. They have the effect of creating two-dimensional (2D) slices from which events can be accepted in any transaxial direction. Thus, for a system with 18 rings of detectors, 18 direct imaging planes are established. To increase sensitivity, coincidence circuitry can also be used to record interactions occurring in two detectors in adjacent rings resulting in the addition of a new acquisition plane positioned

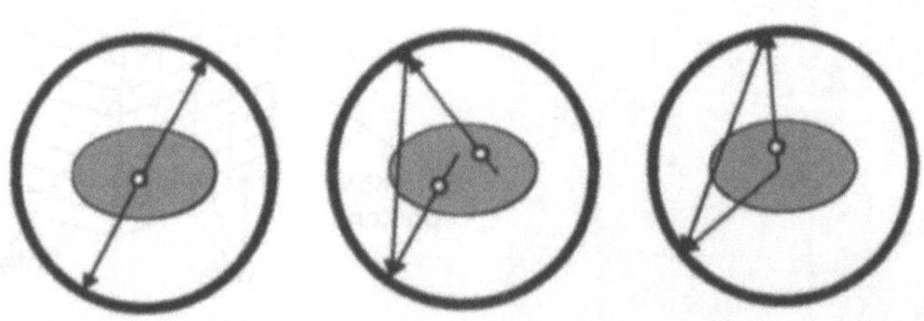

FIGURE 2.7. In coincidence counting, a true coincidence is identified when two photons (two singles events) from a single annihilation process are simultaneously detected in two opposing detectors (A). When two singles events from two separate annihilation processes are detected simultaneously, a random coincidence is identified (B). When one of the two photons from a single annihilation process scatters in the patient but is still detected simultaneously with the unscattered photon, a true coincidence with erroneous positional information is identified (C). Total coincidence events are the sum of true, random, and scatter coincidences.

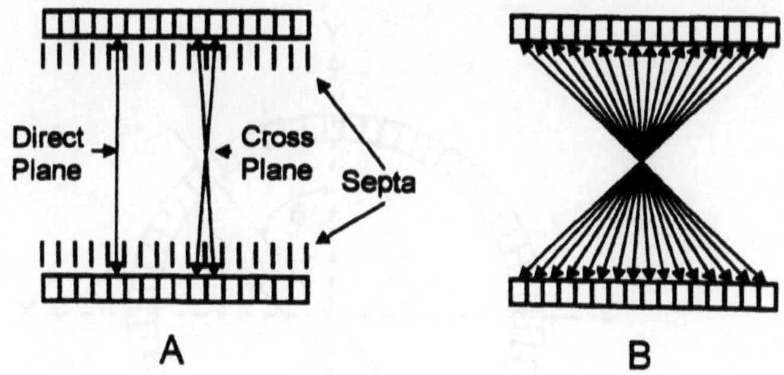

FIGURE 2.8. The use of septa collimators permit 2D acquisition by limiting the detection of coincidence events to detectors within a single ring (direct planes) and detectors in adjacent rings (cross planes) (A). When the septa are withdrawn, 3D acquisition is established by permitting the measurement of a coincidence event in two detectors in any two rings of the system (B).

midway between the adjacent detector rings. Thus, in an 18-ring system, 17 new cross-imaging planes can be added for a total of 35 imaging planes. Additional sensitivity is obtainable by adding adjacent planes to this process. For example, three or five planes of detectors may be electronically grouped so that coincidence events may be measured in any two detectors within these groupings. The localization of the coincidence event in a transaxial imaging plane is typically determined by averaging the axial positions of the two detectors. The axial separation of any two rings that can actually be used in the measurement of the activity in a 2D plane is limited by the length of the septa.

With the septa retracted, detector rings are opened to photons traveling in all directions, and a three-dimensional (3D) imaging geometry is established as shown in Figure 2.8B. This increases the system sensitivity by a factor of 3 to 5 over that of 2D imaging. However, the randoms rate and scatter fraction are increased with this geometry resulting in images with reduced contrast. It is possible to limit the acceptance angle in the axial direction to reduce the effects of randoms and scatter, but this results in a reduction in sensitivity.

Data Acquisition and Image Reconstruction

A coincidence event is recorded when two single events are simultaneously measured in two separate detectors. Thus, the location of the coincidence event is determined by the coordinates of the two detectors as shown in Figure 2.9A. These coordinates are captured by calculating the perpendicular distance from the center of the scan field to a line connecting the two detectors (r) and measuring the angle between this line and the vertical axis (ϕ). These coordinates are then recorded as a data point in a (r,ϕ) plot, or sinogram as shown in Figure 2.9B. Each unit in the final sinogram will consist of the total number of coincidence events recorded by a two-detector pair. The sinogram method of storage is used because it is more efficient than the storing of list mode data that record individual coordinates of detector pairs. In 2D image acquisition, there will be ($2n - 1$) sinograms recorded, one for each direct plane and one for each cross plane, where n is the number of detector rings in the PET system. When the two detectors are in different detector rings, the event is recorded in the sinogram corresponding to the average axial position of the two rings.

Image reconstruction of the 2D data is accomplished by first converting each sinogram of data into a set of planar projections. This is accomplished in a straightforward manner from the sinograms since each horizontal row of data in a sinogram represents events recorded at one angular position. It is also noted that the events from each two-detector pair are uniformly spread across the sinogram. A filtering algorithm is applied to each projection after which the data are projected back along the lines from which they were acquired to generate the final image (that is, filtered back projection). Each sinogram of data is used to generate an image corresponding to the activity distribution rep-

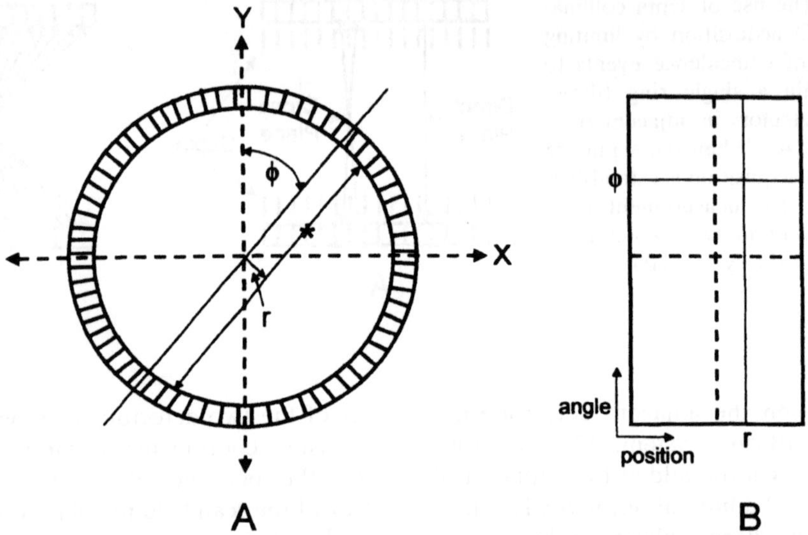

FIGURE 2.9. The coordinates of the two detectors involved in a coincidence measurement are captured by calculating the perpendicular distance from the center of the scan field to a line connecting the two detectors (r) and measuring the angle between this line and the vertical axis (ϕ) (A). These coordinates are then recorded as a data point in an (r,ϕ) plot or sinogram (B). Each unit in the final sinogram will consist of the total number of coincidence events recorded by a two-detector pair.

resented by the sinogram. Iterative algorithms that make use of ordered sets (Ordered Sets Estimation Maximization [OS-EM] can also be used in the 2D reconstruction process to reduce noise and provide high quality images.[5] The use of iterative algorithms also simplifies the process of adding corrections for effects such as attenuation and scatter.

The acquisition and reconstruction of 3D data sets are more complicated than that for 2D applications. First, it is not possible to perform the axial averaging of events recorded from two detectors in different detector rings. The origins of these data must be preserved in the acquisition process, and this results in a significant increase in the size of the acquired data set since n^2 sinograms are now required to accurately acquire the data. In addition, the reconstruction process is complicated by the fact that it is necessary to use a true three-dimensional volume algorithm to accurately locate detected events in axial, as well as transverse directions. Iterative reconstruction algorithms, although very time-consuming and labor-intensive, are well-designed for this application. Currently available systems offer this technique as an option, and it has proven useful in brain imaging because the imaging volume is relatively small and count rates are relatively low. Because of the added sensitivity provided by 3D imaging, a great deal of effort is currently being applied to develop accurate and efficient 3D algorithms and techniques to correct for scatter in order to improve contrast. As improvements are made, it is anticipated that the use of 3D techniques will become more prevalent in the future.

Quantitative Techniques

Because of the block detector technology used with PET systems, there is a deadtime associated with measurements of activity distributions, and corrections for this effect must be implemented so that the measurements are quantitatively accurate. When an interaction occurs in a crystal, a finite length of time is required to collect the light produced and process the resulting signal. If another event occurs in the same block while the first interaction is being processed, the light from the two events will be summed together by the photomultiplier tubes in that block, and the resulting signal will probably fall outside of the pulse height window. This effect will result in an erroneously low measurement of count rate. Modern systems have deadtime correction capability utilizing correction factors determined for the system as a function of count rate. These correction factors adjust for errors in count rate but cannot add the lost events back into the acquired image.

A state-of-the-art PET scanner may have several thousand discrete crystals coupled to hundreds of photomultiplier tubes. Thus, there are inherent differences in sensitivity between detector pairs in the measurement process, and it is necessary to correct for these differences in order for measurements of coincidence events to correspond to the activity distribution being imaged. This correction is generally accomplished by exposing each detector pair to a uniform source distribution, typically created by a rotating rod source of ^{68}Ge, and measuring the response of each detector pair. This data set is called a blank scan, and an example of the sinograms acquired with this process is shown in Figure 2.10. The blank scan can be used to create normalization factors that are stored away and used to correct data subsequently acquired in image acquisition. Blank scans must be acquired frequently (at least weekly) in order to monitor system parameters and adequately correct for small changes in detector responses.

A second factor to be considered is the exponential attenuation of photons within the body. Photons are either absorbed or scattered by tissues based on the attenuation coefficients of these tissues and the distance of travel through the body. The attenuation effects are much more significant in coincidence imaging than in single photon imaging since both photons from a single annihilation process must pass through the body without interaction in order to be detected and counted as a coincidence event. The probability of this occurrence is much less than that for a single photon emitted from the same location to escape the body without interaction. These effects result in nonuniformities, distortions of intense structures, and edge effects. Therefore, it is necessary to correct for attenuation to eliminate these effects, especially in the thorax and abdomen where attenuation is nonuniform due to the presence of different tissue types. Since the brain is relatively uniform, it is possible to perform a calculated attenuation correction. This is accomplished by outlining the outer contour of the head, assuming uniform attenuation within this volume, and calculating correction factors to be applied to the raw projection data.

In the thorax and abdomen, because of the nonuniform attenuation, it is necessary to perform a measured attenuation correction. This approach is very accurate because attenuation of two annihilation photons from an annihilation event is independent of the location of the event since the total distance traveled through the patient is constant as shown in Figure 2.11A–C. Therefore, it is possible to measure the attenuation using an external source as shown in Figure 2.11D. This is typically accomplished by transmission scanning using a rotating rod source of ^{68}Ge as in the acquisition of a blank scan for detector normalization, but with the patient present in the

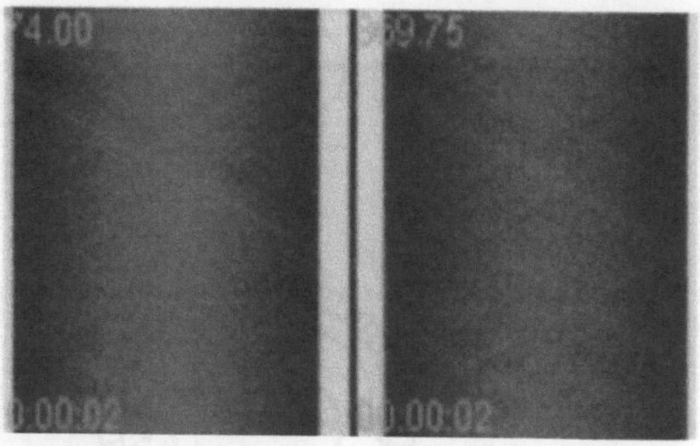

FIGURE 2.10. Two sinograms from adjacent planes acquired using a ^{68}Ge rod source. These sinograms are acquired with nothing in the field of view and provide measurements of sensitivity for each detector pair. These blank scans can then be used to determine normalization factors to be used to eliminate the differences in sensitivity that are seen as lines of varying intensity in the sinograms.

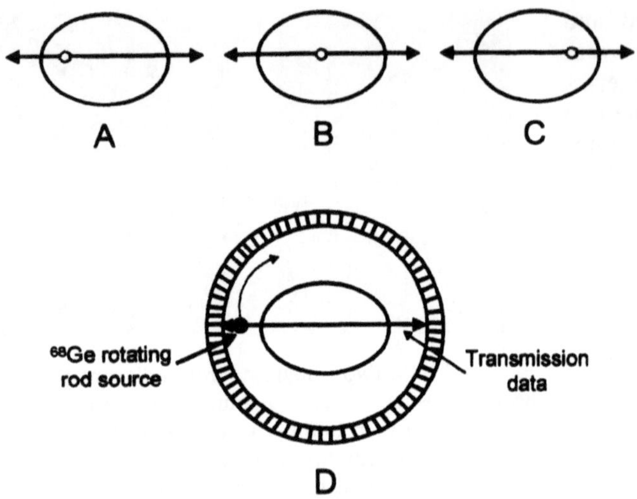

FIGURE 2.11. The attenuation of two annihilation photons is independent of the location from which the two photons were produced, since the photon pair must always travel the same distance within the patient and escape without interaction in order to be detected as a true event (A–C). Thus, attenuation can be measured using a rotating rod source of a positron emitter such as ^{68}Ge (D).

scan field. The rod sources used for detector normalization and transmission scanning in one system (General Electric Advance) are shown in Figure 2.12. The transmission data can then be used to correct the raw projection data during the reconstruction process, and iterative reconstruction algorithms can be easily adapted to handle the attenuation correction process. Transmission scans with high counting statistics are required to prevent the addition of statistical noise in the corrected images. In the past, it was necessary to perform the transmission scan prior to administration of the radiopharmaceutical. This resulted in lengthened studies and the need for careful repositioning of the patient before acquiring the emission scan. Recent improvements in count rate capabilities have made it possible to acquire transmission scans after the patient has been injected with a radiopharmaceutical by increasing the activity in the transmission source. It has also been shown that it is possible to shorten the length of the transmission scan by using a process called segmented attenuation correction. In this process, attenuation coefficients are predetermined (based on certain tissue types) and

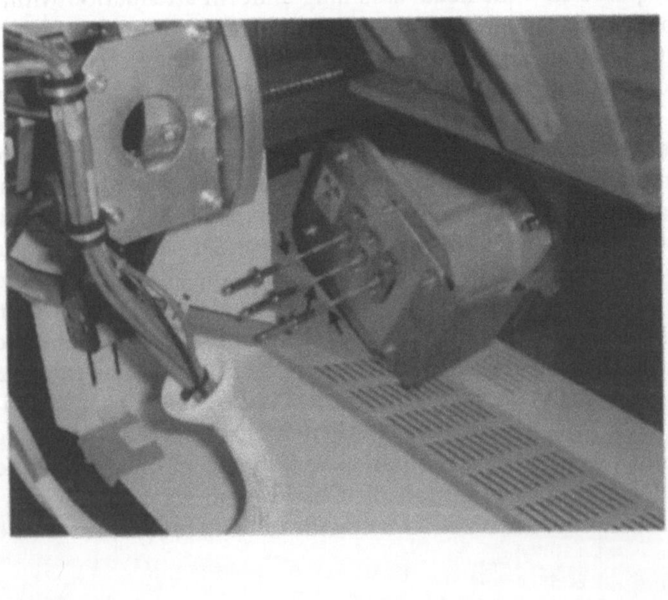

FIGURE 2.12. The ^{68}Ge rod source at the center is a 1.5 mCi source used for detector normalization, and the two sources adjacent to it are 10 mCi sources used for transmission scanning in the General Electric Advance PET scanner. The sources can be selectively extended and withdrawn into a lead housing as necessary.

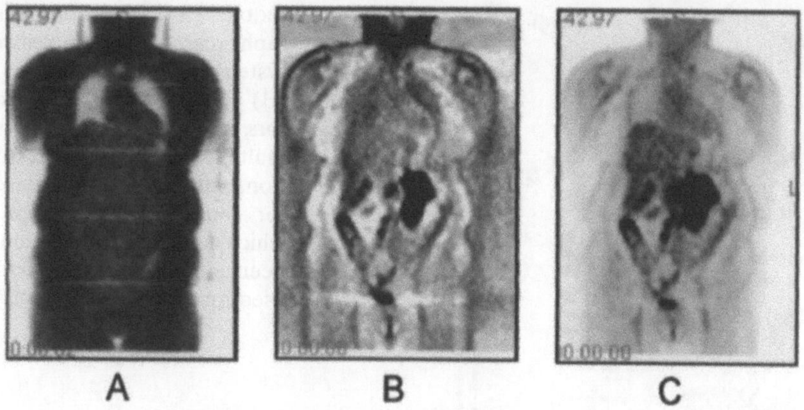

FIGURE 2.13. (A) A coronal view of a transmission data set acquired from a multiring PET scanner. (B) A coronal view of a patient with gastric cancer imaged with ^{18}FDG. The image was reconstructed without attenuation correction using filtered back projection. (C) The same coronal view of the ^{18}FDG distribution reconstructed with attenuation correction from the transmission data set shown in (A) using an iterative reconstruction algorithm (OS-EM).

limited in number. The measured attenuation coefficients from the transmission scan are then modified to match the closest allowed coefficients from the predetermined options. Figure 2.13A–C shows a single coronal view reconstructed from a set of transmission scans, the corresponding view reconstructed from emission data using filtered back projection without attenuation correction, and the same view reconstructed using an OS-EM algorithm with attenuation correction.

The addition of transmission scanning permits accurate delineatione of body contours. This fact limits image reconstruction to the areas defined by the contours. In addition, accurately knowing these contours permits the development of mathematical models for determining the contribution to the images of random and scatter events and subsequently, the implementation of correction methods to eliminate their effects. Work is ongoing in this area.

In order to make absolute measurements of activity in a region of the body, one additional calibration is necessary. A cylindrical phantom containing a very accurately known distribution of activity is scanned, and total counts (after attenuation correction) are determined. A quantitative calibration factor is then determined by dividing the measured counts per unit time by the concentration of activity in the phantom. This results in a calibration factor of counts/sec/μCi/cc. To determine activity in a specific region, a region of interest is identified, the counts in the region are determined and converted to a count rate using the scan time, and the calibration factor is then used to calculate μCi/cc in the region. Current systems have the capability of measuring absolute activity to within 5%. In practice, the same acquisition and reconstruction algorithms (and filters) should be used in acquiring and processing the phantom data and the patient data to obtain accurate quantitative data. A quantitative measurement that has proven to be of use in clinical applications is the standard uptake value (SUV). This factor is determined by normalizing the measured activity in a region to the administered activity per unit of patient weight. Using the SUV, regions of abnormal uptake can be compared to those of normal regions, and lesion uptake in serial scans can be compared.

Categories of PET Systems

The high-end dedicated PET system has been used to describe the physical principles of coincidence detection. This system consists of mul-

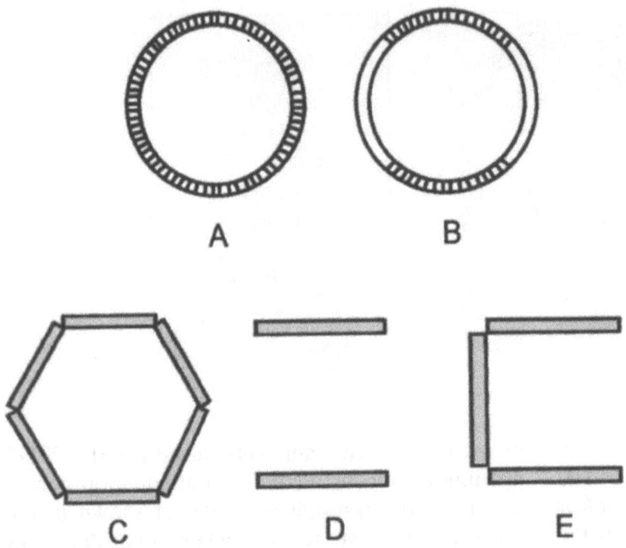

FIGURE 2.14. Positron emission tomography can be accomplished using (A) systems with complete rings of detectors, (B) systems with partial rings of detectors, and (C) camera-type systems with multiple large-area detectors. In addition, multihead scintillation cameras used for routine single photon imaging to which coincidence detection circuitry has been added (hybrid cameras) can also be used for this purpose (D–E).

tiple complete rings of small crystals with 2D imaging with septa in place and 3D imaging with septa retracted. This is the approach taken with the Siemens-CTI EXACT series of scanners and the General Electric Advance system. However, there are other, less expensive, mid-range dedicated PET systems commercially available, as shown in Figure 2.14A. Characteristics and specifications of several commercially available systems are summarized in Table 2.3. One approach to reducing cost is to reduce the number of detectors and detector rings and eliminate the septa as shown in Figure 2.14B. This is the approach taken with the Siemens-CTI ART system. This system consists of 24 rings of dual-opposed arcs (60 degrees) of detectors. Crystal thickness is reduced to 20mm, and complete sampling in transaxial planes is accomplished by rotating the detector rings at 30rpm. Since the septa have been eliminated, only 3D acquisition and image reconstruction are used with this system.

Another approach is to replace the discrete crystals with large-area, camera-type NaI(Tl) detectors as shown in Figure 2.14C.[6] To increase detection efficiency, the crystal thickness has been increased to 1 inch (25.4mm), compared to 3/8 inch (9.5mm) for conventional single photon camera systems. To improve system sensitivity, six detector heads are used in a

TABLE 2.3. Characteristics of PET imaging systems.

	EXACT	HR+	ART	Advance			ADAC
	2D	3D	3D	2D	3D	C-PET	MCD
Crystal material	BGO		BGO	BGO	—	NaI (Tl)	NaI (Tl)
Crystal size (mm)	4.05 × 4.4 × 30	—	6.75 × 6.75 × 20	4 × 8 × 30	—	500 × 256 × 25.4	508 × 381 × 15.9
Crystals/block	64	—	64	32	—	NA	NA
No. of crystals	18,432	—	4,224	12,096	—	6	2
No. of detector rings	32	—	24	18	—	NA	NA
No. of slices	63	—	47	35	—	NA	NA
Axial fov (mm)	15.5	—	16.2	15.2	—	256.0	380.0
FWHM at center of fov:							
axial	4.2	3.5	4.9	4.0	6.0	6.5	5.3
transaxial	4.6	4.6	6.2	4.5	4.5	4.9	5.0
Sensitivity (cps/Bq/cc)	5.4	24.3	7.5	5.7	27.6	10.8	3.2
Scatter fraction (%)	17.0	33.0	37.0	10.0	35.0	30.0	32.0
Transmission source	^{18}Ge	—	^{18}Ge	^{18}Ge	—	^{137}Cs	^{137}Cs

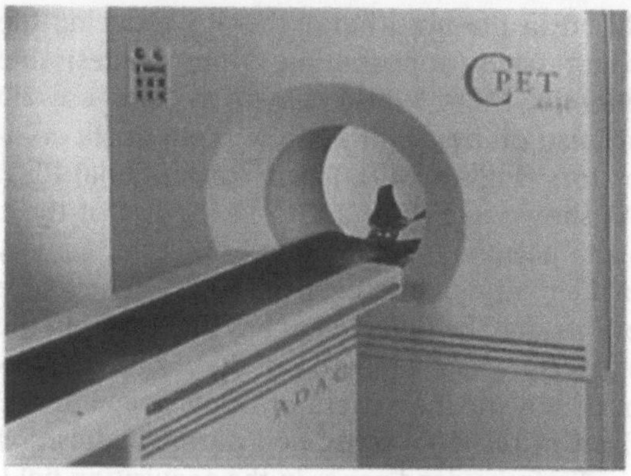

FIGURE 2.15. C-PET system manufactured by ADAC/Philips. (Courtesy of ADAC Labs, Milpitas, CA.)

hexagonal arrangement to completely surround the patient. Complete sampling in transaxial planes is accomplished by rotating the system during image acquisition. Septa are not used with these systems, and therefore, these systems are limited to 3D acquisitions. Since large-area, camera-type detectors are used, the axial field of view is increased over that of ring-type systems. The first of these systems to be commercially available was the C-PET system (Figure 2.15), and it was manufactured by ADAC/Philips.[7,8] The C-PET uses a unique curved crystal design to improve the acquisition geometry. Count rate capability is enhanced by the use of a parallel processing technique provided by limiting the measurement of light produced by a photon interaction to the photomultiplier tubes closest to the interaction and clipping of the voltage pulses that result from this measurement. This process is made possible by the relatively large amount of light produced from a 511 keV photon interaction in the crystal and permits the simultaneous measurement of multiple photon interactions in different locations of the crystal.

Hybrid Camera Systems

Coincidence imaging capability is also available on multihead scintillation camera systems used for routine nuclear medicine imaging procedures (Figure 2.14D–E and Figure 2.16).[9] To make these hybrid systems possible, conventional camera systems have been modified by the addition of detector shielding, the extension of the pulse height energy range, and the implementation of high-energy sensitivity and linearity corrections. To increase sensitivity, crystal thickness has been increased to $\frac{5}{8}$ to $\frac{3}{4}$ inch (15.8 to 19 mm), the maximum crystal thickness that can be used while preserving spatial resolution in the conventional single photon energy range. Even with $\frac{5}{8}$ inch (15.8 mm) thick crystals, the photopeak detection efficiency is only increased to approximately 17%, and the coincidence photopeak detection efficiency is only 2.9%. Coincidence circuitry has been added to establish a possible line of coincidence between any two positions in opposing heads. The most significant improvement in scintillation camera technology making it possible to perform coincidence imaging is the development of high count rate capability. As in the dedicated PET camera systems previously described, the relatively high light

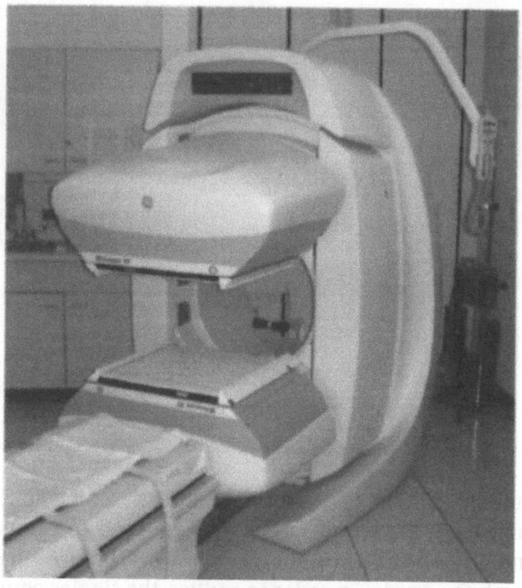

FIGURE 2.16. Hybrid multipurpose scintillation camera (General Electric). The camera can be operated in either a single photon mode for routine nuclear medicine procedures or a coincidence detection mode for positron imaging.

output resulting from 511 keV photon interactions makes it possible to clip the electrical pulses resulting from these interactions, even before all of the light has been collected. This results in a shortening of the duration of signals to 40 to 200 nanoseconds instead of the approximately 1 microsecond signals that have been typically used for routine single photon imaging. One manufacturer (ADAC/Philips) uses the photomultiplier tube grouping technique to permit the simultaneous measurement of multiple interactions.

Due to the extremely high count rates from singles events inherent in coincidence imaging, some manufacturers have made use of graded absorbers to reduce the count rate as shown in Figure 2.17A. These are thin sheets of materials of decreasing atomic number (lead > tin > copper) which absorb low energy photons resulting from multiple scatter in the region of interest (and also characteristic X rays produced in the absorbers), thereby reducing the count rate contribution from undesirable photons. Most hybrid camera systems use 2D acquisition by making use of septa or slit collimators (Figure 2.17B) as in conventional PET. As shown in Figure 2.17C–D, the use of these septa permits the definition of slices of activity in the region of interest from which coincidence events may be detected at any angle within the slice. The exact geometry of these slits is determined by the manufacturer. They may either be fixed in place or translated during acquisition to eliminate dead zones in the acquisition field. Although the acquisition with slit collimators is referred to as 2D, some of the acquired events deviate substantially from the perpendicular in the axial direction, although much less than is the case without the use of septa.

Additional sensitivity can be obtained by removing the septa and increasing the acceptance angle in the axial direction to the full field

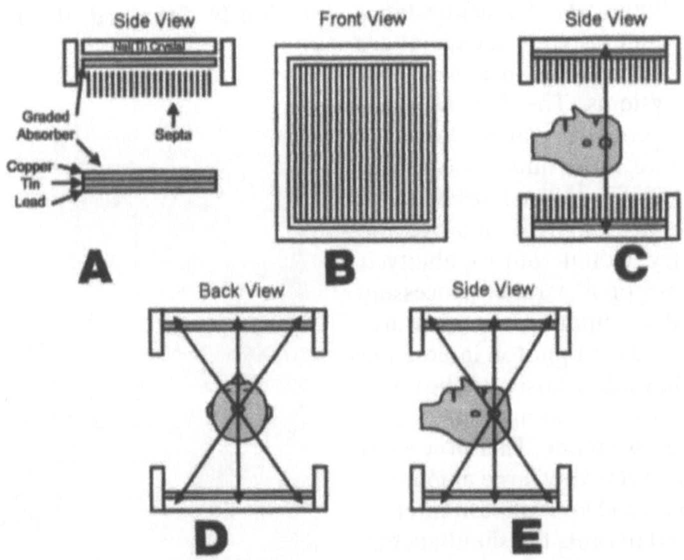

FIGURE 2.17. In hybrid camera coincidence imaging, a graded absorber may be used to preferentially absorb low-energy photons before they reach the crystal in order to reduce the singles count rate (A). In 2D coincidence imaging, parallel lead slits (septa) are used to define the transaxial imaging slices (B). These slits limit the acceptance of annihilation photons in the axial direction to small angles (C) while permitting acceptance of photons from any angle in the transaxial direction (D). In 3D coincidence imaging, the parallel lead slits (septa) (A) are removed so that annihilation photons may be accepted at any angle in both the transaxial (D) and axial (E) directions. (Reprinted with permission from the Society of Nuclear Medicine from Patton JA, Turkington TG: Coincidence imaging with a dual-head scintillation camera. J Nucl Med 1999;40:432–441.)

of view as shown in Figure 2.17E. This mode permits the acceptance of coincidence events from any angle, and thus, a true 3D acquisition is accomplished. As with dedicated PET systems, this mode of acquisition results in a factor of 3 to 5 increase in sensitivity at the cost of increased scatter and randoms contribution (and reduced image contrast) to the image. Most manufacturers do not use this method of acquisition, although one (ADAC/Philips) makes use of short septa at a 45-degree angle with respect to the axial direction, permitting 3D acquisition. Complete transaxial sampling of the region of interest is accomplished by rotating the camera system around the patient as in conventional single photon tomography. This is accomplished in a single rotation using either a step-and-shoot mode, a continuous rotation mode, or by using multiple rotations in systems with slip ring technology.

Because of the low photopeak detection efficiencies of the NaI(Tl) crystals currently used in hybrid coincidence imaging systems, other methods have been sought to increase efficiency. One approach is to include Compton interactions in the crystal that only result in partial absorption of the annihilation photons. This is acceptable since the origin of the annihilation event, and hence, the location of the positron emission is determined by interactions in each of the two detectors, and thus, a coincidence event may be recorded by measuring a photopeak interaction in one detector and a Compton interaction in the other detector. These Compton interactions can be recorded with one or more pulse height analyzer windows (W3), covering the range from 100 to 350keV. Some manufacturers use a single window to include the total energy range, others use a single window to include only part of the range (for example, 200 to 350keV), and still others provide multiple windows for added versatility in pulse height analysis.

Attenuation correction in hybrid systems is more practical using single photon imaging techniques because of low photon detection efficiency issues with NaI(Tl) crystals. In addition, the preferred source, ^{137}Cs, emits 662keV photons, which are resolved above the 511keV photopeak, thereby allowing transmission scanning after injection of the radiotracer. The design currently in use involves a point source in a fan-beam geometry that is translated across the field of view of one of the camera heads and the collection of multiple projections as the camera heads are rotated around the patient.

Reconstruction of coincidence images from hybrid camera systems was originally performed using filtered back projection. However, because of the relatively low count rates from these systems, iterative reconstruction techniques using OS-EM are now being used in most systems because of the ability of these algorithms to reduce noise in the reconstructed images.

Some interesting comparisons can be made between hybrid camera systems and full ring dedicated PET systems. Both systems have approximately the same spatial resolution (4 to 5mm) and yield approximately the same scatter fraction measurements (15 to 25% in 2D mode). The larger size of the scintillation camera provides an increased axial field of view which is approximately 2.5 times greater than the dedicated PET systems. However, the dedicated systems have an advantage in measured sensitivity by a factor of 8 to 12 over hybrid systems. Differences in measured count rates from patients are even more significant. This significant difference in sensitivity is due to the differences in photopeak detection efficiencies at 511keV for NaI(Tl) (~17% for 5/8 inch crystals) and BGO (~90% for 30mm crystals) and the fact that ring systems completely surround the patient with detectors, whereas the camera systems must rotate around the patient for complete sampling. This difference in sensitivity translates into difficulty in reliably detecting lesions smaller than 1.5cm in diameter.[10]

One approach to increasing sensitivity is to add detectors, an approach taken by Marconi[11] with the production of a three-detector system (Figure 2.14E) with the detectors grouped in pairs electronically for coincidence imaging. A second approach is to increase the crystal thickness. However, this would result in unacceptable imaging characteristics for conventional single photon imaging. An innovative solution to this problem has been introduced by Siemens and General Electric and makes use of

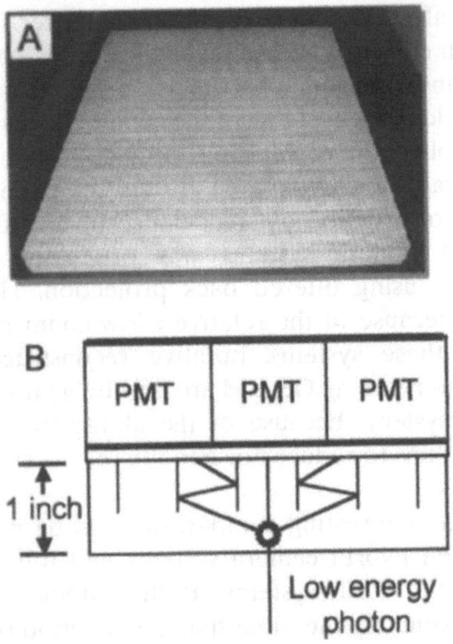

FIGURE 2.18. (A) One-inch thick NaI(Tl) crystal with orthogonal grooves cut partially through the crystal. (B) The grooves reflect light from scintillations produced in the front half of the crystal by low-energy photon interactions.

a thick NaI(Tl) crystal with a pattern of orthogonal grooves cut partially through the crystal as shown in Figure 2.18A. Using this technique, the crystal thickness can be increased to 1 inch, approximately doubling the efficiency at 511 keV. Acceptable spatial resolution can also be obtained at low single photon energies because the presence of the grooves limits the dispersion of scintillations produced by interactions in the crystal as shown in Figure 2.18B. A third approach is to change detector materials. Solid-state detectors such as cadmium-zinc-telluride (CZT) are being evaluated for single photon imaging applications and may eventually have applications in high energy imaging. Another approach under study is to couple LSO and NaI(Tl) in a detector sandwich for both low and high photon imaging with improved efficiency at high energies. If many small detectors are used instead of single, large-area detectors as with current scintillation cameras, significant gains in count rate capabilities could be obtained by parallel signal detection and processing. This approach is currently being evaluated by Siemens-CTI.

Image Fusion

PET scans of ^{18}FDG distributions in oncologic applications provide high resolution images that measure tissue metabolism at the time of the study. However, interpretation of these emission scans is often complicated by the absence of detailed anatomy in the emission data. In practice, interpretation is accomplished by visually comparing the emission scans to high quality anatomical maps such as those provided by clinical CT scanners. In these situations, it is often difficult for the interpreting physician to visually integrate the two image sets to precisely locate a region of increased uptake on the CT scan that was identified on the PET scan. To aid in image interpretation, several techniques have been developed to register the emission scans with the high resolution anatomical maps provided by CT.[12] One of these techniques requires the generation of three-dimensional surface maps of the two distributions and the use of iterative algorithms to find parameters that optimize the alignment of the two distributions. These parameters are then used to transform one of the two acquired data sets so that it is registered with the second set. This technique provides the best registration for a small, rigid body in which the surface is well-defined by both modalities, such as the brain.[13]

A second method involves the use of automated algorithms which assume that corresponding pixels in the two images are directly related by a common factor, and iterative optimization algorithms are used to determine this factor by minimizing the variance of the ratio of the adjusted-to-reference images. The application of this technique must be limited to the actual tissue distributions by the use of tissue masks that can be determined by edge detection algorithms and is best suited for registering images from a common modality.[14]

The third technique is an iterative interaction procedure in which a knowledgeable observer uses an interactive mathematical registration algorithm that permits the identification of an initial set of trial transformation parameters, an algorithm that performs the transformation, and techniques for image correlation that permit control and evaluation of the accuracy of the transformation. This technique is the most versatile of the three algorithms and has a wide variety of applications, assuming sufficient anatomical markers are present in both image sets. However, it is somewhat subjective and depends on the skills of the observer.[15] After registration has been accomplished using one of these techniques, images of corresponding anatomical slices can then be overlaid (fused) to provide precise anatomical location of detected abnormalities. However, these methods often suffer from registration errors due to difficulties in patient repositioning and movement of internal organs between scanning sessions.

PET-CT Integrated Systems

To address these problems, a commercial CT scanner and a commercial dedicated PET scanner have recently been integrated and mounted on a single support system with a common imaging table as shown in Figure 2.19.[16] The PET scanner used in this configuration was a Siemens-CTI ART scanner (Figure 2.19A), a partial ring system described previously. The CT scanner used was a Siemens third generation, single-slice, helical scanner (Figure 2.19B). The CT scanner was mounted on the front of a rotational support gantry, and the PET scanner was mounted on the back of the same gantry (Figure 2.19C–D). The combined gantry has a rotational speed of 30 rpm. The centers of the two imaging systems are offset axially by 60 cm. A common imaging table is positioned at the front of the gantry and permits an axial travel range of 180 cm. Because of the offsets between the two imaging systems, the system is limited to a maximum axial distance of 100 cm that can be imaged by both systems without moving the patient.

A similar PET-CT system is being manufactured by General Electric. With these integrated systems, a diagnostic CT scan and a PET scan can be acquired sequentially with the patient lying on the imaging table and simply being translated between the two systems. Accurate calibration of the position of the imaging table and the use of common parameters in data acquisition and image reconstruction permit the fusion of images of anatomy and metabolism from the same region of the body that are registered in space and only slightly offset in time. Since the CT scan is actually a high-resolution

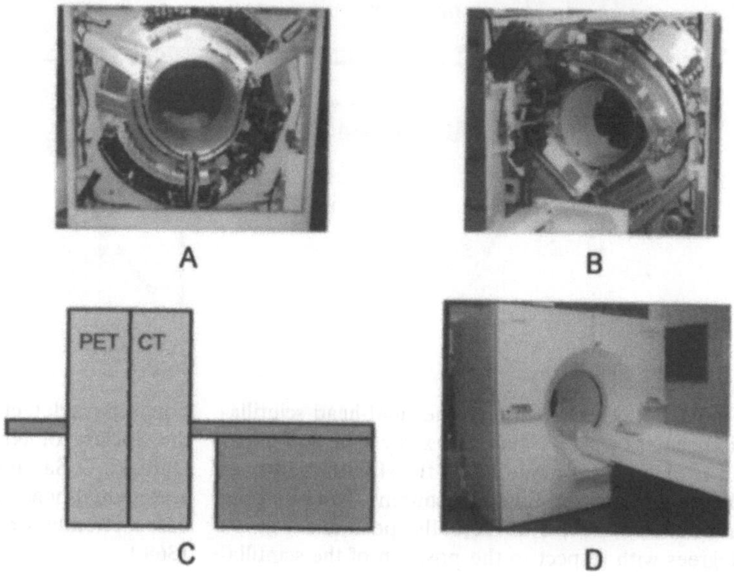

FIGURE 2.19. A partial ring PET scanner (Siemens-CTI ART) (A) and a diagnostic CT Scanner (Siemens single slice, helical scanner) (B) have been coupled to a single rotational gantry and a common imaging table (C) to produce an integrated PET-CT scanner (D). (Courtesy of David Townsend, PhD, University of Pittsburgh, Pittsburgh, PA.)

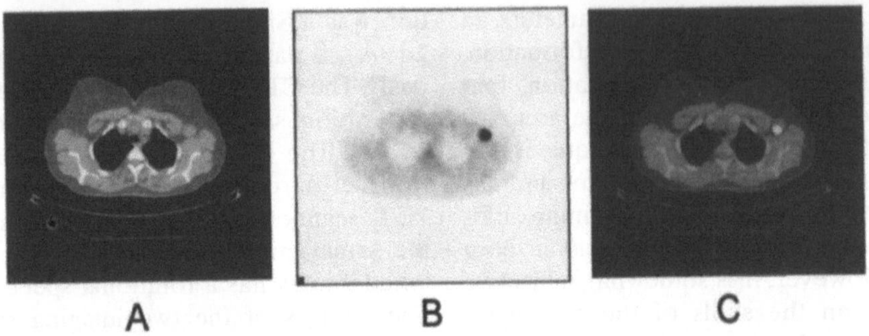

FIGURE 2.20. Patient with recurrent lymphoma imaged with ^{18}FDG on an integrated multiring PET/CT system (General Electric). (A) Transmission scan from the CT system. (B) PET scan with attenuation correction from (A) of the ^{18}FDG distribution. (C) Fused image of (A) and (B) demonstrating the correlation of anatomy and metabolic activity. (Courtesy of General Electric Medical Systems and Rambam Medical Center, Haifa, Israel.)

transmission map, these data can be used to perform a high quality attenuation correction during image reconstruction of the emission data. An example of a fused image acquired with this system is shown in Figure 2.20.

In addition, a new PET-CT system, the PosiTRACE, is being produced by SMV/General Electric. This system consists of six camera heads with $^3/_4$ inch thick NaI(Tl) crystals arranged in a hexagonal array and integrated with a diagnostic CT scanner. This system acquires coincidence data in 3D mode with complete sampling obtained by rotating the detector system around the patient.

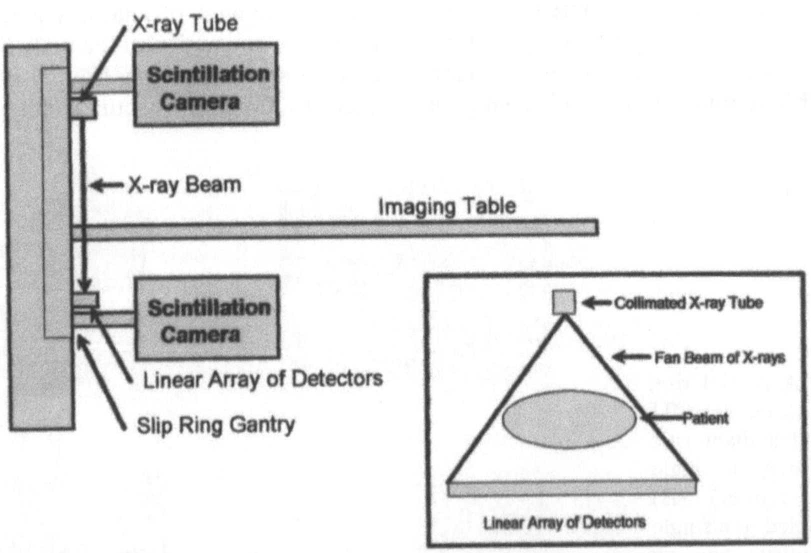

FIGURE 2.21. Schematic of the dual-head scintillation camera with a collimated x-ray tube and linear array of detectors mounted on the slip ring gantry of the camera for transmission scanning. Note that the transmission device is actually positioned at 90 degrees with respect to the position of the scintillation camera detectors. (Reprinted with permission of the Society of Nuclear Medicine from Patton JA, Delbeke D, Sandler MP: Image fusion using an integrated dual-head coincidence camera with x-ray tube based attenuation maps. J Nucl Med 2000;41:1364–1368.)

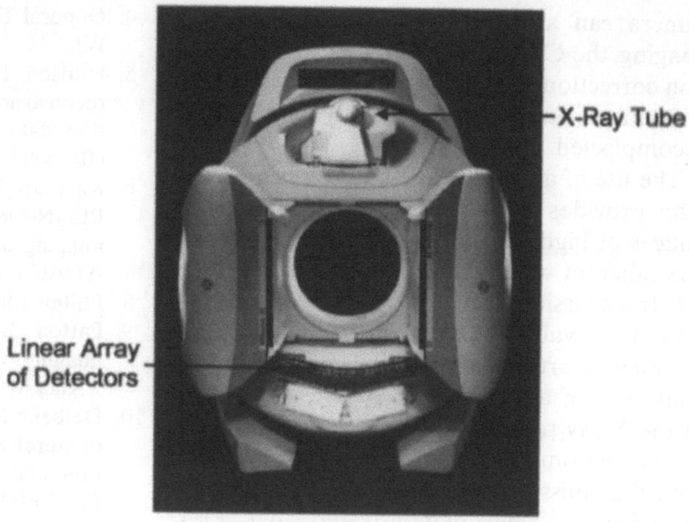

FIGURE 2.22. General Electric Hawkeye, an integrated CT/dual-head scintillation camera with coincidence imaging capability.

Similar advancements have been made in hybrid camera technology. General Electric has installed an X-ray tube and linear detector array on a dual-head scintillation camera with coincidence imaging capability to provide attenuation maps and anatomical localization, as shown in Figures 2.21 and 2.22.[17] The X-ray tube and linear detector array are mounted on the slip ring gantry of the camera and continuously rotate together with the detector heads around the patient in a fixed geometry for data acquisition. The X-ray tube is a low output tube, and the detector array consists of 384 solid-state detectors (each 1.8 × 28 mm). The X-ray tube is collimated to provide a fan beam of photons expanding to fill the field of view of the linear array in the transverse direction (see insert in Figure 2.21) and with a beam width of 1 cm at the center of the scan field in the axial direction. Since the fan beam is wide enough to cover the full width of the patient and the X-ray tube and detector array are in a fixed geometry and rotate together, this system has the characteristics of a low-end, third generation CT scanner. One CT slice is acquired in 13.6 seconds. As with the integrated PET-CT system, anatomical and metabolic images are acquired sequentially, and the high photon flux CT images are used for high quality attenuation correction of the emission data. The CT images and the emission images can also be fused to provide functional images to accurately locate regions of increased metabolic activity. An example of a clinical study acquired with this integrated system is shown in Figure 2.23A–C. Since this

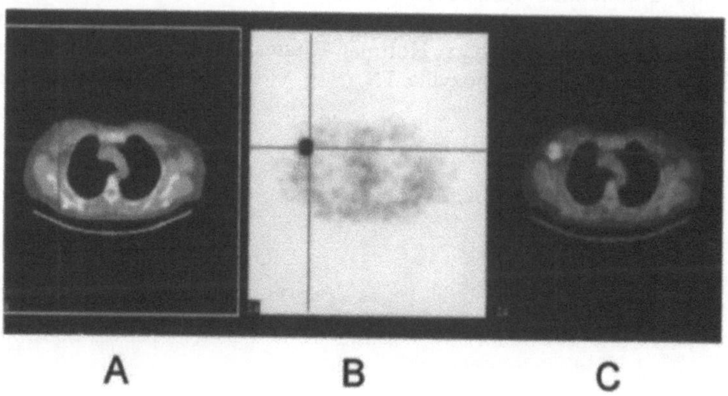

FIGURE 2.23. Patient with breast cancer imaged with ^{18}FDG on an integrated hybrid scintillation camera/CT system. (A) Transmission scan from the CT system. (B) Emission coincidence scan with attenuation correction from (A) of the ^{18}FDG distribution. (C) Fused image of (A) and (B) demonstrating the correlation of anatomy and metabolic activity.

camera can also be used for single photon imaging, the CT scans can be used for attenuation correction of SPECT images, and fusion of anatomical and SPECT images can also be accomplished.

The use of an X-ray tube-based transmission scan provides attenuation-corrected emission images of high quality due to the high photon flux inherent with this technique. Using the X-ray transmission scan for attenuation correction adds value due to the elimination of attenuation artifacts and improvement in image contrast. An added benefit of the availability of the X-ray transmission scan is the provision of an anatomical map for correlation/fusion with the emission images. Although numerous investigators have demonstrated that PET imaging provides increased sensitivity/specificity versus CT in differentiating benign from malignant lesions, staging primary cancer with metastatic disease, and monitoring therapeutic response of radiation and chemotherapy, the inability of PET to provide anatomical localization remains a significant impairment in maximizing its clinical utility. However, fusion of anatomical maps and FDG images obtained sequentially in time and registered in an integrated system without patient movement allows precise anatomic localization of lesions that have increased metabolism and provides a valuable new tool for diagnostic and therapeutic applications.

References

1. Schmand M, Dahlbom M, Eriksson L, et al.: Performance of a LSO/NaI(Tl) phoswich detector for a combined PET/SPECT imaging system. J Nucl Med 1998;39:9P.
2. Siemens Medical Systems, Hoffman Estates, IL.
3. CTI PET Systems, Knoxville, TN.
4. General Electric Medical Systems, Milwaukee, WI.
5. Hudson HM, Larkin RS: Accelerated image reconstruction using ordered subsets of projection data. IEEE Trans Med Imaging 1994;13: 601–609.
6. Karp JS, Muehllehner G, Mankoff DA, et al.: PENN-PET: A positron tomograph with volume imaging capability. J Nucl Med 1990;31:617–627.
7. ADAC Laboratories, Milpitas, CA.
8. Philips Medical Systems, Best, The Netherlands.
9. Patton JA: Instrumentation for coincidence imaging with multihead scintillation cameras. J Nucl Med 2000;30:239–254.
10. Delbeke D, Martin WH, Patton JA, et al.: Value of iterative reconstruction, attenuation correction, and image fusion in the interpretation of FDG PET images with an integrated dual-head coincidence camera and x-ray-based attenuation maps. Radiology 2001;218:163–171.
11. Marconi Medical Systems, Cleveland, OH.
12. Berger C, Berthold T: Image Fusion, in von Schulthess GK (ed): Clinical Positron Emission Tomography (PET). Philadelphia: Lippincott Williams & Wilkins, 2000, pp 41–48.
13. Pelizzari CA, Chen GT, Spelbring DR, et al.: Accurate three-dimensional registration of CT, PET, and/or MR images of the brain. J Comput Assist Tomogr 1989;13:20–26.
14. Woods RP, Cherry SR, Mazziotta JC: Rapid automated algorithm for aligning and reslicing PET images. J Comput Tomogr 1992;16:620–633.
15. Pietrzyk U, Herholz K, Fink G, et al.: An interactive technique for three-dimensional image registration: Validation for PET, SPECT, MRI, and CT brain studies. J Nucl Med 1994;35:2011–2018.
16. Beyer T, Townsend DW, Brun T, et al.: A combined PET/CT scanner for clinical oncology. J Nucl Med 2000;41:1369–1379.
17. Patton JA, Delbeke D, Sandler MP: Image fusion using an integrated dual-head coincidence camera with x-ray tube based attenuation maps. J Nucl Med 2000;41:1364–1368.

3
FDG Production and Distribution

Jeff Clanton

FDG is an extremely versatile diagnostic radiopharmaceutical used in PET imaging. In 1998, demand for the clinical use of fluorodeoxyglucose (^{18}FDG) began to rise at an astonishing rate. There were several factors in the driving force behind this growth. One factor was the availability of lower cost gamma camera SPECT systems with coincidence imaging capability. Another factor was the limited approval by private insurers, as well as Medicare, to pay for specific clinical uses of ^{18}FDG. Another significant contributor to the increasing demand was the emergence of regional cyclotron facilities that produce and distribute ^{18}FDG. As these regional centers began to network across the United States, ^{18}FDG became widely available, even in areas perceived unreachable by previous models.

Regional Cyclotron Facilities

In the 1970s and 1980s, the original planners for PET imaging centers incorporated a cyclotron with ancillary equipment and personnel into their pro forma before completing a budget for the project. This would have been a logical conclusion as ^{18}F has a half-life of only 109 minutes, with other cyclotron-produced positron emitters having significantly shorter half-lives. As experience grew with cyclotron centers producing short-lived positron emitters, it became apparent that a facility of this type was expensive and difficult to operate in a reliable and efficient manner. In the mid-1990s, through the efforts of several companies operating independently, the concept of the regional cyclotron facility/pharmacy was born. Once this model comes to fruition (potentially by 2005), virtually all PET imaging centers desiring the use of ^{18}FDG should be within a 4-hour drive of a cyclotron facility across the United States (Figure 3.1, see color plate).

The Cyclotron

Many factors must be considered prior to the selection of a cyclotron. These include (1) negative versus positive ion machines, (2) proton energy, (3) self-shielding versus the construction of a vault for shielding, (4) local versus regional distribution, (5) desired isotopes to be produced, (6) local regulations, (6) construction site limitations, and (7) cyclotron reliability.

Cyclotrons can accelerate virtually any charged particle. The two general classes of cyclotrons used for isotope production are positive and negative ion machines. The most common particle required for PET isotope production is the proton.

Positive ion machines accelerate only protons. Proton-only cyclotrons have historically been used for higher energy (>30 MeV) applications such as radioisotope production for standard nuclear medicine and physics research. The high-energy proton will activate the interior components of the cyclotron as well as areas of the concrete vault used for shielding. The result is maintenance difficulties

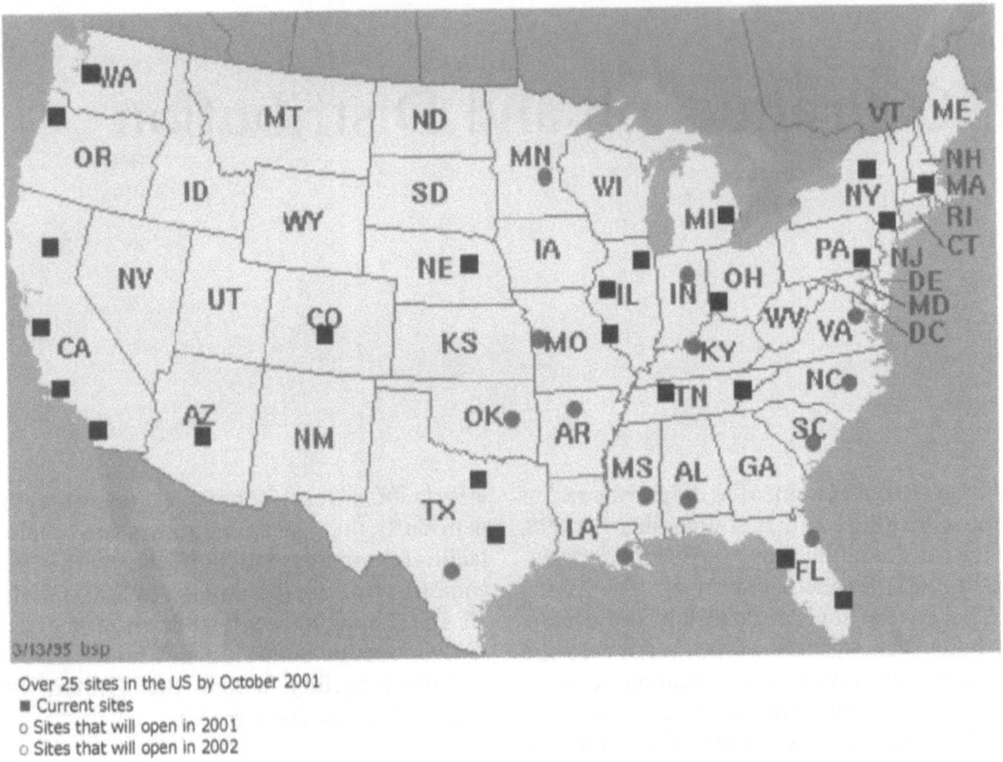

FIGURE 3.1. United States map depicting current and proposed cyclotron facilities of the largest ^{18}FDG production company, PETNet, Knoxville, TN (October 2000). (Courtesy of PETNet, Knoxville, TN.) (See color plate)

and high decommissioning costs. Negative ion machines accelerate an ion comprised of two electrons combined with one proton. This ion has a net negative charge. For isotope production, the two electrons are removed during acceleration leaving the proton for target bombardment.

Cyclotron manufacturers (for example, CTI, Ebco, GE, and IBA) have developed competitive products for the PET market. Generally, these devices were designed a decade or more ago with the idea that every hospital or clinic desiring PET imaging would own and operate its own cyclotron. These cyclotrons all have a relatively small footprint allowing them to be sited in an area less than 1,500 square feet. Depending on the model, the protons can be accelerated to a potential energy between 11 and 18 MeV, and many are available as self-shielded units (Figure 3.2, see color plate). Virtually all the cyclotrons in this class are negative ion machines.

Negative ion machines have several advantages operating in the aforementioned energy range for ^{18}F production. Unlike the positive ion machine, which accelerates only the proton, the negative ion does not activate internal components of the cyclotron. This allows the cyclotron to be serviced more quickly after operation without the risk of inordinate amounts of radiation exposure to personnel. It also helps minimize activation of ancillary shielding and surrounding walls.

The negative ion machine affords several convenient methods to efficiently extract the proton beam to the desired target. A popular method of beam extraction is accomplished by rotating a thin carbon foil into the negative ion beam under computer control. Once the foil is in the beam, the foil strips two electrons from the negative ion, leaving only the proton. The proton is then repelled down a beam tube to the target to produce the desired isotope. Most isotopes produced in this fashion are formed by

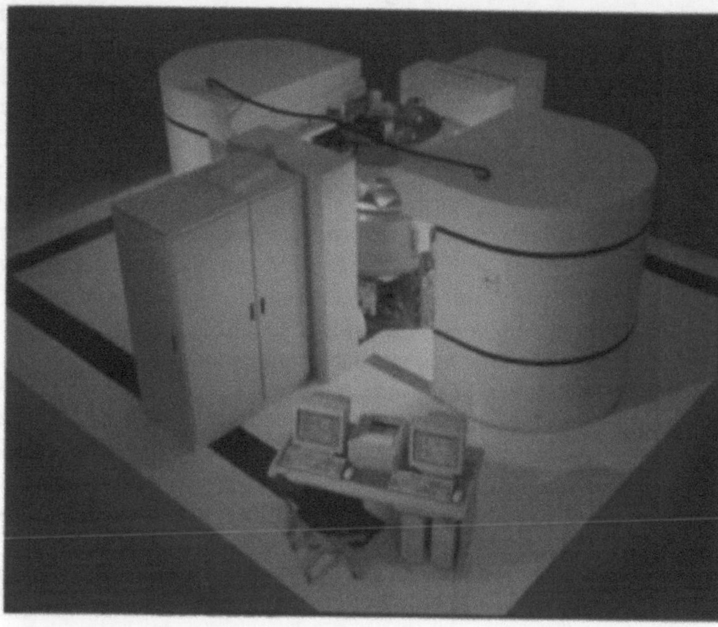

FIGURE 3.2. RDS-111 PET cyclotron manufactured by CTI in Knoxville, TN. (Courtesy of CTI, Knoxville, TN.) (See color plate)

a proton hitting the nucleus of the desired precursor, expelling a neutron, and remaining in the nucleus. This is commonly referred to as a "p,n" reaction.

The drawback to the negative ion machine is the requirement for a vacuum that is at least tenfold lower than the vacuum required for a positive ion machine. Because the negative ion machine accelerates two electrons with a proton, should this species strike any atom during acceleration it has the potential of losing one or more electrons on impact, rendering the ion neutral or positive in charge and unavailable for acceleration.

Consideration must also be given to proton energy. Of the mini cyclotrons available today for PET, there are two basic energies to choose from: 11 or 18 MeV. Basically, the higher the proton energy in this range, the greater the amount of ^{18}F that can be produced per unit time.

The 11 MeV cyclotrons range in energy from 10.5 to 11.5 MeV and have a slightly smaller footprint than the 18 MeV (16.5 to 19.5 MeV) machines since the potential energy imparted to the proton is directly related to the radius of the cyclotron. The primary advantage of the 11 MeV cyclotron is its ability to be self-shielded. Self-shielding translates to lower construction and decommissioning costs. Two principle disadvantages of the 11 MeV cyclotron are lower energy and difficulty in accessing the cyclotron for service because of the shielding surrounding the unit. Generally, 11 MeV machines with shielding are priced 10 to 20% less than the 18 MeV cyclotrons without shielding.

At least one manufacturer offers an 18 MeV cyclotron that is self-shielded. Unfortunately, the cost of self-shielding is almost equivalent in cost to the construction of a concrete vault to shield the cyclotron. The advantage of a vault is the ease with which the cyclotron can be serviced. When choosing the energy, one must consider the quantity of ^{18}F that will be required for a particular installation. Per unit time, the 18 MeV cyclotrons are capable of producing approximately twice the ^{18}F that 11 MeV machines produce. Independent of the cyclotron energy, service and reliability should be a principal concern when purchasing equipment of this type.

After the selection of the cyclotron is complete, the final installation must provide an environment for reliability. Cyclotron reliability is directly related to the following factors: the availability of repair parts, accessibility to experienced cyclotron service personnel, and consistent performance of preventative maintenance. For a successful program, all of these factors must be in place and managed effectively.

^{18}F Production

The most common method of ^{18}F production is proton bombardment of ^{18}O-water. For reasonable yields of ^{18}F with mini PET cyclotrons, the water used must be 95% enriched with ^{18}O. ^{18}O is a natural isotope of oxygen that occurs at about 0.3% abundance in nature. A molecular still is required to enrich the water to 95% ^{18}O-water. The process from natural water to 95% ^{18}O enrichment requires approximately ten months under carefully controlled conditions. Today, the world's requirement for ^{18}O enriched water is met from four facilities. Two distillation facilities are located in the United States, one is located in Israel, and one is located in Georgia (formerly part of the U.S.S.R.). Because the water is difficult to produce and obtain, this ingredient tends to be the single most expensive component of ^{18}F-FDG production at $150 to $200 per gram.

For ^{18}F production, approximately 1 to 2 grams of ^{18}O-water is loaded into a target; the target is then sealed and bombarded with protons. The result is ^{18}F as HF in ^{18}O-water. At the completion of bombardment, the ^{18}F in water is transferred to an automated synthesis unit for ^{18}FDG production.

^{18}FDG Production

The most common method of ^{18}FDG production is a nucleophilic synthesis described by Hamacher et al.[1] Basically, the ^{18}F is separated from the ^{18}O-water using an anion exchange resin. The ^{18}F is then eluted from the resin with aqueous potassium carbonate (K_2CO_3). An aminopolyether, 4,7,13,16,21,24-Hexaoxa-1,10-Diazabicyclo[8,8,8]Hexacosane (known as Krytofix 222 or K-222), is introduced, and the aqueous solution is evaporated with dry acetonitrile. In the absence of water, potassium made available from the added potassium carbonate is sequestered within the cagelike structure of the aminopolyether (K-222) forming a weak ion pair with 18-F. In this chemical state, 18-F is available for nucleophilic substitution. The nucleophilic substitution is performed with a protected sugar (1,3,4,5-tetra-O-acetyl-2-[^{18}F]fluoro-B-D-manno-pyranose). The protective acetyl groups are then hydrolyzed in aqueous medium following the evaporation of all remaining organic solvents with acid (1N HCl) or base (2N NaOH). Acid hydrolysis requires approximately 12 minutes at 100°C, whereas alkaline hydrolysis may be accomplished in 90 seconds at room temperature. The resulting product is 2-[^{18}F]-fluoro-2-deoxy-D-glucose in aqueous solution. After hydrolysis, the aqueous reaction mixture is passed through disposable chromatographic cartridges for removal of any remaining impurities and pH adjustment followed by a 0.22 micron filter to ensure sterility.

There are several manufacturers of computer-controlled ^{18}FDG synthesis modules. The synthesis modules on the market currently are manufactured by Coincidence, CTI, and Nuclear Interface (Figure 3.3, see color plate). The Coincidence module utilizes patented chemistry that incorporates alkaline hydrolysis. The QuadRX module (CTI) can perform up to four runs with one setup and uses acid or base hydrolysis. The Nuclear Interface unit utilizes acid hydrolysis. All of these modules accomplish the synthesis of ^{18}FDG in an automated fashion.

Other unique methods of ^{18}FDG production, including an electrophilic synthesis[2], have been attempted but have not proven practical in a routine production environment.

^{18}FDG Quality Control

The United States Pharmacopeia (USP) describes in detail product standards for ^{18}FDG, as well as the quality control (QC) methods that must be utilized to test the final product. The methods that may be required for ^{18}FDG quality control prior to patient administration include the following tests: pH, isotonicity, chemical purity, radiochemical purity, radionuclidic purity, sterility, bacterial endotoxin testing, and organic volatiles.

FIGURE 3.3. Automated synthesis units currently available for ^{18}FDG production—(A) Coincidence, (B) QuadRx, and (C) Nuclear Interface. ((A) Courtesy of Bioscan, Washington, DC; (B) Courtesy of CTI, Knoxville, TN; (C) Courtesy of Nuclear Interface, Berlin, Germany.) (See color plate)

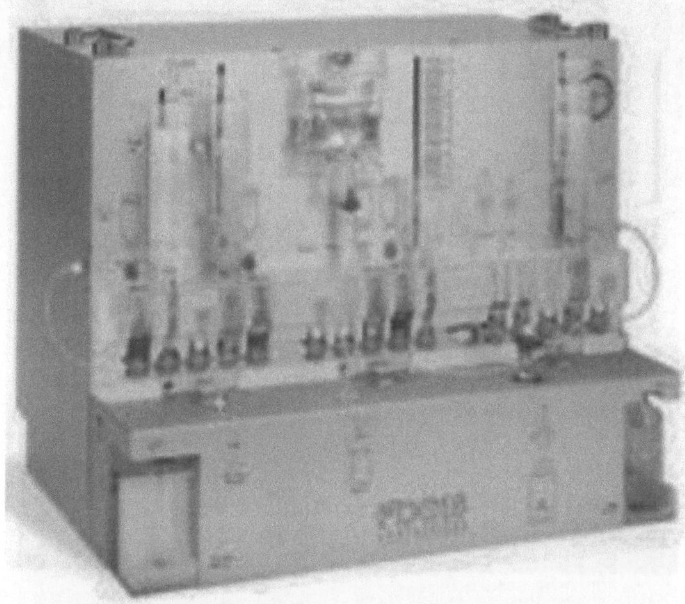

A

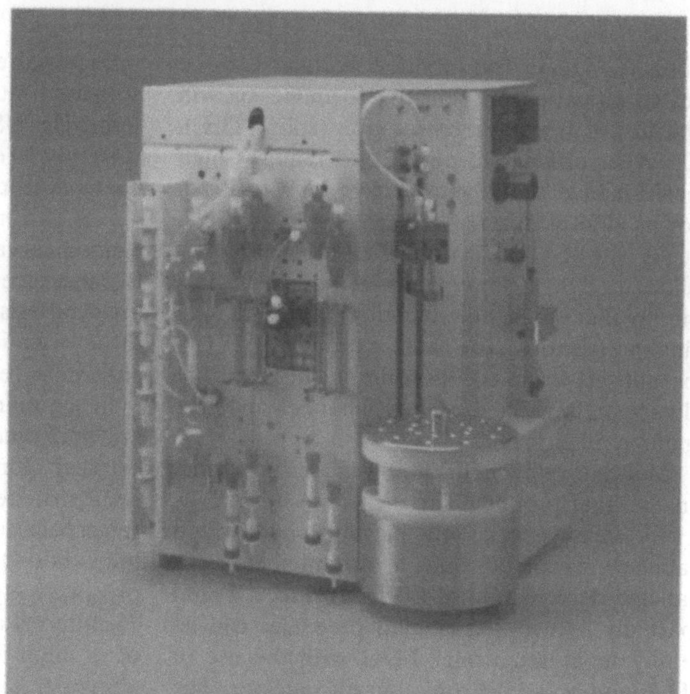

B

Because the primary component of ^{18}FDG is normal saline (0.9% NaCl in sterile water), the USP standard for pH is the same as that required for normal saline, 4.5 to 7.0. Due to the small volume of ^{18}FDG produced in each batch or lot, pH testing is normally accomplished with standardized pH paper. Chemically, the significant byproducts that could appear in the final product are the aminopolyether (K-222) and chloride-labeled deoxyglu-

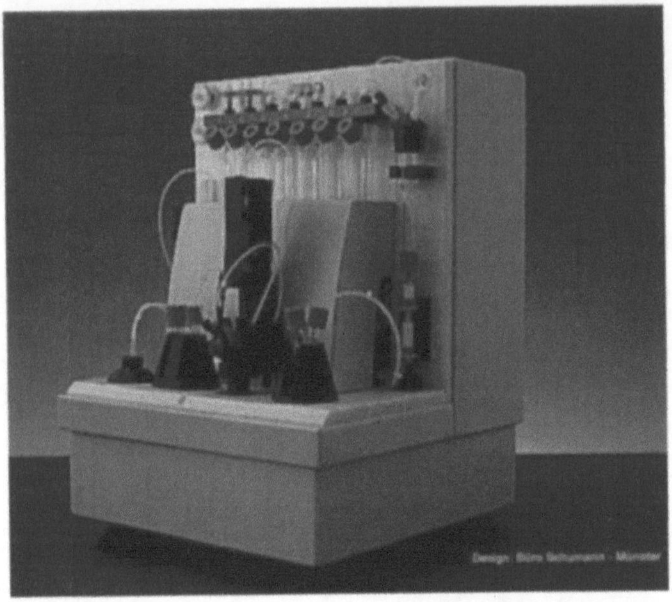

C

FIGURE 3.3. *Continued*

cose (Cl-DG). The aminopolyether can be tested with a reagent sensitive to amines or with the use of thin layer chromatography (TLC). Cl-DG is difficult to detect and requires high performance liquid chromatography (HPLC) for its identification.

As with the production of all other radionuclides used in nuclear medicine, there is the possibility that other radionuclides may exist in the final preparation. The same methodologies can be utilized to detect these impurities, half-life determinations, and/or multichannel analyzer gamma fingerprints.

Multiple radiochemical impurities may exist in the final product. These include free ^{18}F as H^{18}F, three species of partially hydrolyzed labeled precursor, and a potential for ^{18}F labeled deoxymannose (^{18}FDM). Free ^{18}F and partially hydrolyzed labeled precursor can be easily separated from ^{18}FDG with the use of TLC and a radiochromatogram detector. The detection of ^{18}FDM is more complex, requiring the use of HPLC.

Sterility is tested in the same fashion as all other radiopharmaceuticals, utilizing two types of inoculated growth media to detect aerobic and anaerobic bacteria. The USP sterility test requires 14 days for completion.

Bacterial endotoxin testing is accomplished utilizing limulus amebocyte lysate (LAL) reagents. The USP limit for bacterial endotoxins is currently 10 endotoxin units per ml of injectate, not to exceed 175 endotoxin units per injection.

Gas chromatography is required to test for residual organic solvents in the final product. Because acetonitrile and ethanol are used in the synthesis of ^{18}FDG, the suggested limits for these organics in the final product are 0.04% and 0.5%, respectively.

In summary, several quality control measures are performed prior to releasing the pharmaceutical for administration. Although the results of sterility testing are available only in retrospect due to the short half-life of the drug, the other QC measures can be accomplished prospectively in a matter of approximately 75 minutes and are able to provide assurance of a high quality product safe for human administration.

Regulatory Impact

The greatest impact on the production of PET radiopharmaceuticals will occur in the next several years when the Food and Drug Administration (FDA) develops new regulations regarding PET pharmaceuticals. Currently most PET drugs, including ^{18}FDG, are compounded and distributed under the right to practice medicine and pharmacy granted by individual states within the United States.

In November 1997, the Food and Drug Administration Modernization Act (FDAMA) was passed in the United States. Part of FDAMA was targeted directly toward the PET community. This portion of legislation allotted a four-year time line for all cyclotron facilities in the United States to become registered as drug manufacturers. The first two years were to be utilized by the FDA to work with the PET community to develop Good Manufacturing Practices (GMP) that applied to the unique characteristics of PET. (As of March 2001, the time frame has been exceeded by more than one year without PET-specific GMPs in the immediate future.) The remaining two-year period, which begins on GMP completion, is granted to allow all existing and new cyclotron facilities adequate time to comply with the new PET GMPs and register as a drug manufacturer.

Following its mandate to protect the public, the FDA decided to develop regulations and control PET radiopharmaceuticals as if these small local facilities were large wholesale drug manufacturers. The difficulties in developing GMPs for the PET industry include the following: drug lots and production runs that consist of only one vial, half-lives of two minutes, and existing facilities in academic institutions that lack adequate space for required GMP upgrades. The added bureaucracy afforded by the FDA may not improve drug quality. The additional paperwork will possibly make the ^{18}FDG more expensive and difficult to deliver to the patient in a reliable fashion.

Delivery

Shipment of ^{18}FDG in the United States is regulated by the Department of Transportation (DOT). Because ^{18}FDG is radioactive, ^{18}FDG is classified as a hazardous material under the Code of Federal Regulations (CFR). To legally ship ^{18}FDG, several conditions must be met by the shipper. First, approved shipping containers designed and tested to transport ^{18}FDG (DOT-7A containers) must be utilized. Second, all personnel involved in the shipping process must be trained in accordance with 49 CFR part 172. Should the shipper (in this case the cyclotron facility) decide to transport the hazardous material instead of using an approved courier service, additional regulations must be met.

The challenges encountered with ^{18}FDG delivery in the United States are twofold. One is the short half-life of ^{18}FDG (109 minutes), and the second is the expansive area that exists in the United States (approximately 3.7 million square miles). To provide controlled, reliable, and economic delivery, the PET imaging site should be located within 200 miles of a cyclotron facility. Once this distance is exceeded, air transport must be utilized.

Air transport can be utilized to ship ^{18}FDG, but reliability decreases due to increased complexity. To effectively ship ^{18}FDG by air, dedicated charter aircraft must be used. Currently, qualified air couriers charge approximately $1.75 per mile flown for a small twin engine aircraft. Generally, the cost of air charter delivery is three to four times that of ground transportation.

Ground transportation, while slower than aircraft, is more reliable. Weather problems that affect air transportation often have little to no effect on ground transport. When using air transportation, ground transport must deliver the ^{18}FDG from the cyclotron facility to the airport and be used once again to pick up the ^{18}FDG at the destination airport and deliver it to the PET site. Scheduling and flight delays can cause havoc with this scenario. Most important is the fact that should a problem occur at the cyclotron facility that causes a decreased yield in ^{18}FDG production, it is economically feasible to provide multiple ground transports during the day to meet imaging needs. This is a luxury that cannot be afforded using air transport.

Due to the increasing demand of ^{18}FDG as a diagnostic tool for PET imaging, its production and distribution will continue to grow and mature as a unique local/regional pharmaceutical industry.

References

1. Hamacher K, Coenen HH, Stocklin G: Efficient stereospecific synthesis of no-carrier added 2-[^{18}F]-fluoro-2-deoxy-D-glucose using aminopolyether supported nucleophilic substitution. J Nucl Med 1996;27:235–238.
2. Bida GT, Satyamurthy N, Barrio JR: The synthesis of 2-[^{18}F]-fluoro-2-deoxy-D-glucose using glycals: A reexamination. J Nucl Med 1984;25: 1327–1334.

4 Clinical Applications for the Central Nervous System

Dominique Delbeke

The glucose metabolism of the brain can be evaluated using the glucose analog, ^{18}F-fluorodeoxyglucose (FDG). FDG is transported into the cells by the same mechanism as glucose. FDG is then phosphorylated by a hexokinase into FDG-6-phosphate. As brain tissue does not have a glucose-6-dephosphatase, FDG-6-phosphate cannot progress into further glycolytic pathways, so it accumulates proportional to the glycolytic rate of the cells. The cortex of the brain normally only uses glucose as its substrate; therefore, FDG accumulation is high. Because dedicated PET systems with full rings of bismuth germanate oxide (BGO) detectors provide for soft tissue attenuation and are calibrated with an external source of known activity of ^{68}germanium, true count rates can be measured over a region of interest. Dynamic scanning after injection of FDG and dynamic arterial blood sampling to obtain both tissue and plasma tracer concentrations over time permit quantification of the actual metabolic rate using kinetic modeling. True quantitative measurements are extremely useful in the investigation of the physiopathological mechanisms of neuropsychiatric diseases and can be performed not only with FDG, but also with a variety of other radiopharmaceuticals labeled with positron emitters. This approach is time-consuming, cumbersome, and more invasive than obtaining a static image after FDG reaches a plateau, usually 45 minutes following intravenous injection. Measurement of the absolute metabolic rate is rarely performed clinically. Semiquantitative evaluation with asymmetry indices or ratios to reference structures of the brain is usually satisfactory for clinical diagnostic purposes. Correction for attenuation can be performed using transmission maps, obtained from external radioactive sources (measured attenuation correction), or using calculated attenuation correction. Correction for attenuation effects can be performed using calculated geometric attenuation for uniform structures that are predictable in shape and content, such as the brain. Calculated attenuation correction can be used very accurately and is patient-independent.

To interpret tomographic cerebral images, it is critical to utilize software capable of reorienting the images along the anterior commissure-posterior commissure (AC-PC) line. The images should be viewed on a monitor in all three projections (axial, coronal, and sagittal), utilizing color scales and gray scale with appropriate intensity settings. If two sets of images must be compared (ictal and interictal, baseline and activation, pre- and post-therapy or intervention), similar orientation, section thickness, and windowing is critical. Comparison with current MRI or CT images is also critical to correlate with structural abnormalities.

Normal Distribution and Variants

Perfusion and glucose metabolic images of the brain have a similar appearance, except in pathologic circumstances when there is decoupling of perfusion and metabolism. The adult pattern of uptake is established by age two. The normal perfusion of the gray matter is approximately 70 ml/min/100 g, and that of the white matter is 20 ml/min/100 g. In the newborn, the perfusion and metabolism of basal ganglia, visual cortex, and sensory-motor cortex are similar to that of an adult, but there is relative decreased perfusion to the frontal and parietotemporal cortices, giving an immature pattern of perfusion and metabolism.[1] This must be recognized to accurately interpret metabolic PET images in children under age two.

The weight of the brain decreases approximately 10% between the ages of 30 and 75, and the cerebral blood flow decreases by 20%, probably because of neuronal loss and replacement by gliosis. On CT and MRI, this is demonstrated by progressive cortical atrophy with age.

In normal individuals, cerebral perfusion and metabolism are both influenced by certain drugs. Sedatives decrease the cerebral blood flow and metabolism. If a patient requires sedation for the scanning period, sedatives should be administered no earlier than 30 minutes after administration of the radiopharmaceutical. It is important to be aware of the medications taken by patients and their effects on the pattern of cerebral perfusion and metabolism.

Cerebral Vascular Disease

The etiologies of a cerebral infarction are multiple: thrombotic, embolic, and hemorrhagic, among others. Functional images are usually abnormal before anatomical images because the physiological dysfunction of an organ precedes the resulting anatomical changes. Positron emitters include ^{15}oxygen (half-life = 2 minutes), ^{13}nitrogen (half-life = 10 minutes), ^{11}carbon (half-life = 20 minutes), and ^{18}fluorine (half-life = 110 minutes) and require coincidence detection with a PET scanner for imaging. These radioisotopes have the advantage of being innate to the molecular structure of endogenous substrates. PET studies using $^{15}O\text{-}H_2O$ to evaluate perfusion, $^{15}O\text{-}O_2$ to evaluate oxygen metabolism, and ^{18}F-FDG to evaluate glucose metabolism have contributed to the understanding of the physiopathology of cerebral infarction. Because of the short half-life of positron emitters, these PET radiopharmaceuticals are not practical for clinical use, except for ^{18}F-FDG.

Within the first hours to days after a stroke, there is decreased relative perfusion compared to glucose and oxygen metabolism, a phenomenon called "misery perfusion." Twenty-four hours to one week after infarction, the perfusion usually improves, but the symptoms and crossed cerebellar diaschisis persist. There is decoupling of metabolism and perfusion, a phenomenon called "luxury perfusion," that may last from one to ten days and is thought to be due to local accumulation of free radicals. The "luxury perfusion" usually resolves one month after the acute event. In addition, there exists a "penumbral zone" surrounding the infarcted area, which is ischemic and demonstrates decreased perfusion but increased oxygen extraction fraction. If perfusion to the "penumbral zone" can be restored in a timely manner, irreversible damage will not occur.

There are regions that show decreased perfusion and metabolism that are distant to the region of infarction. For example, cortical infarcts are usually associated with decreased uptake in the contralateral cerebellar hemisphere (crossed cerebellar diaschisis) due to deafferentiation, a phenomenon that occurs when the impulses through the cortico-ponto-cerebellar fibers fail to be transmitted and stimulate the contralateral cerebellar hemisphere. Other areas that can demonstrate decreased perfusion and metabolism are the ipsilateral thalamus and caudate nucleus, probably also related to deafferentiation. Infarction of specific thalamic nuclei results in cortical hypometabolism, while infarction of others do not, due to specific thalamocortical tracts.

Seizures

Seizures may be due to idiopathic epilepsy or the presence of an irritating focus, such as a neoplasm or an infectious process. There are two types of epilepsy: (1) generalized seizures (grand mal and petit mal) thought to be due to abnormal impulses between the neocortex and the thalamic reticular system and (2) partial seizures due to sudden depolarization of a focal group of neurons. The partial seizures are called complex if the patient looses awareness or simple if awareness is preserved. Most partial seizures arise from the temporal lobe. More than half of the patients with partial seizures become refractory to medical therapy. If the seizure focus can be localized and resected surgically, the symptoms improve or are cured in most patients. MRI scanning is helpful if a structural lesion that may be responsible for the seizure can be localized or if hippocampal sclerosis is demonstrated. However, both the MRI and electroencephalogran (EEG) often fail to localize the seizure focus. Functional imaging using both SPECT and PET radiopharmaceuticals has been demonstrated to be highly predictive of the postsurgical outcome of these patients.[2] Both regional cerebral perfusion and metabolism are increased during the ictal period and decreased during the interictal period. FDG PET imaging is more sensitive for demonstration of the seizure focus in the interictal state, but ^{99m}Tc-HMPAO or ^{99m}Tc-ECD SPECT is more suitable for ictal administration because of its rapid first pass uptake.

Brain Tumors

Following treatment of high-grade brain tumors with a combination of surgery, radiation therapy, and chemotherapy, patients often develop neurological symptoms that may be related to edema and radiation necrosis or to recurrent tumor. The changes on CT and MRI are very similar for both etiologies. In the early 1980s, Di Chiro and collaborators[3,4] were the first investigators to demonstrate the potential of metabolic imaging with FDG PET for differentiation of recurrent high-grade tumor from radiation necrosis. An excellent review has been published by Langleben et al.[5] FDG PET imaging can also differentiate high-grade (uptake well above level of white matter) from low-grade glioma (uptake similar to that of white matter).[6–9] Lesions located within the gray matter that have uptake similar to that of physiologic gray matter uptake should be considered high-grade lesions. The appearance of foci of high FDG uptake in low-grade gliomas indicates malignant transformation and worsening of the prognosis.[10] A high degree of uptake in high-grade gliomas is a poor prognostic factor.[11–13] In HIV positive patients with brain lesions, FDG PET imaging can differentiate lymphoma (high FDG uptake) from toxoplasmosis (low FDG uptake),[14–16] greatly affecting therapy and outcome.

Brain metastases can be hypometabolic or hypermetabolic; therefore, the sensitivity of FDG PET imaging for detection of brain metastases is relatively low (68%).[17] In a study of patients with lung carcinoma, the sensitivity of FDG PET imaging for detection of brain metastases was 82%, but the specificity was only 38%.[18] In a larger population of 273 patients with suspected malignancy, FDG PET imaging detected brain metastases in 0.7%, whereas cerebral metastases were found in 1.5% by other modalities.[19] Although it is not uncommon to detect cerebral metastases on FDG PET imaging, MRI remains the most sensitive imaging modality and the standard of care for detection of brain metastases.

Dementias and Neuropsychiatric Diseases

In degenerative dementia, structural imaging with CT and MRI will either be normal or demonstrate nonspecific cortical atrophy. Functional imaging will either be normal (in pseudodementia/depression) or demonstrate a pattern of hypometabolism that correlates with the various syndromes. In the preliminary assessment of dementia, patients must first be separated on the basis of whether or not signs and symptoms of motor dysfunction are present (subcortical dementias) or not (cortical dementias). In cortical dementia, the subcortical structures are spared; the patients do not have motor dysfunction but present with apraxia, aphasia, memory loss, and abnormal affect (Alzheimer's disease or Pick's disease).

In subcortical dementias, the basal ganglia, thalami, and brain stem are affected; the patients have motor dysfunction (disorder of posture and tone, tremor, gait disturbance) as well as abnormal cognitive dysfunction. These disorders include extrapyramidal syndromes (for example, Parkinson's disease and syndromes, Huntington's disease, and Wilson's disease), white matter disease (for example, multiple sclerosis), HIV encephalopathy, and normal pressure hydrocephalus. A mixed category includes conditions that involve both cortical and subcortical structures such as vascular dementias (for example, multi-infarct dementia and Biswanger's disease), infectious dementias (for example, Creutzfeldt-Jakob), and hypoxic encephalopathy.[20,21]

Alzheimer's disease accounts for 75% of the dementias in the elderly. These patients present with short-term memory loss and visuospatial problems. However, clinically the diagnosis is unclear in a large proportion of these patients, especially early in the course of the disease. In advanced disease, CT and MRI demonstrate more pronounced atrophy in the temporoparietal and anterior frontal cortex; occasionally severe hippocampal atrophy is also seen. On FDG PET images, there is a characteristic pattern of decreased uptake in the posterior parietotemporal cortex, probably related to neuronal depletion in these areas, with perservation. These functional changes precede the atrophy seen on structural imaging, sometimes by years, and are more specific. Thirty percent of the patients present initially with a unilateral abnormality (often the left), but symmetrically decreased activity is present in most. Later in the disease, there is also decreased uptake in the frontal cortex.[22,23] Alzheimer's disease can occur in conjunction with Parkinsonism and Lewy body disease. In these cases, the imaging findings are indistinguishable from Alzheimer's disease, and histopathologically, the findings are those of Alzheimer's disease in addition to Parkinson's or Lewy body disease. The sensitivity and specificity of posterior parietal perfusion defect for Alzheimer's disease are in the range of 90%. Posterior parietal perfusion defects mimicking Alzheimer's disease can be seen in other entities such as normal pressure hydrocephalus, Creutzfeldt-Jakob disease, and AIDS encephalopathy, among others.

Frontal metabolic and perfusion deficits are a landmark for Pick's disease but can also be found in multiple system atrophy, progressive supranuclear palsy, nonspecific frontal gliosis, and chronic alcoholism. Pick's disease presents clinically with personality changes, emotional disturbances, and deterioration in behavior and judgment.

In Huntington's disease, there is decreased flow and metabolism in the caudate nucleus. These findings are present not only in symptomatic patients, but also in asymptomatic gene carriers. Therefore, functional imaging may be helpful in identifying those family members with the disease who have not yet expressed the gene clinically.

FDG PET images of multi-infarct dementia usually show multiple cortical defects. The large defects follow a vascular distribution. Sometimes vascular dementia and Alzheimer's disease may coexist in an individual patient.

Numerous studies have been published to investigate various neuropsychiatric diseases such as affective disorders, schizophrenia, obsessive-compulsive disorder, chronic fatigue syndrome, and chronic pain syndrome, mainly with PET using FDG and ^{18}F-labeled receptor ligands. To date, there are few clinical applications, but preliminary reports are promising.

Imaging Protocols for Evaluation of the Brain

Patients are instructed to fast for four hours and drink plenty of clear fluids. The serum glucose level is measured just before FDG administration to document euglycemia. The emission images are acquired 45 to 60 minutes after intravenous administration of 370 MBq (10 mCi) of FDG. During the distribution phase, the patients are required to rest in a quiet room with dimmed light and are instructed to keep their eyes closed. Sedatives, if necessary, are administered no earlier than 30 minutes after FDG administration.

The FDG images displayed in this chapter were acquired using either of two different dedicated tomographs with full rings of germanate bismuth oxide (BGO) detectors: Siemens ECAT 933 (CTI, Knoxville, TN) and GE Advance (General Electric Medical Systems, Milwaukee, WI). The acquisition protocols were the following:

Siemens ECAT 933

Emission scan: 2D mode, 15 minutes per bed position in two interleaved bed positions to provide sections of 4 mm in thickness.

Image reconstruction: filtered back projection with calculated attenuation correction.

GE Advance

Emission scan: 2D mode, 20 minutes in one bed position with sections of 4.5 mm in thickness.

Transmission scan: 2D mode, after the emission scan, 10 minutes in one bed position.

Image reconstruction: iterative reconstruction with segmented attenuation correction.

Hybrid Coincidence Imaging Systems

Due to the lower sensitivity of hybrid dual-head coincidence imaging systems as compared to full ring detector dedicated PET systems, the use of these hybrid systems for central nervous system applications is strongly discouraged because of the need for higher quality images that cannot be provided by these systems at this time.

References

1. Chugani HT, Phelps ME, Mazziotta JC: Positron emission tomography study of human brain development. Ann Neurol 1987;22:487–497.
2. Delbeke D, Lawrence SK, Abou-Khalil BW, Blumenkopf B, Kessler RM: Postsurgical outcome of patients with uncontrolled complex partial seizures and temporal lobe hypometabolism on ^{18}FDG positron emission tomography. Investigative Radiology 1996;31:261–265.
3. Patronas NJ, Di Chiro G, Brooks RA, et al.: Work in progress: [^{18}F] fluorodeoxyglucose and positron emission tomography in the evaluation of radiation necrosis of the brain. Radiology 1982;144:885–889.
4. Di Chiro G, Oldfield E, Wright DC, et al.: Cerebral necrosis after radiotherapy and/or intra-arterial chemotherapy for brain tumors: PET and neuropathologic studies. AJR 1988;150:189–197.
5. Langleben DD, Segall GM: PET in differentiation of recurrent brain tumor from radiation injury. J Nucl Med 2000;41:1861–1867.
6. Di Chiro G, DeLapaz RL, Brooks PA, et al.: Glucose utilization of cerebral gliomas measured by [^{18}F] fluorodeoxyglucose and positron emission tomography. Neurology 1982;32:1323–1329.
7. Patronas NJ, Brooks RA, DeLaPaz RI, Smith BH, Kornblitz PL, Di Chiro J: Glycolytic rate (PET) and contrast enhancement (CT) in human cerebral gliomas. AJNR 1983;4:533–535.
8. Kim CK, Alvi JB, Alavi A, Reivich M: New grading system of cerebral gliomas using positron emission tomography with F-18-fluorodeoxyglucose. J Neurooncol 1991;10:85–91.
9. Delbeke D, Meyerowitz C, Lapidus RL, et al.: Optimal cut-off level of F-18-fluorodeoxyglucose uptake in the differentiation of low grade from high grade brain tumors with PET. Radiology 1995;195:47–52.
10. De Witte O, Levivier M, Violon P, et al.: Prognostic value positron emission tomography with [18F]fluoro-2-deoxy-D-glucose in the low-grade glioma. Neurosurgery 1996;39(3):470–476; discussion 476–477.
11. Patronas NJ, Di Chiro G, Kufta C, et al.: Prediction of survival in glioma patients by means of positron emission tomography. J Neurosurg 1985;62:816–822.
12. Alavi JB, Alvai A, Chawluk J, et al.: Positron emission tomography in patients with gliomas: A predictor of prognosis. Cancer 1988;62:1074–1078.
13. Barker FJ, Chang SM, Valk PE, Pounds TR, Prados MD: 18-Fluorodeoxyglucose uptake and survival of patients with suspected recurrent malignant glioma. Cancer 1997;79:115–126.
14. Rosenfeld SS, Hoffman JM, Coleman RE, Glantz MJ, Hanson MW, Schold SC: Studies of primary central nervous system lymphoma with fluorine-18-fluorodeoxyglucose positron emission tomography. J Nucl Med 1992;33:532–536.
15. Hoffman JM, Waskin HA, Schifter T, et al.: FDG-PET in differentiating lymphoma from non-malignant central nervous system lesions in patients with AIDS. J Nucl Med 1993;34:567–575.

16. Kessler RM, Pierce M, Maciunas R, Allen G: Accuracy of FDG PET studies in distinguishing cerebral infections from lymphoma in patients with AIDS. J Nucl Med 1993;34:37P.
17. Griffeth LK, Rich KM, Dehdashti F, et al.: Brain metastases from non-central nervous system tumors: Evaluation with PET. Radiology 1993; 186(1):37–44.
18. Palm I, Hellwig D, Leutz M, et al.: Brain metastases of lung cancer: Diagnostic accuracy of positron emission tomography with fluorodeoxyglucose (FDG-PET) (German). Med Klin 1999;94(4):224–227.
19. Larcos G, Maisey MN: FDG-PET screening for cerebral metastases in patients with suspected malignancy. Nucl Med Commun 1996;17(3):197–198.
20. Tien RD, Felsberg GJ, Ferris NJ, Osumi AK: The dementias: Correlation of clinical features, pathophysiology, and neuroradiology. AJR 1993;161: 245–255.
21. Mazziotta JC, Frackowiak RSJ, Phelps ME: Positron emission tomography in the clinical assessment of dementia. Semin Nucl Med 1992;22:233–246.
22. Friedland RP, Budinger TF, Ganz E, et al.: Regional cerebral metabolic alterations in dementia of the Alzheimer type: Positron emission tomography with F-18-fluorodeoxyglucose. J Computer Assist Tomograph 1983;7(4):590–598.
23. Reiman EM, Caselli RJ, Yun LS, et al.: Preclinical evidence of Alzheimer's disease in persons homozygous for the E4 allele for apolipoprotein E. N Engl J Med 1996;334:752–758.

Case Presentations

Case 4.1

History

A 16-year-old male with intractable seizures refractory to medical treatment presented for evaluation of possible temporal lobe resection. A cerebral MRI was normal. The ictal scalp EEG shows discharges predominantly in the left posterotemporal region. He was referred for FDG PET imaging of the brain (Figure 4.1). The patient was monitored with EEG during

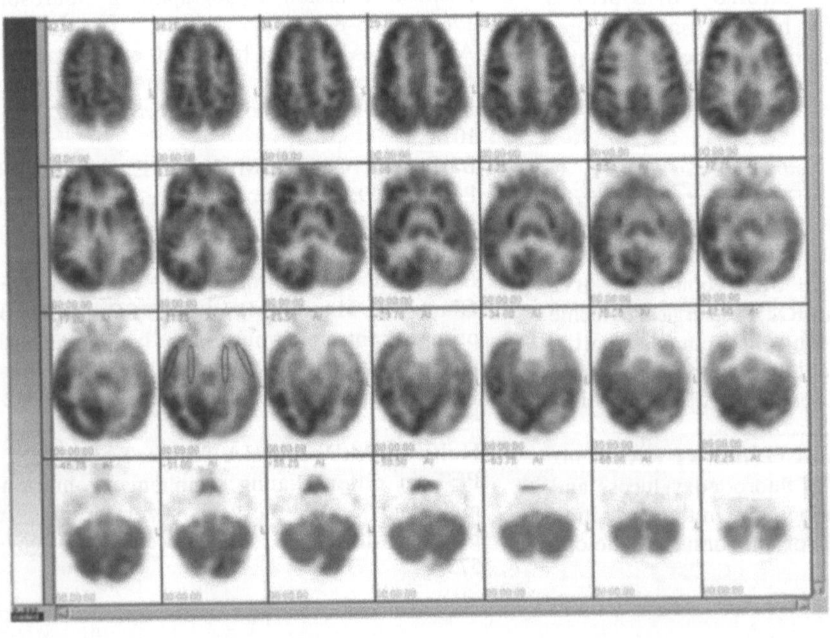

FIGURE 4.1.

the distribution phase of FDG, and there was no evidence of ictal discharges. The FDG images were acquired with a dedicated PET tomograph (GE Advance) in the 2D mode and reconstructed with iterative reconstruction and measured segmented attenuation correction. For the semiquantitative analysis, the PET images were reoriented along the temporal lobe axis of the brain. Regions of interest (ROI) were drawn to assess the activity in the mesial and lateral portion of the temporal lobes, using mirror image for left and right, as shown in the figure. The asymmetry index was calculated as follows: asymmetry index = (left – right)/0.5 (left + right)

Findings

The FDG images demonstrate marked hypometabolism in the entire left temporal cortex compared to the right, more severe laterally and involving the posterior temporal cortex as well, correlating with the EEG. The asymmetry indices were 47% in the lateral and 7% in the mesial temporal cortex.

Discussion

In the clinical setting of this patient, these findings are consistent with an interictal seizure focus in the left temporal cortex. An asymmetry index greater than 15% is considered significant.[1]

Epilepsy affects 1% of the population in the United States. The seizures can be partial or generalized. If the patient does not loose awareness, the seizures are called "simple partial," and if they do loose awareness, they are called "complex partial." When the seizures become refractory to medical therapy, surgical removal of the seizure focus can be curative. In patients considered for surgery, precise localization of the seizure focus is critical. CT and MRI can identify focal lesions responsible for the seizure in 40 to 60% of the patients, most commonly low-grade astrocytoma, hamartomas, and ganglioglioma/neuroma. In the remainder of the patients, correlation of functional imaging using radiopharmaceuticals with the clinical presentation of the seizure and the EEG findings plays a pivotal role in identifying patients who will improve following surgery. The temporal lobe is the most common focus of partial seizures, and mesial temporal sclerosis is the most common pathologic lesion.

During a seizure, both metabolism and perfusion are increased at the seizure focus, and between seizures both are decreased. The uptake of FDG in the brain occurs slowly, reaching a maximum between 30 and 50 minutes after intravenous injection. Because seizure activity is usually of short duration compared to the distribution time of FDG, FDG imaging should be performed in the interictal state. Therefore, patients are usually instructed to take their antiseizure medications, and EEG monitoring can be performed during the distribution time to document the absence of epileptiform activity during FDG uptake.

Functional imaging in combination with other noninvasive techniques has made monitoring with invasive intracranial electrodes unnecessary in 50% or more of the patients with temporal lobe epilepsy. Identification of a single focus of interictal temporal lobe hypometabolism on FDG PET images (asymmetry index greater than 15%) is an excellent predictor of seizure control after surgery. The sensitivity of interictal FDG PET to detect temporal lobe epileptic foci is in the range of 80%, greater than interictal ^{99m}Tc-HMPAO SPECT that is in the range of 60%. If a first-pass perfusion radiopharmaceutical is injected at the onset of EEG-detected seizure activity, ictal SPECT imaging will detect an additional 20 to 30% temporal seizure foci compared to interictal SPECT. The combination of increased flow during an ictal injection and decreased flow during an interictal injection is highly predictive for a seizure focus, with a sensitivity in the 75 to 90% range.

Diagnosis

Seizure focus in the left temporal lobe.

Reference

1. Rowe CC, Bercovic SF, Sia STB, et al.: Localisation of epileptic foci with postictal single photon emission computed tomography. Ann Neurol 1989;26:660–668.

Case 4.2

History

A 53-year-old female presented with progressive memory loss. MRI was normal. She was referred for FDG PET imaging of the brain (Figure 4.2). The FDG images were acquired with a dedicated PET tomograph (Siemens ECAT 933) and reconstructed with filtered back projection and calculated attenuation correction.

Findings

Markedly decreased uptake is seen in the posterior parietotemporal cortex bilaterally and to a lesser extent in the frontal cortex. The uptake is preserved in the sensorimotor cortex, subcortical gray matter (basal ganglia and thalami), and cerebellum.

Discussion

This pattern is typical for Alzheimer's disease.

Decreased uptake in the posterior parietotemporal cortex is consistent with a degenerative disorder, most likely Alzheimer's disease. Ten percent of the population over 65 year of age is demented, and 50% of those are evaluated in hospitals. The cost of long-term care is tremendous. Over half of these demented patients have Alzheimer's disease. These patients present with memory loss accompanied by visual and spatial skills impairment. From the physiopathologic point of view, there is accelerated neuronal death affecting mainly the hippocampus and the posterior parietal and temporal cortices. Recently, it has been demonstrated that a variant of the apolipoprotein E allele is associated with many of the cases of late onset of Alzheimer's disease.

FDG is a glucose analog labeled with a positron emitter allowing direct evaluation of glucose metabolism. This functional imaging technique allows diagnosing degenerative neurological diseases that do not show typical findings on CT or MRI images. Although there is a large overlap between the patterns of uptake of different degenerative dementias, this patient has a pattern typical for advanced Alzheimer's

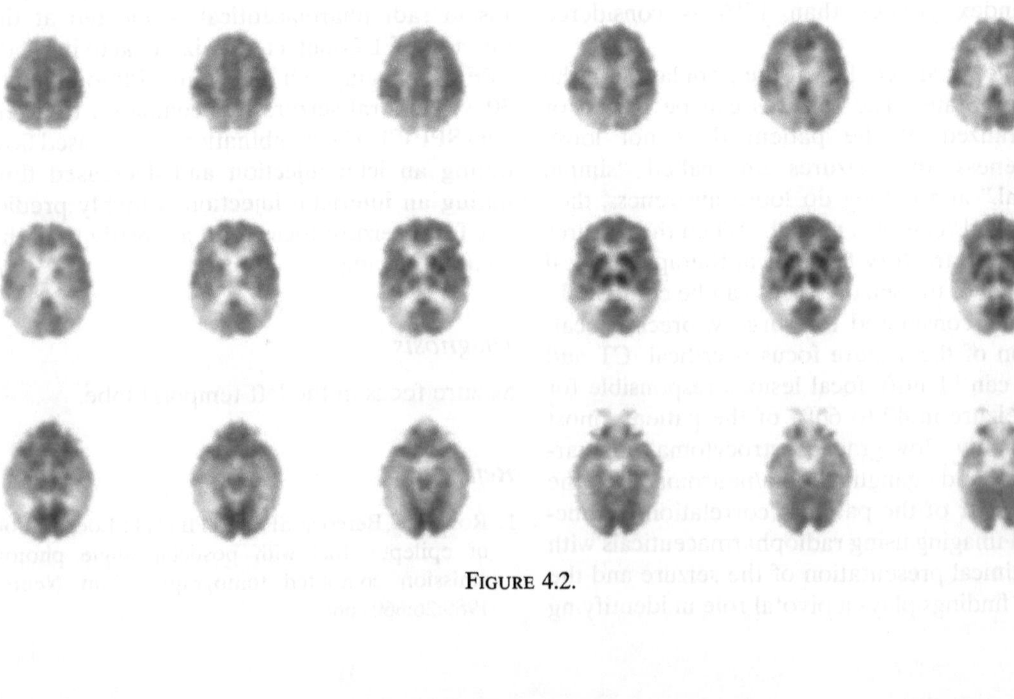

FIGURE 4.2.

disease. The degree of decreased FDG uptake seems to correlate with the severity of the symptoms. Histopathological observation of postmortem brains from patients with Alzheimer's disease have revealed the presence of abundant senile plaques and neurofibrillary tangles in the regions with decreased FDG uptake.

This pattern of uptake, however, is not pathognomonic for Alzheimer's disease; it may also be seen in patients with Parkinson's disease, bilateral parietal subdural hematomas, bilateral parietal stroke, bilateral parietal radiation therapy, and normal pressure hydrocephalus. The symptoms characterizing Parkinson's disease are bradykinesia, rigidity, and tremor, and it affects 1% of the population over 60 years of age. The disease is caused by degeneration of dopaminergic neurons in the substantia nigra and locus coerulus, leading to decreased dopamine production, decreased dopamine storage, and nigrostriatal dysfunction. About 10 to 30% of patients with Parkinson's disease develop dementia, and their pattern of FDG uptake is indistinguishable from the Alzheimer's pattern. The difficulty of making a diagnosis clinically early in the disease and overlap of pattern of uptake in patients with other dementing syndromes on functional FDG imaging is illustrated in a recent report by Hoffman et al.[1,2] In a series of patients with pathologically verified dementia (biopsy or autopsy), the sensitivity and specificity for the clinical diagnosis were 75% and 100% respectively, and the pattern of bilateral temporoparietal metabolism of PET images were 93% and 63%. The accuracy for both the clinical and FDG PET imaging diagnosis were in the same range of 82%. However, FDG PET imaging was more sensitive, and the clinical diagnosis was more specific.

In the differential diagnosis of dementias, multi-infarct dementia represents only about 10 to 15% of the dementias. It is characterized clinically by a stepwise progression of the symptoms, attributable to repeated episodes of infarction. Sometimes, the stepwise progression of the symptoms is subtle, and the clinical presentation is similar to that of Alzheimer's disease. Alzheimer's disease and vascular dementia can also coexist. Usually patients with multi-infarct dementia have evidence of infarcts on CT or MRI, and the presence of infarcts of different age is highly suggestive of that diagnosis. On functional scans, their global cerebral perfusion and glucose metabolism are reduced to a greater extent than in patients with Alzheimer's disease. In multi-infarct dementia, the sensorimotor cortex can be involved while it is almost invariably spared in Alzheimer's disease.

Diagnosis

Alzheimer's disease.

References

1. Hoffman JM, Welsh-Bohmer KA, Hanson M, et al.: FDG PET imaging in patients with pathologically verified dementia. J Nucl Med 2000;41: 1920–1928.
2. Silverman DHS, Phelps ME: Invited commentary: Evaluating dementia using PET: How do we put into clinical perspective what we know to date? J Nucl Med 2000;41:1929–1932.

Case 4.3

History

A 40-year-old HIV-positive male presented with mental status changes. He was referred for MRI (Figure 4.3A) and FDG PET imaging of the brain (Figure 4.3B). The FDG images were acquired with a dedicated PET tomograph (Siemens ECAT 933) and reconstructed with filtered back projection and calculated attenuation correction.

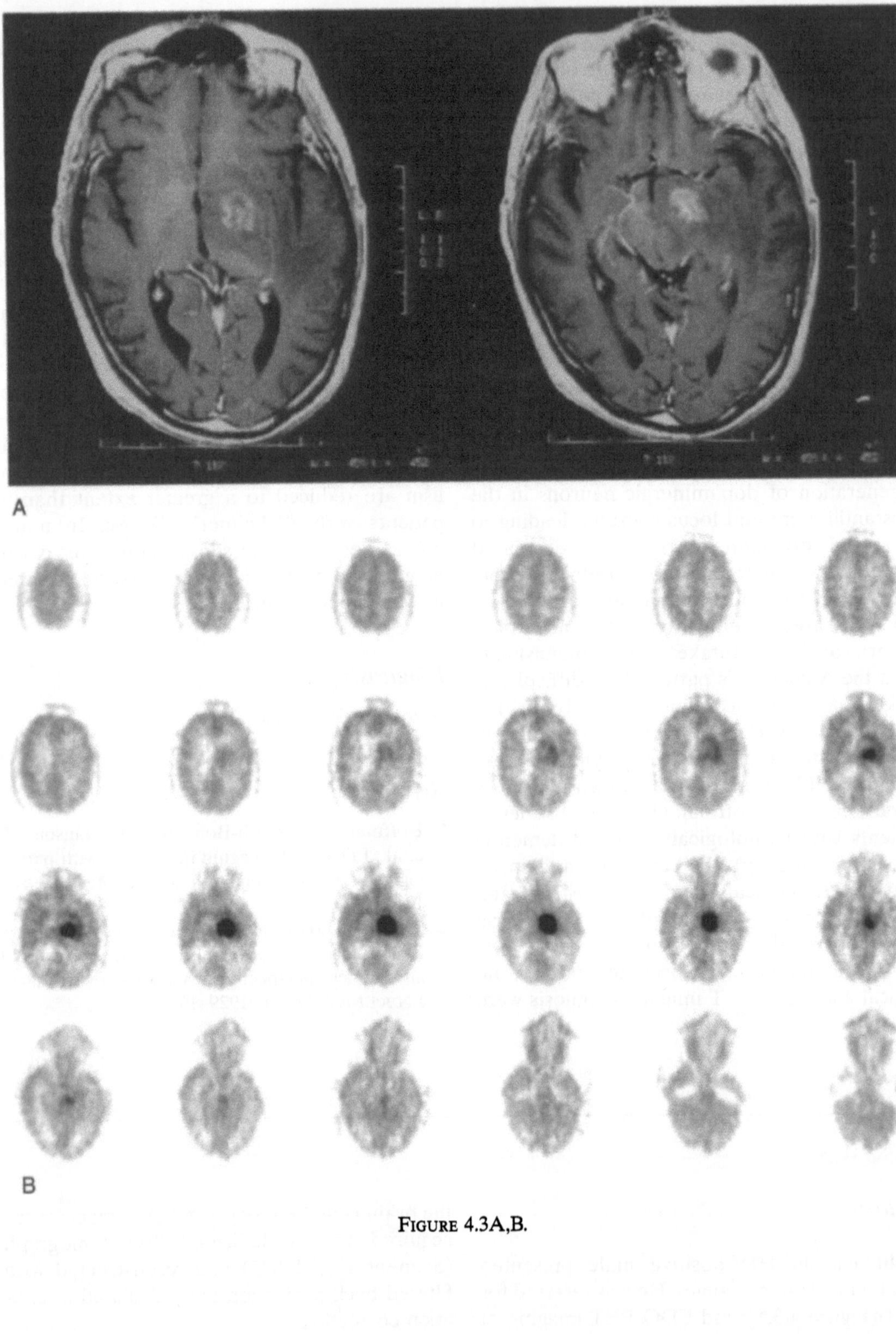

FIGURE 4.3A,B.

Findings

Post-gadolinium T1-weighted MRI images show a 2 cm enhancing lesion in the left basal ganglia. On the PET images, there is FDG uptake in the enhancing lesion. The uptake is more than twice that of uninvolved cortex.

Discussion

These findings indicate a high-grade tumor, such as lymphoma. The patient was treated with radiation therapy, and a follow-up CT scan showed improvement of the lesion.

In a patient with acquired immunodeficiency syndrome (AIDS), cerebral lesions are most frequently related to infection by toxoplasmosis or high-grade lymphoma. High FDG uptake in the lesion indicates that the lesion is most likely a lymphoma, whereas low uptake favors the diagnosis of toxoplasmosis. Another pathologic process in the differential diagnosis is progressive multifocal leucoencephalopathy (PML), which is most often hypometabolic but may appear hypermetabolic. Fungal infections are most commonly hypermetabolic but are uncommon in HIV-positive patients.

HIV-positive patients are immunosuppressed and have a tendency to develop malignant tumors such as lymphoma and opportunistic infections. Primary lymphoma of the central nervous system is a rare tumor but occurs in 2 to 6% of patients with AIDS. In the immunocompromised patients, lymphoma typically presents as multiple ring-enhancing lesions on CT and MRI. The most common opportunistic infection involving the central nervous system is toxoplasma gondii. This infection may produce a diffuse meningoencephalitis or cause focal lesions appearing as multifocal ring-enhancing lesions on CT and MRI. Therefore, it is not possible to differentiate toxoplasmosis from lymphoma on the basis of CT or MRI findings. These two diseases have different treatment and prognosis. Because toxoplasmosis is more frequent than lymphoma, these patients are typically treated with antitoxoplasmosis therapy, but it takes approximately two weeks before clinical improvement becomes apparent. Lymphoma is rapidly progressive and has a very poor prognosis. Early diagnosis improves the response to therapy of these patients. Primary lymphoma of the central nervous system demonstrates increased accumulation of FDG to the same degree as high-grade gliomas, while lesions due to toxoplasmosis are usually hypometabolic. Therefore, FDG PET is an accurate imaging modality to differentiate these two entities without the need of a biopsy.[1]

Fungal infections are usually associated with granulomatous inflammation, and inflammatory cells (particularly macrophages) are known to have high levels of glucose utilization. Therefore, active granulomatous processes such as fungal and yeast infections (especially aspergillosis, nocardia, and candida), tuberculosis, and sarcoidosis have been reported to accumulate high levels of FDG and cause false-positive scans in the evaluation of malignancy. Aspergillosis involving the central nervous system is rarely encountered and usually affects immunosuppressed patients and those debilitated by neoplasms or collagen vascular diseases, drug addiction, or alcoholism. The gross appearance is often that of a necrotic and hemorrhagic abscess with central cavitation. Sixty percent of HIV-positive patients with cerebral lesions have toxoplasmosis, 30 percent have cerebral lymphoma, and only 10 percent will have another pathological process. Therefore, a cerebral lesion with high FDG uptake is likely a lymphoma in the HIV-positive patient and a high-grade glioma in the HIV-negative patient. In debilitated or immunosuppressed patients that are HIV-negative, granulomatous abscesses should be considered in the differential diagnosis.

AIDS-related dementia is another frequent complication of HIV infection and is sometimes difficult to distinguish from the simple depression or psychiatric problems that these patients experience. It is the result of direct HIV infection of the brain, and multinucleated giant cells can be found in the white matter and to a lesser extent in the gray matter. The viral infection can also result in demyelination. Patients with AIDS-related dementia have global decrease of cortical uptake compared to basal ganglia and thalami. This pattern of FDG uptake is helpful in the differential diagnosis with the limitation that these patients are often polydrug abusers, and there is some overlap between the pattern of uptake due to HIV infection, cocaine abuse, and alcohol abuse, among others.

Diagnosis

AIDS-related primary lymphoma of the central nervous system.

Reference

1. Roelcke U, Leenders KL: Positron emission tomography in patients with primary CNS lymphomas. J Neurooncol 1999;43(3):231–236. Review.

Case 4.4

History

A 59-year-old female presented with behavioral problems and memory impairment. A cerebral MRI was normal for age. FDG PET imaging of the brain was performed to evaluate the etiology of her cognitive disorder (Figure 4.4). The FDG images were acquired with a dedicated PET tomograph (GE Advance) in the 2D mode and reconstructed with iterative reconstruction and measured segmented attenuation correction.

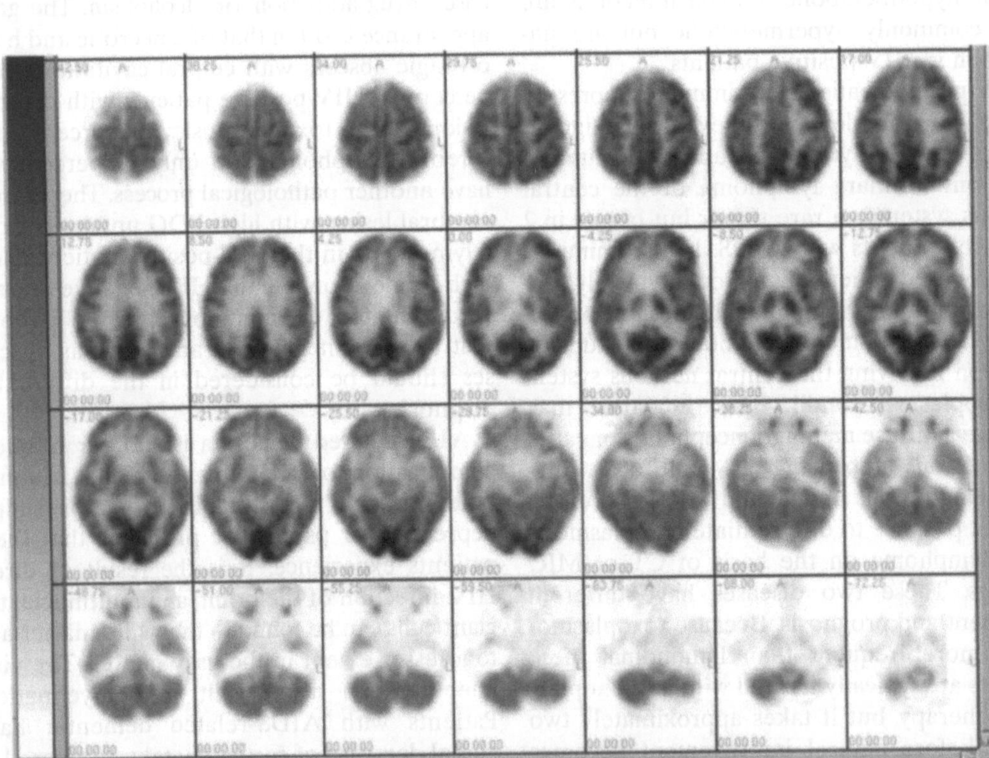

FIGURE 4.4.

Findings

On the FDG PET images, there is severely decreased uptake in the frontal cortex bilaterally, as well to a lesser degree in the basal ganglia. Uptake in the parietotemporal cortex is preserved.

Discussion

The finding of marked decreased uptake in the frontal cortex suggests Pick's disease or frontal lobe dementia.

Alzheimer's disease and Pick's disease are very difficult to differentiate clinically. As Alzheimer's disease is more prevalent, a clinical diagnosis of Alzheimer's disease is usually made rather than Pick's disease. Pathologically, the two diseases are very different. Alzheimer's disease is characterized by the presence of tangles and plaques primarily in the cortex. Pick's disease is characterized by swollen neurons and neurons containing Pick's bodies in the cortex, basal ganglia, thalami, and sometimes other regions of the brain. Alzheimer's disease tends to present with general cortical atrophy, and Pick's disease demonstrates more circumscribed atrophy located in the frontal and sometimes temporal cortex. On functional imaging with FDG or HMPAO, Alzheimer's disease typically shows decreased uptake in the posterior parietotemporal cortex, whereas Pick's disease affects the frontal cortex and anterior temporal cortex. However, there is some overlap of pattern of uptake between degenerative dementias, and occasionally patients with Alzheimer's disease demonstrate hypometabolism limited to the frontal cortex. In Pick's disease, the degree of decreased metabolism correlates better with the degree of gliosis than the concentration of Pick's bodies.[1]

Studies suggest that Pick's disease may be one member of a larger clinicopathologic syndrome called frontal lobe dementia.[2,3] In frontal lobe dementia, the pattern of uptake is the same as in Pick's disease. These patients typically present with early symptoms of social withdrawal and behavioral inhibition followed several years later by the development of progressive dementia. Pathological examination of the brain demonstrates frontal lobe atrophy with various degrees of frontal gliosis and neuronal loss. One type of frontal lobe dementia presents in association with clinical features of motor neuron disease. This type progresses more rapidly and pathologically demonstrates mild frontal gliosis and spongiform changes.

Other dementing conditions such as amyotrophic lateral sclerosis may involve the frontal lobes but can usually be differentiated from frontal lobe dementia on clinical grounds.

Diagnosis

Pick's disease or frontal lobe dementia.

References

1. Kamo H, McGeer PL, Harrop R, et al.: Positron emission tomography and histopathology in Pick's disease. Neurology 1987;37:439–445.
2. Kumar A, Shapiro MB, Haxby JV, Grady CL, Friedland RP: Cerebral metabolic and cognitive studies in dementia with frontal lobe behavioral features. J Psyched Res 1990;24:97–109.
3. Miller BL, Cummings JL, Villanueva-Meyer J, et al.: Frontal lobe degeneration: Clinical, neuropsychological, and SPECT characteristics. Neurology 1991;41:1374–1382.

Case 4.5

History

An 8-year-old female presented with a history of intractable multifocal partial seizures since age three. During admission for EEG-CCTV monitoring, she had more than 50 seizures characterized by drop attacks. The EEG suggested generalized ictal discharges predominantly from the right hemisphere. MRI (Figure 4.5A) and FDG PET imaging of the brain (Figure 4.5B) were performed for pre-surgical evaluation. EEG monitoring was performed during the distribution phase of FDG. The FDG images were acquired with a dedicated PET tomograph (Siemens ECAT 933) and reconstructed with filtered back projection and calculated attenuation correction.

Findings

The MRI images show cortical dysplasia with polymicrogyria and pachygyria diffusely in the right hemisphere. The FDG PET images demonstrate increased uptake in the right hemicortex, predominantly in the right frontal cortex, compared to the left, with an asymme-

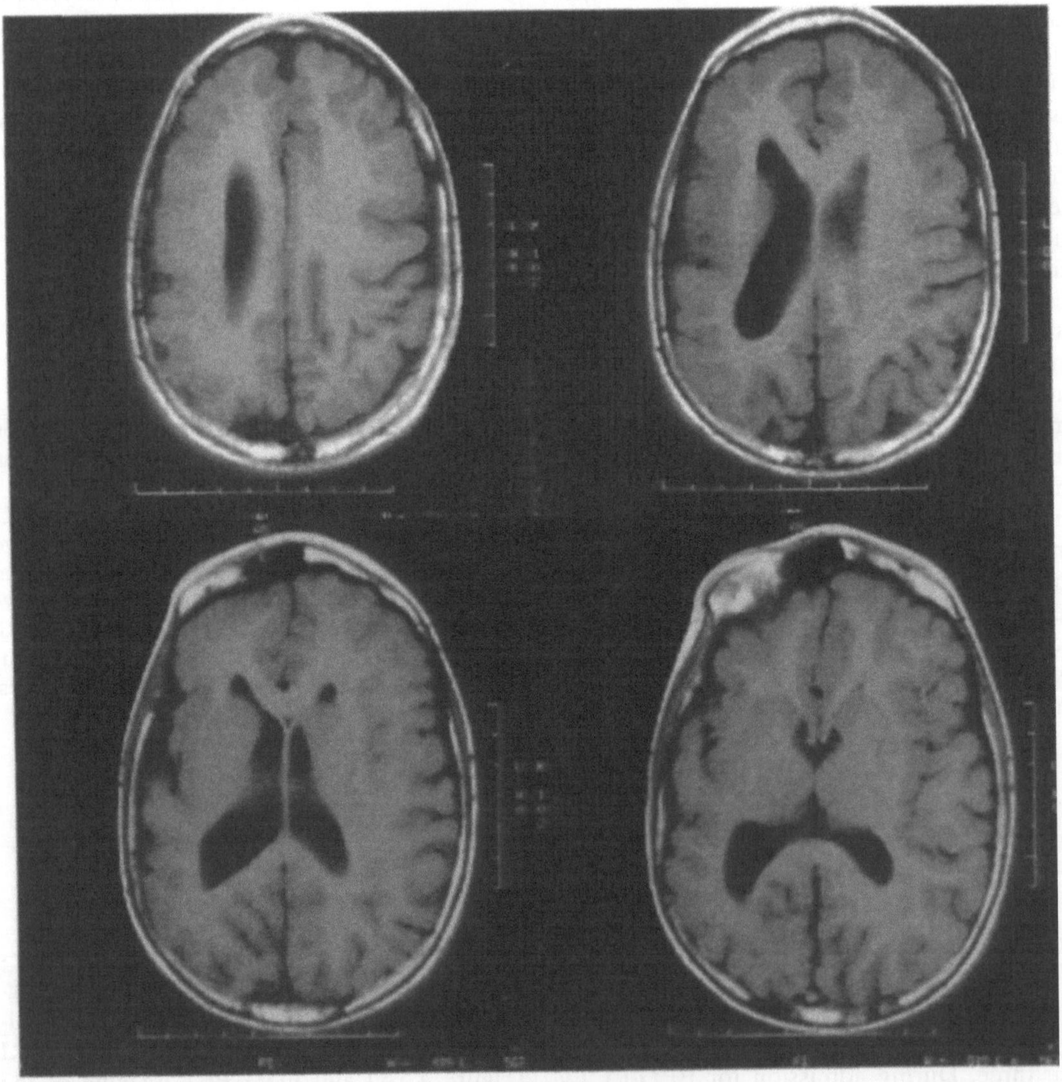

FIGURE 4.5A.

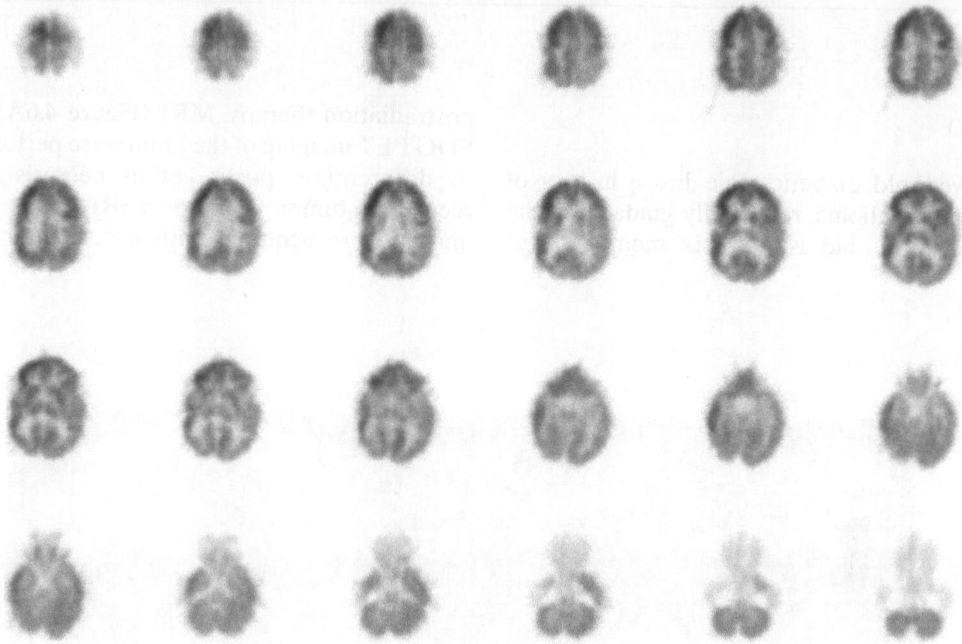

FIGURE 4.5B.

try index of 44%. The pattern of uptake in the right hemisphere correlates with the pattern of cortical dysplasia seen on the MRI. The EEG obtained during the distribution phase of FDG demonstrated frequent ictal discharges.

Discussion

These findings indicate ictal discharges from the region with cortical dysplasia predominantly in the right frontal cortex.

FDG PET imaging in patients with seizures is usually performed during the interictal state because the uptake of FDG occurs over a period of 30 to 45 minutes, while the duration of a seizure is usually for a period of a few minutes, as discussed in Case 4.1. Therefore, a short period of increased FDG uptake (ictal period) during a longer period of decreased uptake (postictal period) does not result in a change of FDG uptake on the images. If the patient is having frequent discharges during the FDG distribution phase, however, the images will demonstrate increased FDG uptake in the region of the seizure focus.

In this patient with frequent ictal discharges on the EEG performed during the uptake phase, the findings of increased FDG uptake are consistent with a seizure focus arising from the cortical dysplasia. The localization of the seizure focus in a region of cortical dysplasia or heterotopia is extremely useful for surgical planning in these patients.[1] In this case because of the extensive nature of the process and high degree of generalization of her seizures, resulting in frequent drop attacks throughout the day, it was felt that the patient would benefit from complete corpus callosotomy. This procedure would convert her generalized seizures into focal ones.

Diagnoses

1. Cortical dysplasia.
2. Seizure focus arising from the cortical dysplasia.

Reference

1. Gelfand MJ, Delbeke D, Lawrence SK: Pediatric brain imaging, in Sandler MP et al. (eds): Diagnostic Nuclear Medicine, 3d ed. Baltimore: Williams & Wilkins, 1996, pp 1465–1492.

Case 4.6

History

A 69-year-old diabetic male has a history of multicentric glioma, reportedly grade II on the initial biopsy, and is now six months status postradiation therapy. MRI (Figure 4.6A) and FDG PET imaging of the brain were performed to differentiate postradiation necrosis from recurrent tumor (Figure 4.6B). The FDG images were acquired with a dedicated PET

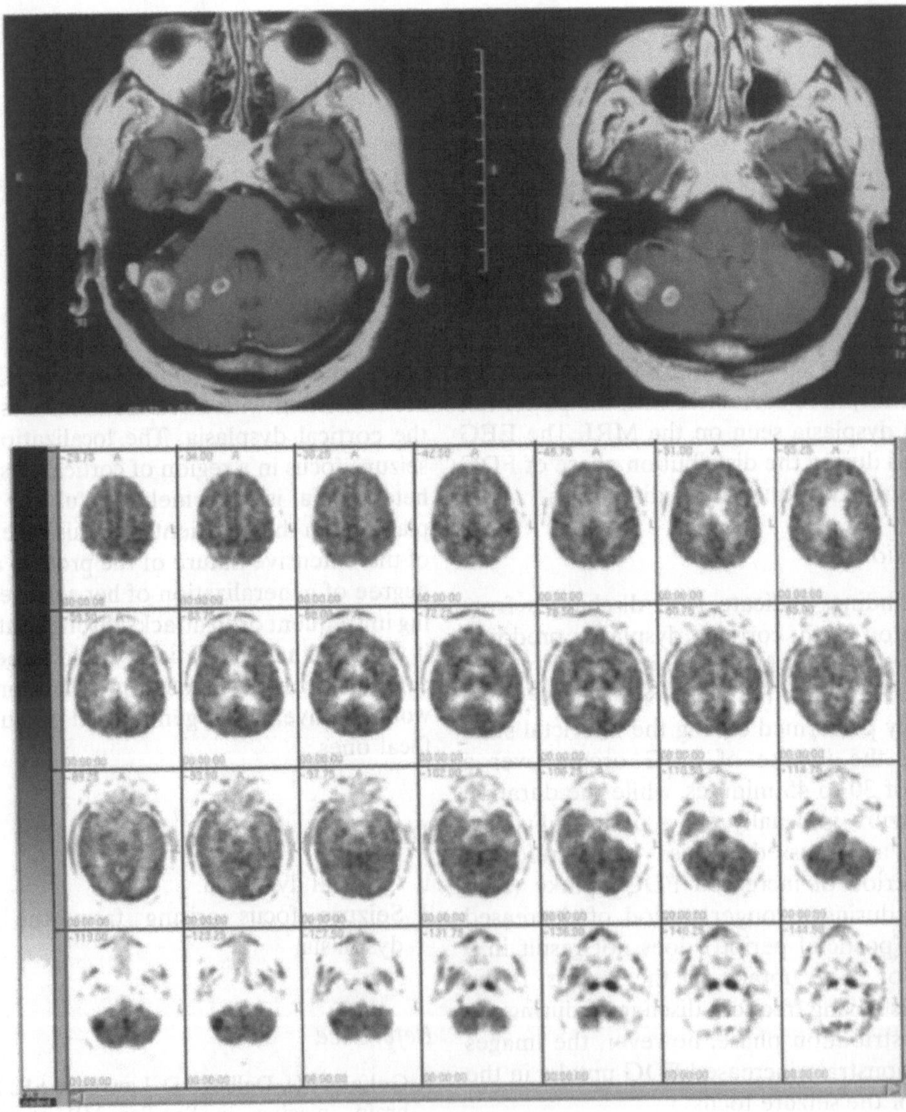

FIGURE 4.6A,B.

tomograph (GE Advance) and reconstructed with iterative reconstruction and measured segmented attenuation correction.

Findings

The post-gadolinium T1-weighted MRI images show areas of enhancement in the right cerebellum that have slightly increased in size compared to the previous study. On the FDG PET images, there is increased FDG uptake corresponding to the area of enhancement on MRI. The degree of FDG uptake is above the level of uninvolved cortex. The second finding is decreased uptake globally in the cortex. One clue to global decreased cortical uptake is noisy images; another clue is visualization of the scalp and lymphoid tissue of the head and neck. Poor uptake can be confirmed by measuring the standard uptake value (SUV) that is the absolute activity in a region of interest normalized for the dose administered and the weight of the patient.

Discussion

These findings indicate high-grade tumor recurrence. The poor uptake in the cortex is probably due to hyperglycemia in a diabetic patient. Poor uptake makes the images suboptimal for evaluation, although they were diagnostic in this patient.

High-grade (III and IV) gliomas (anaplastic astrocytoma and glioblastoma multiforme) are usually treated by resection when possible, followed by a combination of radiation and chemotherapy. The evaluation of the response to therapy and tumor recurrence is a clinical challenge. Necrosis of the tumor and surrounding brain tissue occurs with conventional radiation therapy and in a large proportion of patients following stereotactic radiosurgery. These areas of necrosis have the appearance of edematous masses on CT and MRI that enhance because there is increased permeability of the blood brain barrier; this typically occurs 6 to 18 months after therapy and may cause symptoms indistinguishable from those caused by tumor recurrence. Similar changes follow intra-arterial infusion of chemotherapy and high-dose methotrexate therapy given intravenously after radiation. These changes on CT and MRI are indistinguishable from residual or recurrent high-grade tumor.

Metabolic imaging with FDG can differentiate recurrent brain tumor from radiation necrosis. As most tumors recur as high-grade, they demonstrate marked FDG uptake. However, radiation injury leads to tissue necrosis that does not accumulate FDG.

FDG PET imaging may also help provide guidance at the site which is the more metabolically active, as some tumors such as cerebral gliomas may be well-differentiated in some regions and contain highly atypical cells in others. Biopsy sampling error is not a rare occurrence. PET is an accurate imaging modality differentiating a low-grade process from high-grade tumors based on the glucose metabolism. It is particularly helpful when the access to the lesion for biopsy is difficult or to provide guidance for the biopsy at the site of maximum activity.

Several investigators have demonstrated that the degree of FDG uptake in high-grade tumors has prognostic importance. Patients with tumors that have a lesion/cortex FDG uptake ratio greater than 1.4 have an extremely poor prognosis, with death occurring within six months.

Since FDG competes with glucose for cellular transport, high levels of plasma glucose will competitively inhibit FDG transport into all cells, including the neurons. This is one reason why patients have to fast for four hours prior to FDG injection. Taking the history is important, too, to identify patients with diabetes who may benefit from administration of insulin before FDG administration. The glycemia should be measured to assess both the fasting state and identify patients with glucose intolerance. Administration of sedating medications prior to FDG injection will also result in global hypometabolism.

Diagnoses

1. Recurrent high-grade tumor.
2. Poor FDG uptake in the cerebral cortex due to hyperglycemia.

Case 4.7

History

A 4-month-old male presented with intractable seizures. The EEG suggested a left temporal origin. The cerebral MRI was normal. He was referred for FDG PET imaging of the brain (Figure 4.7A and B, see color plate). The FDG images were acquired with a dedicated PET tomograph (Siemens ECAT 933) and reconstructed with filtered back projection and calculated attenuation correction.

Findings

The FDG PET images demonstrate decreased uptake in the frontal and posterior parietotemporal cortex bilaterally, with preservation of metabolism in the sensorimotor cortex, visual cortex, subcortical gray matter, and cerebellum. There is slightly more decreased uptake in the left temporal cortex than the right, with an asymmetry index of 10%. This degree of decreased uptake is sometimes difficult to appreciate visually on gray scale images, but often can be seen on color scales, and can be confirmed with semiquantitative measurements in the region of interest.

Discussion

This pattern of uptake is normal for the age of the patient. The adult pattern of perfusion and metabolism is established by age two. In the newborn, perfusion and metabolism of the basal ganglia, thalami, sensorimotor cortex, visual cortex, brain stem, and cerebellum are similar to that of an adult. The other regions of the cerebral cortex are immature with lower

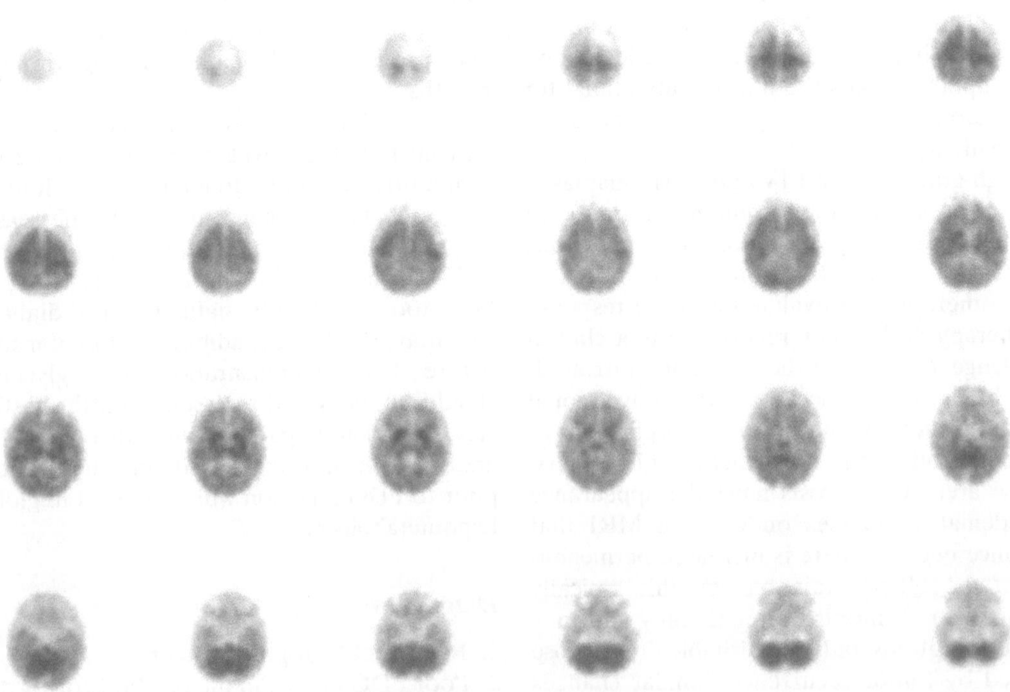

FIGURE 4.7A.

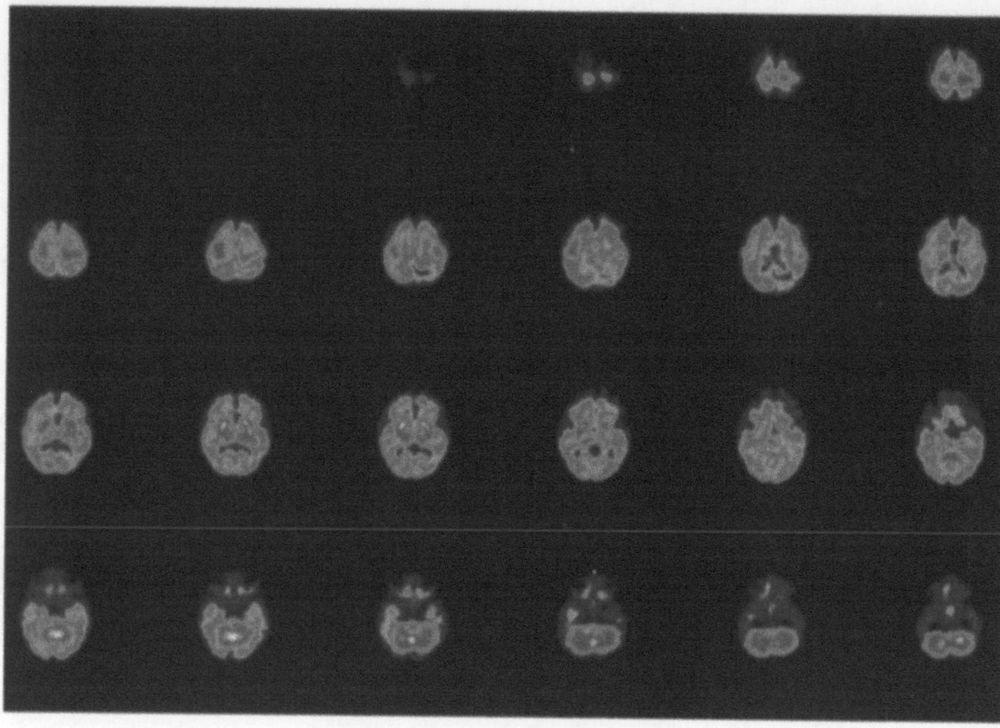

FIGURE 4.7B. (See color plate)

perfusion and metabolism. These regions progressively mature over time, reaching an adult pattern of perfusion and metabolism around age two.

There is only mild decreased uptake in the left temporal cortex compared to the right. An asymmetry index greater than 15% is considered significant and correlates best with surgical results. However, in the appropriate clinical setting and in combination with the results of other diagnostic testing, a milder degree of asymmetry supports localization of the seizure focus and may obviate the need for EEG monitoring via deep electrodes or surface grid electrodes.

Diagnoses

1. Physiologic immature pattern of metabolism in a 4-month-old infant.
2. Supportive of a left temporal lobe seizure focus.

Case 4.8

History

A 16-year-old-male presented with a six-month history of seizures. The clinical pattern suggested onset from the right hemisphere. The cerebral CT scan showed a questionable hypodensity in the posterior right frontal lobe on the images without contrast. The CT images with contrast were normal. A cerebral MRI scan could not be performed because of a metallic

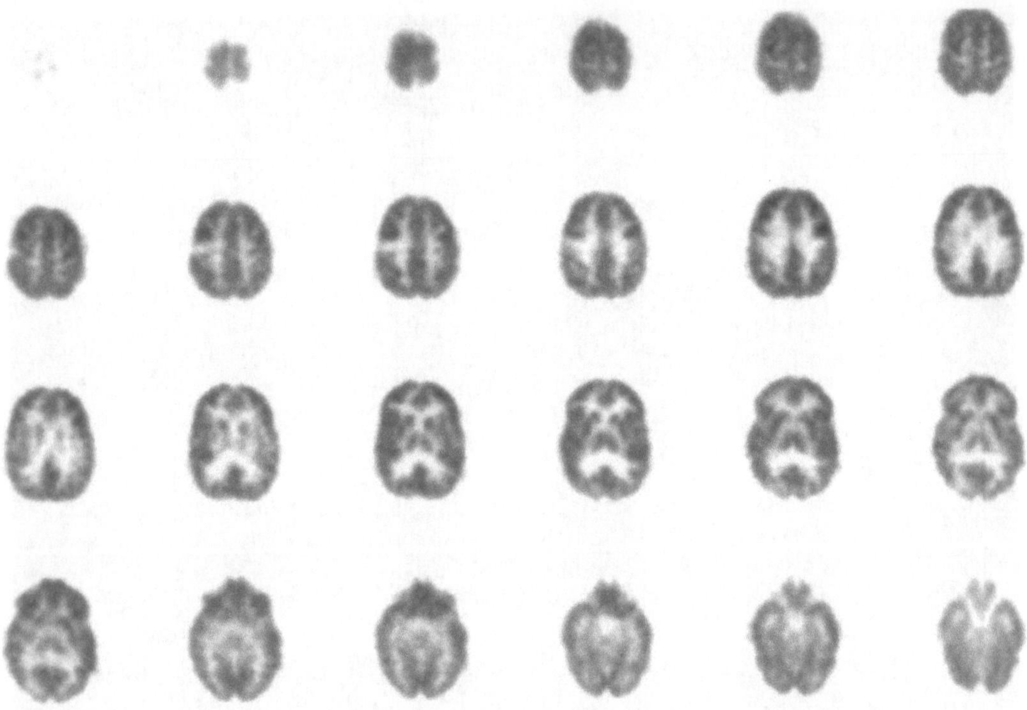

FIGURE 4.8.

cochlear implant. He was referred for FDG PET imaging of the brain (Figure 4.8). The FDG images were acquired with a dedicated PET tomograph (Siemens ACAT 933) and reconstructed with filtered back projection and calculated attenuation correction.

Findings

On the FDG PET images, there is a focus of marked decreased uptake in the right frontal cortex posteriorly. The degree of uptake is similar to that of physiologic white matter.

Discussion

The focus of decreased cortical uptake confirms the presence of a lesion that was difficult to see on the CT image. In a young patient with recent onset of seizures, the low degree of FDG uptake indicates a low-grade neoplasm, most likely a low-grade glioma. The lesion was resected, and pathologic examination of the surgical specimen demonstrated an oligodendroglioma.

Intracranial neoplasms represent approximately 10% of all neoplasms, cerebral metastases represent 25 to 30% of intracranial neoplasms, and primary brain tumors represent 70 to 75%. Fifty percent of primary brain tumors are gliomas (60% of which are low-grade and 40% are high-grade), 12 to 15% are meningiomas, and 1 to 2% are lymphomas. When a patient presents with personality changes, seizures, or a neurologic deficit suggesting a brain lesion, CT or MRI imaging is usually performed first to assess the presence of a structural abnormality. Enhancement of the lesion after intravenous administration of a contrast agent indicates increased permeability of the blood-brain barrier and is usually a feature of high-grade tumors, whereas low-grade tumors can be more conspicuous but tend not to enhance. As most high-grade gliomas develop in the setting of low-grade gliomas, there is debate in the literature about the therapeutic approach to presumably low-grade astrocytomas. Some oncologists favor early biopsy and treatment with resection when possible, followed by radiation therapy. Others favor a more conservative approach, until the lesion enlarges or enhances on CT and MRI images indicating degeneration into high-grade glioma, which are treated with resection when possible, followed by radiation and chemotherapy.

One of the first clinical applications that emerged for FDG PET imaging in the early 1980s was its ability to differentiate low-grade from high-grade gliomas. For semiquantitative analysis, different regions of the brain have been used for reference. As gliomas are tumors arising from the white matter, it is logical to use the white matter as reference to evaluate the degree of uptake. Most low-grade gliomas accumulate FDG at the same level as white matter. Most high-grade gliomas accumulate FDG to a level greater than twice that of white matter. As perfusion and metabolism of gray matter is two to four times that of white matter, the level of uptake of high-grade gliomas can be below, equal to, or above the level of cortical uptake.

Many other pathologic entities affecting the brain do not accumulate FDG, and on FDG PET imaging alone, low-grade gliomas cannot be differentiated from some benign lesions such as hemangiomas, infectious foci, or small areas of infarctions.

Diagnosis

Low-grade glioma.

Case 4.9

History

A 14-year-old male presented with intractable seizures since age three. Subsequently, he developed mild mental retardation and a mild left hemiparesis. The cerebral MRI showed a nonspecific temporal lobe abnormality on the right but no focal lesion. He underwent FDG PET imaging of the brain (Figure 4.9). The FDG images were acquired with a dedicated PET tomograph (Siemens ECAT 933) and reconstructed with filtered back projection and calculated attenuation correction.

Findings

The FDG PET images show mild global decreased uptake and multiple focal areas of increased uptake in the right hemisphere.

Discussion

These findings are most compatible with multiple right hemispheric ictal foci. This can be seen in Rasmussen's encephalitis. A cerebral biopsy was performed in this patient demonstrating gliosis suggestive of Rasmussen's encephalitis. There was no evidence for viral infection.

Rasmussen's encephalitis is a chronic, progressive inflammation of the brain of unclear pathogenesis. It occurs most commonly in childhood and is characterized by severe epilepsy, progressive hemiparesis, mental deterioration, inflammation of one cerebral hemisphere, and brain atrophy. The atrophy is usually more predominant in the temporoinsular cortex. Recent advances in the understanding of this syndrome suggest an autoimmune etiology. Early diagnosis and treatment with immunoreactive agents and/or hemispherec-

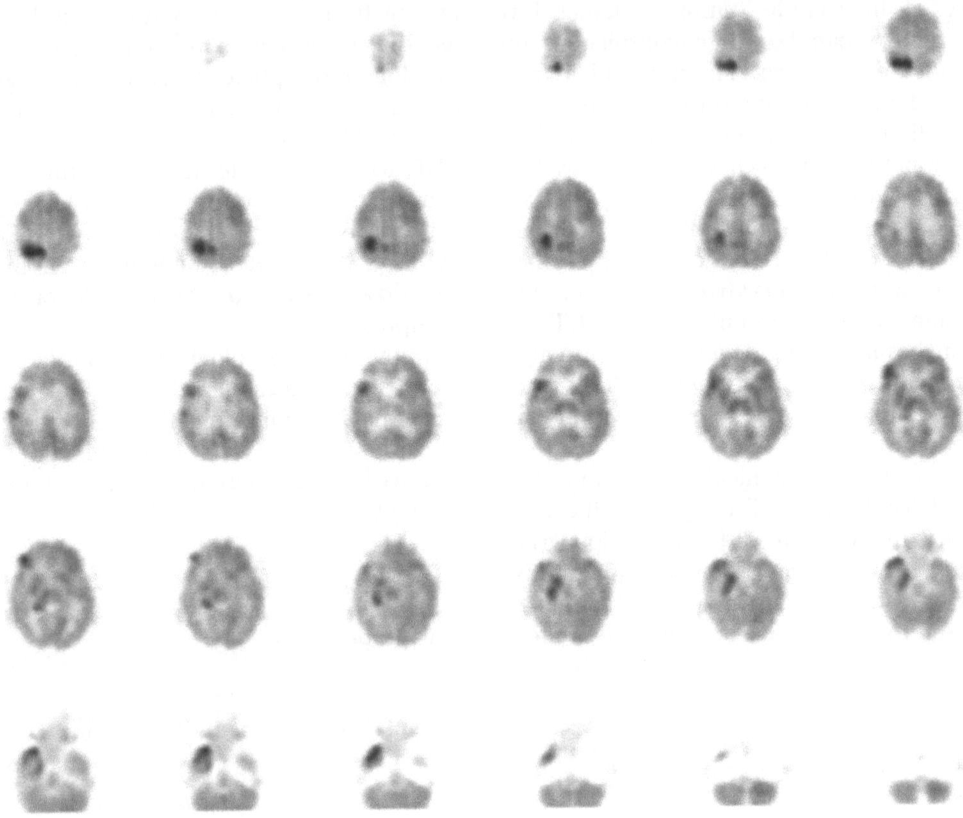

FIGURE 4.9.

tomy seem to improve seizure control and prevent progressive cognitive decline. If hemispherectomy is performed in early childhood, the capacity of the developing brain for compensatory reorganization has been demonstrated.[1] Neuroradiological examinations are important in the diagnosis of Rasmussen's encephalitis but are frequently normal or show only nonspecific findings early in the disease. FDG PET imaging shows decreased uptake in the affected hemisphere or focal regions or increased uptake if the patient is in the ictal state. Hypometabolism in the affected hemisphere usually precedes severe atrophy that becomes apparent on structural imaging later in the course of the disease.[2–4] Combined anatomic and functional imaging is helpful to hasten brain biopsy for definitive diagnosis. The addition of functional PET imaging to conventional anatomic imaging allows a definitive diagnosis to be made earlier when therapy may be more effective.[5]

The differential diagnosis is viral encephalitis. Patients with viral infections of the brain usually present with global deficits such as seizures, confusion, coma, or delirium. Focal deficits such as involuntary movements or ocular palsies may also occur. A variety of viral agents can cause encephalitis. They can be classified in six broad categories: (1) arbovirus (Eastern and Western equine encephalitis, often lethal), (2) enterovirus (poliomyelitis), (3) respiratory virus, (4) virus from childhood infections (measles, mumps, rubella, and chickenpox), (5) other virus (cytomegalovirus, herpes simplex and Zoster, and Epstein-Barr virus), and (6) slow virus. The true slow viruses include subacute sclerosing panencephalitis often preceded by measles, progressive rubella panencephalitis, and progressive multifocal encephalopathy occurring in patients that are chronically debilitated (tuberculosis, sarcoidosis, and rheumatoid arthritis) or immunosuppressed (including AIDS). The unconventional slow viruses include Kuru and Creutzfeldt-Jakob that cause spongiform changes in the gray matter.

Herpes simplex can produce a number of diseases according to the organ involved. Both herpes simplex I (labialis) and II (genitalis) can caused encephalitis in neonates often involving the entire brain. Herpes simplex I is also responsible for most cases of encephalitis (acute necrotizing encephalitis) in older children and adults which typically involve the temporal lobes and orbitofrontal cortex. Untreated, many cases are fatal, and some patients survive with severe dementia and memory deficits. The recently discovered effective therapy with arabinoside A (acyclovir) has generated a need for early diagnosis.

The blood-brain barrier is often abnormal in viral infections of the brain, and blood-brain barrier imaging is often abnormal several days before the CT or MRI. There is increased uptake on the dynamic images and extensive areas of diffusely increased uptake on the delayed images. Functional cerebral images of perfusion and glucose metabolism demonstrate increased uptake in the temporal lobes in acute herpes encephalitis. These changes also precede by several days the changes on CT and MRI. In the chronic phase, when damage to the brain has occurred, the uptake may be decreased.

Diagnosis

Multiple ictal seizure foci in Rasmussen's encephalitis.

References

1. Muller RA, Chugani HT, Muzik O, Mangner TJ: Brain organization of motor and language functions following hemispherectomy: A [(15)O]-water positron emission tomography study. J Child Neurol 1998;13:16–22.
2. Yacubian EM, Marie SK, Valerio RM, Jorge CL, Yamaga L, Buchpiguel CA: Neuroimaging findings in Rasmussen's syndrome. J Neuroimaging 1997;7:16–22.
3. Geller E, Faerber EN, Legido A, et al.: Rasmussen encephalitis: Complementary role of multitechnique neuroimaging. Am J Neuroradiol 1998;19: 445–449.
4. Kaiboriboon K, Cortese C, Hogan RE: Magnetic resonance and positron emission tomography changes during the clinical progression of Rasmussen's encephalitis. J Neuroimaging 2000;10: 122–125.
5. Leach JP, Chadwick DW, Miles JB, Hart IK: Improvement in adult-onset Rasmussen's encephalitis with long-term immunomodulatory therapy. Neurology 1999;52:738–742.

Case 4.10

History

A 62-year-old female presented with progressive cognitive dysfunction, weakness, sensory deficits, and speech disorder. The cerebral MRI showed mild frontal atrophy. She was referred for FDG PET imaging of the brain (Figure 4.10, see color plate). The FDG images were acquired with a dedicated PET tomograph in the 2D mode and reconstructed with iterative reconstruction and measured segmented attenuation correction.

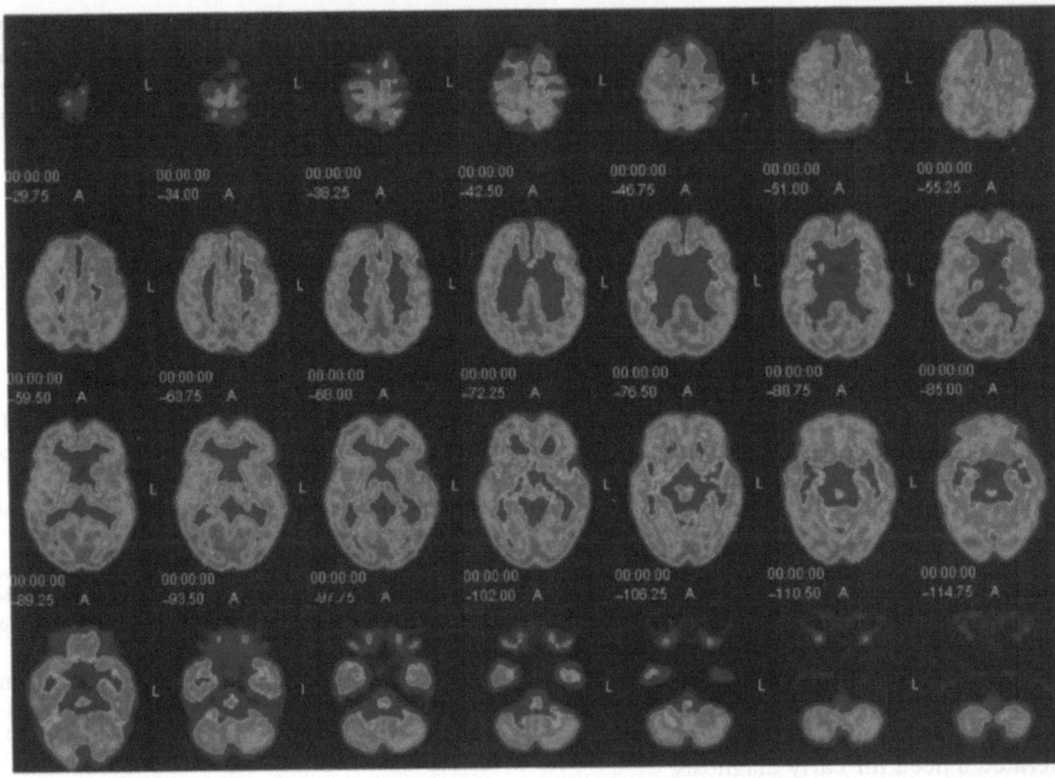

FIGURE 4.10. (See color plate)

Findings

The FDG PET images show moderately decreased FDG uptake in the head of the caudate nuclei, putamen, and thalami, as well as hypometabolism in the frontal cortex.

Discussion

The differential diagnosis of decreased perfusion and metabolism in the basal ganglia include Huntington's disease, Wilson's disease, and some of the Parkinsonian syndromes, including progressive supranuclear palsy and multisystem atrophy.

Huntington's disease is an autosomal dominant disorder that in most cases presents in the third or fourth decade by progressive cognitive deterioration and extrapyramidal or choreiform movements, as well as psychiatric abnormalities. The genetic anomaly is located in the short arm of chromosome 4. The more profound pathological changes are in the putamen and caudate nuclei. In advanced disease, atrophy of the caudate nuclei can be demonstrated on CT and MRI. FDG PET imaging is able to identify decreased metabolism in the caudate nuclei in subjects with symptomatic Huntington's disease and in asymptomatic gene carriers. Similar findings may be seen in symptomatic patients using ^{99m}Tc-HMPAO SPECT. Imaging dopamine receptor activity using both PET and SPECT ligands has been found useful in the evaluation of Huntington's disease patients, both before and after the appearance of symptoms.

Wilson's disease is an autosomal recessive disorder of copper metabolism that can lead to movement and psychiatric disorder due to accumulation of copper in the brain. Patients with Wilson's disease have decreased glucose metabolism in the striatum and cerebellum.

Patients with progressive supranuclear palsy present with paralyzed gaze, dystonia, axial rigidity, and sometimes dementia. On functional images, the most striking finding is decreased uptake in the frontal cortex, but uptake in the basal ganglia and thalami is also decreased.

Multisystem atrophy (Shy-Drager syndrome) includes syndrome of striatonigral degeneration, pallidopyramidal degeneration, olivopontocerebellar atrophy, and pure autonomic dysfunction. FDG PET images usually show decreased metabolism in the striatum. The striatonigral degeneration variant clinically resembles Parkinson's disease but without tremor. On FDG PET images, there is striatal and prefrontal hypometabolism. The olivopontocerebellar atrophy variant begins clinically with gait disturbances and progresses to dysarthria and limb ataxia. There is degeneration of the neurons from the cerebellar cortex, pons, and inferior olives, which demonstrate hypometabolism on FDG images.

The differential diagnosis of decreased uptake in the basal ganglia also includes atypical Parkinson's disease, atypical Creutzfeldt-Jakob disease, prior viral encephalopathy (particularly Herpes Zoster), toxic encephalopathies (such as ethylene glycol), and a variety of other degenerative neurological diseases.

Diagnosis

Probable multisystem atrophy.

Case 4.11

History

A 19-year-old white female presented with mental status changes. She was referred for MRI (Figure 4.11A) and FDG PET imaging of the brain (Figure 4.11B). Figure 4.11A shows a sagittal T1-weighted image without gadolinium enhancement (left) and a transaxial T2-weighted image (right). The FDG images were acquired with a dedicated PET tomo-

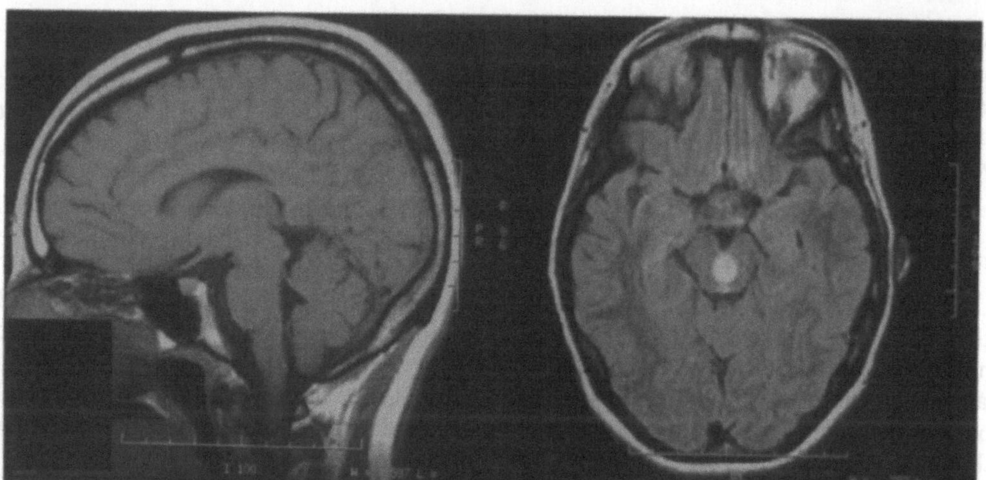

FIGURE 4.11A.

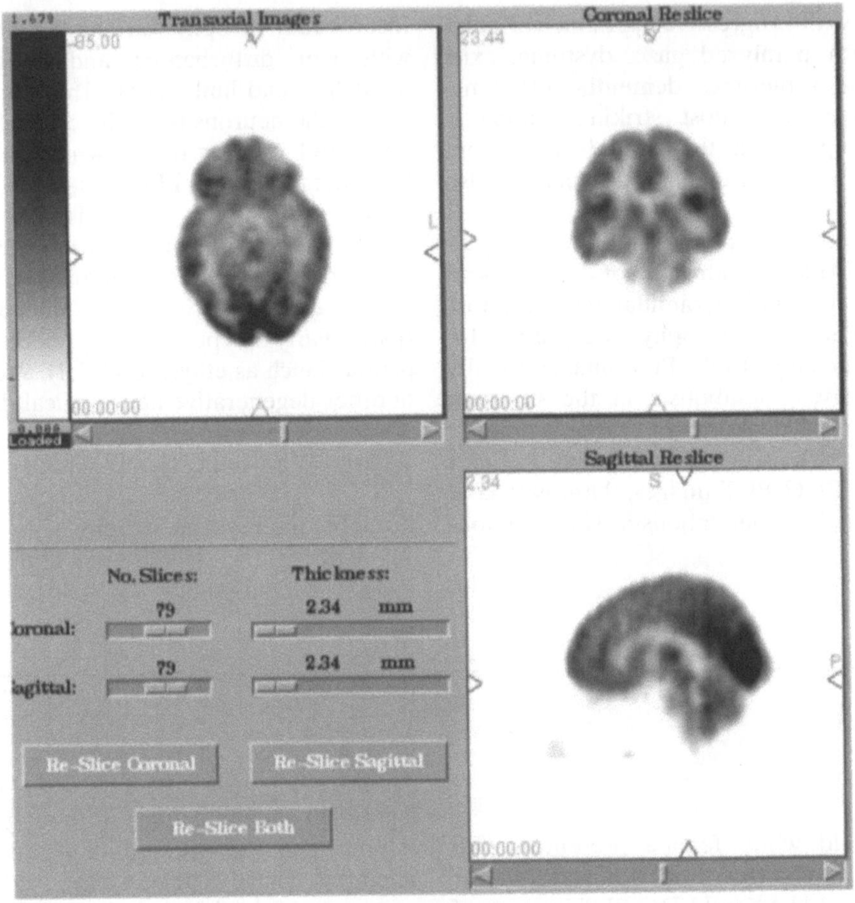

FIGURE 4.11B.

graph (GE Advance) in the 2D mode and reconstructed with iterative reconstruction and measured segmented attenuation correction. Orthogonal images through the brain stem are shown.

Findings

The sagittal T1-weighted MRI image reveals a subtle area of decreased signal in the midbrain (Figure 4.11A on the left). The lesion was not enhancing on the post-gadolinium image. The lesion was best demonstrated on T2-weighted MRI image (Figure 4.11A on the right). On FDG PET images, the lesion demonstrates increased FDG uptake.

Discussion

The absence of enhancement on the MRI images suggests a low-grade tumor, but the increased FDG uptake on PET images suggests a high-grade tumor. Pilocytic astrocytoma, usually found in children, has a distinct histology and biologic behavior compared to the forms of astrocytoma found in adults. They represent approximately 10% of pediatric brain tumors and are usually located in the posterior fossa. Although they behave like low-grade tumors, they usually demonstrate marked FDG accumulation. Some pilocytic astrocytomas also demonstrate contrast enhancement on CT and MRI.[1–3] The significance of this finding is not understood. One explanation is that the fenestrated epithelial cells of this tumor may be hyperplastic and hypermetabolic.

Other low-grade tumors of the brain can demonstrate high levels of FDG uptake. Ependymomas represent 2 to 8% of pediatric brain neoplasms and have variable FDG uptake.[2] Ganglioglioma is another low-grade glioma that is usually hypometabolic but can have hypermetabolic foci.[4,5] The normal pituitary gland does not accumulate FDG, but the most common intrasellar tumors, pituitary adenoma and craniopharyngioma, do accumulate FDG to a high degree, even though they are benign.[6,7]

Diagnosis

Probable pilocytic astrocytoma.

References

1. Fulham MJ, Melisi JW, Nishimiya J, Dwyer AJ, Di Chiro G: Neuroimaging of juvenile pilocytic astrocytomas: An enigma. Radiology 1993;189: 221–225.
2. Hoffman JM, Hanson MW, Friedman HS, et al.: FDG-PET in pediatric fossa brain tumors. J Comput Assist Tomogr 1992;16:62–68.
3. Roelcke U, Radu EW, Hausmann O, Vontobel P, Maguire RP, Leenders KL: Tracer transport and metabolism in a patient with juvenile pilocytic astrocytoma. A PET study. J Neurooncol 1998; 36(3):279–283.
4. Kincaid PK, El-Saden SM, Park SH, Goy BW: Cerebral gangliogliomas: Preoperative grading using FDG-PET and 201Tl-SPECT. Am J Neuroradiol 1998;19(5):801–806.
5. Provenzale JM, Arata MA, Turkington TG, McLendon RE, Coleman RE: Gangliogliomas: Characterization by registered positron emission tomography-MR images. Am J Roentgenol 1999; 172(4):1103–1107.
6. De Souza B, Brunetti A, Fulham MJ, et al.: Pituitary microadenomas: A PET study. Radiology 1990;177:39–44.
7. Bergstrom M, Muhr C, Lundberg PO, Langstrom B: PET as a tool in the clinical evaluation of pituitary adenomas. J Nucl Med 1991;32:610–615.

Case 4.12

History

A 52-year-old man presented with a past history of glioma in the left temporal lobe two years ago and was treated with surgical resection, followed by chemotherapy and radiation therapy. He was referred for MRI (Figure 4.12A) and FDG PET imaging of the brain (Figure 4.12B). Figure 4.12A shows post-gadolinium T1-weighted MRI images. The FDG images were acquired with a dedicated PET tomograph (GE Advance) in the 2D mode and reconstructed with iterative reconstruction and measured segmented attenuation correction.

Findings

The post-gadolinium T1-weighted MRI images demonstrate an area of enhancement in the subcortical white matter of the left frontal lobe. There is no corresponding FDG uptake on the PET images. However, there is a focus of marked FDG uptake in the left mesial temporal cortex adjacent to the resection site, where there is no corresponding abnormality on MRI.

Discussion

These findings indicate that the enhancement on MRI in the left frontal white matter is related to increased permeability of the blood-brain barrier, secondary to radiation necrosis rather than tumor recurrence. In the absence of a structural abnormality on MRI, the focus of uptake in the left temporal lobe is likely related to ictal activity occurring during FDG distribution. Follow-up imaging three months later confirmed the absence of FDG uptake in the white

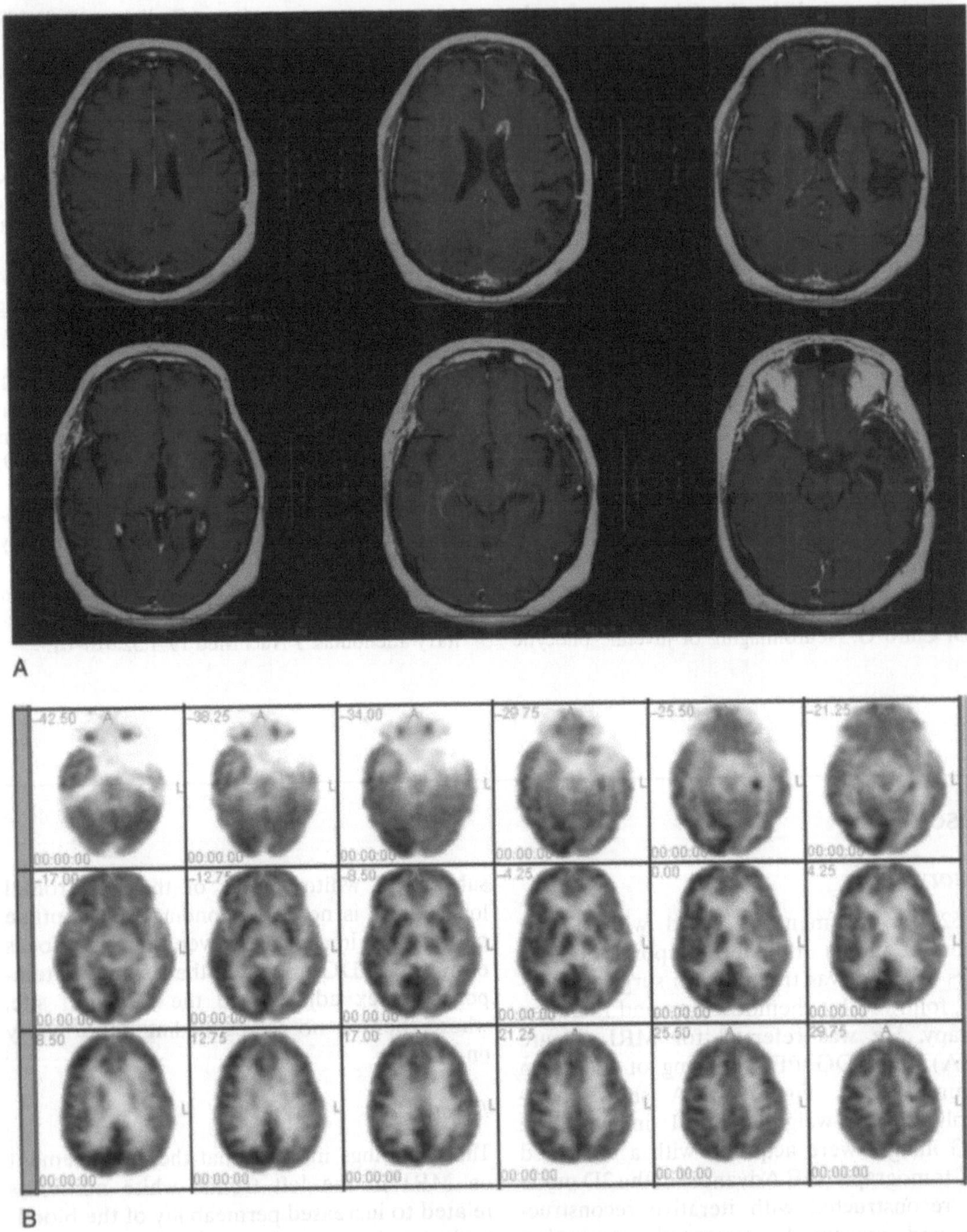

FIGURE 4.12A,B.

matter of the frontal lobe, whereas the area of enhancement had increased in size on MRI (Figure 4.12C), and the focus of increased FDG uptake in the left temporal cortex was no longer present (Figure 4.12D). This confirms that the focus of hypermetabolism seen on the first scan, but not on the second scan, was related to ictal activity rather than neoplasm.

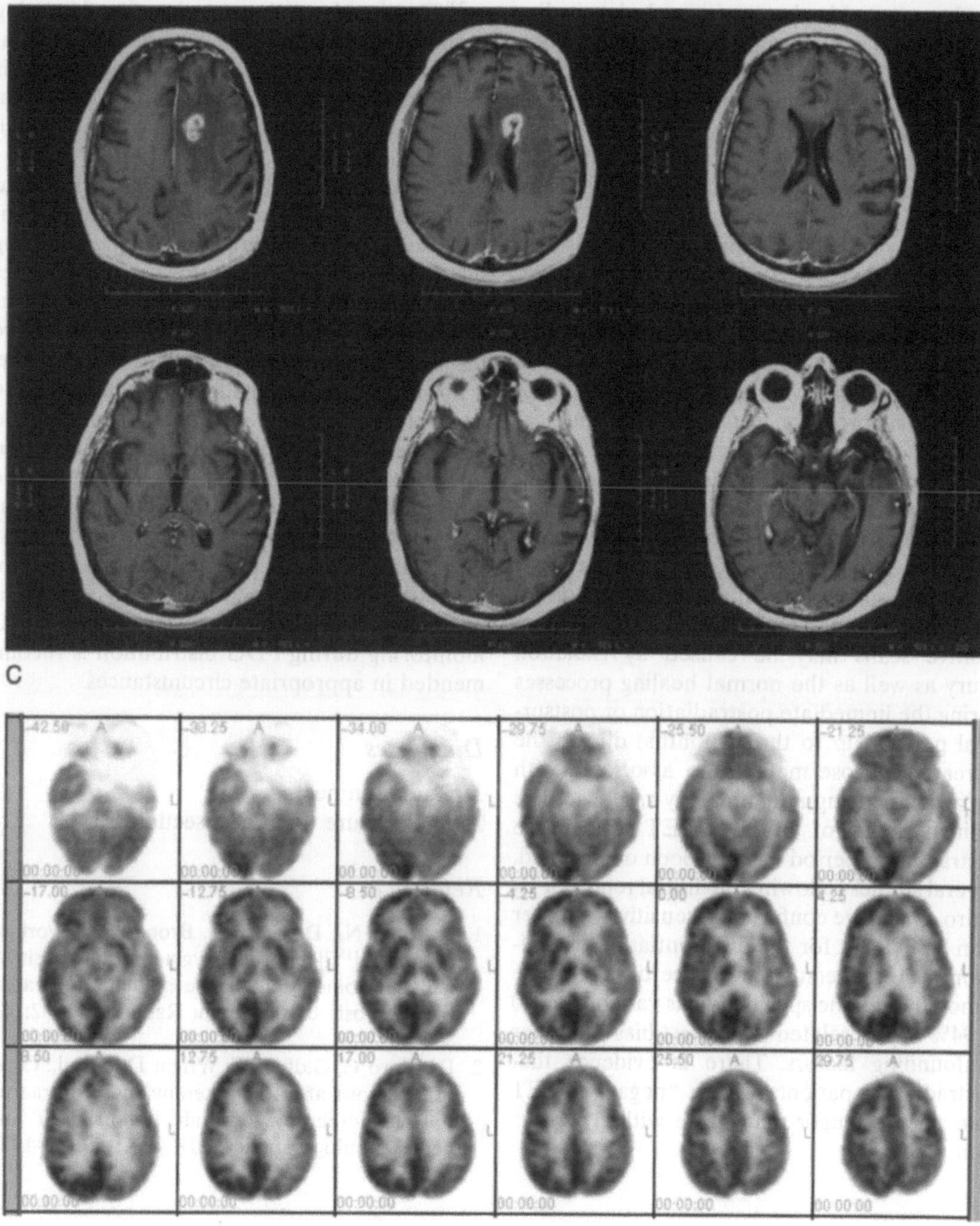

FIGURE 4.12C,D.

Patients who receive high dose radiation therapy are at risk for development of radiation necrosis. Cerebral radiation injury has been classified according to the time of appearance of symptoms after therapy. Acute injury appears at the time of therapy, and the symptoms are usually transient. Early radiation injury occurs from a few weeks to three months posttherapy and is also transient. In late radiation injury, the symptoms occur between four months and ten years after therapy, although 70% occur within two years. The incidence of late-delayed radiation injury is 5 to 37%. Two forms of late radiation injury may occur: focal injury and diffuse white matter disease. They can occur together or separately. Focal radiation injury presents as a mass lesion with focal neurologic deficits. Symptoms of radiation necrosis and recurrent tumor are similar, and the clinical course of each is indistinguishable. Treatment of late-delayed radiation necrosis ranges from conservative measures to control intracranial pressure to aggressive surgical resection of the edematous mass.

The typical radiographic appearance of brain tumors as well as radiation necrosis is a contrast-enhancing mass surrounded by edema and mass effect. Areas of radiation necrosis have lower glucose metabolism than a normal brain because they are less cellular. False-positive scans may be caused by radiation injury as well as the normal healing processes during the immediate postradiation or postsurgical period (up to three months) due to the increased glucose metabolism associated with the accompanying inflammatory response. The optimal timing of an FDG PET scan in the postradiation period has not been determined. Several studies following the initial report of Di Chiro et al. have confirmed a sensitivity greater than 80 percent for the differentiation of radiation necrosis versus recurrence of high-grade tumor, though the specificity has varied from 40 to 94% in part related to posttest bias and other confounding factors. There is evidence that postradiation patients with a "negative" PET scan survive longer than those with a positive scan.[1,2]

^{201}Thallium is an alternate functional imaging radiopharmaceutical allowing the differentiation of recurrent tumor from radiation necrosis using the SPECT technique with conventional gamma cameras that are more available than PET tomographs.

Lesions (both benign and malignant) located in the region of the temporal lobe can present with seizures. If seizures are frequent during the FDG uptake phase (the first 20 minutes after injection of FDG), the ictal seizure focus will have increased FDG uptake usually above the level of cortical uptake. This high uptake, if not recognized as due to seizure, may lead to an erroneous interpretation of high-grade tumor. Therefore, it is important to recognize that interpretative errors may occur without the appropriate clinical information, as well as correlation with anatomical images. The interpreter must evaluate precisely in what anatomical structure the abnormal FDG uptake is present. Correlation with continuous EEG monitoring during FDG distribution is recommended in appropriate circumstances.

Diagnoses

1. Radiation necrosis.
2. Ictal seizure focus at resection site.

References

1. Patronas NJ, Di Chiro G, Brooks RA: Work in progress: [^{18}F] fluorodeoxyglucose and positron emission tomography in the evaluation of radiation necrosis of the brain. Radiology 1982;144: 885–889.
2. Di Chiro G, Oldfield E, Wright DC, et al.: Cerebral necrosis after radiotherapy and/or intraarterial chemotherapy for brain tumors: PET and neuropathologic studies. AJR 1988;150:189–197.

5

Cardiac Applications of FDG Imaging with PET and SPECT

Jeroen J. Bax, Chris Y. Kim, Don Poldermans, Abdou Elhendy, Eric Boersma, A.F.L. Schinkel, Gerrit W. Sloof, and Martin P. Sandler

Positron emission tomography (PET) using ^{18}F-fluorodeoxyglucose (FDG) has been used to evaluate cardiac glucose utilization in different cardiac diseases, including hypertrophic cardiomyopathy,[1] acute ischemic syndromes (infarction and unstable angina),[2,3] and chronic ischemic left ventricular (LV) dysfunction.[4,5] Most studies have evaluated patients with ischemic cardiomyopathy with the aim of assessing myocardial viability. Currently, the only clinically accepted application of cardiac FDG imaging is the assessment of viability in this subset of patients. Using FDG imaging for the assessment of viability makes prediction of improvement of LV function, heart failure symptoms, and long-term prognosis after revascularization possible.[6,7] In the 1980s, FDG imaging could only be performed with PET equipment, but with the introduction of 511 keV collimators in the 1990s, FDG imaging is now feasible with single photon emission computed tomography (SPECT).[6] Particularly with the increasing demand and the relative unavailability of PET equipment, the development of high-energy SPECT imaging was welcomed in the field of nuclear cardiology. Finally, with the development of dual-head coincidence imaging, the resolution of gamma camera PET imaging further approaches that of full view PET imaging. This chapter describes different aspects of cardiac FDG imaging. Following a discussion of the clinical relevance of viability assessment and the details of data acquisition and analysis, the evidence supporting cardiac FDG imaging is summarized. In particular, the studies focusing on prediction of outcome after revascularization and long-term prognosis are highlighted.

Viability Assessment and Clinical Relevance

Heart failure is becoming the most comprehensive problem in clinical cardiology, in terms of affected patients. Approximately five million Americans have chronic heart failure, and 400,000 new cases are diagnosed each year.[8,9] Based on pooled analysis of the 13 multicentered heart failure trials published over the past ten years in the *New England Journal of Medicine*, coronary artery disease was the underlying etiology in almost 70% of the 20,000 patients involved in these trials.[8,9] The prognosis of patients with ischemic cardiomyopathy remains poor, despite recent progress in medical therapy.[8,9] The treatment of choice is heart transplantation, but the number of donor hearts does not match the enormous demand.[10] An alternative modality of treatment may be coronary revascularization.[11] Following revascularization, the left ventricular function of some patients improves, and this improvement in LV function may translate to superior survival.[3,4] However, not all patients improve in LV function postrevascularization; in a recent study, approximately 35% of the patients improved significantly (that is, improvement in (LVEF) 5% or more) in LV function postrevascularizaton.[12] Revascularization procedures are associated with a substantially higher risk in this category of patients.[11] Therefore, a careful evaluation is mandatory for optimal patient management and risk stratification.

In order to explain the postoperative improvement in LV performance and prognosis, the concept of viability has been proposed.[13–17] Patients with viable myocardium have been demonstrated to improve in LV function, heart failure symptoms, and prognosis following revascularization.[13–17] Conversely, patients without viable myocardium do not benefit.[13–17] Another study has shown that preoperative viability testing results in improved perioperative risk stratification.[18] Finally, retrospective analyses have demonstrated that the presence of viable myocardium in patients with ischemic cardiomyopathy, who were treated medically, was associated with an extremely high event rate.[19] The exact prevalence of viability among patients presenting with heart failure secondary to poor LV function in the presence of chronic coronary artery disease is currently not clear. Auerbach et al. evaluated 283 patients with ischemic cardiomyopathy with FDG PET and demonstrated that 156 (55%) had viable myocardium.[20] Schinkel et al.[21] evaluated 104 patients (all chronic coronary artery disease, LVEF <35%) with FDG SPECT and demonstrated viability in 54% of the patients (Figure 5.1). Although these data were obtained in tertiary referral centers (and may not be applicable to the community), it appears that a substantial percentage of patients with ischemic cardiomyopathy have viable myocardium. This does not necessarily mean that all of these patients are suitable candidates for revascularization; other factors, including comorbidity, quality of target vessels, and severe LV dilatation, also influence the decision whether revascularization should take place. Still, considering the enormous number of patients with ischemic cardiomyopathy and the lack of optimal treatment for these patients, preoperative viability testing will help to guide patient management.

Currently, a variety of techniques are available for the assessment of myocardial viability, including nuclear imaging and stress echocardiography. Cardiac FDG imaging is considered the most accurate technique for the assessment of viability.

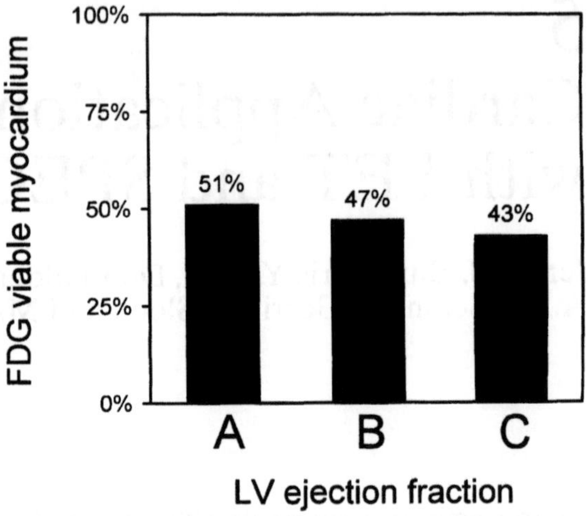

FIGURE 5.1. Bar graph showing the presence of viability according to FDG SPECT in 104 patients with ischemic cardiomyopathy. Group A: patients with LVEF <20%; Group B: patients with LVEF 20 to 30%; Group C: patients with LVEF 30 to 35%. Substantial viability was observed in 54% of the patients. (Data based on Reference 21.)

Protocols

First, information on contractile function is needed, since assessment of viability is predominantly important in regions with akinesia or severe hypokinesia. This information is currently provided noninvasively by echocardiography, radionuclide ventriculography, or gated perfusion SPECT or invasively in the catheterization laboratory.

Second, information on perfusion is needed. With PET imaging, a variety of tracers have been used to assess perfusion, including ^{82}Rb, $^{13}NH_3$, ^{11}C-acetate, and ^{15}O-water. Since the half-life of these PET perfusion tracers is too short for SPECT imaging, SPECT tracers are used to assess perfusion, that is, ^{201}Tl and ^{99m}Tc-labeled agents.

Third, when FDG uptake is evaluated, the patient's metabolic conditions are extremely important in determining cardiac FDG uptake.[22] The perfusion and FDG data can be acquired sequentially or simultaneously. With PET and gamma camera based dual-head coincidence imaging, only sequential acquisition is possible. With SPECT imaging, both sequential and simultaneous acquisitions are possible. The initial FDG SPECT studies used ^{201}Tl as a perfusion tracer and were thus acquired sequentially.[6,7] This approach has been validated extensively over time and has been proven comparable to FDG PET in terms of prediction of improvement of function postrevascularization.[6,7] The more recent SPECT studies have used a dual-isotope simultaneous acquisition (DISA) protocol.[6,7] Important advantages of the DISA protocol are the reduction in acquisition time and the perfect alignment between the perfusion and FDG data. With gated SPECT imaging (performed mainly with ^{99m}Tc-labeled agents), the information on regional contractile function (to identify the dysfunctional regions) can also be provided by SPECT, thus avoiding misalignment between 2D echocardiography or radionuclide ventriculography and SPECT. Preliminary data indicate that the DISA protocol has similar accuracy in predicting functional outcome postrevascularization.[6,7] Some studies have used FDG imaging in isolation,[23,24] without the use of a perfusion tracer. In these studies, cutoff criteria for FDG uptake are used to classify dysfunctional segments as viable or nonviable. Although the use of a single tracer appears attractive, the accuracy for predicting functional outcome after revascularization is suboptimal, mainly due to overestimation of functional recovery (see following).

For the data analysis, different approaches have been reported, including absolute quantification requiring dynamic imaging, semiquantitative analysis using static imaging, and visual analysis.[6,7]

Viability Criteria

Over the years, many different viability criteria have been used.

Perfusion-FDG Match and Mismatch

Based on the concept of "hibernation,"[25] segments with reduced perfusion but preserved FDG uptake (perfusion-FDG mismatch) are classified as viable. Indeed, many studies have indicated that these segments frequently improve in function following adequate revascularization.[26–34] In contrast, segments with reduced perfusion and concordantly reduced FDG uptake (perfusion-FDG match) are considered scar tissue and only rarely improve in function following revascularization.[26–34] Additional studies have demonstrated that dysfunctional segments with near normal perfusion and preserved FDG uptake also frequently improve in function. These segments may represent areas of repeated stunning.[35]

Normalized FDG Uptake

Cutoff values of normalized FDG uptake are applied when FDG is used without a perfusion tracer. Most frequently, a cutoff value of ≥50% of normal (or maximum) is used to identify viable myocardium.[23] However, this approach may not be accurate in the prediction of functional recovery, since segments with severely reduced perfusion may still have increased FDG uptake although less than 50% of normal or maximum. Also, segments with a mild reduction in perfusion and concordantly reduced FDG uptake (but still ≥50% of normal or maximum) are likely to represent areas of subendocardial necrosis and will not improve in function following revascularization;[32,36] these segments have been referred to as "mild match" in some studies.[32,36] Indeed, the superiority of combined assessment of perfusion and FDG uptake over the use of FDG alone for prediction of functional outcome has been demonstrated.[36] Finally, if normalized FDG uptake is used, the optimal cutoff value has not been defined adequately. Some studies[23] have used a 50% cutoff value, whereas other studies using receiver operating characteristics curve analysis (ROC-curve analysis) showed that the optimal cutoff value for prediction of functional recovery was 85 to 90% of maximum uptake.[37]

Absolute Glucose Utilization

Another option is the use of absolute quantification of regional glucose utilization. Fath-Ordoubadi et al. have used ROC-curve analysis and identified the cutoff value of regional glucose utilization ≥0.25 μmol/min/g as the optimal predictor of improvement of regional LV function postrevascularization.[38] Applying this cutoff value in a subsequent study, a sensitivity of 99% and a specificity of 33% for predicting improvement of LV function were obtained.[24] Similar to using normalized FDG uptake, the specificity is suboptimal, indicating that some segments defined as viable by FDG imaging do not improve in function after revascularization. Again, this is most likely caused by nontransmural scars that contain a certain amount of viable nonischemic myocardium, which cannot improve in function with revascularization.

Patient Preparation

Under normal resting conditions, cardiac metabolism is mainly oxidative with free fatty acids (FFA) and glucose being the major sources of energy.[39] In the presence of ischemia, however, oxidative metabolism of free fatty acids is decreased, and glucose becomes the preferred substrate for the myocardium. Depending on the degree of residual oxygen availability, glucose may predominantly be metabolized anaerobically. The amount of energy produced by anaerobic glycolysis may not be adequate to maintain contractility but sufficient to preserve the cellular integrity. This explains the situation in dysfunctional but viable myocardium: Contraction is severely reduced or absent while glucose utilization and viability are maintained. Since the 1980s, FDG has been used to evaluate myocardial glucose utilization.[5–7] FDG closely resembles glucose, with the exception that one hydroxyl group has been replaced by an ^{18}F-particle. The initial trans-sarcolemmal uptake of FDG is identical to that of glucose. FDG competes with glucose for uptake and phosphorylation to FDG-6-phosphate (FDG-6-PO4), mediated by the enzyme hexokinase. Unlike glucose-6-PO4, FDG-6-PO4 does not undergo further metabolism and remains trapped in the myocyte, providing a strong tracer for cardiac imaging. FDG uptake in the myocardium is highly dependent on the dietary conditions (that is, plasma levels of FFA, glucose, and insulin).[22] High insulin levels with the resultant suppression of FFA promote FDG uptake, whereas high FFA levels inhibit FDG uptake. Several protocols are available to promote cardiac FDG uptake, including oral glucose loading, hyperinsulinemic euglycemic clamping, and the administration of nicotinic acid derivatives.[22] Oral glucose loading is the most frequently used approach, although it often results in uninterpretable images in patients with impaired glucose tolerance or diabetes (that is, fasting serum glucose >115 mg/dl).[22] To circumvent this problem, both the addition of intravenous insulin or the use of hyperinsulinemic euglycemic clamping have been proposed.[40–42] The clamping procedure is the most rigorous procedure which allows perfect regulation of metabolic substrates and insulin levels, ensuring excellent image quality in all patients. However, the procedure is laborious and time-consuming and may not be feasible in busy nuclear medicine departments. Martin et al.[42] have adapted the clamping protocol and described a rather elegant and less extensive protocol: A fixed glucose-insulin-potassium (GIK) solution was infused over 30 minutes, followed by FDG injection, which resulted in excellent image quality with 99% of the images being interpretable.

Finally, Knuuti et al. have recently demonstrated that oral administration of a nicotinic acid derivative (acipimox) may be an alternative to clamping.[43] Acipimox inhibits peripheral lipolysis, thus reducing plasma free fatty acid levels and indirectly stimulating cardiac FDG uptake.[44] Bax et al.[45] compared the different patient preparations in a small group of patients; all patients underwent three cardiac FDG studies following oral glucose loading, acipimox administration, or during hyperinsulinemic euglycemic clamping. The image quality was expressed as a myocardium-to-background ratio, being 2.2 ± 0.3 with oral glucose loading ($P < 0.05$ versus acipimox and clamping), 2.9 ± 0.7 with acipimox administration, and 2.8 ± 0.8 with clamping. Visually, the FDG images were superior with clamping and after acipimox administration as compared to oral glucose loading.

Since acipimox is unavailable in the United States, a 30-minute infusion of a fixed glucose-insulin solution is the most practical yet effective technique for stimulating myocardial FDG uptake.

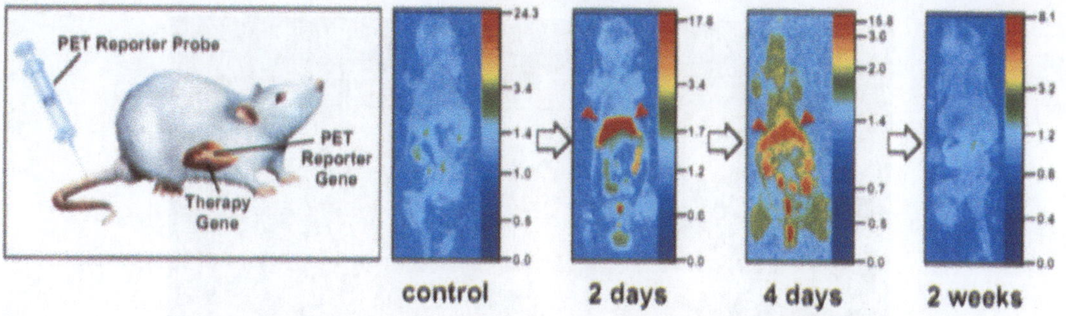

FIGURE 1.10. Images of gene expression with microPET in a living mouse. Mice were intravenously injected with an adenovirus that localizes greater than 90% to the liver. In the control mouse, the virus did not contain a PET reporter gene. The image was taken after intravenous injection of a PET reporter probe. Since there is no PET reporter gene expression to report, the image shows uniform activity through the section shown. A mouse was then injected with an adenovirus containing a PET reporter gene. Repeated images were taken at 2 days, 4 days, and 2 weeks in the same mouse after injecting the mouse with a PET reporter probe that will image expression of the PET reporter gene. Images were taken 60 minutes after injection of the probe. At 2 days, the image shows high gene expression in the liver, with lower expression at 4 days and loss of expression at 2 weeks due to termination of the virus by the immune system. The color scale is proportional to gene expression, with red being the highest. Descriptions of this technique for imaging gene expression in vivo with PET is provided elsewhere.[5,6,43,44]

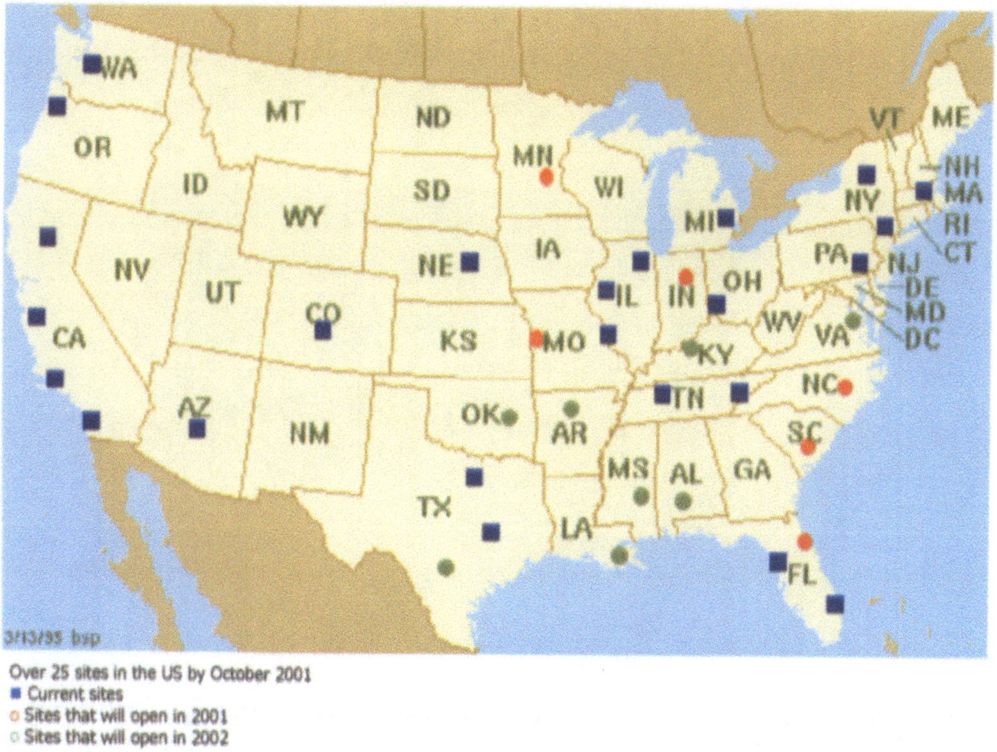

FIGURE 3.1. United States map depicting current and proposed cyclotron facilities of the largest ^{18}FDG production company, PETNet, Knoxville, TN (October 2000). (Courtesy of PETNet, Knoxville, TN.)

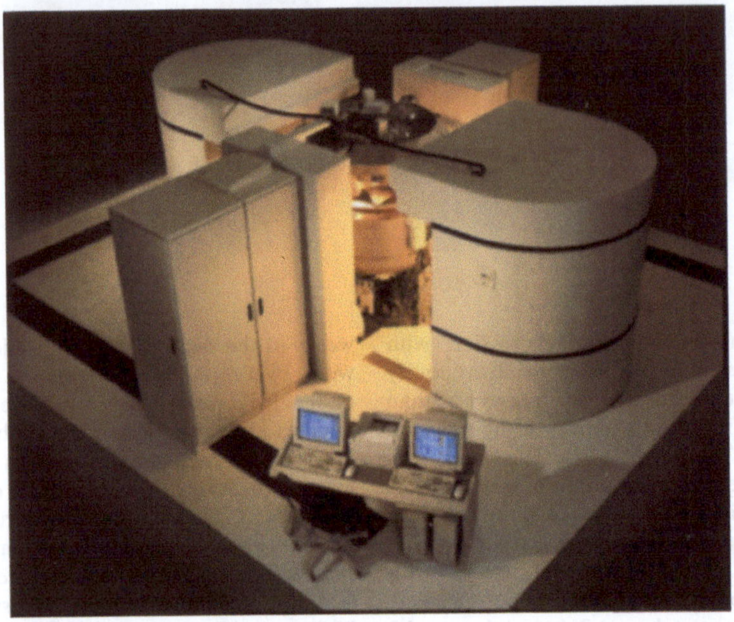

FIGURE 3.2. RDS-111 PET cyclotron manufactured by CTI in Knoxville, TN. (Courtesy of CTI, Knoxville, TN.)

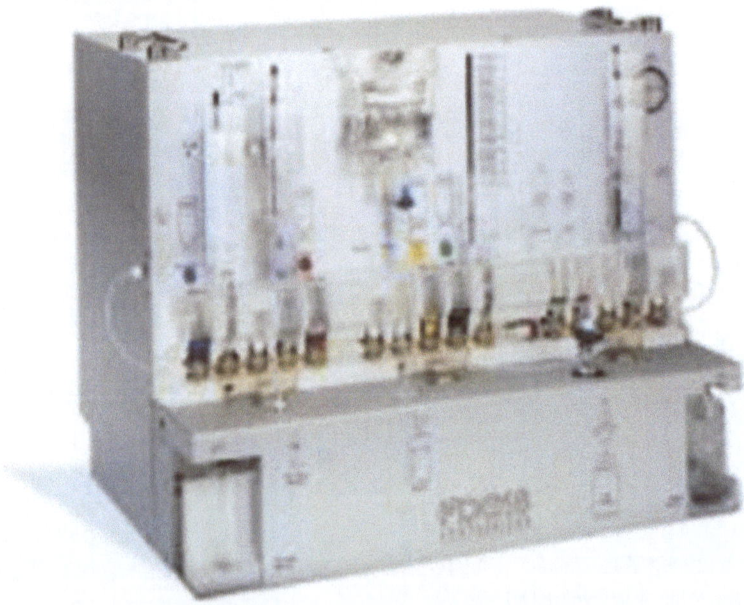

FIGURE 3.3. Automated synthesis units currently available for ^{18}FDG production—(A) Coincidence, (B) QuadRx, and (C) Nuclear Interface. ((A) Courtesy of Bioscan, Washington, DC; (B) Courtesy of CTI, Knoxville, TN; (C) Courtesy of Nuclear Interface, Berlin, Germany.)

COLOR PLATE III

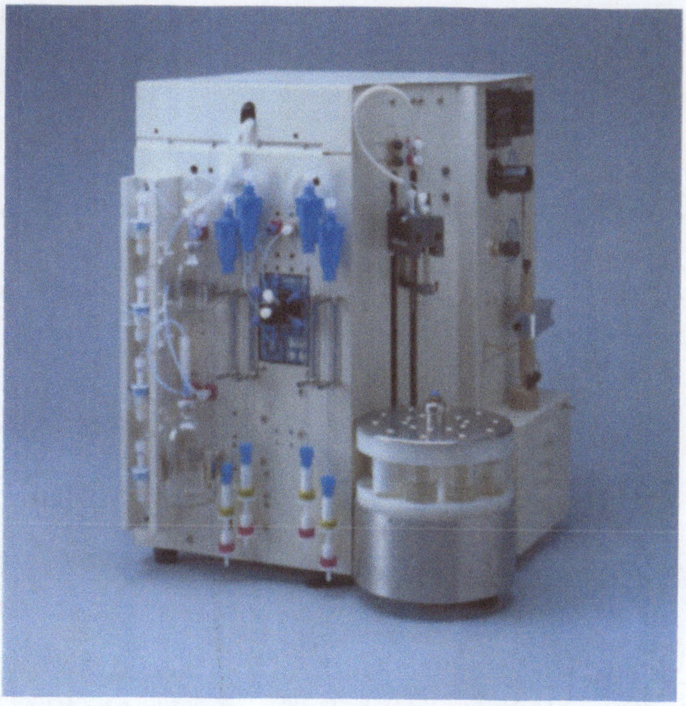

FIGURE 3.3B.

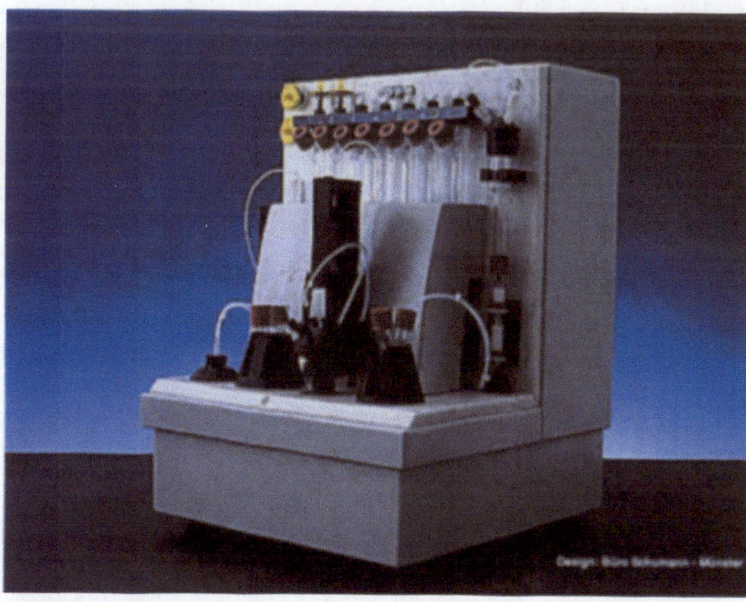

FIGURE 3.3C.

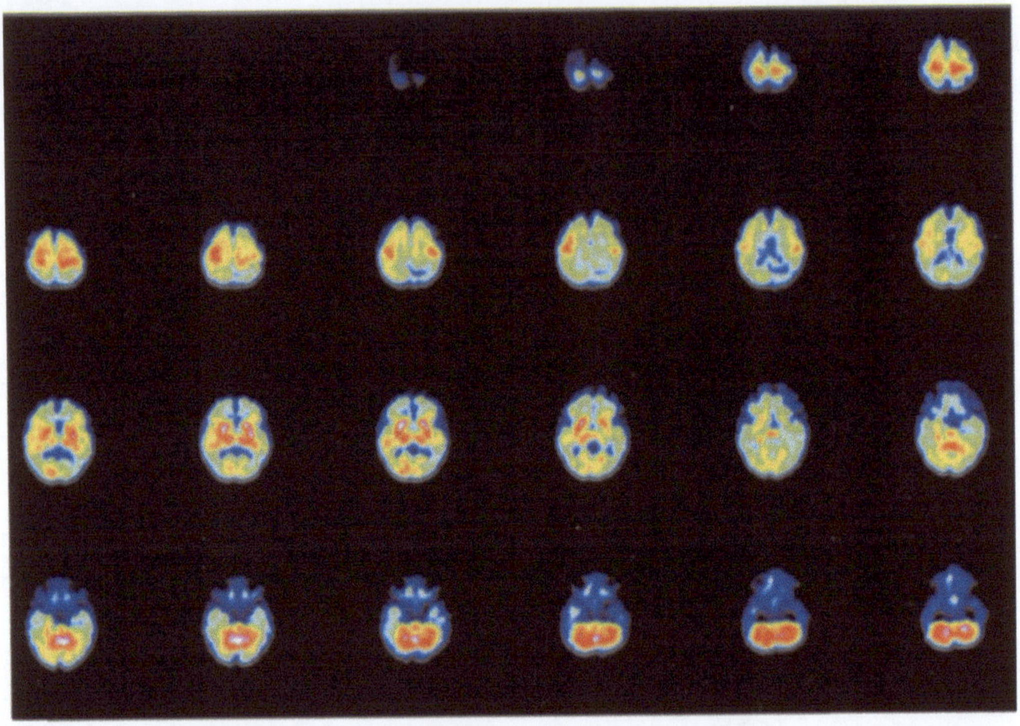

FIGURE 4.7B.

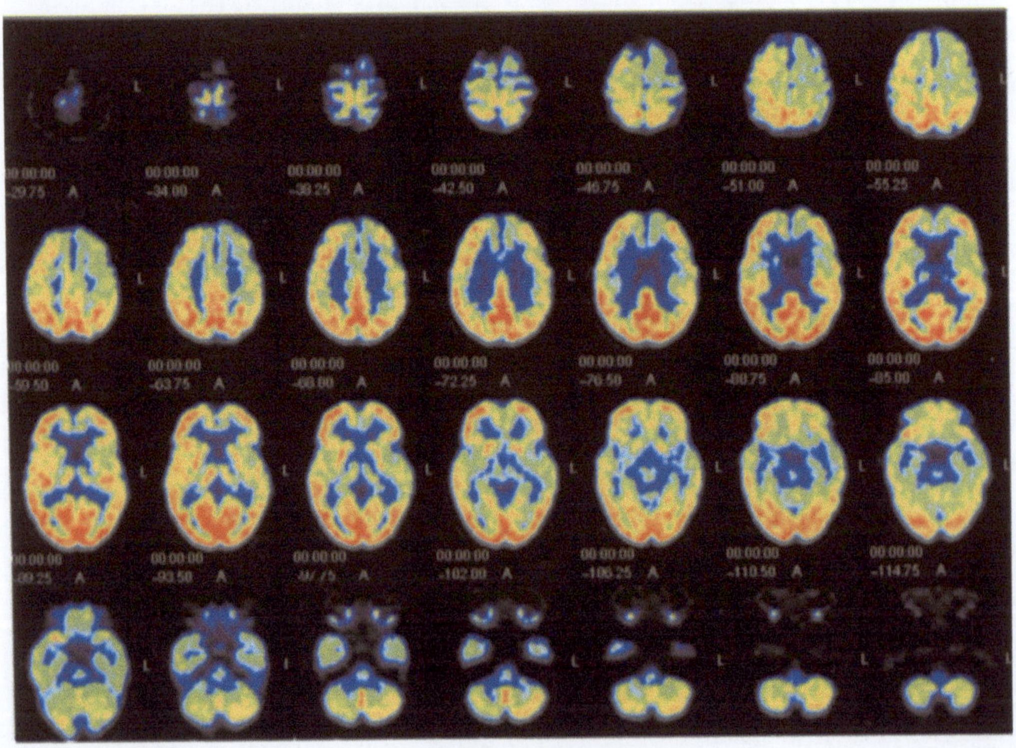

FIGURE 4.10.

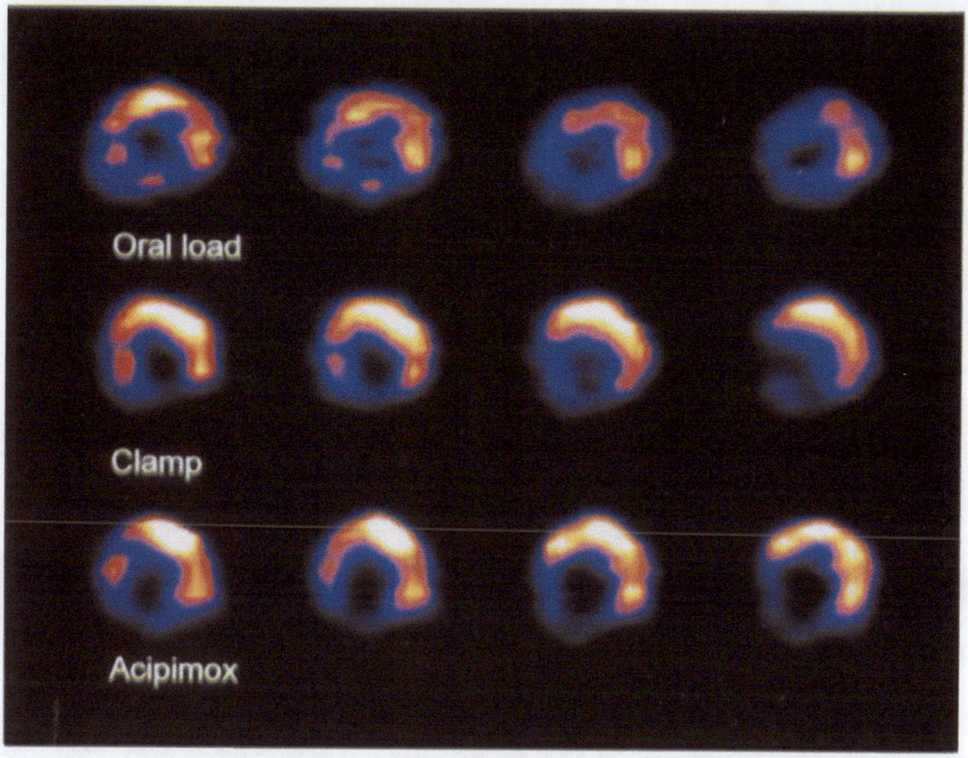

FIGURE 5.5.

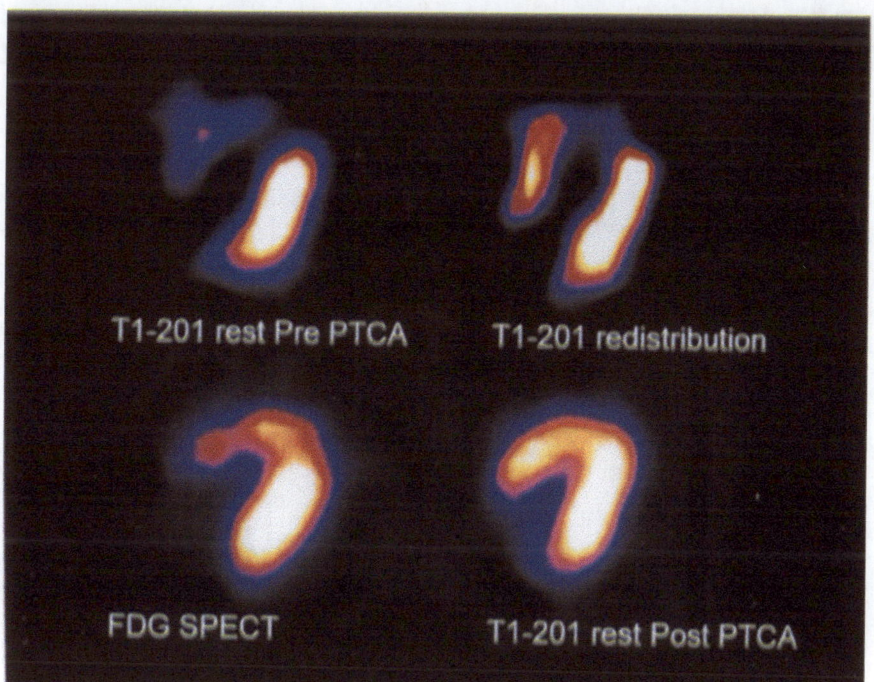

FIGURE 5.6.

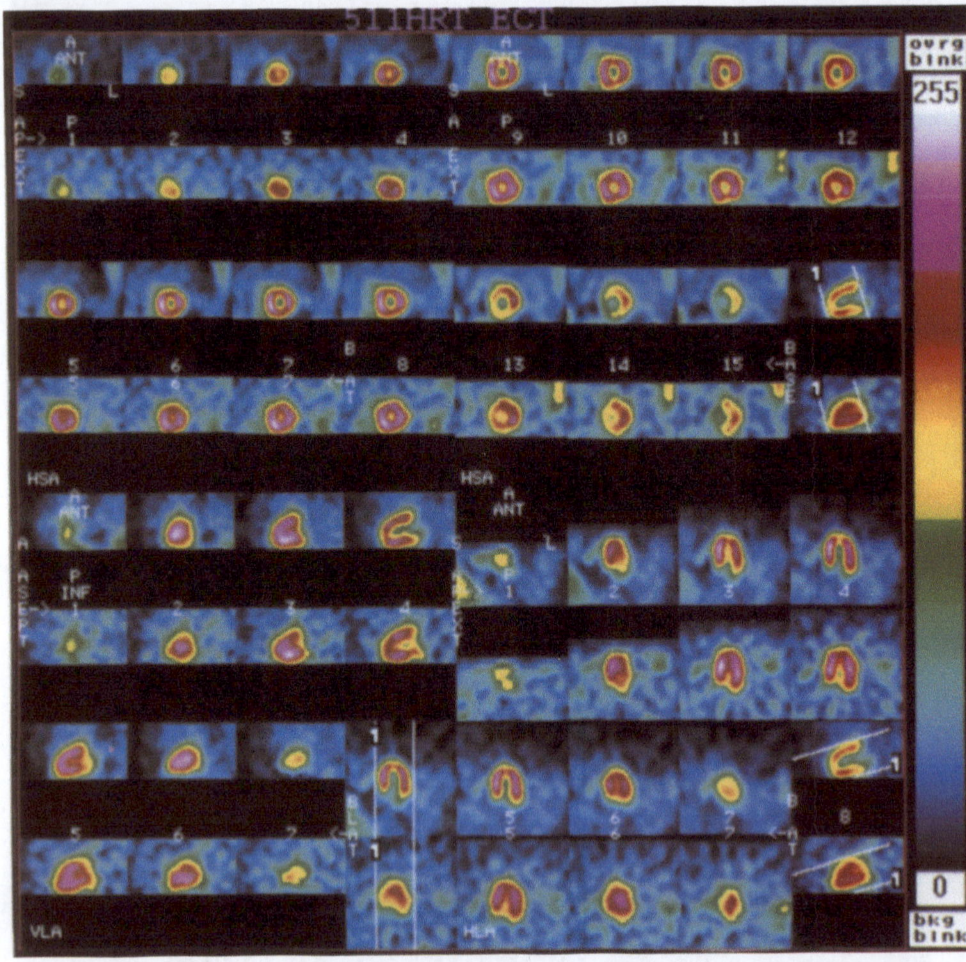

FIGURE 5.8A.

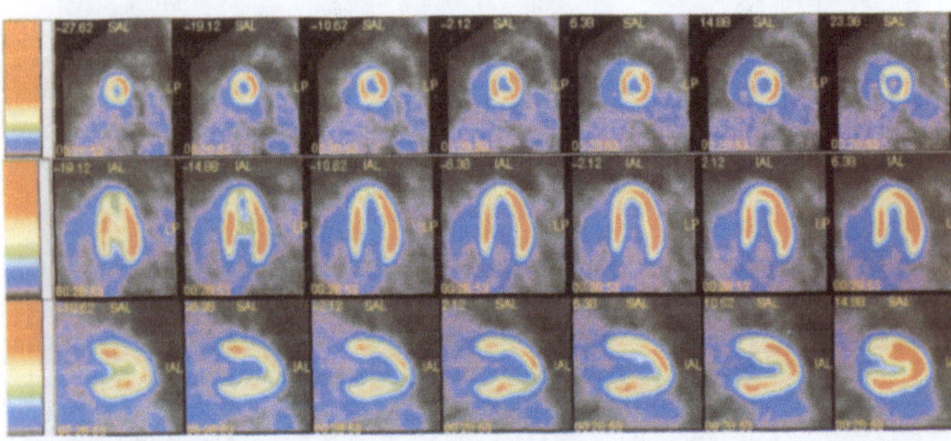

FIGURE 5.8B.

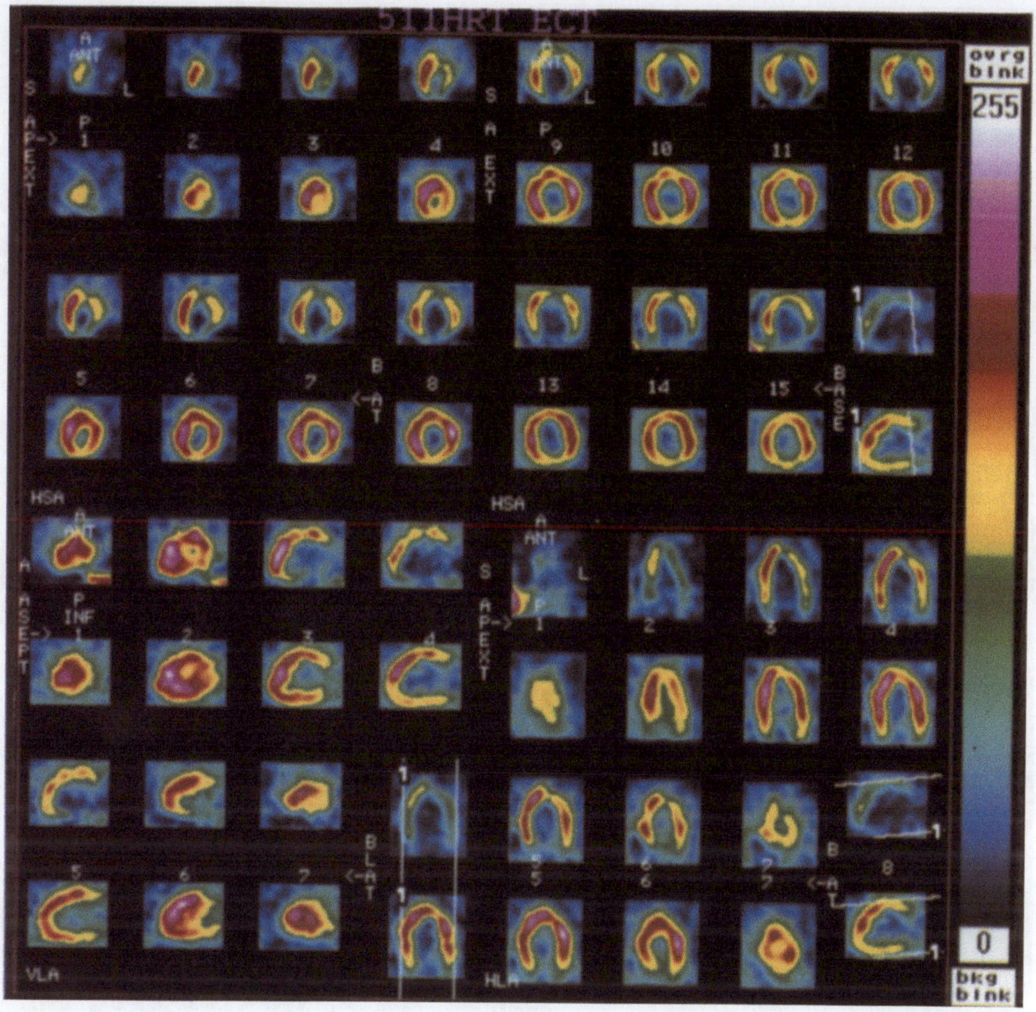

FIGURE 5.9.

COLOR PLATE VIII

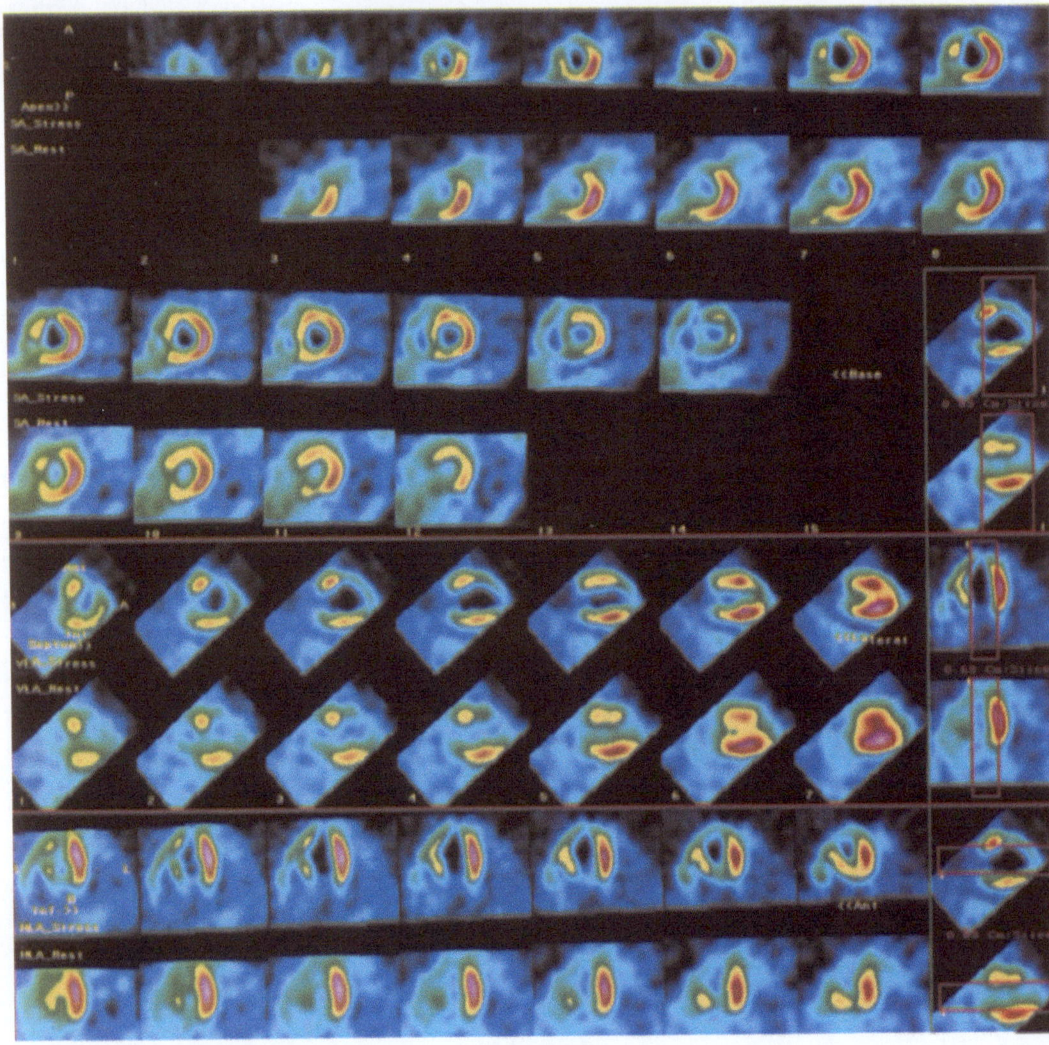

FIGURE 5.10.

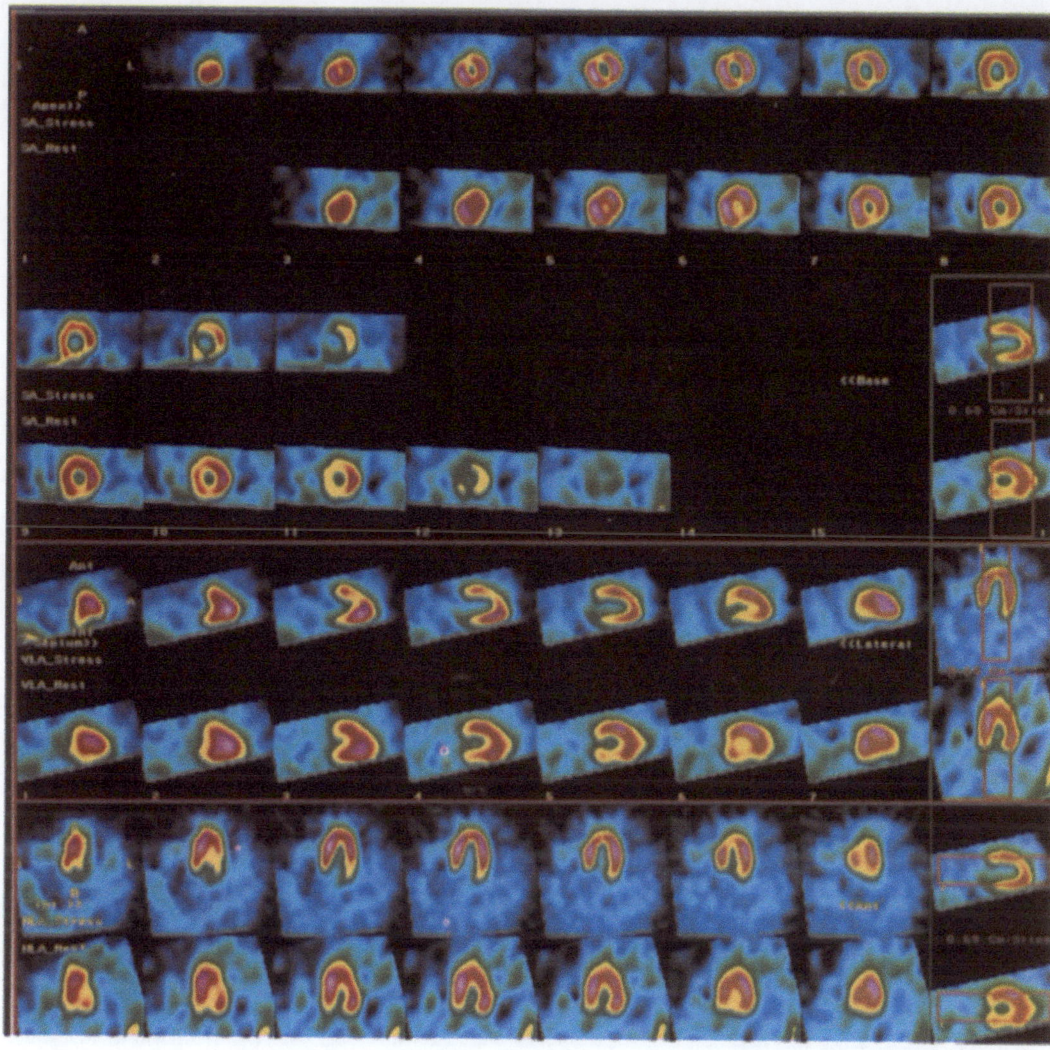

FIGURE 5.11A.

COLOR PLATE X

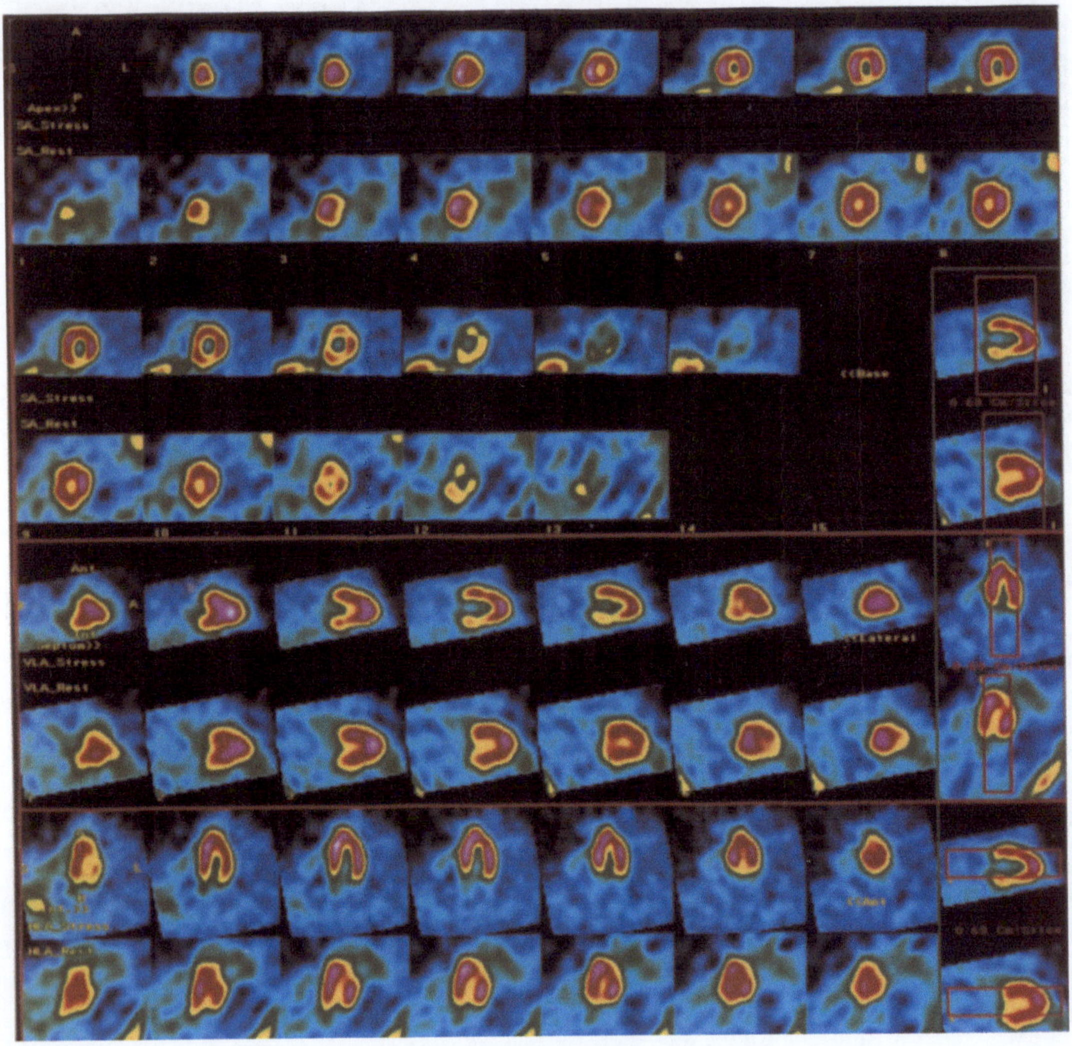

FIGURE 5.11B.

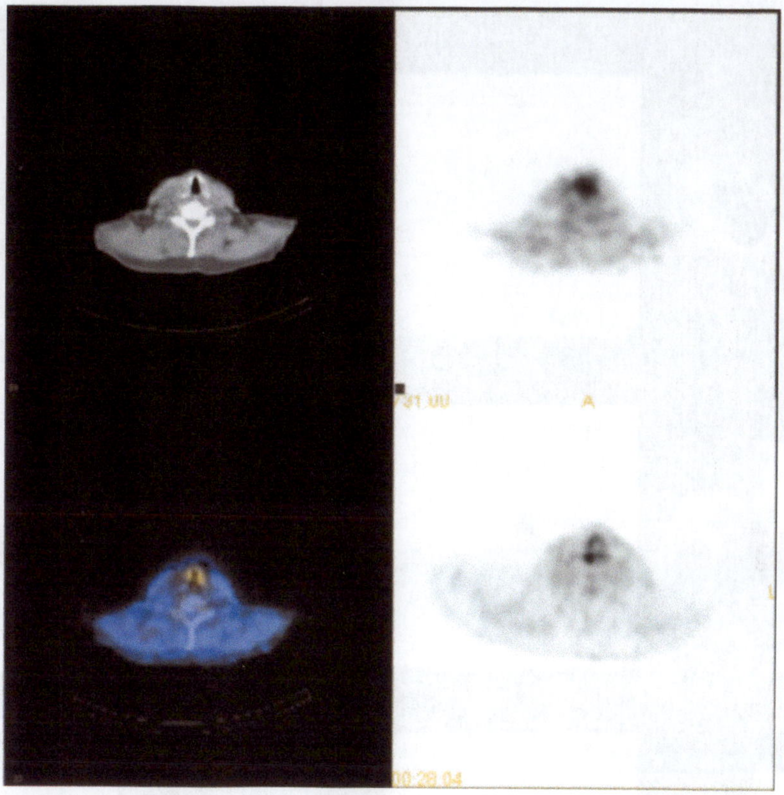

FIGURE 6.1.5C.

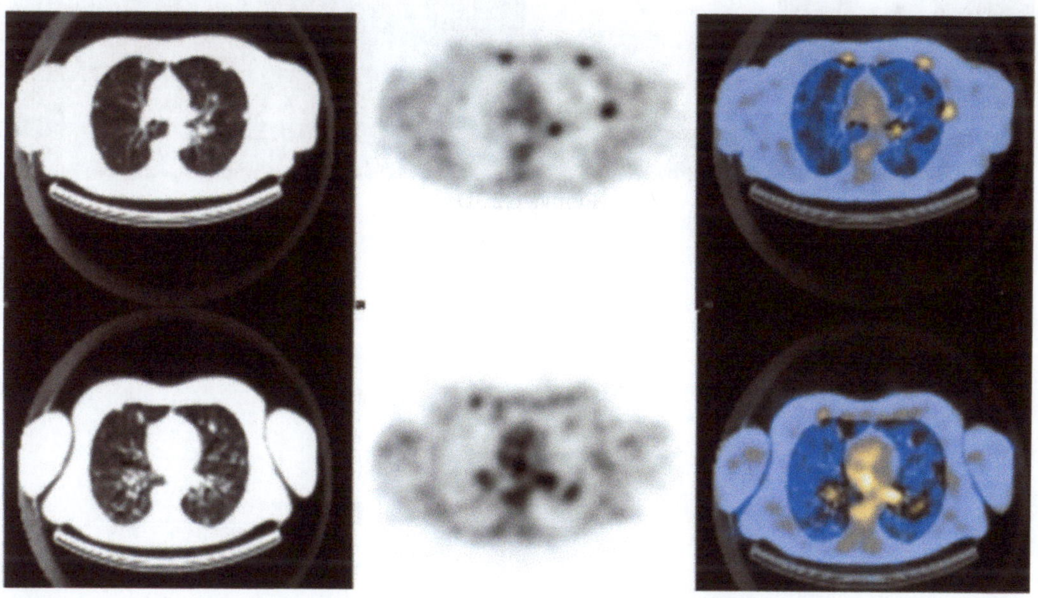

FIGURE 6.2.1C.

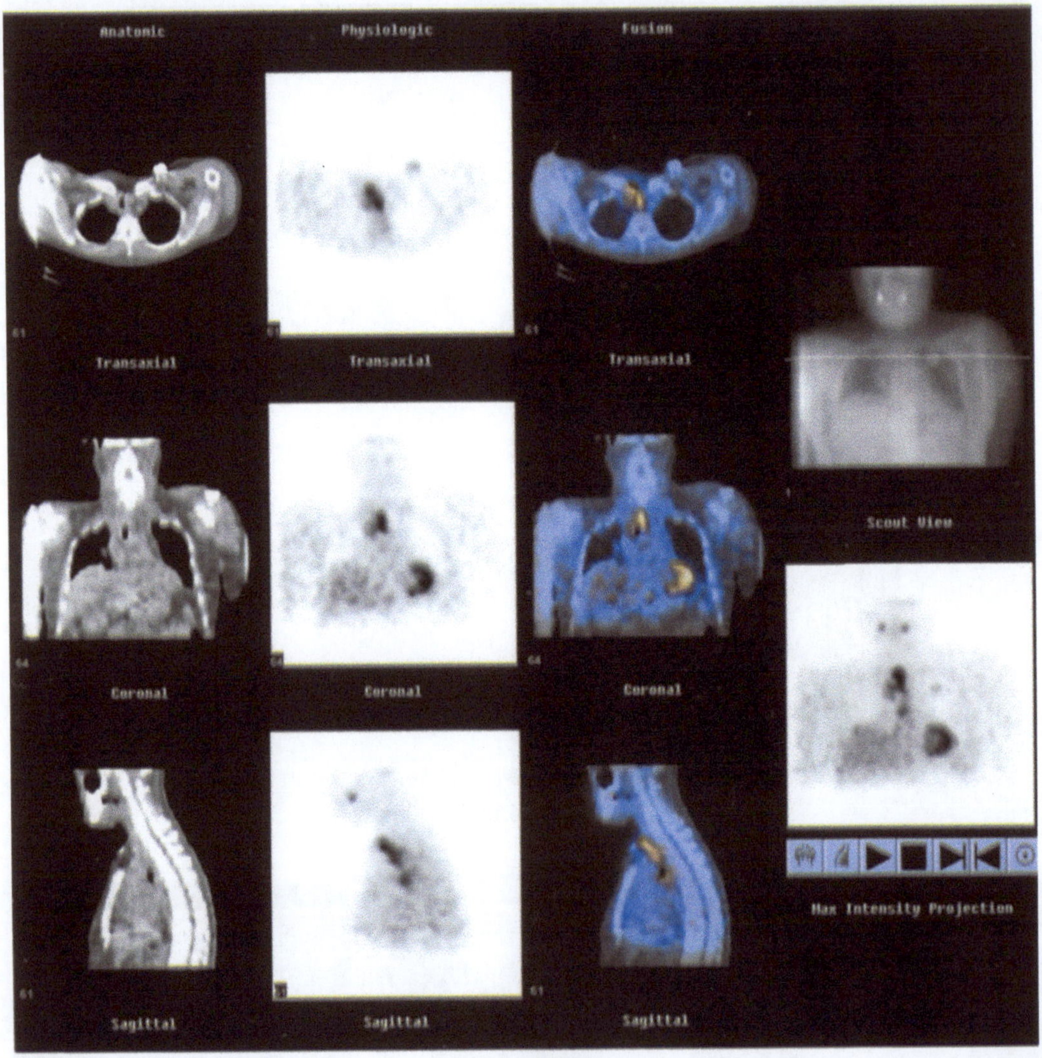
Anatomic
Physiologic
Fusion
Transaxial
Transaxial
Transaxial
Scout View
Coronal
Coronal
Coronal
Max Intensity Projection
Sagittal
Sagittal
Sagittal

FIGURE 6.2.3D.

COLOR PLATE XIII

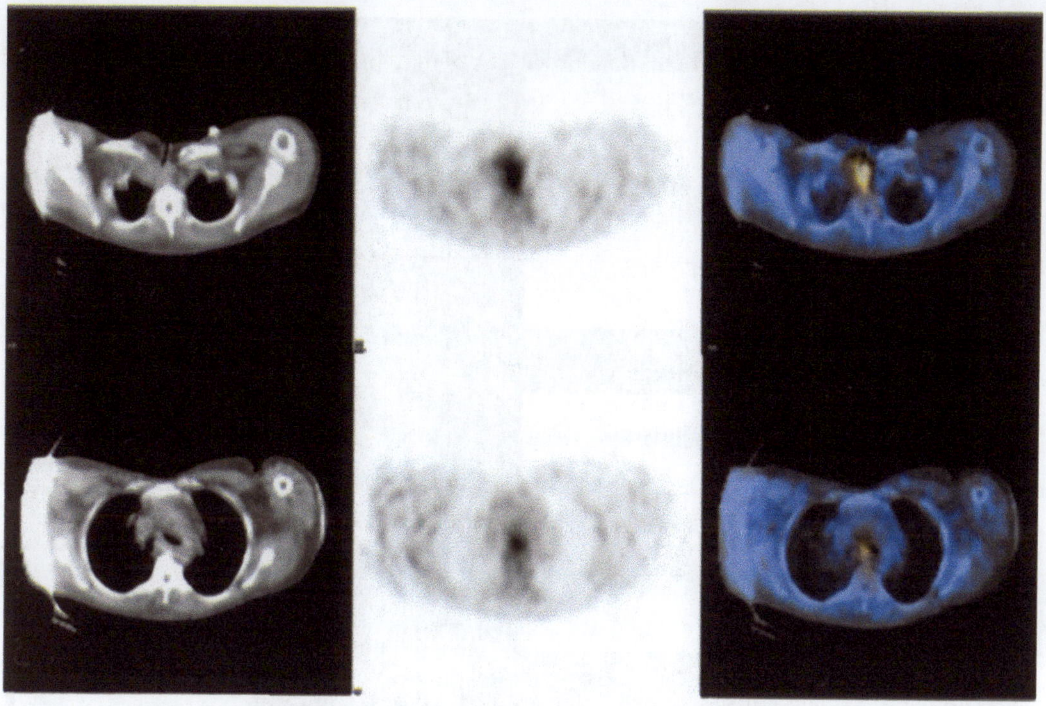

FIGURE 6.2.3E.

COLOR PLATE XIV

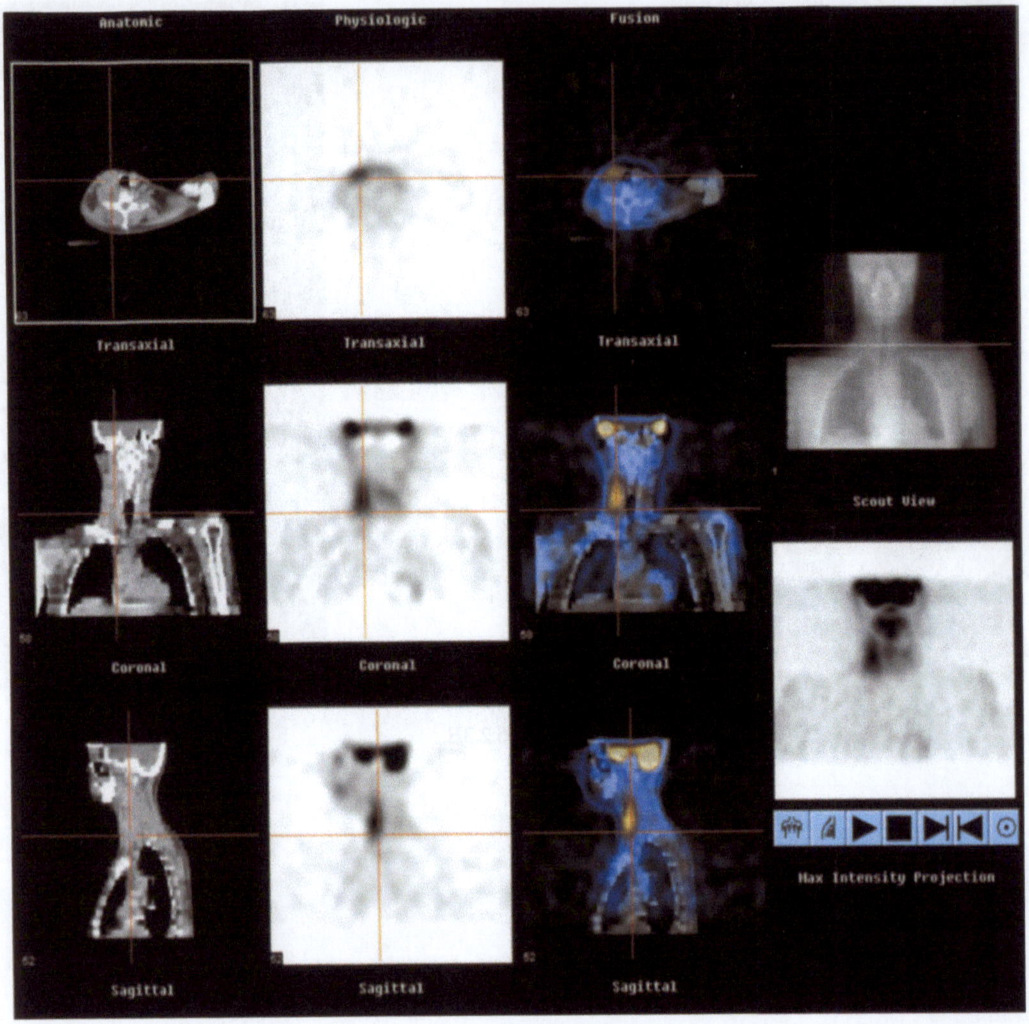

FIGURE 6.2.5C.

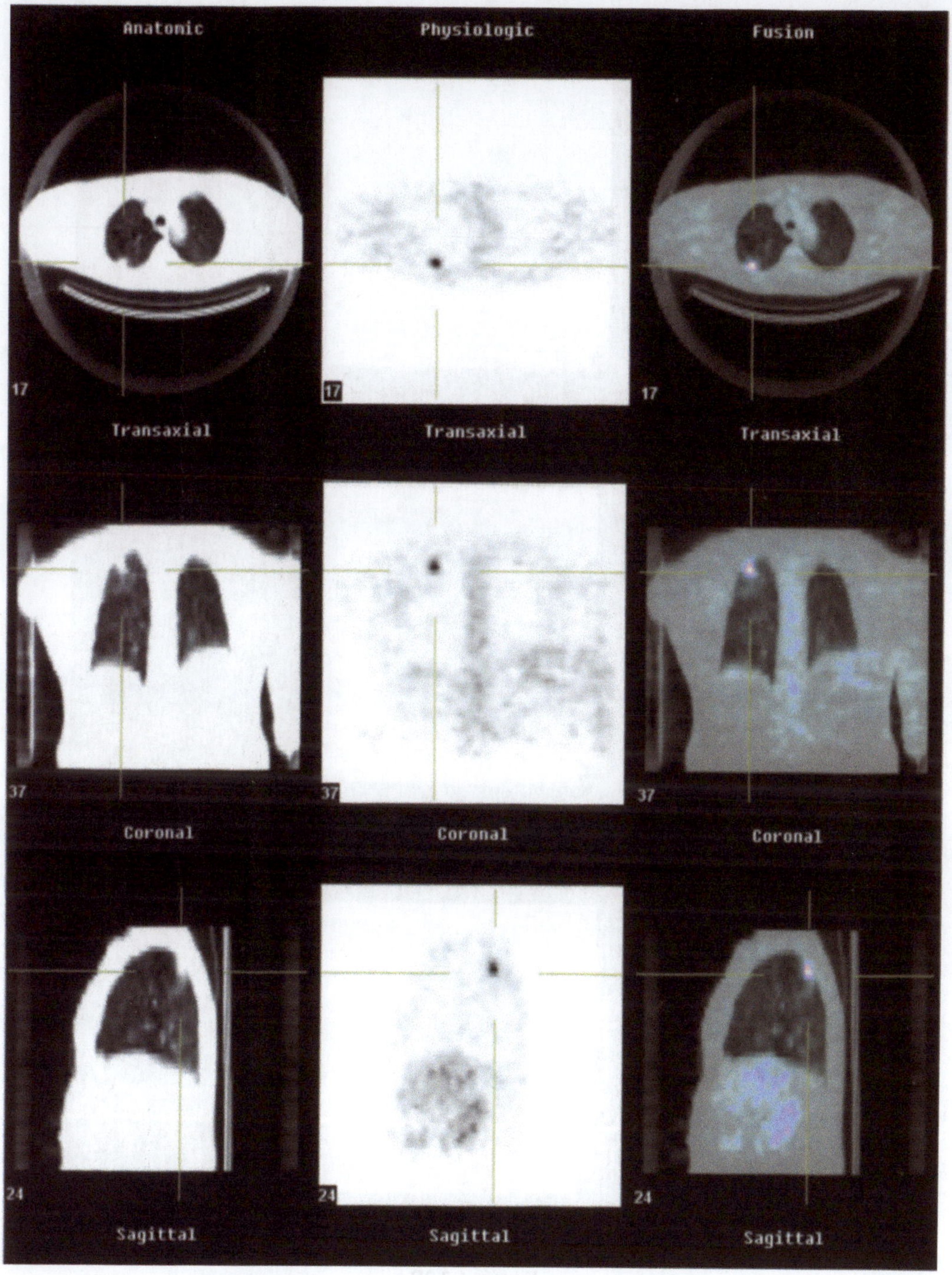
Anatomic
Physiologic
Fusion
17
17
17
Transaxial
Transaxial
Transaxial
37
37
37
Coronal
Coronal
Coronal
24
24
24
Sagittal
Sagittal
Sagittal

FIGURE 6.3.1C.

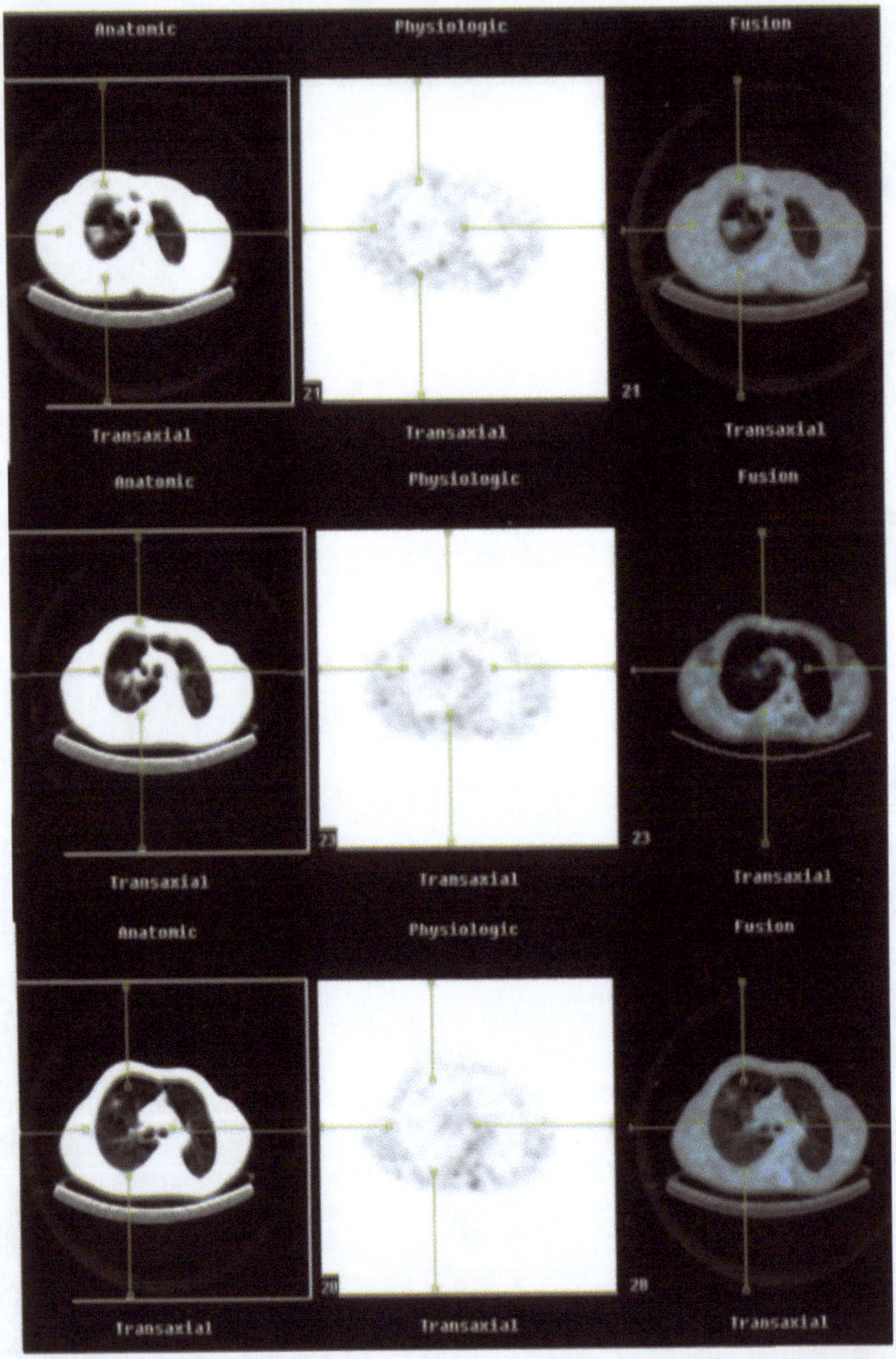
Anatomic
Physiologic
Fusion
21
21
Transaxial
Transaxial
Transaxial
Anatomic
Physiologic
Fusion
23
23
Transaxial
Transaxial
Transaxial
Anatomic
Physiologic
Fusion
20
20
Transaxial
Transaxial
Transaxial

FIGURE 6.3.2B.

COLOR PLATE XVII

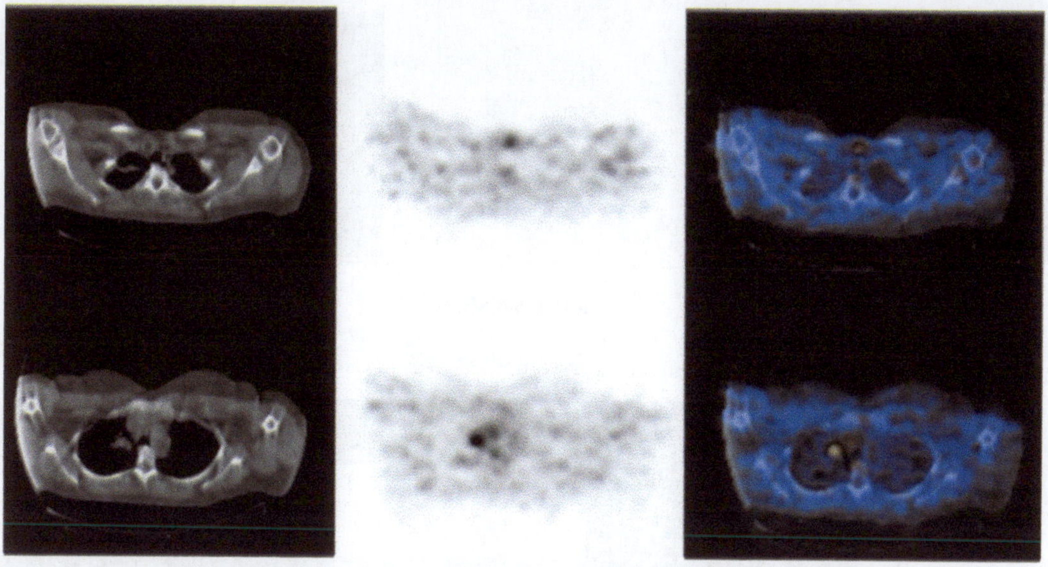

Figure 6.3.11E.

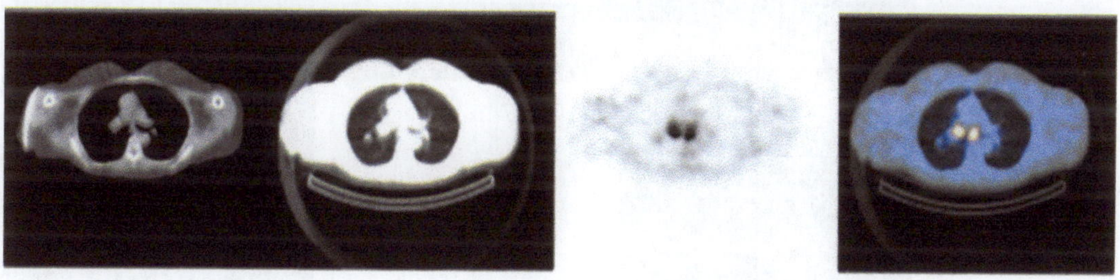

Figure 6.5.4C.

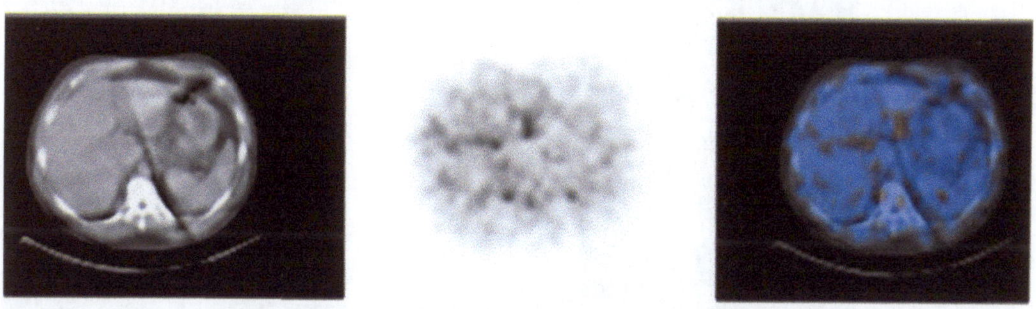

Figure 6.5.7D.

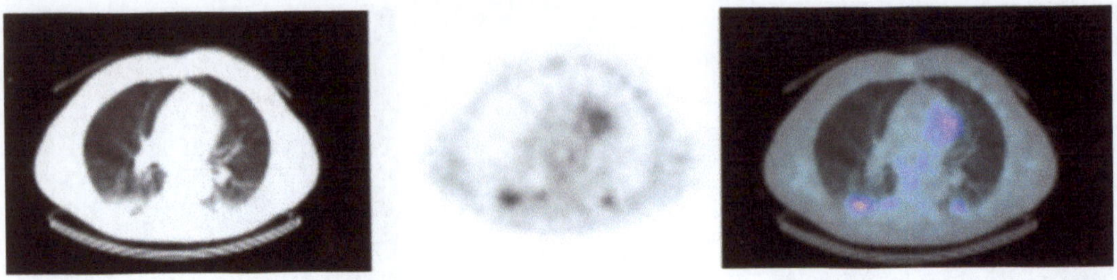

FIGURE 6.6.8B.

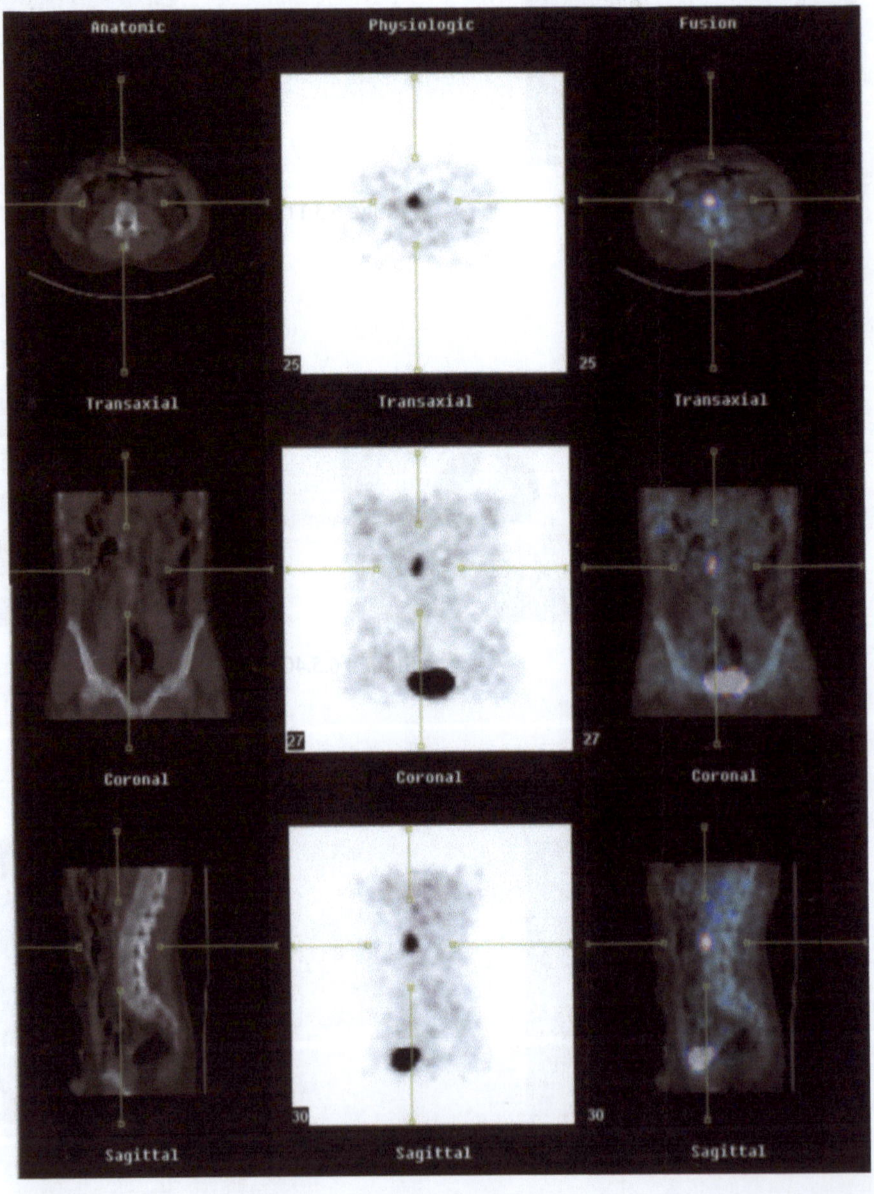

FIGURE 6.7.1B.

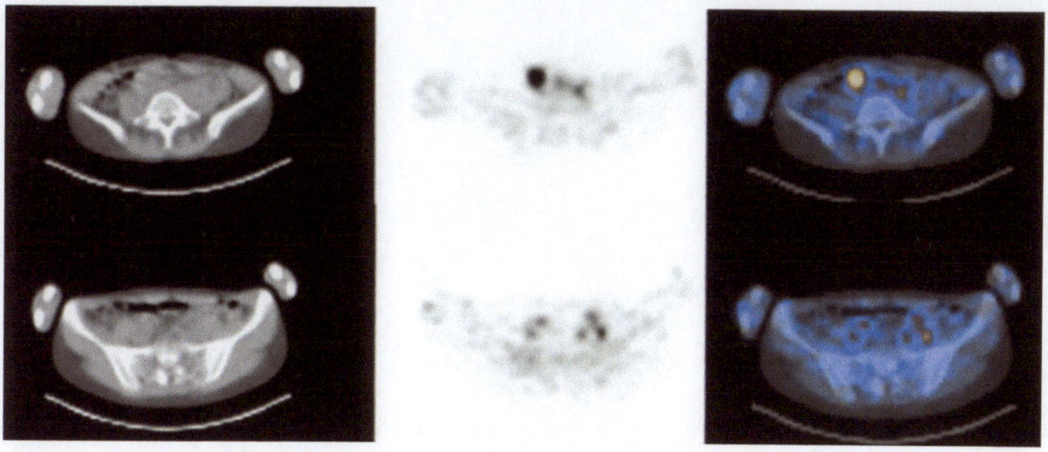

FIGURE 6.8.1B.

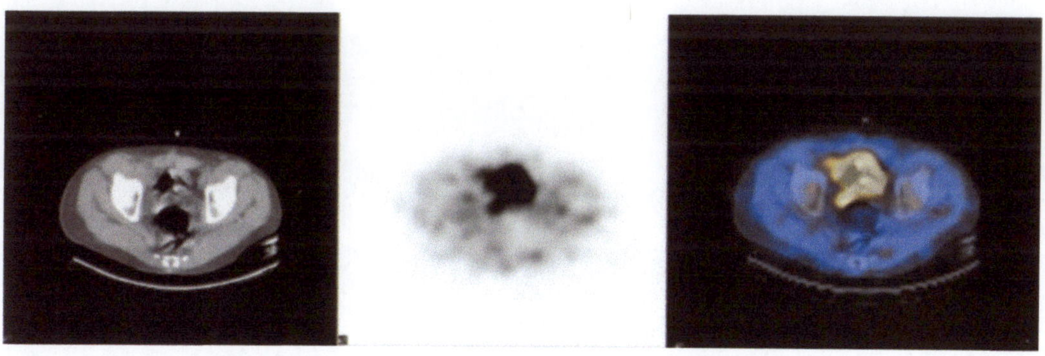

FIGURE 6.9.7C.

Assessment of Viability

FDG PET

Over the past 15 years, numerous studies have used FDG PET to evaluate tissue viability in patients with chronic coronary artery disease and severely depressed LV function. The initial work in patients was performed by the University of California at Los Angeles (UCLA) group and demonstrated the existence of matches and mismatches.[46] Subsequently, Brunken et al. demonstrated that 40% of the regions with Q-waves on the electrocardiogram (ECG) and severe wall-motion abnormalities showed persistent FDG uptake, indicating residual viability.[47] Moreover, Brunken et al. demonstrated in additional studies that FDG PET was capable of detecting residual viability in a significant proportion of fixed defects on ^{201}Tl imaging.[48]

FDG SPECT

Driven by the increased demand for FDG PET studies to assess viability, considerable effort has been invested in the development and optimization of 511 keV collimators to allow FDG imaging without a PET system. The technical details of these collimators are discussed by Van Lingen et al.[49] Following initial experience with planar imaging,[50] several centers have evaluated the use of SPECT to detect myocardial FDG uptake.[51–57] Five studies, with a total of 113 patients, have compared FDG PET with FDG SPECT, showing a good agreement between PET and SPECT (ranging from 76 to 100%) for the assessment of viable myocardium (Table 5.1).[52–56] The NIH-group studied 28 patients with chronic coronary artery disease and a mean LVEF of 33 ± 15%.[56] These patients underwent both FDG PET and FDG SPECT following oral glucose loading. Regional LV function was evaluated by radionuclide ventriculography or gated SPECT imaging. When a 50% FDG uptake threshold was used to distinguish between viable and nonviable tissue, both techniques provided comparable information in 920 of 977 segments, yielding an agreement of 94%. When the analysis was restricted to 41 akinetic segments, FDG PET and SPECT yielded concordant information in 80% of the segments (Figure 5.2). The other comparative studies also demonstrated a good agreement between both modalities. However, a comparative study between FDG PET and SPECT in patients undergoing revascularization (with recovery of function postrevascularization as an independent measurement for viability) is still lacking.

TABLE 5.1. Head-to-head comparisons between FDG PET and FDG SPECT for the evaluation of myocardial viability (113 patients, 5 studies) (data based on References 52–56.)

Study	Patients (n)	LVEF (%)	Patients with MVD (%)	Patients with previous MI (%)	Agreement (%)
Burt[52]	20	NA	NA	NA	93
Martin[53]	9	NA	NA	NA	100
Bax[54]	20	39 ± 16	83	100	76
Chen[55]	36	NA	NA	NA	90
Srinivasan[56]	28	33 ± 15	93	64	94

Note:
FDG: F18-fluorodeoxyglucose
LVEF: left ventricular ejection fraction
MI: myocardial infarction
MVD: multivessel disease
NA: not available
PET: positron emission tomography
SPECT: single photon emission computed tomography

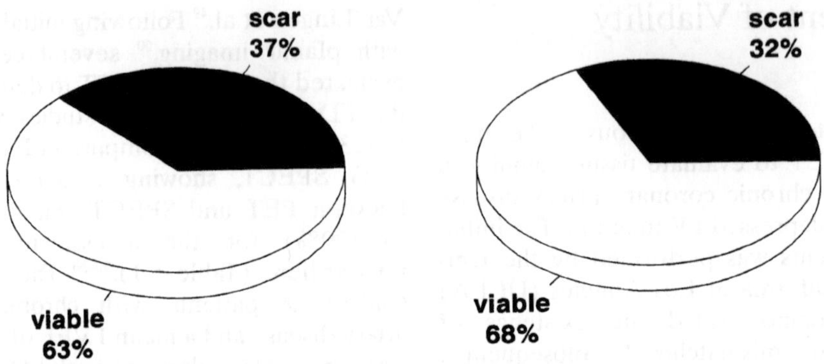

FIGURE 5.2. Agreement between FDG PET and FDG SPECT in 41 akinetic segments in 18 patients with ischemic cardiomyopathy (LVEF 33 ± 15%). Left: distribution according to FDG PET; right: distribution according to FDG SPECT. (Data based on Reference 56.)

Outcome after Revascularization: Improvement of Regional LV Function

FDG PET

Many studies have employed FDG PET to evaluate tissue viability and predict improvement of function after revascularization. This first study, by the UCLA group, involved 17 patients with a depressed LVEF (32 ± 14%) who were scheduled for surgical revascularization.[26] Perfusion was assessed by ^{13}N-ammonia PET, and FDG PET was performed following oral glucose loading. Regional LV function was evaluated before revascularization and three months after revascularization, and 37 segments improved in function postrevascularization, with 35 being classified as viable on PET. Conversely, 30 segments did not improve in function, with 24 classified as nonviable by PET. Thus, the sensitivity and specificity to predict improvement of regional LV function postrevascularization were 95% and 80%, respectively. Recently, the results of 12 FDG PET studies (with a total of 322 patients) were pooled to determine the value of FDG PET for the prediction of improvement of regional LV function following revascularization.[17] Pooling of the results yielded a sensitivity of 88% with a specificity of 73% and a negative predictive value of 86% with a positive predictive value of 76%.

Although it is interesting to pool these studies to provide an estimation of the diagnostic accuracy of FDG PET to predict improvement of function, these data should be interpreted with caution; some shortcomings are summarized in Table 5.2. These observations emphasize the need for standardization of metabolic conditions, protocols, and viability criteria of FDG PET studies to assess myocardial viability.

TABLE 5.2. Limitations of pooling FDG PET studies to predict improvement of regional LV function postrevascularization.

1. Variation in patient characteristics between studies
2. Substantial variation in metabolic conditions among studies
3. Different protocols: FDG alone and FDG-perfusion with different perfusion agents
4. Viability criteria not uniform
5. Differences in data-analyses

Note:
FDG: F18-fluorodeoxyglucose
LV: left ventricular
PET: positron emission tomography

FDG SPECT

The available evidence in the literature on FDG SPECT for prediction of improvement of regional LV function is less extensive than that for PET. One study evaluated 55 patients with severe coronary artery disease and depressed LV function (LVEF 39 ± 14%) with FDG SPECT prior to revascularization.[58] Data were acquired sequentially: ^{201}Tl SPECT was used to assess resting perfusion, and FDG SPECT was performed during hyperinsulinemic euglycemic clamping. Echocardiography was performed before and three months after revascularization to assess regional wall motion. Of the 281 segments with abnormal contraction, improved function occurred in 94 segments, with 80 being viable on FDG SPECT. Conversely, 187 segments did not improve in function, and 141 of these were classified nonviable by FDG SPECT. Accordingly, the sensitivity and specificity to predict improvement of regional LV function postrevascularization were 85% and 75%, which is virtually identical to the pooled data for FDG PET imaging.

Outcome after Revascularization: Improvement of Global LV Function

FDG PET

Improvement of LVEF is clinically more relevant than improvement of individual segments, since LVEF is an important prognostic parameter of survival. It is likely that the improvement of LVEF translates to improvement of heart failure symptoms, exercise capacity, and survival. In the study by Tillisch et al., global LVEF was evaluated before and three months after revascularization.[26] The authors demonstrated that a significant improvement in LVEF occurred (from 30 ± 11% to 45 ± 14%) in patients with a substantial volume of viable myocardium as defined by FDG PET. Currently, 11 studies have evaluated LVEF before and after revascularization and related the findings to the FDG PET data[7] (Figure 5.3). In 10 of 11 studies, the average LVEF improved significantly in patients with viable tissue on FDG PET, ranging from 7 to 18% absolute increase in LVEF. In the patients without viable tissue (included in seven FDG PET studies), however, the LVEF did not increase significantly, ranging from 4% absolute increase to 12% absolute decrease in LVEF. Moreover, data from the Hammersmith group in the United Kingdom have shown that a linear relation existed between the extent of viable myocardium and the absolute change in LVEF.[59]

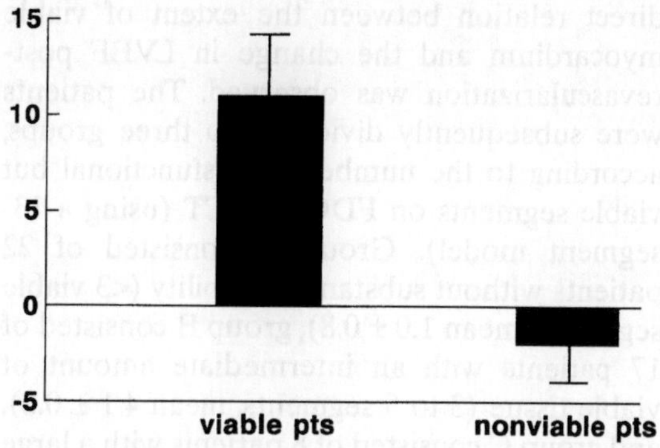

FIGURE 5.3. Average changes in LVEF following revascularization in FDG PET studies. Eleven studies included patients with viable myocardium (n = 322), and seven of these studies also included patients with nonviable myocardium (n = 205) (defined according to FDG PET results). In patients with viable myocardium, the average LVEF increased 11 ± 4%, whereas the average LVEF decreased 2 ± 2% in patients with nonviable myocardium. (Data based on Reference 7.)

FDG SPECT

Prediction of improvement of global LV function has also been evaluated using FDG SPECT. Forty-seven patients with ischemic cardiomyopathy (LVEF 30 ± 6%) were studied with the sequential SPECT protocol prior to surgical revascularization.[60] Most of these patients presented with heart failure symptoms instead of angina pectoris. LVEF was assessed before and three to six months after revascularization by radionuclide ventriculography. A direct relation between the extent of viable myocardium and the change in LVEF post-revascularization was observed. The patients were subsequently divided into three groups, according to the number of dysfunctional but viable segments on FDG SPECT (using a 13-segment model). Group A consisted of 22 patients without substantial viability (<3 viable segments, mean 1.0 ± 0.8), group B consisted of 17 patients with an intermediate amount of viable tissue (3 to 5 segments, mean 4.1 ± 0.8), and group C consisted of 8 patients with a large amount of viable tissue (>5 segments, mean 7.4 ± 1.4). The largest increase in LVEF was observed in group C (from 30 ± 5% to 44 ± 10%, P = 0.001); seven of eight (88%) patients showed a significant increase in LVEF (mean increase 16 ± 6%). Patients in group B showed a moderate increase in LVEF (28 ± 7% to 32 ± 9%, P = 0.002), while patients in group A did not show improvement in LVEF.

Outcome after Revascularization: Improvement of Symptoms

FDG PET

Few studies have focused on prediction of improvement of symptoms. Both DiCarli et al.[61] and Eitzman et al.[62] demonstrated a significant improvement of heart failure symptoms following revascularization, which was most evident in patients with viable tissue on FDG PET. In these studies, heart failure symptoms were scored according the New York Heart Association (NYHA) classification, which is a rather subjective measurement; still, it is the most frequently used measurement in the clinical setting. Two additional studies have focused on prediction of improvement of exercise capacity.[63,64] Marwick et al. evaluated 23 patients with FDG PET, prior to revascularization.[63] The results indicated that patients with two or more viable segments (>29% of the LV) experienced a significant improvement in peak rate-pressure product, percentage of maximal heart rate, and an improvement in exercise capacity (from 5.6 ± 2.7 to 7.5 ± 1.7 METS [metabolic equivalents]). Similarly, DiCarli et al. showed a direct relation between the preoperative amount of viable tissue and the improvement in exercise capacity (expressed in METS) postrevascularization.[64]

FDG SPECT

The change in heart failure symptoms in relation to preoperative viability was assessed in the same 47 patients, as described in the previously.[60] Using FDG SPECT, the patients were divided into three groups. Group A included patients without substantial viability, group B included patients with an intermediate extent of viable tissue, and group C comprised patients with a large amount of viable myocardium. Heart failure symptoms were graded before and three months after revascularization using the NYHA classification. The average NYHA score before revascularization was comparable among the three groups. The largest improvement in NYHA score was again observed in group C (from 3.4 ± 0.5 to 1.7 ± 0.8, P = 0.001). Patients in group B showed slightly less improvement in NYHA score (from 3.3 ± 0.5 to 2.2 ± 1.0, P = 0.003). Patients in group A showed no improvement in symptoms (3.1 ± 0.5 versus 2.9 ± 0.8, ns) (Figure 5.4).

Long-Term Prognosis

FDG PET

It has been hypothesized that the presence of viable tissue protects the patients from perioperative events, and the postoperative improvement of LV function, symptoms, and exercise capacity may translate into improvement of long-term survival. Several studies provide evidence for these hypotheses. It should be emphasized, however, that these are all retrospective and nonrandomized studies, and a prospective randomized study is needed to draw definitive conclusions. The first issue, assessment of risk perioperatively, was addressed by

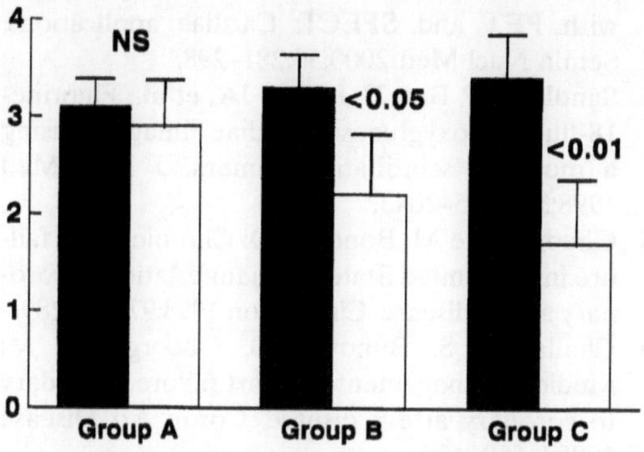

FIGURE 5.4. Changes in New York Heart Association score after revascularization in the three groups with different degrees of viability. The largest improvement in NYHA score was observed in Group C, slightly less improvement was observed in Group B, and no improvement was observed in Group A. (Based on data from Reference 60.) NS = not significant.

Haas et al.[18] The authors analyzed 76 patients with chronic coronary artery disease and depressed LV function; 35 patients underwent surgical revascularization on the basis of clinical presentation and results of coronary angiography only. Another 41 patients underwent preoperative FDG PET, and patients were referred to surgical revascularization on the basis of the extent of viable tissue on FDG PET, in addition to the clinical and angiographic data. Small areas of viable tissue and large areas of scar tissue were deciding factors against surgery. Accordingly, seven patients were treated medically or underwent heart transplantation, and 34 were revascularized. In the patients who did not undergo FDG PET, a higher perioperative event rate was observed, accompanied by a higher short-term (30 days) and long-term (12 months) mortality. The patients who did undergo FDG PET needed catecholamine support less frequently and had a significantly higher rate of uncomplicated recovery. Five studies specifically addressed the long-term prognostic value of FDG PET.[61,62,65–67] In these studies, a total of 549 patients were included. The patients were grouped according to treatment (revascularization/medical) and viability status (absent/present). The mean follow-up varied from 12 to 29 months. All studies included hard events (for example, death and infarction), and four studies also considered soft events (for example, late revascularization and unstable angina pectoris). Pooling from the results showed that the highest event-rate (42%) was observed in the "viable patients" who were treated medically. In contrast, the lowest event-rate (9%) was observed in the "viable patients" who underwent revascularization. The other groups also had relatively low event-rates. These results suggest that residual viability in patients with chronic coronary artery disease and depressed LV function is an unstable set prone to future events. Following this hypothesis, timely revascularization may be favored. There are currently two reports that have demonstrated the benefit of timely revascularization in patients with viable myocardium on FDG PET.[68,69] Beanlands et al. evaluated 35 patients with chronic coronary artery disease and depressed LVEF. Eighteen patients underwent early revascularization (<12 ± 9 days), and 17 patients underwent late revascularization (145 ± 97 days).[68] In the "early group," the preoperative mortality rate was lower, more patients improved in LVEF postoperatively, and the event-free survival was higher. Similar findings were observed by Schwarz et al.[69]

FDG SPECT

To date, no prognostic FDG SPECT studies have been published, but two centers have reported preliminary data on this topic. In a large cohort of 135 patients with depressed LV function undergoing FDG SPECT and a follow-up of 28 ± 11 months, Bax et al.[70] demonstrated that the event-rate was highest (60%) in the patients with viable myocardium treated medically, and the lowest event-rate (4%) was observed in the patients with viable myocardium undergoing revascularization. Intermediate event-rates were observed in the patients with nonviable myocardium who were revascularized (16%) or treated medically (9%). Similar findings have been reported by Wijffels et al.[71] These data are very similar to the aforementioned FDG PET data.

Summary

FDG imaging with either PET or SPECT allows accurate assessment of myocardial viability in patients with ischemic cardiomyopathy. This is currently the only clinical indication for cardiac FDG imaging. Over the past 15 years, FDG PET (and more recently FDG SPECT) has been proven to be a very powerful tool in the prediction of recovery of (regional and global) LV function postrevascularization. In addition, viability as detected by FDG imaging is predictive of improvement in heart failure symptoms and exercise capacity. The patients with viable myocardium have fewer complications during coronary bypass surgery and have excellent long-term survival. In contrast, the patients with viable myocardium who are treated medically experience an extremely high event-rate. These data confirm the role of FDG imaging in the diagnostic and prognostic workup of patients with ischemic cardiomyopathy.

References

1. Grover-McKay M, Schwaiger M, Krivokapich J, et al.: Regional myocardial blood flow and metabolism at rest in mildly symptomatic patients with hypertrophic cardiomyopathy. J Am Coll Cardiol 1989;13:317–324.
2. Camici P, Araujo L, Spinks T, et al.: Increased uptake of 18-F-fluorodeoxyglucose in postischemic myocardium of patients with exercise-induced angina. Circulation 1986;74:81–88.
3. Schwaiger M, Brunken R, Grover-McKay M, et al.: Regional myocardial metabolism in patients with acute myocardial infarction assessed by positron emission tomography. J Am Coll Cardiol 1986;8:800–808.
4. Camici PG: PET and myocardial imaging. Heart 2000;83:475–480.
5. Schelbert HR: Measurements of myocardial metabolism in patients with ischemic heart disease. Am J Cardiol 1998;82:61K–67K.
6. Bax JJ, Patton JA, Poldermans D, Elhendy A, Sandler MP: 18-Fluorodeoxyglucose imaging with PET and SPECT: Cardiac applications. Semin Nucl Med 2000;30:281–298.
7. Sandler MP, Bax JJ, Patton JA, et al.: Fluorine-18-fluorodeoxyglucose cardiac imaging using a modified scintillation camera. J Nucl Med 1998;39:2035–2043.
8. Gheorghiade M, Bonow RO: Chronic heart failure in the United States. A manifestation of coronary artery disease. Circulation 1998;97:282–289.
9. Challapalli S, Bonow RO, Gheorghiade M: Medical management of heart failure secondary to coronary artery disease. Coron Art Disease 1998;9:659–674.
10. Evans RW, Manninen DL, Garrison LP, et al.: Donor availability as the primary determinant of the future of heart transplantation. JAMA 1986; 255:1892–1898.
11. Baker DW, Jones R, Hodges J, et al.: Management of heart failure. III. The role of revascularization in treatment of patients with moderate or severe left ventricular systolic dysfunction. JAMA 1994;272:1528–1534.
12. Bax JJ, Poldermans D, Elhendy A, et al.: Improvement of left ventricular ejection fraction, heart failure symptoms and prognosis after revascularization in patients with chronic coronary artery disease and viable myocardium detected by dobutamine stress echocardiography. J Am Coll Cardiol 1999;34:163–169.
13. Wijns W, Vatner SF, Camici PG: Hibernating myocardium. N Engl J Med 1998;339:173–181.
14. Beller GA: Noninvasive assessment of myocardial viability. N Engl J Med 2000;343:1488–1490.
15. Dilsizian V, Bonow RO: Current diagnostic techniques of assessing viability in patients with hibernating and stunned myocardium. Circulation 1993;87:1–20.
16. Marwick TH: The viable myocardium. Epidemiology, detection, and clinical implications. Lancet 1998;351:815–819.
17. Bax JJ, Wijns W, Cornel JH, et al.: Accuracy of currently available techniques for prediction of functional recovery after revascularization in patients with left ventricular dysfunction due to chronic coronary artery disease: Comparison of pooled data. J Am Coll Cardiol 1997;30:1451–1460.
18. Haas F, Haehnel CJ, Picker W, et al.: Preoperative positron emission tomographic viability assessment and perioperative and postoperative risk in patients with advanced ischemic heart disease. J Am Coll Cardiol 1997;30:1693–1700.
19. Bax JJ, Wijns W: FDG imaging to assess myocardial viability: PET, SPECT or gamma camera

coincidence imaging? J Nucl Med 1999;40:1893–1895.
20. Auerbach MA, Schoder H, Gambhir SS, et al.: Prevalence of myocardial viability as detected by positron emission tomography in patients with ischemic cardiomyopathy. Circulation 1999;99: 2921–2926.
21. Schinkel AFL, Bax JJ, Sozzi FB, et al.: Prevalence of myocardial viability assessed by SPECT in patients with chronic ischemic left ventricular dysfunction. J Nucl Cardiol 2001 [Abstract, in press].
22. Gropler RJ: Methodology governing the assessment of myocardial glucose metabolism by positron emission tomography and fluorine 18-labeled fluorodeoxyglucose. J Nucl Cardiol 1994;1:S1–S14.
23. Baer FM, Voth E, Deutsch HJ, et al.: Predictive value of low dose dobutamine transesophageal echocardiography and fluorine-18 fluorodeoxyglucose PET for recovery of regional left ventricular function after successful revascularization. J Am Coll Cardiol 1996;28:60–69.
24. Pagano D, Bonser RS, Townend JN, Ordoubadi F, Lorenzoni R, Camici PG: Predictive value of dobutamine echocardiography and positron emission tomography in identifying hibernating myocardium in patients with postischaemic heart failure. Heart 1998;79:281–288.
25. Rahimtoola SH: Hibernating myocardium has reduced blood flow at rest that increases with low-dose dobutamine. Circulation 1996;94:3055–3061.
26. Tillisch J, Brunken R, Marshall R, et al.: Reversibility of cardiac wall-motion abnormalities predicted by positron tomography. N Engl J Med 1986;314:884–888.
27. Marwick TH, MacIntyre WJ, Lafont A, et al.: Metabolic responses of hibernating and infarcted myocardium to revascularization. Circulation 1992;85:1347–1353.
28. Gropler RJ, Geltman EM, Sampathkumaran K, et al.: Comparison of carbon-11-acetate with fluorine-18-fluorodeoxyglucose for delineating viable myocardium by positron emission tomography. J Am Coll Cardiol 1993;22:1587–1597.
29. Knuuti MJ, Saraste M, Nuutila P, et al.: Myocardial viability: Fluorine-18-deoxyglucose PET in prediction of wall motion recovery after revascularization. Am Heart J 1994;127:785–796.
30. Depr C, Vanoverschelde JLJ, Melin JA, et al.: Structural and metabolic correlates of the reversibility of chronic left ventricular ischemic dysfunction in humans. Am J Physiol 1995;268: H1265–H1275.
31. Tamaki N, Kawamoto M, Tadamura E, et al.: Prediction of reversible ischemia after revascularization. Perfusion and metabolic studies with positron emission tomography. Circulation 1995; 91:1697–1705.
32. Vom Dahl J, Altehoefer C, Sheehan FH, et al.: Recovery of regional left ventricular dysfunction after coronary revascularization. Impact of myocardial viability assessed by nuclear imaging and vessel patency at follow-up angiography. J Am Coll Cardiol 1996;28:948–958.
33. Gerber BL, Vanoverschelde J-LJ, Bol A, et al.: Myocardial blood flow, glucose uptake and recruitment of inotropic reserve in chronic left ventricular ischemic dysfunction. Implications for the pathophysiology of chronic hibernation. Circulation 1996;94:651–659.
34. Maes AF, Borgers M, Flameng W, et al.: Assessment of myocardial viability in chronic coronary artery disease using technetium-99m sestamibi SPECT. Correlation with histologic and positron emission tomographic studies and functional follow-up. J Am Coll Cardiol 1997;29:62–68.
35. Vanoverschelde JLJ, Wijns W, Depre C, et al.: Mechanisms of chronic regional postischemic dysfunction in humans. New insights from the study of noninfarcted collateral-dependent myocardium. Circulation 1993;87:1513–1523.
36. Bax JJ, Visser FC, Elhendy A, et al.: Prediction of improvement of regional left ventricular function after revascularization using different perfusion-metabolism criteria. J Nucl Med 1999;40: 1866–1873.
37. Knuuti MJ, Nuutila P, Ruotsalainen U, et al.: The value of quantitative analysis of glucose utilization in detection of myocardial viability by PET. J Nucl Med 1993;34:2068–2075.
38. Fath-Ordoubadi F, Pagano D, Marinho NVS, Keogh BE, Bonser RS, Camici PG: Coronary revascularization in the treatment of moderate and severe postischemic left ventricular dysfunction. Am J Cardiol 1998;82:26–31.
39. Camici P, Ferrannini E, Opie LH: Myocardial metabolism in ischemic heart disease: Basic principles and application to imaging by positron emission tomography. Prog Cardiovasc Dis 1989;32:217–238.
40. Knuuti J, Nuutila P, Ruotsalainen U, et al.: Euglycemic hyperinsulinemic clamp and oral glucose load in stimulating myocardial glucose utilization during positron emission tomography. J Nucl Med 1992;33:1255–1262.

41. Vom Dahl J, Hermann WH, Hicks RJ, et al.: Myocardial glucose uptake in patients with insulin-dependent diabetes mellitus assessed by positron emission tomography. Circulation 1993; 88:395–404.
42. Martin WH, Jones RC, Delbeke D, et al.: A simplified intravenous glucose loading protocol for fluorine-18 fluorodeoxyglucose cardiac single-photon emission tomography. Eur J Nucl Med 1997;24:1291–1297.
43. Knuuti MJ, Yki-J, Rvinen H, Voipio-Pulkki LM, et al.: Enhancement of myocardial [fluorine-18] fluorodeoxyglucose uptake by a nicotinic acid derivative. J Nucl Med 1994;35:989–998.
44. Musatti L, Maggi E, Moro E, et al.: Bioavailability and pharmacokinetics of acipimox, a new antilipolytic and hypolipidaemic agent. J Int Med Res 1981;9:381–386.
45. Bax JJ, Veening MA, Visser FC, et al.: Optimal metabolic conditions during fluorine-18 fluorodeoxyglucose imaging: A comparative study using different protocols. Eur J Nucl Med 1997;24:35–41.
46. Marshall RC, Tillisch JH, Phelps ME, et al.: Identification and differentiation of resting myocardial ischemia and infarction in man with positron computed tomography, 18F-labeled fluorodeoxyglucose and N-13 ammonia. Circulation 1983;67:766–778.
47. Brunken R, Tillisch J, Schwaiger M, et al.: Regional perfusion, glucose metabolism, and wall motion in patients with chronic electrocardiographic Q wave infarctions: Evidence for persistence of viable tissue in some infarct regions by positron emission tomography. Circulation 1986;73;5:951–963.
48. Brunken R, Schwaiger M, Grover-McKay M, et al.: Positron emission tomography detects tissue metabolic activity in myocardial segments with persistent thallium perfusion defects. J Am Coll Cardiol 1987;10:557–567.
49. Van Lingen A, Huijgens PC, Visser FC, et al.: Performance characteristics of a 511-keV collimator for imaging positron emitters with a standard gamma-camera. Eur J Nucl Med 1992;19: 315–321.
50. Huitink JM, Visser FC, Bax JJ, et al.: Predictive value of planar 18F-fluorodeoxyglucose imaging for cardiac events in patients after acute myocardial infarction. Am J Cardiol 1998;81:1072–1077.
51. Stoll HP, Helwig N, Alexander C, et al.: Myocardial metabolic imaging by means of fluorine-18 deoxyglucose/technetium-99m sestamibi dual-isotope single-photon emission tomography. Eur J Nucl Med 994;21:1085–1093.
52. Burt RW, Perkins OW, Oppenheim BE, et al.: Direct comparison of fluorine-18-FDG SPECT, fluorine-18-FDG PET and rest thallium-201 SPECT for the detection of myocardial viability. J Nucl Med 1995;36:176–179.
53. Martin WH, Delbeke D, Patton JA, et al.: FDG-SPECT: Correlation with FDG-PET. J Nucl Med 1995;36:988–995.
54. Bax JJ, Visser FC, Blanksma PK, et al.: Comparison of myocardial uptake of F18-fluorodeoxyglucose imaged with positron emission tomography and single photon emission computed tomography. J Nucl Med 1996;37: 1631–1636.
55. Chen EQ, MacIntyre J, Go RT, et al.: Myocardial viability studies using fluorine-18-FDG SPECT: A comparison with fluorine-18-FDG PET. J Nucl Med 1997;38:582–586.
56. Srinivasan G, Kitsiou AN, Bacharach SL, et al.: [18F]fluorodeoxyglucose single photon emission computed tomography. Can it replace PET and thallium SPECT for the assessment of myocardial viability? Circulation 1998;97:843–850.
57. Sandler MP, Videlefsky S, Delbeke D, et al.: Evaluation of myocardial ischemia using a rest metabolism/stress perfusion protocol with fluorine-18 deoxyglucose/technetium-99m MIBI and dual-isotope simultaneous-acquisition single-photon emission computed tomography. J Am Coll Cardiol 1995;26:870–888.
58. Bax JJ, Cornel JH, Visser FC, et al.: Prediction of improvement of contractile function in patients with ischemic ventricular dysfunction after revascularization by F18-fluorodeoxyglucose SPECT. J Am Coll Cardiol 1997;30:377–384.
59. Pagano D, Townend JN, Little WA, et al.: Coronary artery bypass surgery as treatment for ischemic heart failure: The predictive value of viability assessment with quantitative positron emission tomography for symptomatic and functional outcome. J Thorac Cardiovasc Surg 1998; 115:791–799.
60. Bax JJ, Visser FC, Poldermans D, et al.: Relationship between preoperative viability and postoperative improvement in LVEF and heart failure symptoms. J Nucl Med 2001;42:79–86.
61. DiCarli M, Davidson M, Little R, et al.: Value of metabolic imaging with positron emission tomography for evaluating prognosis in patients with coronary artery disease and left ventricular dysfunction. Am J Cardiol 1994;73:527–533.

62. Eitzman D, Al-Aouar ZR, Kanter HL, et al.: Clinical outcome of patients with advanced coronary artery disease after viability studies with positron emission tomography. J Am Coll Cardiol 1992;20:559–565.
63. Marwick TH, Nemec JJ, Lafont A, et al.: Prediction by postexercise FDG PET of improvement in exercise capacity after revascularization. Am J Cardiol 1992;69:854–859.
64. DiCarli MF, Asgarzadie F, Schelbert HR, et al.: Quantitative relation between myocardial viability and improvement in heart failure symptoms after revascularization in patients with ischemic cardiomyopathy. Circulation 1995;92: 3436–3444.
65. Tamaki N, Kawamoto M, Takahashi N, et al.: Prognostic value of an increase in fluorine-18 deoxyglucose uptake in patients with myocardial infarction: Comparison with stress thallium imaging. J Am Coll Cardiol 1993;22:1621–1627.
66. Lee KS, Marwick TH, Cook SA, et al.: Prognosis of patients with left ventricular dysfunction, with and without viable myocardium after myocardial infarction. Relative efficacy of medical therapy and revascularization. Circulation 1994;90:2687–2694.
67. Vom Dahl J, Altehoefer C, Sheehan FH, et al.: Effect of myocardial viability assessed by technetium-99m-sestamibi SPECT and fluorine-18-FDG PET on clinical outcome in coronary artery disease. J Nucl Med 1997;38:742–748.
68. Beanlands RSB, Hendry PJ, Masters RG, et al.: Delay in revascularization is associated with increased mortality rate in patients with severe left ventricular dysfunction and viable myocardium on fluorine 18-fluorordeoxyglucose positron emission tomography. Circulation 1998; 98:II-51–II-56.
69. Schwarz ER, Schoendube FA, Kostin S, et al.: Prolonged myocardial hibernation exacerbates cardiomyocyte degeneration and impairs recovery of function after revascularization. J Am Coll Cardiol 1998;31:1018–1026.
70. Bax JJ, Visser FC, Poldermans D, et al.: Long-term prognostic value of FDG SPECT in patients with ischaemic left ventricular dysfunction. Abstracted, Eur Heart J 1999;20:257.
71. Wijffels E, Wijns W, Verheye S, et al.: Prognostic value of FDG imaging using SPECT in patients with severe left ventricular dysfunction. J Am Coll Cardiol 1999;33:416A.

Case Presentations

Case 5.1

History

A 64-year-old male with extensive three-vessel coronary artery disease, LVEF of 32 percent, and a remote inferior infarction was referred for FDG imaging. The patient did not have a history of diabetes mellitus. Three sets of images (Figure 5.5, see color plate) were obtained to evaluate the influence of metabolic conditions during FDG imaging on image quality: following oral glucose loading (top), following hyperinsulinemic euglycemic clamping (middle), and following oral administration of acipimox (a nicotinic acid derivative, bottom).

Findings

In all three sets of short-axis slices a clear defect is observed in the inferior and inferoseptal walls, indicating scar tissue and compatible with the known inferior infarction. FDG uptake is preserved in the other regions. The images obtained following clamping and acipimox demonstrate homogenous FDG uptake in these other regions and provide similar clinical information. The images obtained following oral glucose loading, however, show heterogeneous FDG uptake, which makes clinical interpretation difficult.

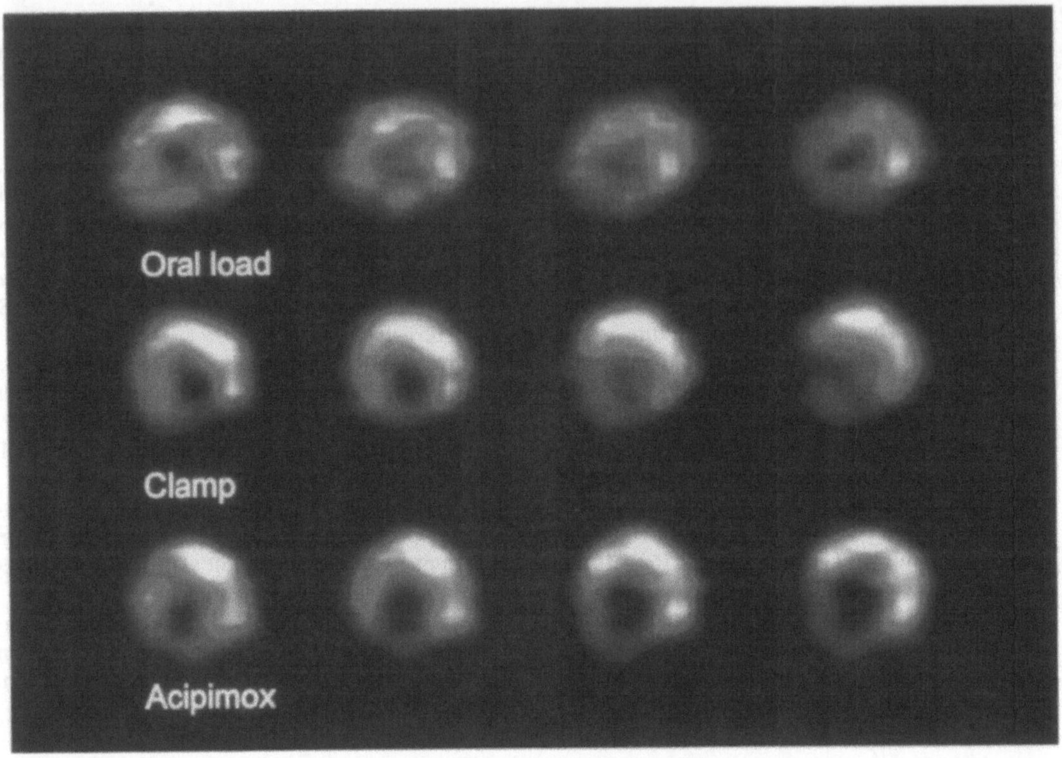

FIGURE 5.5. (See color plate)

Discussion

The metabolic conditions during FDG imaging are extremely important; they determine myocardial FDG uptake and thus image quality. High insulin levels accompanied by suppressed FFA levels promote FDG uptake, whereas high FFA levels inhibit FDG uptake. The low insulin levels and elevated FFA levels seen in the fasting patients result in uninterpretable FDG images in approximately 50% of fasting patients. Several protocols are available to promote cardiac FDG uptake. Oral glucose loading is the most frequently used approach, although it often results in uninterpretable images in patients with impaired glucose tolerance or diabetes mellitus (that is, fasting serum glucose >115 mg/dl). The hyperinsulinemic euglycemic clamp allows near perfect regulation of metabolic substrates and insulin levels, ensuring excellent image quality in all patients. However, the procedure is laborious and time-consuming. Oral administration of a nicotinic acid derivative (acipimox) may be an alternative to clamping. Acipimox inhibits peripheral lipolysis, thus reducing plasma free fatty acid levels and indirectly stimulating cardiac FDG uptake. Initial data suggest that good image quality can be obtained using this approach.

Diagnosis

Myocardial infarction of the inferior wall: comparison of the quality of FDG images under different metabolic conditions. (Based on Bax JJ, et al.: *Eur J Nucl Med* 1997;24:35–41; images reprinted with permission).

Case 5.2*

History

A 69-year-old male with congestive heart failure was referred for FDG imaging (Figure 5.6, see color plate). The patient had a history of a prior anterior infarction but no current symptoms of angina. Coronary angiography showed a subtotal occlusion of the left anterior descending coronary artery; the other coronary arteries showed no significant stenoses. Left ventricular ejection fraction was 23%. Echocardiography showed akinesia in the anteroseptal wall and apex.

Findings

Viability was evaluated by ^{201}Tl rest-redistribution SPECT (upper panel, transaxial slices), showing a resting perfusion defect in the anteroseptal wall and apex with only a little redistribution at the septum, indicating a small area of viable tissue. The FDG SPECT images (bottom, left) obtained following hyperinsulinemic euglycemic clamping show preserved glucose utilization in the anteroseptal wall and apex.

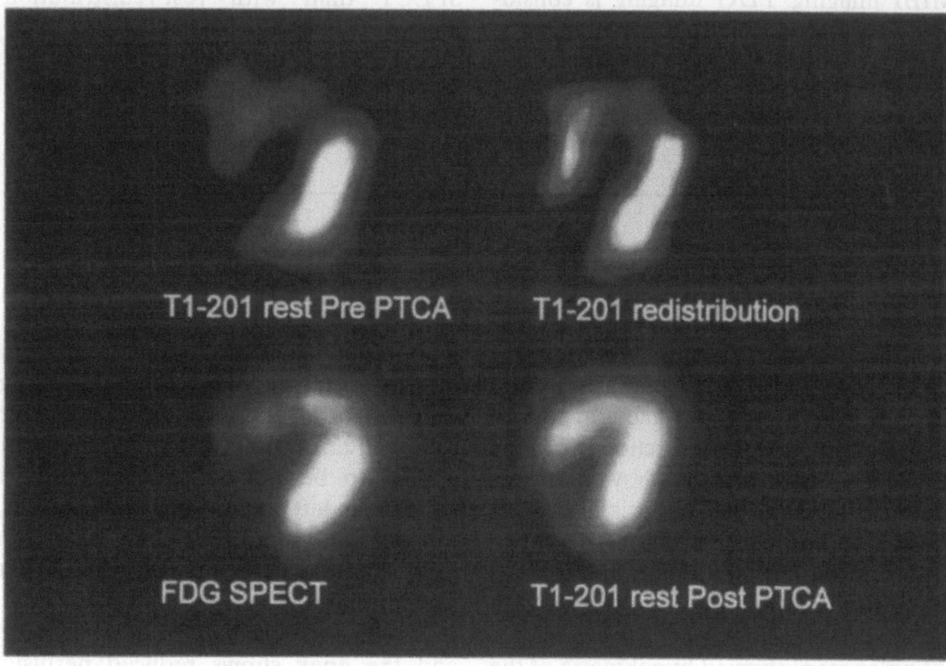

FIGURE 5.6. (See color plate)

* Based on Bax JJ, Visser FC, Cornel JH, van Lingen A, Fioretti PM, Visser CA: Improved detection of viable myocardium with fluorodeoxyglucose-labeled single-photon emission computed tomography in a patient with hibernating myocardium: comparison with rest-redistribution thallium 201-labeled single-photon emission computed tomography. J Nucl Cardiol 1997;4(2 Pt 1):178–179. No abstract available; images reprinted with permission.

Discussion

Assessment of viability in patients with ischemic cardiomyopathy has become an important tool both in the diagnostic and prognostic workup of these patients. Improvement of function following revascularization is possible when viable tissue is present in the dysfunctional region, whereas improvement of contractile function will not occur in the absence of viability. Revascularization in patients with ischemic cardiomyopathy has a high risk for periprocedural adverse events. Different techniques are available for detection of viable tissue; the most frequently applied nuclear techniques include FDG imaging (with PET or SPECT), ^{201}Tl imaging (using either a rest-redistribution or reinjection protocol), and ^{99m}Tc-MIBI imaging. FDG imaging is considered highly accurate for assessment of viability, as demonstrated in the current case. ^{201}Tl rest-redistribution could only demonstrate viability in a small region, whereas FDG SPECT demonstrated viability in a much larger region. The patient underwent percutaneous transluminal coronary angioplasty procedure of the left anterior descending artery. Four months after revascularization, echocardiography showed improvement of wall motion in the anteroseptal region, and the left ventricular ejection had increased to 38%. Perfusion following the procedure (bottom, right) had normalized.

Diagnosis

Viable myocardium in the anteroseptal wall and apex demonstrated better with FDG SPECT than with rest-redistribution ^{201}Tl images.

Case 5.3

History

A 61-year-old male was evaluated for recurrent episodes of congestive heart failure in the absence of angina. The patient had a history of an inferolateral myocardial infarction two years ago. Coronary angiography showed three-vessel disease: a 50 to 70% stenosis in the left anterior descending coronary artery, a 90 to 99% lesion in the left circumflex, and a 90 to 99% lesion in the right coronary artery. LVEF was 21%. Echocardiography (using a 13-segment polar map) showed hypokinesia of the septal segments and akinesia of the lateral, inferior, and apical segments (Figure 5.7, left panel). Myocardial viability was evaluated with dobutamine echocardiography (Figure 5.7, second panel from left) and FDG SPECT (Figure 5.7, third panel from left); the results are schematically presented in 13-segment polar maps. FDG SPECT was performed in combination with early resting ^{201}Tl SPECT (for assessment of perfusion).

Findings

Dobutamine echocardiography shows viability in the septal segments; the other segments (apical, lateral, and inferior) do not exhibit systolic wall thickening with dobutamine and thus appear to be nonviable (Figure 5.7, second panel from left). The scintigraphic results are as follows: The septal segments exhibit normal perfusion and FDG uptake, whereas the inferior and lateral walls exhibit decreased perfusion with increased FDG uptake (mismatch), and the apex shows reduced perfusion and matching reduced FDG uptake (Figure 5.7, third panel from left).

The patient underwent complete surgical revascularization. Three months after revascularization, the septal segments showed normal wall motion (and were thus improved in function), and the other segments remained unchanged (Figure 5.7, right panel). LVEF had improved slightly from 21 to 25%. Resting echocardiography was repeated 14 months

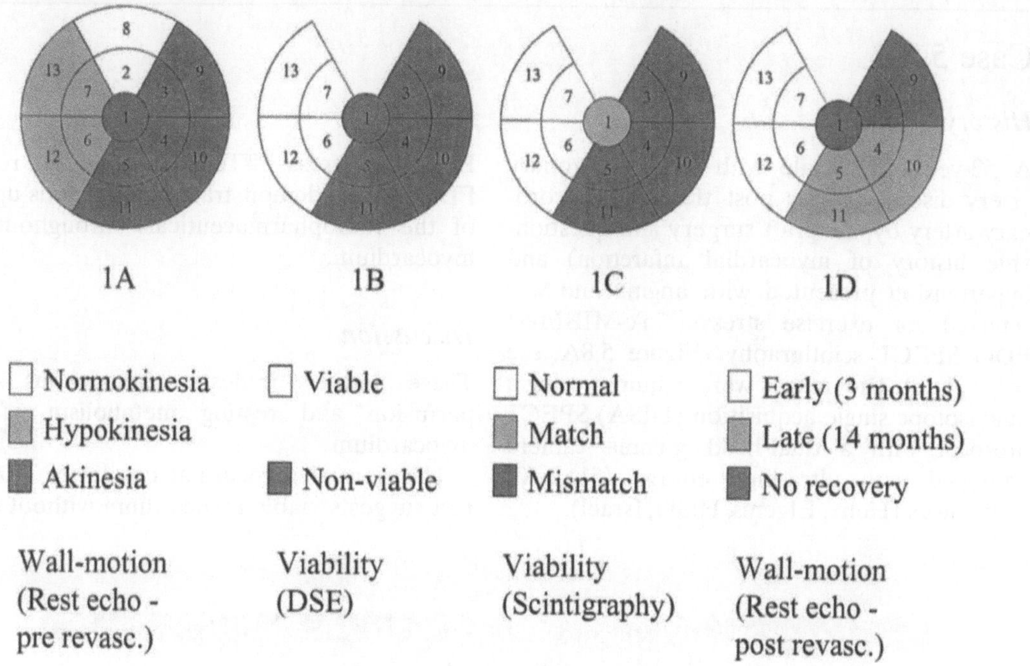

FIGURE 5.7.

after the revascularization. By then, the inferior wall and part of the lateral wall had also improved in wall motion; the rest of the lateral wall and the apex remained unchanged. LVEF was 32%. Thus, at long-term follow-up, additional improvement occurred in the segments that were classified viable by FDG SPECT and nonviable by dobutamine echocardiography. The segmental improvement resulted in further improvement of global LVEF.

Discussion

Dobutamine echocardiography and FDG imaging are frequently used for assessment of viability. However, FDG imaging detects myocardial glucose utilization, whereas dobutamine echocardiography detects contractile reserve. It is likely that some severely damaged (long-term hibernating) segments no longer exhibit contractile reserve but still have intact glucose metabolism, thus making FDG imaging more sensitive for detection of viable tissue. As demonstrated in this case, these segments may take longer time to improve in function postrevascularization. This is an important principle in the interpretation of many of the short-term reports of the results of revascularization. Full functional recovery of dyskinetic myocardial segments may require 6 to 12 months rather than the 1 to 3 months often reported.

Diagnosis

Viable myocardium in the inferolateral wall demonstrated better with FDG SPECT than with dobutamine echocardiography. (Based on Bax JJ, Poldermans D, Visser FC, et al.: Delayed recovery of hibernating myocardium after surgical revascularization: implications for discrepancy between metabolic imaging and dobutamine echocardiography for assessment of myocardial viability. *J Nucl Cardiol* 1999;6(6): 685–687; images reprinted with permission.)

Case 5.4

History

A 52-year-old female with known coronary artery disease (status post three-vessel coronary artery bypass graft surgery and questionable history of myocardial infarction) and hypertension presented with angina and was referred for exercise stress ^{99m}Tc-MIBI/rest FDG SPECT scintigraphy (Figure 5.8A, see color plate). The images were acquired using a dual isotope single acquisition (DISA) SPECT protocol with a dual-head gamma camera equipped with ultra-high energy (511 keV) collimators (Helix, Elgems, Haifa, Israel).

Findings

Both the stress ^{99m}Tc-MIBI and the resting FDG images demonstrate homogenous uptake of the radiopharmaceuticals throughout the myocardium.

Discussion

These findings indicate homogenous stress perfusion and resting metabolism of the myocardium.

The normal myocardial uptake of FDG at rest suggests viable myocardium without areas

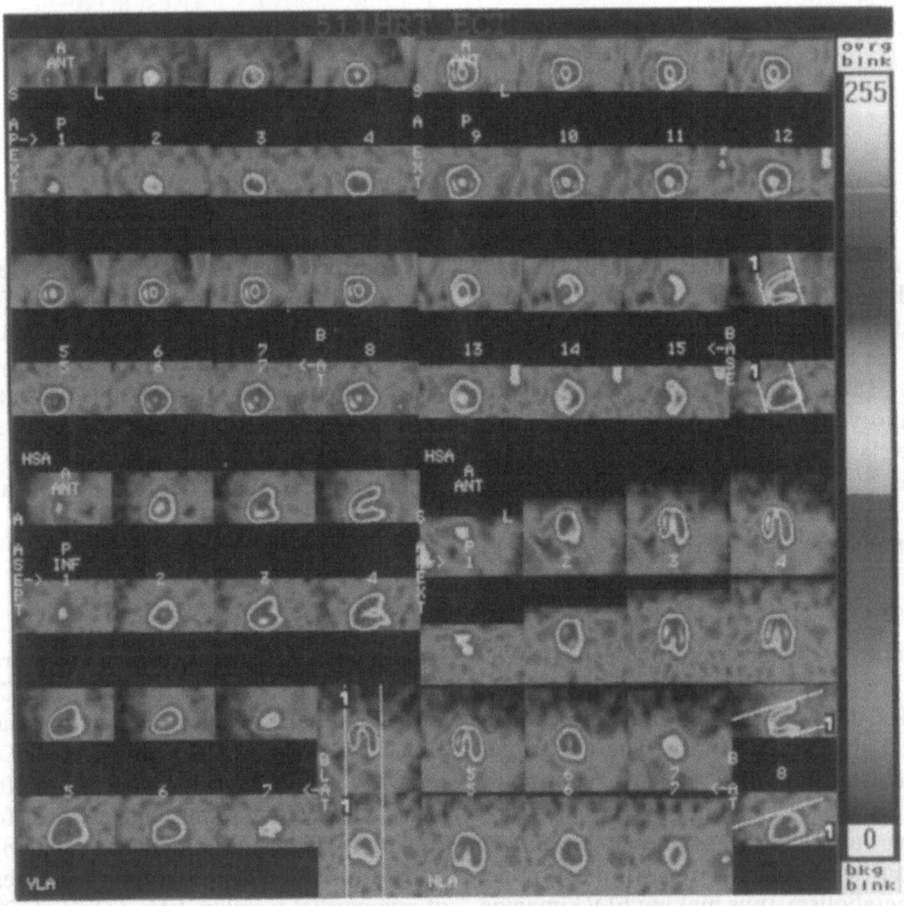

FIGURE 5.8A. (See color plate)

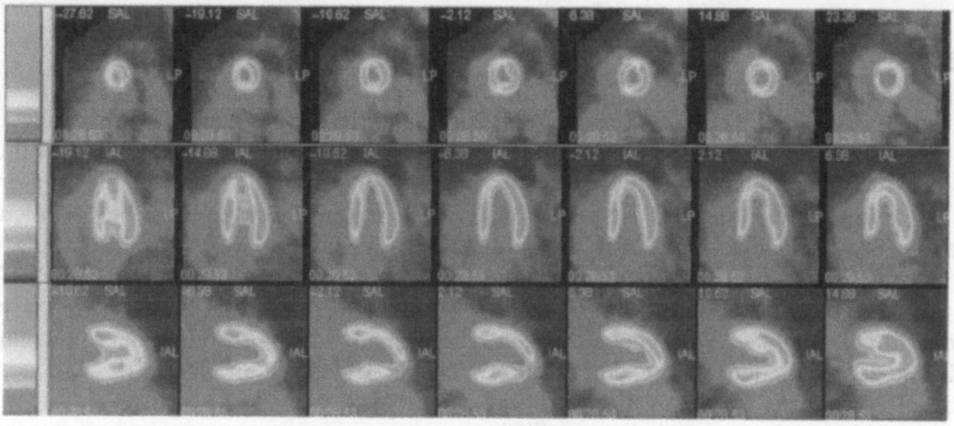

FIGURE 5.8B. (See color plate)

of infarction, whereas the matching homogeneous uptake of ^{99m}Tc-MIBI at stress denotes no evidence of stress-induced ischemia. Modified SPECT gamma camera systems capable of imaging 511 keV photons are now commercially available, thereby allowing FDG metabolic SPECT imaging to be combined with (MIBI) perfusion imaging to provide information regarding perfusion and metabolism using sequential or dual-isotope simultaneous acquisition. Ultra-high energy collimators are necessary to shield the 511 KeV photons. These collimators are in place for both acquisitions of ^{99m}Tc-MIBI and ^{18}F-FDG images if a dual-isotope single acquisition protocol is used for imaging, as in this case. This case illustrates the high quality of both sets of images using such a protocol. The myocardial wall appears thickened and the ventricular chamber is smaller on the FDG images compared to the MIBI images due to the limited resolution of the gamma camera for FDG versus ^{99m}Tc using the SPECT technique. For comparison, normal cardiac FDG images acquired with a dedicated PET tomograph with full rings of BGO detectors (GE advance) and reconstructed with attenuation correction are shown in Figure 5.8B, see color plate.

FDG evidence of viability has been reported in as many as 50% of segments with matched perfusion defects using stress/rest MIBI protocols as well as in 40 to 50% of fixed ^{201}Tl defects with stress-redistribution protocols.[1] The prognosis of a patient with a normal stress perfusion SPECT scan using ^{201}Tl or MIBI is excellent with an annualized cardiac event rate of 0.1% for cardiac death and 0.6% for nonfatal myocardial infarction. This is true regardless of age, gender, symptoms, stress or resting ECG findings, prior revascularization procedure (more than three months), or even the presence of angiographically proven coronary artery disease.[2] Therefore, a normal metabolic/perfusion study in this patient places her at a very low likelihood of myocardial infarct or death in the ensuing two years, thus obviating the need for any further invasive studies such as cardiac catheterization. The past history of myocardial infarction is not confirmed by the scintigraphic findings.

Diagnosis

Normal exercise stress ^{99m}Tc-MIBI/rest FDG cardiac SPECT scintigraphy using a DISA protocol.

References

1. Bergmann SR: Positron emission tomography of the heart, in Gerson MC (ed): Cardiac Nuclear Medicine, ed. 3. New York, McGraw-Hill, 1997, pp 267–299.
2. Brown KA: Prognostic value of nuclear cardiology techniques, in Gerson MC (ed): Cardiac Nuclear Medicine, ed. 3. New York, McGraw-Hill, 1997, pp 619–654.

Case 5.5

History

A 49-year-old obese male with hypertension and a history of chronic tobacco use presented with a cerebrovascular accident. For the past three months, he had been experiencing symptoms of congestive heart failure and progressive exertional angina. An echocardiogram revealed a depressed left ventricular ejection fraction of 20 to 30%. Cardiac catheterization showed significant three-vessel disease (75% left anterior descending artery, 100% left circumflex, and 100% right coronary artery) with diminished LVEF. He was referred for resting ^{99m}Tc-MIBI/FDG SPECT scintigraphy (Figure 5.9, see color plate) for evaluation of the presence of injured but viable hibernating myocardium prior to possible revascularization. The images were acquired using a dual isotope single acquisition (DISA) SPECT protocol using a dual-head gamma camera equipped with ultra-high energy collimators (Helix, Elgems, Haifa, Israel).

Findings

The resting perfusion MIBI images demonstrate large, severe perfusion defects involving

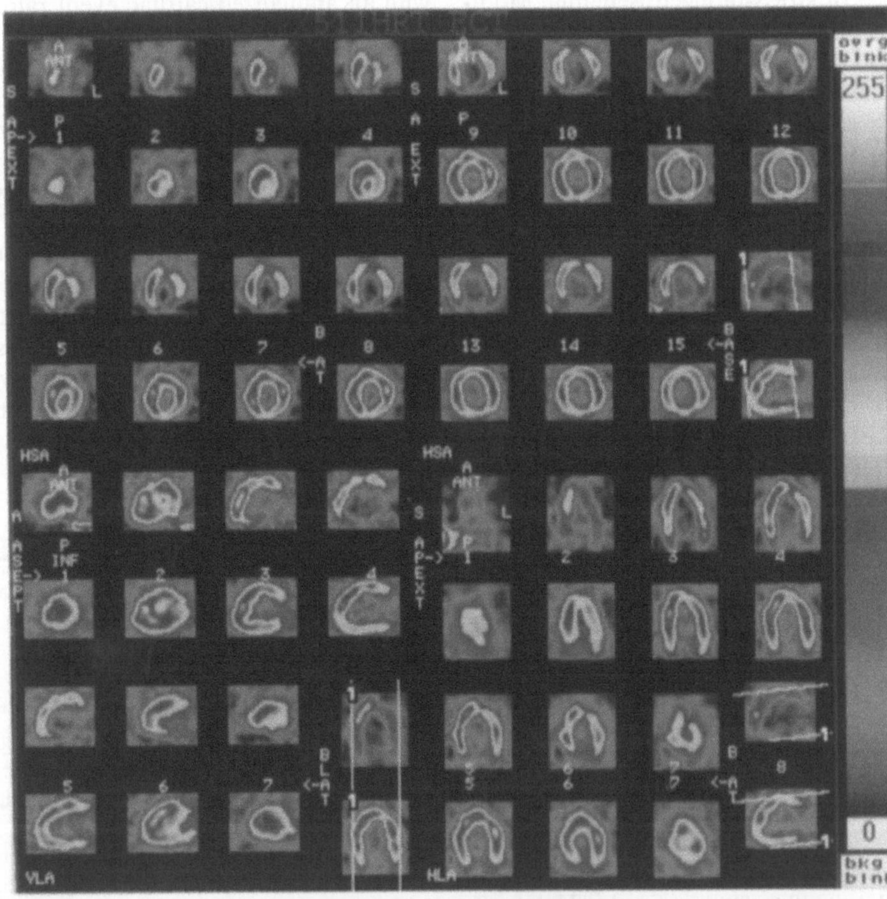

FIGURE 5.9. (See color plate)

both the anterior and inferior myocardial walls. The FDG images demonstrate the presence of metabolism in these segments.

Discussion

The perfusion/metabolism mismatch seen in this patient is consistent with ischemia. Given the cardiac catheterization findings along with the extensive volume of viable myocardium demonstrated by FDG SPECT, the patient was referred for cardiac artery bypass graft surgery. A postoperative echocardiogram revealed an LVEF of 45%.

This patient is an example of ischemic cardiomyopathy with a large volume of hibernating myocardium. Hibernating myocardium refers to a state of persistently impaired left ventricular dysfunction in the resting basal state that is attributable to a chronic reduction in coronary artery blood flow. Ischemic pain may or may not be present, as is the case here. Hibernating myocardium implies that if regional blood flow is restored, myocardial function will improve. Only 25 to 40% of unselected patients with severe coronary artery disease and left ventricular dysfunction demonstrate improvement in global LVEF with revascularization. Therefore, the need for assessment of viability is imperative, as substantial gain can be achieved in such patients if revascularization can be accomplished. At present, FDG imaging is considered the most accurate modality for viability determination.[1]

With rest-redistribution ^{201}Tl imaging, only 68% of myocardial segments with redistribution demonstrate improvement in regional function after revascularization, whereas with MIBI/FDG imaging, 82% of mismatched segments demonstrate functional improvement. Using MIBI/FDG imaging in a series of 146 patients, mean global left ventricular ejection fraction increased from 33 to 47% in patients with a mismatch but decreased from 36 to 32% in patients with matched defects.

Diagnosis

Severe myocardial ischemia and hibernating myocardium.

Reference

1. Bax JJ, Patton JA, Poldermans D, Elhendy A, Sandler MP: 18-Fluorodeoxyglucose imaging with positron emission tomography and single photon emission computed tomography: cardiac applications. Semin Nucl Med 2000 Oct;30(4): 281–298.

Case 5.6

History

A 64-year-old woman with known coronary artery disease presented with unstable angina. The patient had a history of cardiac artery bypass graft surgery seven years earlier, complicated by left internal mammary artery graft failure resulting in a large anteroseptal myocardial infarction. After medical stabilization, she was referred for an adenosine stress ^{99m}Tc-MIBI/rest FDG cardiac SPECT scan (Figure 5.10, see color plate) for evaluation of the presence of injured but viable myocardium prior to possible revascularization. The images were acquired using a dual isotope single acquisition (DISA) SPECT protocol using a dual-head gamma camera equipped with ultra-high energy collimators (VG Millenium, General Electric Medical Systems Inc., Milwaukee, WI). The patient experienced chest discomfort during the adenosine infusion but without accompanying ECG changes suggestive of ischemia.

Findings

The images demonstrate severely decreased uptake of both MIBI and FDG in the anterior wall, septum, and apex of the heart. Gated SPECT images revealed a left ventricular ejection fraction of 20%.

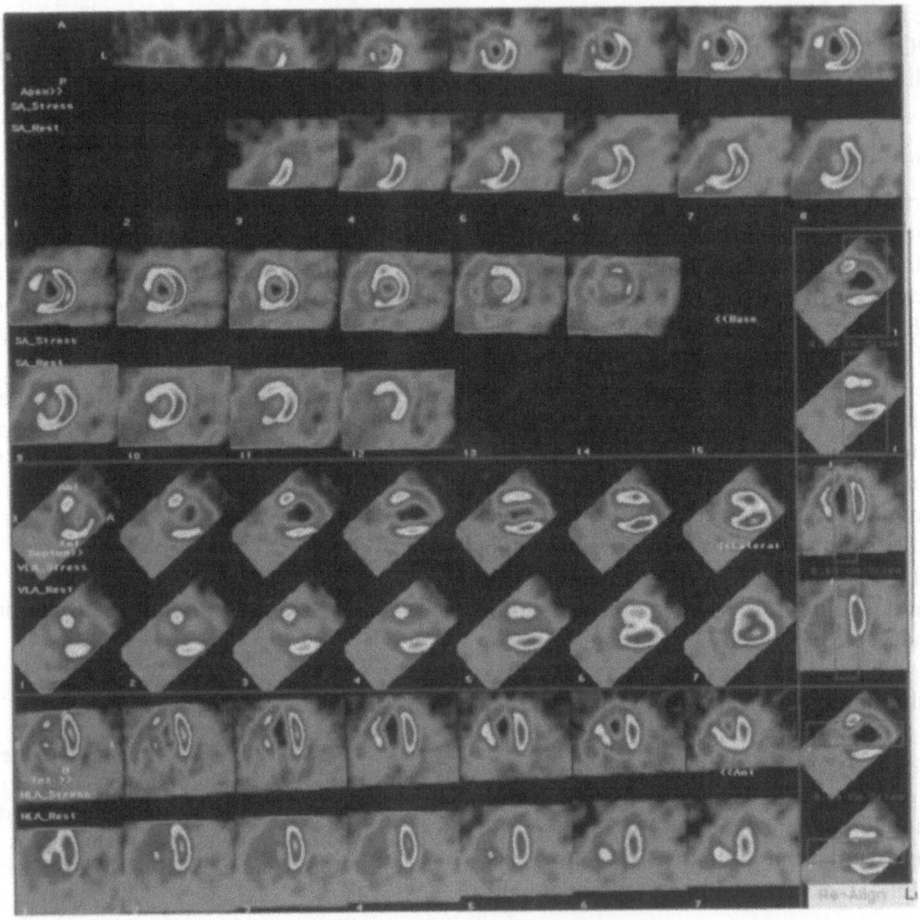

FIGURE 5.10. (See color plate)

Discussion

These findings indicate myocardial infarction in these segments. FDG metabolic SPECT imaging can be combined with MIBI perfusion imaging to give information regarding perfusion and metabolism using sequential imaging or a dual-isotope simultaneous acquisition protocol. In this case, the matched MIBI/FDG defects confirmed the large anteroseptal infarct without evidence of ischemia, obviating the need for further evaluation, that is, cardiac catheterization.

The occurrence of chest pain during adenosine infusion is a nonspecific finding and may occur in as many as 40% of patients without significant coronary artery disease. However, if typical ischemic electrocardiogram (EKG) abnormalities occur during adenosine stress, there is a relatively high incidence of significant coronary artery disease.

Diagnosis

Large anteroseptal and apical myocardial infarction.

Case 5.7

History

A 79-year-old woman with hypertension and hyperlipidemia presented with typical angina. The patient had a past history of coronary artery bypass graft surgery. Recent cardiac catheterization revealed a patent left internal mammary artery graft to the left anterior descending artery and an occluded saphenous vein graft to the left circumflex system. The native coronaries were severely diseased with a total occlusion of the mid-left circumflex. She was referred for adenosine stress ^{99m}Tc-MIBI/rest FDG SPECT scintigraphy (Figure 5.11). The images were acquired both in the supine (Figure 5.11A, see color plate) and prone (Figure 5.11B, see color plate) positions using a dual isotope single acquisition (DISA) SPECT protocol with a dual-head gamma camera equipped with ultra-high energy 511 keV collimators (VG Millenium, General Electric Medical Systems Inc., Milwaukee, WI).

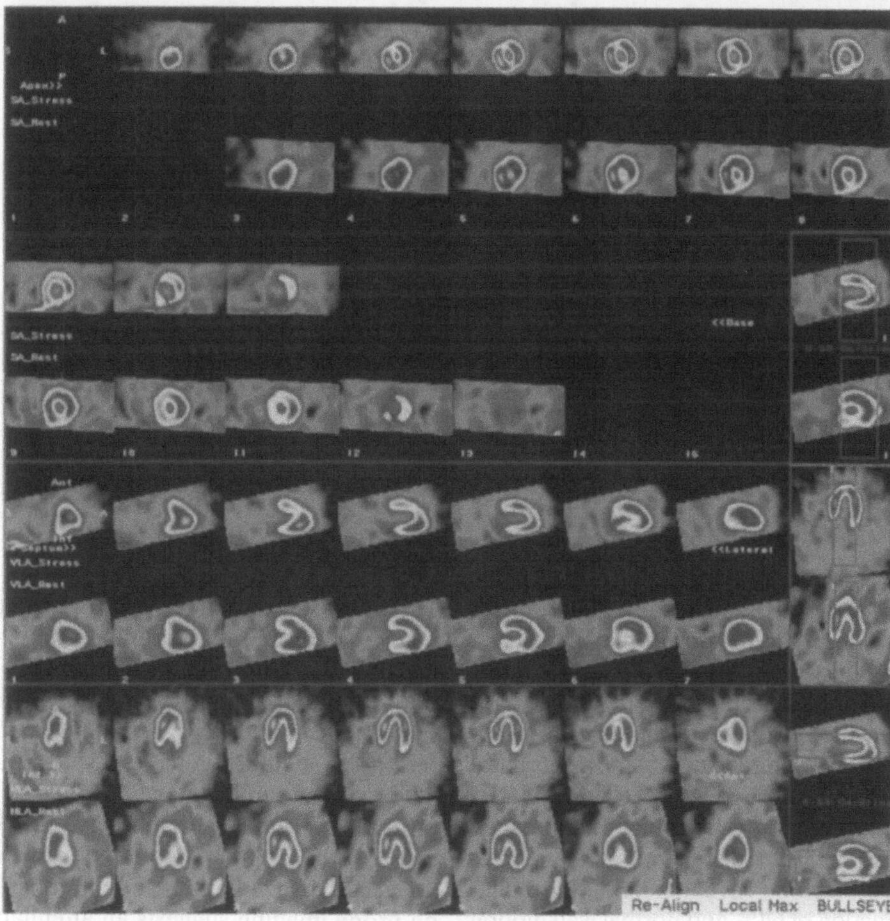

FIGURE 5.11A. (See color plate)

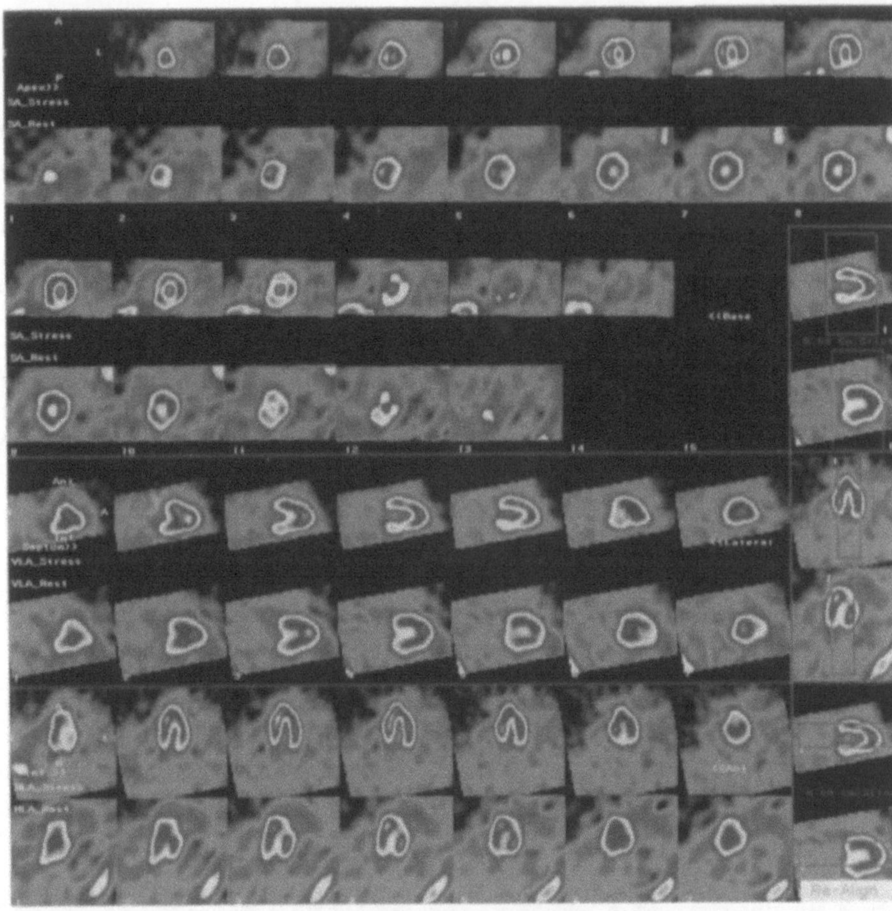

FIGURE 5.11B. (See color plate)

Findings

Both the stress MIBI and resting FDG images obtained in the supine position demonstrate moderately decreased uptake along the anteroseptal and inferobasal walls. On the images obtained in the prone position, the anteroseptal defect is no longer seen. The inferobasal defect partially improves on the prone MIBI images and resolves on the prone FDG images. The gated images displayed in a three-dimensional format reveal a left ventricular ejection fraction of 64% and normal wall motion with normal systolic wall thickening (not shown).

Discussion

The anteroseptal defect is not present on the images acquired in the prone position, suggesting that the anteroseptal abnormality seen in the supine position is due to a breast attenuation artifact rather than actual myocardial perfusion (or metabolic) deficit. The anteroseptal defect on the supine images is better delineated on the MIBI images than on the FDG images due to the better resolution of the MIBI images. Improvement of the inferobasal defect on prone imaging suggests an attenuation artifact from the diaphragm. The partial resolution of the inferobasal defect on MIBI images and complete resolution on FDG images may be explained by differential attenuation of the 140 keV photons from ^{99m}Tc and the 511 keV photons from ^{18}F.

A significant problem with cardiac SPECT imaging is the frequent occurrence of artifactual myocardial defects due to photon attenuation by extra-cardiac soft tissues. This problem is magnified with coincidence imaging, making the importance of attenuation correction more important for PET than for SPECT. Anteroseptal defects are seen in women as a result of overlying breast tissue in as many as 35% of cases. The relative decrease in inferior wall activity is a frequent occurrence in normal patients of both sexes due to interposition of the diaphragm and subdiaphragmatic fat between the heart and the detector(s). This results in lower specificity for inferior wall defects than for anterior and lateral wall defects.

Prone imaging may be used as a means of correcting for soft tissue attenuation by altering the position of the soft tissues, breasts or diaphragm, in relation to the position of the heart. In many cases, the breast attenuation artifact seen with supine imaging will improve or resolve with prone imaging because the breast is displaced laterally. Even when it does not resolve, it may be seen to change location, indicative of soft tissue effect. The heart is mobile within the thoracic cavity and will swing up and away from the diaphragm when a patient is imaged in the prone position so that the diaphragm is spatially separated from the myocardium, causing the inferior wall perfusion defect seen in the supine position to improve significantly or resolve. When using ^{201}Tl, there is a significant improvement in inferior counts in the large majority of patients imaged prone versus supine (striking in approximately 25%), with a resultant improvement in inferior wall specificity of approximately 24%. Because of the higher count rates obtained with ^{99m}Tc-labeled radiopharmaceuticals, soft tissue attenuation artifacts may be a less frequent problem, but they remain a dilemma more frequently than initial reports indicated. Because of the high 511 keV energy of ^{18}F, attenuation artifacts may not be as severe with FDG imaging. For that reason, it is recommended that all patients undergoing ^{201}Tl or ^{99m}Tc and FDG cardiac imaging be imaged in both the supine and prone positions to avoid erroneous interpretations of reversibility along the inferior wall.

The high-count density seen with ^{99m}Tc-MIBI and ^{99m}Tc-tetrofosmin imaging allows acquisition of the study gated to the cardiac cycle and viewing as a continuous cine display, even with DISA ^{99m}Tc /FDG imaging. Regional wall motion can be assessed by subjective evaluation of endocardial excursion, and segmental wall thickening can be assessed by changes in color intensification from end-diastole to end-systole. Whereas an infarct would be expected to demonstrate impaired wall motion and thickening, a soft tissue attenuation artifact should be associated with normal wall motion and thickening. Using gated acquisitions has reportedly decreased the incidence of unexplained fixed perfusion defects from 14 to 3%.[1] This should result in improved specificity and allow a measure of viability as well. In this patient, resolution of the perfusion abnormalities with prone imaging combined with the normal wall motion and wall thickening observed on the gated cine images indicate that the perfusion abnormalities are related to soft tissue attenuation artifact rather than myocardial scarring. The myocardium attended by the left circumflex circulation in this patient is perfused by collaterals from the left anterior descending (LAD) and right coronary artery (RCA).

Diagnosis

Soft tissue attenuation artifact anteriorly by breast tissue and inferiorly by diaphragm.

Reference

1. DePuey EG, Rozanski A: Using gated technetium-99m-sestamibi SPECT to characterize fixed myocardial defects as infarct or artifact. J Nucl Med 1995 Jun;36(6):952–955.

Clinical Applications in Oncology

6.1 Normal Distribution of FDG

Marcus V. Grigolon, William H. Martin, and Dominique Delbeke

Normal Distribution of FDG and Physiologic Variations

FDG is an analog of glucose and is used as a tracer of glucose metabolism. Therefore, the distribution of FDG is not limited to malignant tissue. FDG enters into the cells by the same transport mechanism as glucose and is intracellularly phosphorylated by a hexokinase into FDG-6-phosphate (FDG-6-P). In tissues with a low concentration of glucose-6-phosphatase, such as the brain, myocardium, and most malignant cells, FDG-6-P does not enter into further enzymatic pathways and accumulates intracellularly proportionally to the glycolytic rate of the cell. Some tissues such as the liver, kidney, intestine, muscle, and some malignant cells have variable degrees of glucose-6-phosphatase activity and do not accumulate FDG-6-P to the same extent. To interpret clinical FDG images, one should be familiar with the normal distribution of FDG, physiologic variations, and benign conditions that accumulate FDG.[1–3]

The cortex of the brain normally uses glucose as its substrate; therefore, cerebral FDG accumulation is physiologically high.

Thymic uptake can be present in children and patients with rebound thymic hyperplasia after chemotherapy.[4] Its typical "V" shape usually allows differentiation from bulky more nodular and asymmetric residual lymphoma. Marked diffuse bone marrow uptake is frequently seen after chemotherapy and may interfere with evaluation of the bone marrow for malignant involvement. There is evidence that bone marrow is more prominent if a granulocyte-stimulating factor has been administered. The FDG uptake in the bone marrow is sufficiently low one month after completion of chemotherapy to avoid that problem. Diffuse thyroid uptake can be seen in thyroiditis and Graves' disease or may be a normal variant.

However, the myocardium can use various substrates according to substrate availability, hormonal status, and other factors. In a typical fasting state, the myocardium primarily utilizes free fatty acids, but postprandially or after a glucose load it favors glucose. When the chest is evaluated with FDG to assess the presence of malignant lesions, a longer than usual fasting state (12 hours) is preferable to avoid obscuring malignant foci due to adjacent cardiac activity. However, for evaluation of coronary artery disease, a glucose load is usually given to promote cardiac uptake of FDG.

In the resting state, there is low accumulation of FDG in the muscular system, but following exercise significant accumulation of FDG in selected muscular groups may be misleading. For example, in the evaluation of head and neck cancer, uptake in laryngeal muscles or in the muscles used for mastication may mimic metastases. Therefore, it is important to keep the patient in a relaxed, resting state (no eating or talking) during the distribution phase following FDG injection. Hyperventilation may induce uptake in the diaphragm and anxiety-induced muscle tension is often seen in the trapezius and paraspinal muscles. Muscle relaxants such as benzodiazepines (diazepam, 5 to 10mg orally, 30 to 60 minutes before FDG administration) may be helpful in these tense patients,[5] particularly in patients with head and neck primary neoplasms and lymphomas. Increased FDG uptake in recently exercised skeletal muscles has also been observed, so the avoidance of strenuous exercise for 12 hours prior to FDG imaging is advisable.

Unlike glucose, FDG is excreted by the kidneys into the urine. Accumulation of FDG in the renal collecting system may create artifacts that obscure evaluation of that region. This can be avoided by keeping the patient well hydrated to promote diuresis, and the administration of diuretics (furosemide, 20mg intravenously, 20 minutes after FDG administration) may be helpful as well. In addition, hydration and frequent voiding are advised to limit radiation exposure to the genitourinary tract. For adequate visualization of the pelvis, placement of a Foley catheter in the bladder with irrigation may be helpful. Be careful to avoid misinterpreting physiologic ureteral activity on axial images as pathologic nodal uptake; viewing coronal images will usually provide clarification. Activity in the renal pelvis or renal calyces that are adjacent to the liver may be confused with hepatic metastases.

Another source of misinterpretation is uptake in the gastrointestinal tract that can be quite variable from patient to patient. There is usually uptake in the lymphoid tissue of the Waldeyer ring, and prominent uptake in the cecum of many patients may also be related to abundant lymphoid tissue in the intestinal wall. Uptake along the esophagus is also common, especially in the distal portion and when there is esophagitis; esophageal activity is best identified on sagittal views. The wall of the stomach is usually faintly seen and can be used as an anatomical landmark, but occasionally the uptake can be moderately intense, especially if the stomach is contracted. Moderately increased activity at the esophageal-gastric junction should not be interpreted as metastatic adenopathy. FDG uptake along the rectosigmoid colon is common and may appear focal on coronal images because of the anteroposterior orientation of the colon in that location. Careful examination of the transaxial and sagittal images can usually identify the tubular pattern of the colon and avoid misinterpretation as local recurrence, for example in patients with colorectal carcinoma. Another source of confusion is the usual physiologic uptake at colostomy sites.

Benign Processes Accumulating FDG

Inflammation in general can cause FDG uptake that may be severe enough to be confused with malignant lesions, especially when there is granulomatous inflammation such as tuberculosis,[6] sarcoidosis,[7] histoplasmosis, and aspergillosis among others.[8] Any acute injury to soft tissues results in an inflammatory response. In view of the known high uptake of FDG by activated macrophages, it is not surprising that inflamed tissue demonstrates FDG activity. For this reason, a careful history and physical examination is necessary to avoid misinterpretation of FDG images. Mild to moderate FDG activity may be seen along recent incisions, infected incisions, and at biopsy sites including bone marrow. A recent fracture or osteomyelitis may also appear hypermetabolic.[9–12] Increased FDG activity at tumor sites may persist for several weeks following successful chemotherapy and may persist for several months following radiation therapy, including radioimmunotherapy. A postobstructive pneumonitis may be confusing but should not be interpreted as tumor extension.

If the radiopharmaceutical extravasates into the soft tissues at the site of injection, the tracer may accumulate in draining benign lymph nodes due to lymphatic reabsorption. Therefore, when the PET scan is performed for staging malignancies such as melanoma or breast cancer, FDG should be injected through an intravenous catheter in the arm opposite the primary lesion. Regional nodal uptake ipsilateral to the injection site should be interpreted with caution. The axillae are better evaluated with the arms positioned above the head.

Common causes of abnormal and variant accumulation of FDG leading to false-positive and false-negative interpretations are listed in Tables 6.1.1 and 6.1.2.[13,14]

TABLE 6.1.1. **False positive findings with FDG imaging.**

Physiologic uptake

1. Gastrointestinal uptake (esophagus, stomach, bowel, liver)
2. Genitourinary uptake (hydronephrosis, ureteral activity, transplant or ectopic kidney, bladder diverticulum)
3. Skeletal and smooth muscle, including neck, laryngeal, and diaphragm
4. Postresection or XRT of contralateral structure
5. Biliary ductal dilatation
6. Eiphyseal growth plate
7. Periareolar breast uptake
8. Lactation
9. Thymic hyperplasia
10. Thyroid
11. Spleen
12. Bone marrow reactive hyperplasia

Inflammatory processes

1. Postsurgical inflammation/infection/hematoma, biopsy site, amputation site
2. Postradiation
3. Postchemotherapy
4. Granulomatous disease process
    - Fungal and myocobacterial disease
    - Sarcoidosis
    - Aspergilloma
    - Histiocytosis X
    - Eosinophilic granuloma
    - Suture granuloma
    - Pulmonary anthrasilicosis
5. Abscess, osteomyelitis
6. Herpes encephalitis
7. Gingivitis/sinusitis
8. Mastitis
9. Thyroiditis, Graves' disease
10. Empyema
11. Pleural effusion
12. Pneumonitis or alveolits
13. Rheumatoid lung disease
14. Esophagitis
15. Ostomy sites (trachea, colon) and drainage tubes
16. Acute enterocolitis
17. Retroperitoneal fibrosis
18. Pancreatitis, acute or chronic
19. Pancreatic serous cystadenoma
20. Hepatic hydatid cyst
21. Acute cholangitis
22. Biliary stent
23. Insertion tendinitis
24. Recent fracture
25. Inflammatory arthritis/synovitis
26. Joint prosthesis loosening
27. Myositis
28. Lymphadenitis (bacterial, fungal, nonspecific)

Benign neoplasms

1. Pituitary adenoma
2. Meningioma
3. Salivary gland tumors (Warthin's, pleomorphic adenoma, benign mixed tumor)
4. Schwannoma
5. Hurthle cell and follicular thyroid adenoma
6. Parathyroid adenoma
7. Breast fibroadenoma
8. Fibrocystic breast disease
9. Mammary dysplasia
10. Fibrous mesothelioma
11. Colonic adenoma
12. Pancreatic serous cystadenoma
13. Pheochromocytoma
14. Renal pericytoma
15. Renal angiomyolipoma
16. Ovarian thecoma
17. Ovarian cystadenoma
18. Endometrioma
19. Endometrial/follicular cyst
20. Paget's disease
21. Enchondroma
22. Giant cell tumor
23. Aneurysmal bone cyst
24. Fibrous dysplasia
25. Nonossifying fibroma
26. Chondroblastoma
27. Chondromyxoid fibroma
28. Brown's tumor (parathyroid osteopathy)
29. Desmoplastic fibroma

References
1. Schulte M, Brechte-Krauss D, Heymer B, et al.: Grading of tumors and tumorlike lesions of bone: Evaluation by FDG-PET. J Nucl Med 2000;41:1695–1701.
2. Stadalnik RC: Benign causes of 18-FDG uptake on whole body imaging. Semin Nucl Med 1998;28:352–358.

In conclusion, to avoid misinterpretation of FDG images, it is critical to standardize the environment of the patient during the uptake period; examine the patient for postoperative site, tube placement, stoma, and so forth; and time FDG imaging appropriately after invasive procedures and therapeutic interventions. In addition, a 4-hour fasting period is recommended including no consumption of beverages with sugar and no intravenous dextrose. To prevent myocardial uptake, a 12-hour fasting period is preferable if the chest is to be

TABLE 6.1.2. False negative findings with FDG imaging.

Small size (< 2 × resolution of system)
Hyperglycemia
Recent chemotherapy or radiotherapy
Adjacent physiological activity (skeletal muscle, bowel, kidneys, bladder, myocardial)
Tumor necrosis
Hepatoma
Thyroid carcinoma, well-differentiated
Bronchoalveolar carcinoma
Mucinous carcinoma
Sarcoma, low-grade
Lymphoma, low-grade
Lymphomatous splenic involvement
Plasmacytoma
Neuroendocrine tumors
• Carcinoid
• Pheochromocytoma/paraganglioma
• Islet cell carcinoma
• Uveal melanoma, especially uveal
Genitourinary tumors (prostate, renal cell carcinoma, bladder, teratoma, ovarian adenocarcinoma)
Skeletal metastases, osteoblastic/sclerotic and osteosarcoma
Brain neoplasms, especially low-grade

evaluated. Drinking water should be encouraged to keep the patient hydrated and promote diuresis that will limit artifacts from the renal collecting system and radiation exposure to the bladder. During the distribution phase, the patient should be relaxed and avoid talking, chewing, and any muscular activity.

Imaging Protocols for Evaluation of the Body

Historically, FDG PET imaging has been developed to perform quantitative evaluation of various physiologic parameters, for example, perfusion and glucose metabolism. The sensitivity of dedicated PET tomographs allows dynamic scanning of an organ or region of interest after injection of FDG, and dynamic arterial blood sampling to obtain both tissue and plasma tracer concentrations over time permit the quantification of the actual metabolic rate using tracer kinetic modeling. Quantitative evaluation using kinetic modeling requires attenuation correction to measure true count rate in a specified region of interest of the body. Traditionally, PET images have been corrected for attenuation. Quantitative measurements are time-consuming, cumbersome, and more invasive than obtaining a static image after the radiopharmaceutical reaches a plateau of concentration at the time of acquisition, usually 60 minutes after intravenous FDG administration. In oncology, true quantitation of metabolism cannot be performed accurately because the kinetics of many tumors are not known, and dynamic imaging is not possible over the entire body. Static imaging of the entire body offers the advantage of detecting additional unsuspected lesions in addition to evaluating a specific lesion. Evaluation of static PET images can be performed visually or semiquantitatively using the standard uptake value (SUV) or the lesion to background ratio (L/B). The SUV is the activity in the lesion in μCi/ml normalized for the weight of the patient in kg and the dose of FDG in mCi. Semiquantitative evaluation offers a more objective reporting of the uptake in the lesion and allows comparison to the lesional uptake on a prior scan. However, accurate soft tissue attenuation correction is critical.

For the clinical evaluation of FDG images from oncological patients, correction for soft tissue attenuation has significant advantages. The most important advantage is improved anatomic delineation (for example, mediastinum from lungs, lungs from liver). Without attenuation correction, the lungs typically show higher uptake than the chest wall and mediastinum despite the fact that they contain less metabolic active tissue per volume. This is because the pulmonary parenchyma is filled with air (a low density compound), resulting in less photon attenuation. This artifact is corrected when attenuation correction is performed. Therefore, images with attenuation correction are easier to interpret than images without attenuation correction, especially for the inexperienced interpreter, and lesions can be localized more accurately. The second advantage of attenuation correction is the possibility of semiquantitative measurement using the SUV, which may be helpful in some clinical settings. One example is differentiation of benign from malignant pulmonary lesions greater than twice the resolution of the scanner, and another example is monitoring therapy of malignant lesions. In addition, on images with attenuation correction, lesions are not distorted, and lesions located deeply should have an intensity similar to superficial lesions. However, images with attenuation correction are often noisier than images without attenuation correction, and the degree of noise in images with attenuation correction is dependent on the method used for attenuation correction.

For the images shown in this chapter, patients have been instructed to fast for 12 hours and drink plenty of clear fluids. The serum glucose levels have been measured just before FDG administration to document euglycemia. The emission images were acquired 45 to 60 minutes after intravenous administration of 370 MBq (10 mCi) of FDG. During the distribution phase, the patients were resting in a quiet room with dimmed light. The FDG images were acquired with either of two dedicated tomographs with full rings of germanate bismuth oxide (BGO) detectors: Siemens ECAT 933 (CTI, Knoxville, TN) or the newer GE Advance (General Electric Medical Systems, Milwaukee, WI). Some patients underwent a second imaging session with a hybrid dual-head gamma camera operating in the coincidence mode (VG Millenium, General Electric Medical Systems, Milwaukee, WI). The gamma camera is equipped with an X-ray tube and array of detectors mounted on the gantry of the camera functioning basically as a third generation CT scanner. The acquisition protocols were the following:

Siemens ECAT 933: Dedicated PET

Transmission scan: before FDG administration, field of view including neck, chest, abdomen, and pelvis, 5 minutes per bed position.

Emission scan: 2D mode, field of view including neck, chest, abdomen, and pelvis, extremities when indicated, 15 minutes per bed position with sections of 8 mm in thickness.

Image reconstruction: filtered back projection with measured attenuation correction.

GE Advance: Dedicated PET

Emission scan: 2D mode, field of view including neck, chest, abdomen, and pelvis; extremities when indicated; 5 minutes per bed position with sections of 4.25 mm in thickness (coronal and sagittal images shown are summed to 8.5 mm in thickness).

Transmission scan: 2D mode, after the emission scan, 2 minutes per bed position.

Image reconstruction: iterative reconstruction with measured segmented attenuation correction.

VG Millenium: Hybrid PET

Transmission scan: X-ray transmission maps, 9 minutes per bed position.

Emission scan: 2D mode, 20 cm field of view over the region of interest, 35 minutes per bed position.

Image reconstruction: iterative reconstruction with measured attenuation correction.

Image fusion: The X-ray attenuation maps provide hybrid CT images for image fusion and anatomical mapping.

References

1. Cook GJR, Fogelman I, Maisey MN: Normal physiological and benign pathological variants of 18-fluoro-2-deoxyglucose positron emission tomography scanning: Potential for error in interpretation. Semin Nucl Med 1996;26:308–314.
2. Engel H, Steinert H, Buck A, Berthold T, Boni RAH, von Schulthess GK: Whole body PET: Physiological and artifactual fluorodeoxyglucose accumulations. J Nucl Med 1996;37:441–446.
3. Bakheet SM, Powe J: Benign causes of 18-FDG uptake on whole body imaging. Semin Nucl Med 1998;28(4):352–358.
4. Patel PM, Alibazoglu H, Ali A, Fordham E, Lamonica G: Normal thymic uptake of FDG on PET imaging. Clinical Nucl Med 1996;21:772–775.
5. Barrington SF, Maisey MN: Skeletal muscle uptake of fluorine-18-FDG: Effect of oral diazepam. J Nucl Med 1996;37:1127–1129.
6. Bakheet SMB, Powe J, Ezzat A, Rostom Al: F-18-FDG uptake in tuberculosis. Clin Nucl Med 1998;23:739–742.
7. Lewis PJ, Salama A: Uptake of fluorine-18-fluorodeoxyglucose in sarcoidosis. J Nucl Med 1994;35:1647–1649.

8. Kubota R, Yamada S, Kubota K, Ishiwata K, Tamahashi N, Ido T: Intratumoral distribution of fluorine-18-fluorodeoxyglucose in vivo: High accumulation in macrophages and granulocytes studied by microautoradiography. J Nucl Med 1992;33:1972–1980.
9. Kalicke T, Schmitz A, Risse JH, et al.: Fluorine-18 fluorodeoxyglucose PET in infectious bone diseases: Results of histologically confirmed cases. Eur J Nucl Med 2000;27(5):524–528.
10. Sugawara Y, Braun DK, Kison PV, Russo JE, Zasadny KR, Wahl RL: Rapid detection of human infections with fluorine-18 fluorodeoxyglucose and positron emission tomography: Preliminary results. Eur J Nucl Med 1998;25(9):1238–1243.
11. Robiller FC, Stumpe KD, Kossmann T, Weisshaupt D, Bruder E, von Schulthess GK: Chronic osteomyelitis of the femur: Value of PET imaging. Eur Radiol 2000;10(5):855–858.
12. Guhlmann A, Brecht-Krauss D, Suger G, Glatting G, Kotzerke J, Kinzl L, Reske SN: Chronic osteomyelitis: Detection with FDG PET and correlation with histopathologic findings. Radiology 1998;206(3):749–754.
13. Schulte M, Brechte-Krauss D, Heymer B, et al.: Grading of tumors and tumor-like lesions of bone: Evaluation by FDG-PET. J Nucl Med 2000;41:1695–1701.
14. Stadalnik RC: Benign causes of 18-FDG uptake on whole body imaging. Semin Nucl Med 1998; 28:352–358.

Case Presentations

Case 6.1.1

History

A 10-year-old female was diagnosed with Hodgkin's disease and treated with chemotherapy. Four months after completion of therapy, a CT scan (Figure 6.1.1A), ^{67}gallium scintigraphy (Figures 6.1.1B, C, and D), and FDG imaging (Figure 6.1.1E) were performed during the follow-up. For ^{67}gallium scintigraphy, anterior and posterior planar images are shown in Figure 6.1.1B, and coronal and transaxial SPECT images are shown in Figures 6.1.1C and D, respectively. Figure 6.1.1E shows coronal FDG PET images acquired with a dedicated PET tomograph (GE Advance) and reconstructed with iterative reconstruction and measured segmented attenuation correction.

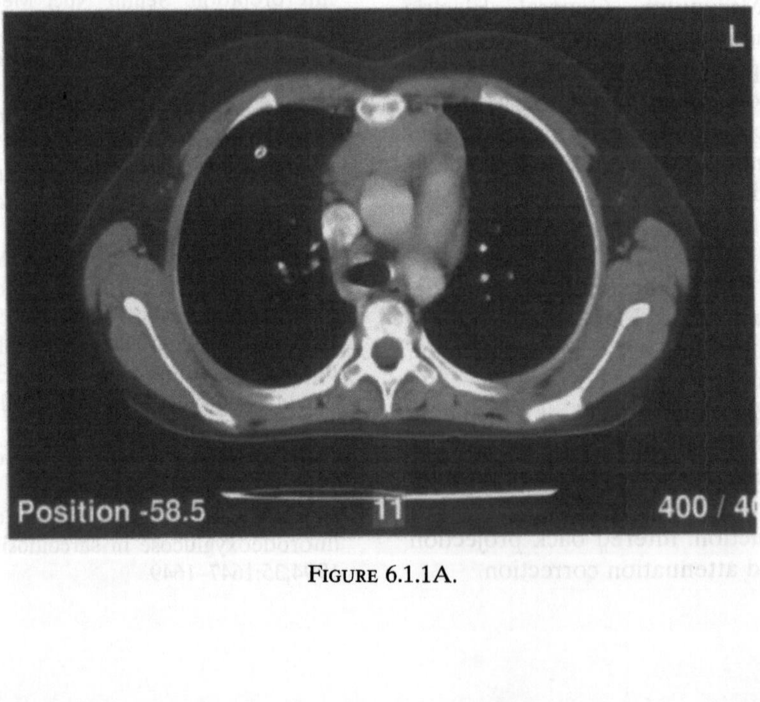

FIGURE 6.1.1A.

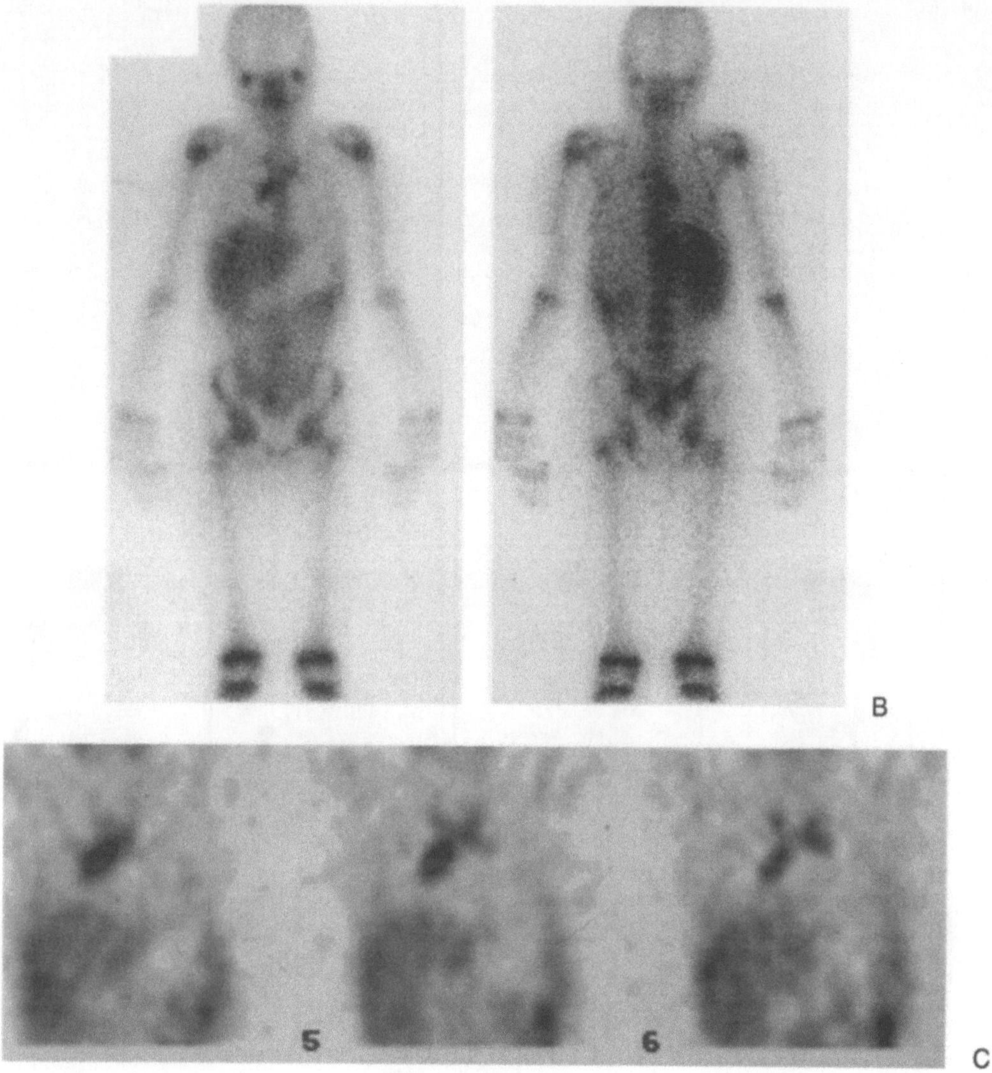

FIGURE 6.1.1B,C.

Findings

The CT scan demonstrates a residual mass in the mediastinum. The ^{67}gallium images show two focal areas of increased uptake in the right hilar area and left paratracheal region of the mediastinum and also an equivocal focus of increased activity in the right pelvis.

The FDG images show mildly increased activity in the anterior mediastinum bilaterally with the configuration of a normal thymus. The standard uptake value (SUV) of this area is 1.1 to 1.3, essentially identical to the SUV within the liver. Mild physiologic myocardial uptake is a useful anatomical landmark. The uptake in the left antecubital fossa is due to dose infiltra-

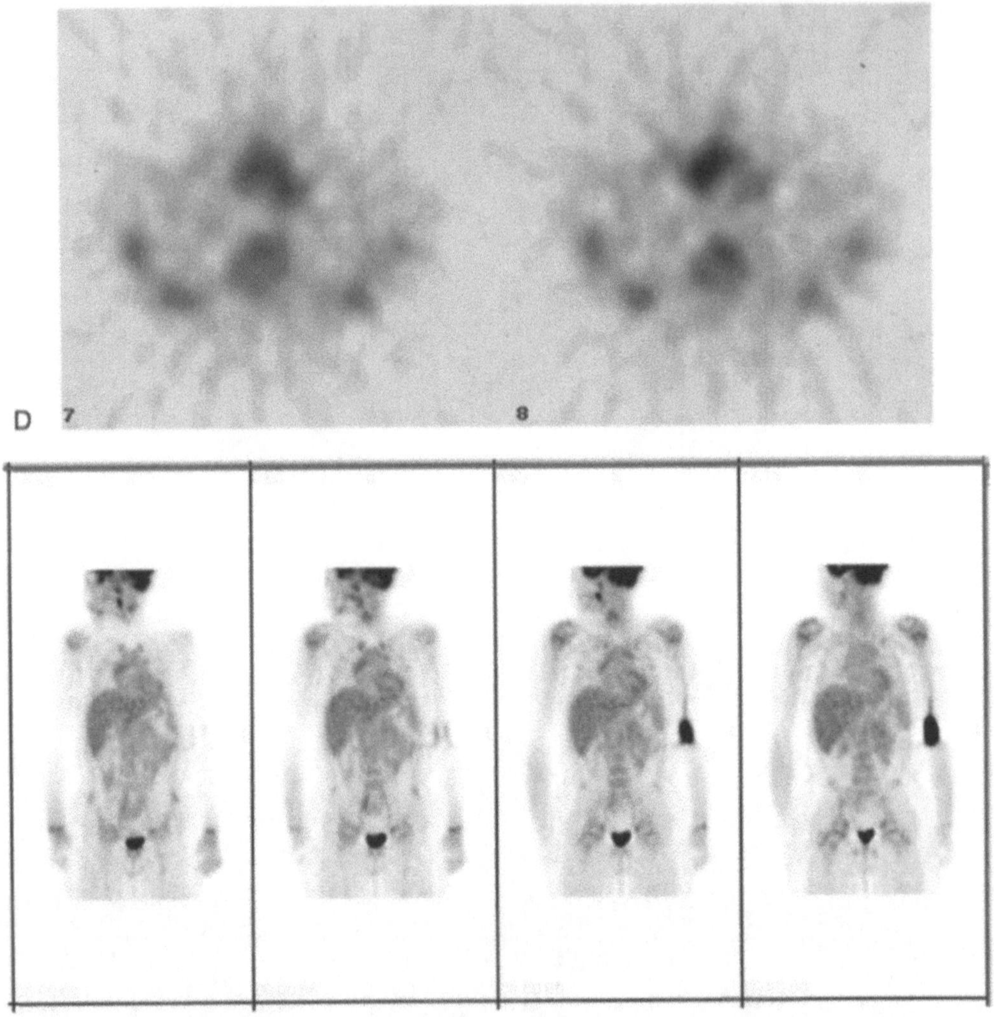

FIGURE 6.1.1D,E.

tion in the subcutaneous tissues. Mild uptake on the midline of the neck probably represents uptake in the laryngeal muscles, and this was verified on the transaxial images. There is also a small, tubular focus of moderately increased activity in the right lower quadrant of the abdomen, thought to be bowel uptake, and not corresponding to the focus of increased activity seen in the pelvis on the ^{67}gallium scan.

Discussion

The thymus is of maximal size and function[1,2] about the time of birth and begins its involution during the first years of life progressing to fatty infiltration around puberty.[3] In children, the thymus demonstrates variable uptake of ^{67}gallium with up to 15% of children under 5 years and 11% of children over 5 years showing ^{67}gallium thymic uptake. Thymic hyperplasia with accompanying increased ^{67}gallium uptake occurs in up to 43% of children (and in some adults) following chemotherapy for lymphoma.[4] The duration of increased activity ranges from 2 to 59 months. Unfortunately, the low resolution of the ^{67}gallium scintigraphy can make it difficult to differentiate homogenous physiologic uptake in the thymus from the irregular or bulky uptake seen in mediastinal malignant lymphadenopathy. Normal thymic tissue can accumulate FDG.[5–7] Physiological thymic FDG uptake has been reported up to the age of 13[5] or even up to the age of 54.[6] Usually, the thymus has a mild to moderate FDG uptake, with SUV values of approximately 1.4.[5] In this case, the superior resolution of the FDG PET images allowed identification of the typical morphology of the thymus, which demonstrated only mildly increased FDG uptake with an SUV of 1.1 to 1.3; no abnormal uptake was observed that would indicate residual or recurrent Hodgkin's disease.

Diagnoses

1. Rebound thymic hyperplasia.
2. No evidence of residual lymphoma.

References

1. Francis IR, Glazer GM, Bookstein FL, et al.: The thymus: Reexamination of age-related changes in size and shape. Am J Roentgenol 1985;145(2): 249–254.
2. Steinmann GG: Changes in the human thymus during aging. Curr Top Pathol 1986;75:43.
3. Baron RL, Lee JKT, Sagel SS, et al.: Computed tomography of the normal thymus. Radiology 1982;142:121.
4. Donahue DM, Leonard JC, Basmadjian GP, et al.: Thymic gallium-67 localization in pediatrics patients. J Nucl Med 1981;22:1043–1048.
5. Patel PM, Alibazoglu H, Ali A, et al.: Normal thymic uptake of FDG on PET imaging. Clin Nucl Med 1996;21:772–775.
6. Alibazoglu H, Alibazoglu B, Hollinger EF, et al.: Normal thymic uptake of 2-deoxy-2[F-18]fluoro-D-glucose. Clin Nucl Med 1999;24:597–600.
7. Rini JN, Leonidas JC, Tomas MB, et al.: FDG uptake in the anterior mediastinum: Physiologic thymic uptake or disease? Clin Pos Imag 2000; 3:115–125.

Case 6.1.2

History

A 78-year-old diabetic white male presented with a CT scan demonstrating three hypodense hepatic lesions suggestive of metastases. He had undergone a colectomy five years ago for colon carcinoma, followed by chemotherapy and radiation therapy. A CT guided biopsy of one of the lesions in the left lobe of the liver was positive for metastasis. FDG PET imaging was performed for staging. Figure 6.1.2 shows coronal FDG images acquired with a dedicated PET tomograph (GE Advance) and reconstructed with iterative reconstruction and measured segmented attenuation correction. Prior to the FDG injection, the patient's serum glucose was over 260 mg/dl. Repeated doses of regular insulin were administered intravenously to a total of 52 units. The FDG was administered when the patient's serum glucose was 135 mg/dl.

Findings

Physiologic activity is identified within the myocardium, bowel, liver, and renal collecting system. There are three foci of increased uptake in the liver corresponding to the lesions identified on CT. The most intense lesion located in the right lobe posteriorly is in the field of view of the images shown. There is diffuse intense muscular uptake bilaterally noted. No extrahepatic focal abnormalities are present.

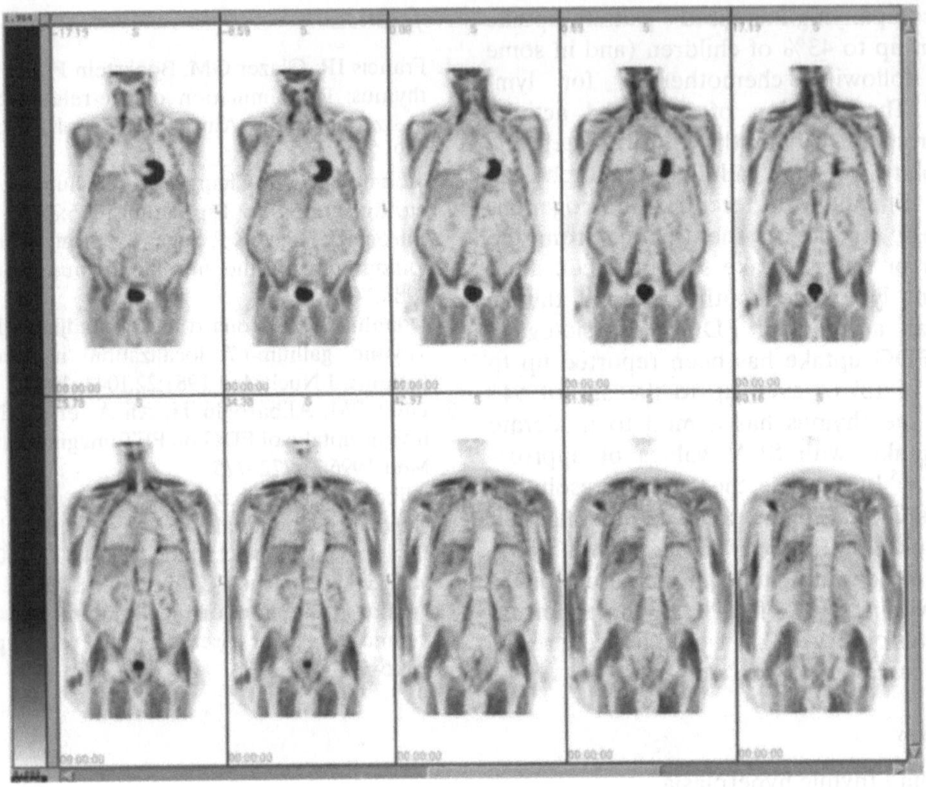

FIGURE 6.1.2.

Discussion

In patients with poorly controlled diabetes, hyperglycemia represents a limitation for the sensitivity of FDG PET imaging because the excess of plasma glucose competes with FDG and consequently reduces FDG uptake in tumors by up to 50%.[1–5] Therefore, control of glycemia in diabetic patients and overnight fasting in normal patients are essential for good quality FDG images. The blood sugar level should always be measured before FDG administration. Commonly, patients with diabetes present with hyperglycemia because they have been instructed to fast overnight and have not appropriately adjusted their therapy. Furthermore, unrecognized diabetes is not uncommon in elderly patients with malignancies. Insulin administration prior to FDG injection promotes FDG uptake by skeletal muscle and myocardium,[6–9] and makes FDG less available for tumor uptake. Therefore, the sensitivity for detection of metastatic disease is decreased. Delaying the FDG injection for several hours after injection of insulin may help but is not practical for patient throughput. Early morning scheduling of diabetic patients for optimal glycemic control prior to the PET appointment is preferable.

Diagnoses

1. Liver metastases.
2. Presence of extrahepatic involvement is suboptimally assessed due to interfering hyperglycemia.
3. Increased muscular uptake of FDG due to insulin administration.

References

1. Torizuka T, Clavo AC, Wahl RL: Effect of hyperglycemia on in vitro tumor uptake of tritiated FDG, thymidine, L-methionine and L-leucine. J Nucl Med 1997;38(3):382–386.
2. Cremerius U, Bares R, Weis J, et al.: Fasting improves discrimination of grade 1 and atypical or malignant meningioma in FDG-PET. J Nucl Med 1997;38(1):26–30.
3. Minn H, Leskinen-Kallio S, Lindholm P, et al.: [18F]fluorodeoxyglucose uptake in tumors: Kinetic vs. steady-state methods with reference to plasma insulin. J Comput Assist Tomogr 1993;17(1):115–123.
4. Lindholm P, Minn H, Leskinen-Kallio S, et al.: Influence of the blood glucose concentration on FDG uptake in cancer—a PET study. J Nucl Med 1993;34(1):1–6.
5. Wahl RL, Henry CA, Ethier SP: Serum glucose: Effects on tumor and normal tissue accumulation of 2-[F-18]-fluoro-2-deoxy-D-glucose in rodents with mammary carcinoma. Radiology 1992;183(3):643–647.
6. Torizuka T, Fisher SJ, Brown RS, et al.: Effect of insulin on uptake of FDG by experimental mammary carcinoma in diabetic rats. Radiology 1998;208(2):499–504.
7. Torizuka T, Fisher SJ, Wahl RL: Insulin-induced hypoglycemia decreases uptake of 2-[F-18]fluoro-2-deoxy-D-glucose into experimental mammary carcinoma. Radiology 1997;203(1):169–172 .
8. Huitink JM, Visser FC, van Leeuwen GR, et al.: Influence of high and low plasma insulin levels on the uptake of fluorine-18 fluorodeoxyglucose in myocardium and femoral muscle, assessed by planar imaging. Eur J Nucl Med 1995;22(10):1141–1148.
9. Shreve PD, Anzai Y, Wahl R: Pitfalls in oncologic diagnosis with FDG PET imaging: Physiologic and benign variants. Radiographics 1999;19:61–77.

Case 6.1.3

History

A 58-year-old male was diagnosed with squamous cell carcinoma of the tongue eight months ago by biopsy. He was treated with chemotherapy and radiation therapy until four months ago. A CT scan performed four months ago was remarkable for a marked interval improvement of the anterior tongue mass and bilateral cervical lymph nodes. Figure 6.1.3 shows coronal FDG PET images acquired with a dedicated PET tomograph (GE Advance) and reconstructed with iterative reconstruction and measured segmented attenuation correction (Figure 6.1.3A) and with filtered back projection without attenuation correction (Figure 6.1.3B).

Findings

FDG PET images show physiologic activity within the myocardium, bowel, liver, and renal collecting system, without focal abnormalities in the head and neck region. Regions of photopenia in the bilateral hips are consistent with bilateral hip prostheses. Increased activity around the bilateral hip prostheses proximally is much less intense on the images obtained without attenuation correction. Physiologic uptake is also noted in the myocardium, the wall of the stomach, and in the renal pelves and ureters bilaterally. Ureteral uptake should not be confused with retroperitoneal lymph node metastases on the transaxial images.

Discussion

Areas of increased activity are identified surrounding both hip prostheses in the images with attenuation correction and to a lesser degree in the images without attenuation correction. This is consistent with inflammatory changes related to prosthetic loosening that may have been amplified on the attenuation-corrected images by slight misregistration artifact due to patient motion.

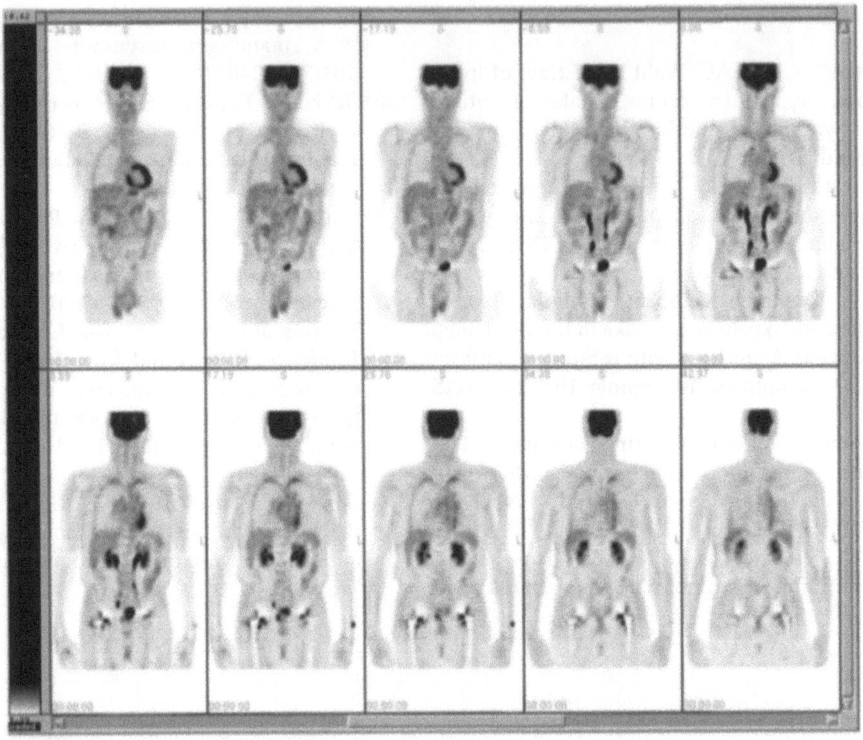

A

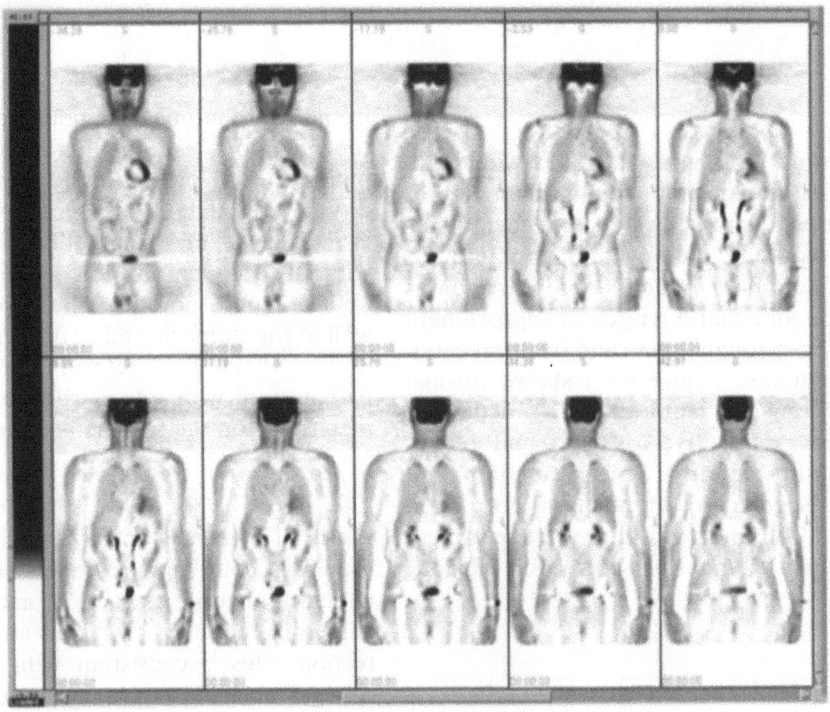

B

FIGURE 6.1.3A,B.

There is recent evidence in the literature that FDG PET may have a role in the evaluation of patients with limb prostheses.[1] Increased uptake at the bone-prosthesis interface suggests an infection. For hip prostheses, if the uptake is limited to an area around the femoral head or neck portion of the prosthesis, loosening is more likely; if the uptake extends to the femoral shaft, infection is more likely. Using these criteria, the sensitivity and specificity of FDG PET imaging for detection of prosthetic infection were 90% and 81%, respectively in a study of 74 prostheses in 62 patients. The final diagnosis was obtained by surgical exploration in 43 patients and one-year follow-up in 19 patients.[1] The absence of FDG activity along the femoral component of the prosthesis in this patient is evidence against a diagnosis of osteomyelitis.

The topic of attenuation correction (AC) has been discussed by R. L. Wahl.[2] It has been demonstrated that attenuation effects are much more significant in coincidence imaging than in SPECT since both photons from an annihilation process must pass through the region without interaction. Attenuation effects in coincidence imaging produce regional nonuniformities, distortions of intense structures, and edge effects. A phantom study comparing FDG imaging of lung nodules with SPECT, camera-based PET, and dedicated PET has demonstrated that correction for these attenuation artifacts improves the quality of the images and increases image contrast.[3]

Correction for attenuation effects can be performed using calculated geometric attenuation for uniform structures that are predictable in shape and content, such as the brain. Calculated attenuation correction can be used very accurately and is patient-independent. This is not the case for body images because of the variability of the body habitus in different patients and the asymmetry of internal organs. For the body, various methods have been developed with measured attenuation using radioactive transmission sources. Measured attenuation correction is commonly performed by direct measurement of 511 keV photon attenuation through the body. It can also be performed using X-ray attenuation maps. The quality of the image corrected for attenuation largely depends on precise registration of the transmission and emission scans. Acquiring a transmission scan prolongs the study and often requires repositioning of the patient in the gantry of the tomograph, which contributes to registration problems and noise in the corrected images. Motion of the patients during long scanning times is a problem as well. With older models of PET scanners (for example, Siemens ECAT 933), the transmission scan had to be acquired prior to FDG injection, necessitating complex laser repositioning systems for emission image acquisition. Therefore, the images with attenuation correction are noisy if there is an error in repositioning the patient, and when this is the case, the findings are more easily seen on images without attenuation correction. In the newer generation of PET scanners (for example, GE Advance), the transmission scan can be acquired sequentially after FDG administration, requiring correction for the FDG activity in the patient but avoiding error when repositioning the patient. In addition, the attenuation correction is based on body segmentation.

The conventional reconstruction algorithm using filtered back projection amplifies the statistical noise that adversely affects image quality. New algorithms using iterative reconstruction have been developed for coincidence imaging that provide good signal to noise ratio in a timely fashion. The emission scan can be reconstructed using an iterative reconstruction algorithm based on the ordered subsets estimation maximization (OSEM) algorithm. State of the art PET scanners and hybrid PET gamma cameras have software allowing reconstruction of the images with an iterative reconstruction algorithm.

To obtain the FDG images shown in this case, transmission images were obtained using rotating pin sources of germanium-68 just after the emission scan without moving the patient from the scanning bed. Perfect registration between the emission images and the transmission images relies on similar positioning of the patient in the gantry of the scanner during the acquisition of the two imaging sessions. Often there is some motion of the patient during the long scanning period, even if the patient is not repositioned between transmission and emission scanning; this is particularly true for the head and neck. If a finding on AC images is equivocal or unexplained, its presence should be confirmed on images not corrected for attenuation.

Diagnoses

1. Bilateral hip prostheses with probable inflammatory changes.
2. No abnormal foci of FDG activity are identified in the oropharynx or otherwise to suggest the presence of recurrent or metastatic disease. These findings are consistent with a good response to therapy.

References

1. Zhuang H, Duarte PS, Pourdehnad M, et al.: The promising role of 18FDG PET in detecting infected lower limb prosthesis implants. J Nucl Med 2001;42:44–48.
2. Wahl RL: To AC or not to AC: That is the question. J Nucl Med 1999;40:2025–2027.
3. Coleman RE, Laymon CM, Turkington TG: FDG imaging of lung nodules: A phantom study comparing SPECT, camera-based PET, and dedicated PET. Radiology 1999;210:823–828.

Case 6.1.4

History

A 46-year-old female presented with a three-month history of left hip pain. She had a malignant melanoma resected from the right upper arm three years earlier, and the sentinel lymph node in the right axilla was not involved by tumor. She was referred for FDG PET imaging (Figure 6.1.4A). The patient was scheduled for another FDG PET scan the following week (Figure 6.1.4B). Both figures show coronal FDG PET images acquired with a dedicated PET tomograph (GE Advance) and reconstructed with iterative reconstruction and measured segmented attenuation correction.

Findings

FDG PET images (Figure 6.1.4A) show dramatically increased FDG accumulation within the skeletal musculature of the neck, upper extremities, shoulder girdle, and lower extremities. Physiological activity is also seen within the renal collecting system and the left ventricular myocardium. No focal abnormalities are identified.

The history obtained after the PET scan indicated that the patient exercises, on a regular basis, both upper and lower extremities as well as the abdomen and back. Due to the markedly increased diffuse muscular uptake, the sensitivity for detection of hypermetabolic foci of neoplasm may be diminished. Therefore, the patient was scheduled for repeat FDG PET imaging. She was instructed not to exercise for 48 hours and was administered 10 mg of diazepam orally, 30 minutes before FDG administration. The second set of FDG images (Figure 6.1.4B) shows resolution of the excessive muscle activity seen on the prior scan, and no evidence of metastatic disease is present. The left ventricular myocardium is now just faintly visualized.

Discussion

These FDG PET images are an extraordinary example of exercise-induced muscular uptake of FDG. The enhanced uptake of glucose into muscle during exercise is well-recognized. The mechanism for the increased uptake is not entirely clear but appears to be distinct from the one involved with the regulation of glucose metabolism by insulin.[1] Possibly, increased blood flow and the translocation and activation of protein carriers in response to calcium

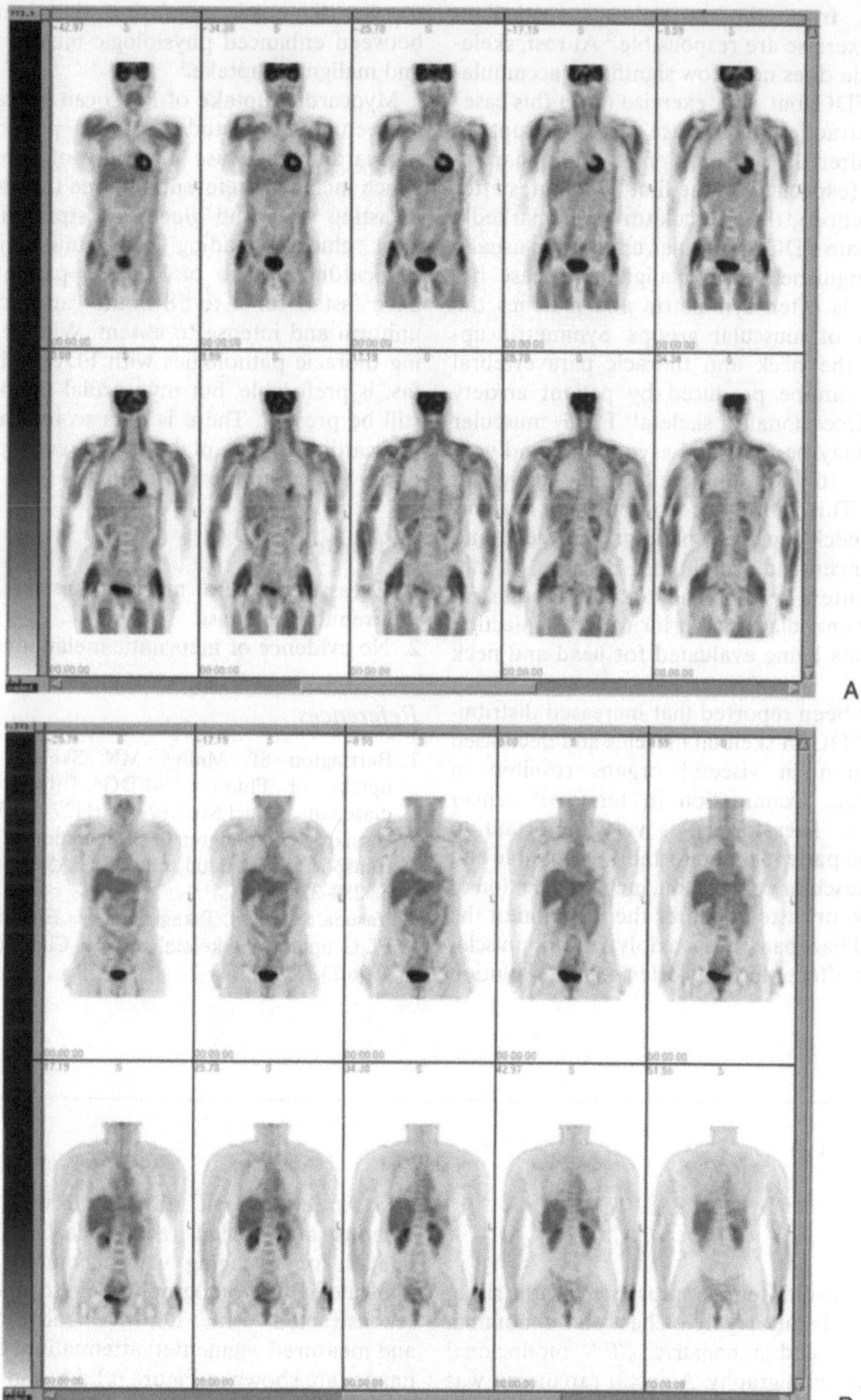

FIGURE 6.1.4A,B.

released from the sarcoplasmic reticulum during exercise are responsible.[2] At rest, skeletal muscle does not show significant accumulation of FDG, but after exercise (as in this case) or if contraction takes place during the uptake period after the injection of the radiopharmaceutical (especially in the first 30 minutes after the injection), the musculature can markedly accumulate FDG.[3] Muscular uptake can usually be distinguished from malignant disease because it is often symmetric and matches the anatomy of muscular groups. Symmetric uptake in the neck and thoracic paravertebral regions can be produced by patient anxiety alone. Occasionally, skeletal FDG muscular uptake may be focal and asymmetric and very difficult to differentiate from malignant lesions.[1] This is of most concern when evaluating the neck region of patients with head and neck cancer and lymphoma. Because of this, some centers recommend routine administration of benzodiazepine prior to FDG injection in patients being evaluated for head and neck cancer.

It has been reported that increased distribution of FDG in skeletal muscles and decreased distribution in visceral organs resulted in incomplete examination in terms of cancer detection. Therefore, it is very important to make the patient as comfortable as possible and avoid muscular contraction, including flexion of the neck, prior to and after the injection of the tracer. Diazepam has anxiolytic and muscle-relaxant effects and may offer a simple solution to the diagnostic confusion that can arise between enhanced physiologic muscle uptake and malignant uptake.[1]

Myocardial uptake of FDG can be variable, as seen in both studies of this patient. The myocardium can use a variety of substrates, which includes preferentially free fatty acids in a fasting state and glucose postprandially or after glucose loading or insulin injection. Myocardial uptake of FDG in patients who have fasted for 4 to 18 hours can vary from uniform and intense to absent. When evaluating thoracic pathologies with FDG, a 12-hour fast is preferable, but myocardial uptake may still be present. There is data to indicate that myocardial FDG uptake is indirectly proportional to the duration of fasting.

Diagnoses

1. Excessive skeletal muscular uptake due to strenuous exercise.
2. No evidence of metastatic melanoma.

References

1. Barrington SF, Maisey MN: Skeletal muscle uptake of Fluorine-18-FDG: Effect of oral diazepam. J Nucl Med 1996;37:1127–1129.
2. Barnard RJ, Youngren JF: Regulation of glucose transport in skeletal muscle. FASEB J 1992; 6:3238–3244.
3. Yasuda S, Ide M, Takagi S, et al.: Elevated F-18 FDG uptake in skeletal muscle. Clin Nucl Med 1998;23:111–112.

Case 6.1.5

History

A 67-year-old female presented with rising CEA levels but negative chest and abdominal CT scans and a negative CEA monoclonal antibody scintigraphy. A rectal carcinoma was resected three years earlier and was followed by neoadjuvant chemotherapy and radiotherapy. An endoscopic ultrasound with biopsy demonstrated rectal recurrence. FDG PET images for restaging were acquired with a dedicated PET tomograph (GE Advance) and reconstructed with iterative reconstruction and measured segmented attenuation. Coronal images are shown in Figure 6.1.5A, and orthogonal images through the neck are shown in Figure 6.1.5B.

A

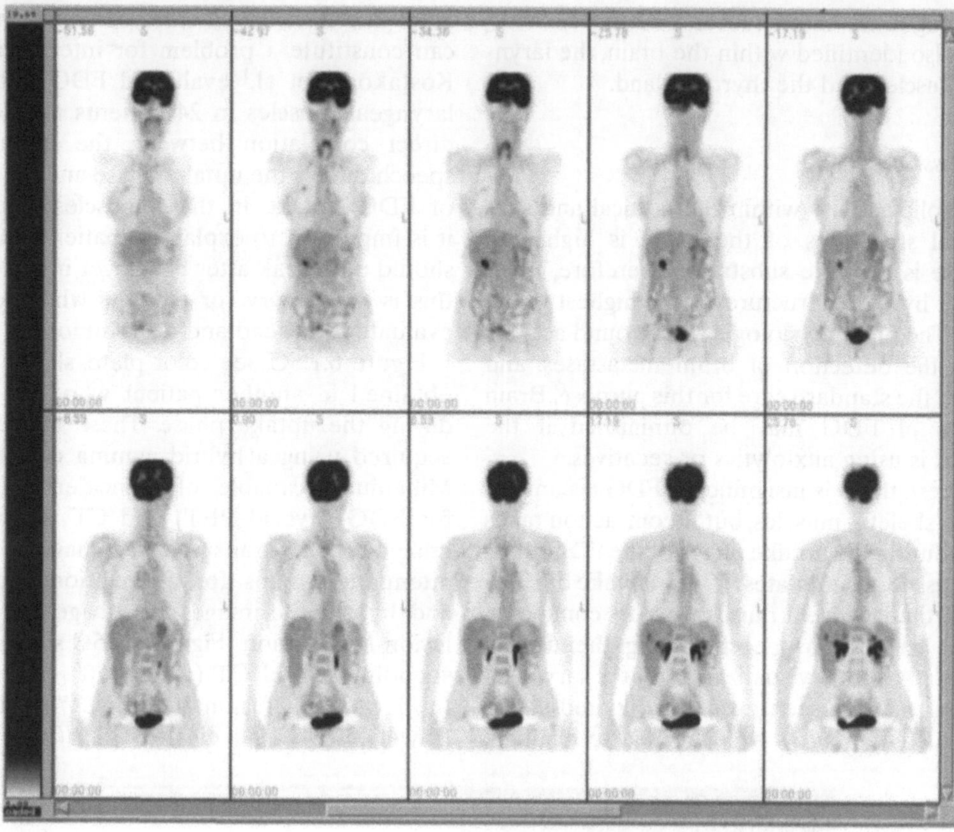

B

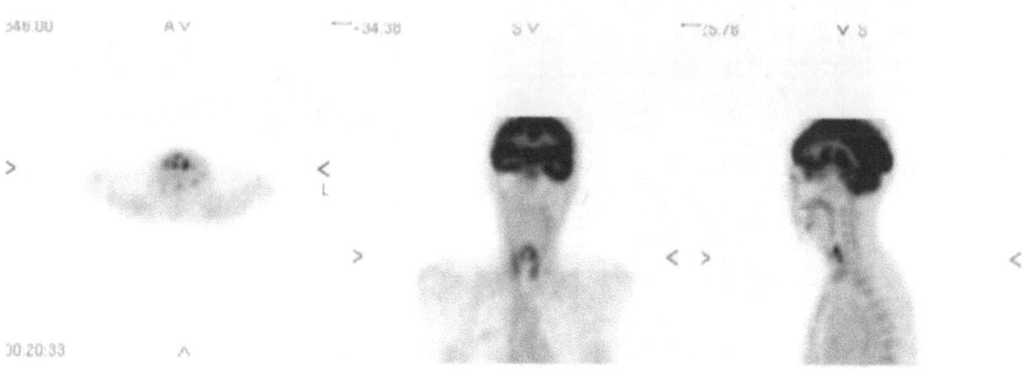

FIGURE 6.1.5A,B.

Findings

The FDG PET images show three foci of increased activity in the liver, one large focus of increased activity anteriorly and two smaller foci in the posterior aspect of the right lobe. Furthermore, there is also a small focus of moderately increased activity in the right anterior mid-lung field. There was also a large focus of intensely increased activity posterior to the bladder in the left pararectal region (not in the field of view of the images shown), corresponding to the known local recurrence. Activity is also identified within the brain, the laryngeal muscles, and the thyroid gland.

Discussion

Metabolic activity within the cortical and subcortical structures of the brain is high, and glucose is the sole substrate. Therefore, FDG uptake by these structures is the highest in the body. The high physiologic background activity limits the detection of brain metastases, and MRI is the standard care for this purpose. Brain uptake of FDG may be diminished if the patient is using anxiolytics or sedatives.

At rest, there is insignificant FDG accumulation in skeletal muscles, but if contraction takes place during the uptake phase of the FDG, muscular tissue accumulates FDG.[1] Uptake of FDG within the laryngeal muscles occurs commonly and is related to speech during the uptake phase.[1,2] A subtle visualization of the laryngeal muscles may be seen even with limited vocalization. If the study is performed to evaluate head and neck carcinomas or lymphoma, this can constitute a problem for interpretation.[1,2] Kostakoglu et al.[1] evaluated FDG uptake by laryngeal muscles in 24 patients and found a direct correlation between the intensity of speech during the uptake phase and the degree of FDG uptake in these muscles. Therefore, it is important to explain to patients that they should not speak after the tracer injection, and this is mandatory for patients who are being evaluated for head and neck tumors.

Figure 6.1.5C, see color plate, shows images obtained in another patient who was talking during the uptake phase. These images were acquired using a hybrid gamma camera (VG Millenium) capable of coincidence imaging for FDG (hybrid PET) and CT transmission imaging. CT transmission images provide attenuation maps for attenuation correction and hybrid CT images for image fusion and lesion localization. Figure 6.1.5C shows corresponding hybrid CT (upper left), hybrid PET (upper right), fusion hybrid CT/hybrid PET (lower left), and dedicated PET (lower right)

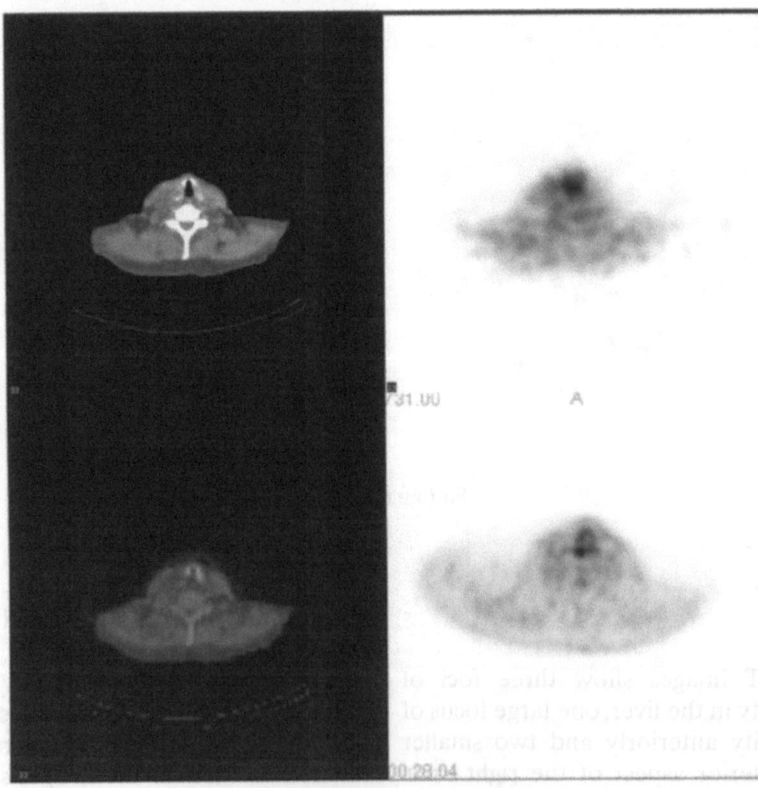

FIGURE 6.1.5C. (See color plate)

images in that patient. The hybrid FDG PET images are noisier than the dedicated PET images, and the characteristic curvilinear shape of uptake cannot be clearly recognized. However, the fusion image demonstrates exact superimposition of the focus of uptake in the neck over the vocal cords on the CT transmission images. This second case demonstrates the advantages of CT transmission images on the hybrid gamma camera to differentiate physiologic from pathologic uptake.

Diffuse thyroid uptake may be a normal variant,[2] but it can also be seen in autoimmune thyroiditis[3] or Graves' disease.[4] It has been reported that one-third of clinically euthyroid patients who were being investigated for other reasons demonstrated FDG uptake in both lobes of the thyroid gland, but other investigators have reported that normal thyroid glands are virtually never visualized by FDG PET. The mechanism of FDG uptake by the thyroid gland is not known. Lymphocytic infiltration is a histological characteristic of chronic thyroiditis, and this may explain FDG uptake in this pathologic process.[4] In Graves' disease, the increased FDG uptake may follow a mechanism similar to that of uptake in chronic thyroiditis, as both are autoimmune diseases, but it may also be impacted by the increased flow seen in these glands and is proportional to the percentage of radioiodine uptake.[4]

Diagnoses

1. Physiologic uptake within the laryngeal muscles, related to talking during the uptake phase.
2. Physiologic uptake in the thyroid gland.
3. Three hypermetabolic areas within the liver are most consistent with metastatic disease. The local recurrence at the resection site is hypermetabolic (not shown).
4. The right middle lobe hypermetabolic lung lesion is most consistent with metastatic disease also, although a second primary neoplasm and granulomatous disease cannot be excluded without biopsy.

References

1. Kostakoglu L, Wong JCH, Barrington SF, et al.: Speech-related visualization of laryngeal muscles with fluorine-18-FDG. J Nucl Med 1996;37:1711–1773.
2. Yasuda S, Shohtsu A, Ide M, et al.: Chronic thyroiditis: Diffuse uptake of FDG at PET. Radiology 1998;207:775–778.
3. Santiago JFY, Jana S, El-Zeftawy H, et al.: Increased F-18 fluorodeoxyglucose thyroidal uptake in Graves' disease. Clin Nucl Med 1999;24(9):714–715.
4. Conti PS, Durski JM, Singer PA, et al.: Incidence of thyroid gland uptake of F-18 FDG in cancer patients, abstracted. Radiology 1997;205(P):220.

Case 6.1.6

History

A 44-year-old male was diagnosed with retroperitoneal lymphoma six months earlier and was treated with chemotherapy but no radiation therapy. He was found to have a residual retroperitoneal mass on CT scan following completion of chemotherapy. FDG PET imaging was performed to differentiate residual viable tumor from scar tissue (Figure 6.1.6). Orthogonal FDG images through the gastric region are shown. These images were acquired with a dedicated PET tomograph (GE Advance) and reconstructed with iterative reconstruction and measured segmented attenuation correction.

Findings

The FDG PET images show physiologic uptake in the myocardium and in the gastrointestinal and genitourinary tracts. Uptake in the wall of

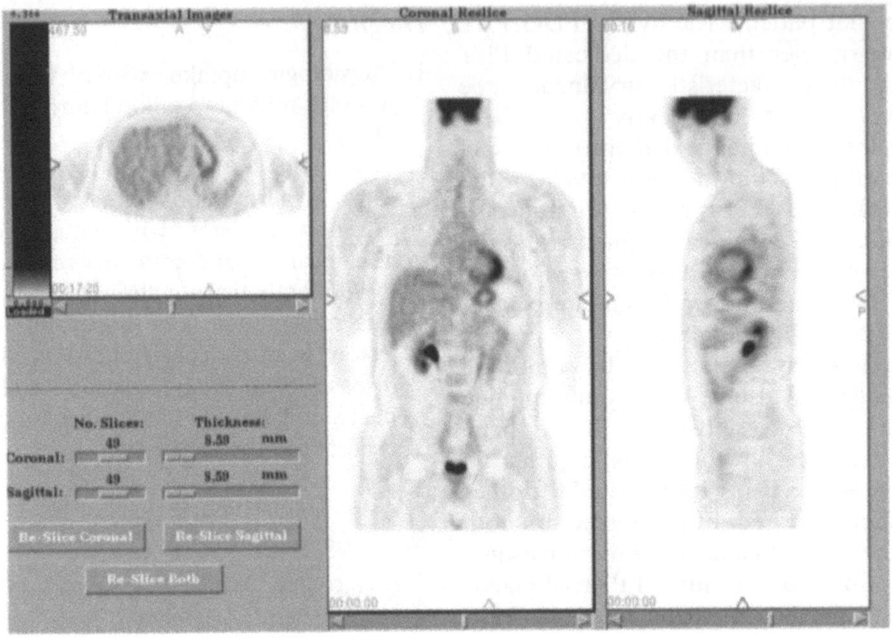

FIGURE 6.1.6.

the stomach is particularly well-demonstrated in this patient. It appears as a doughnut below the heart on the coronal images and is well outlined between the liver and spleen on the transverse image. No abnormal uptake is seen corresponding to the residual mass in the retroperitoneum.

Discussion

The absence of FDG activity congruent with the mass seen on CT is indicative of a good response to therapy and is associated with a good outcome.

As with any other radiopharmaceutical, it is extremely important to be familiar with the biodistribution of FDG, physiologic variations of FDG uptake, and benign conditions that accumulate FDG to perform accurate interpretation of the images. The gastrointestinal tract can have variable FDG uptake, and the wall of the stomach is usually faintly seen and can be used as an anatomical landmark. No luminal activity is seen, and the stomach wall uptake typically gives a ring appearance on coronal images. However, it is not clear whether the FDG uptake accumulates in the smooth muscles or into other layers of the gastric mucosa. This pattern could be confused with lesions with a necrotic center, but the left hypochondrial location and the relatively horizontal position on sagittal views allow correct identification of this organ. Some conditions such as gastritis[1] or nausea and vomiting[2] can lead to a more prominent uptake. Gastric uptake appears more intense when the stomach is contracted.

Due to the high sensitivity of dedicated PET imaging systems and their high resolution, it is relatively simple to discern physiologic gastrointestinal activity from neoplastic activity, as compared to ^{67}gallium scintigraphy and FDG images acquired with hybrid PET gamma cameras that have a lower sensitivity.

Diagnoses

1. Physiologic uptake in the wall of the stomach.
2. No abnormal uptake of FDG, indicating a good response to therapy.

References

1. Nunez RF, Yeung HWD, Macapinlack H: Increased F-18 FDG uptake in the stomach. Clin Nucl Med 2000;25(9):676–678.
2. Abdel-Dayem HM, Naddaf S, El-Zeftawy H: F-18 FDG gastric and anterior muscle uptake secondary to nausea and vomiting. Clin Nucl Med 1998;23(11):769–770.

Case 6.1.7

History

A 14-year-old male diagnosed with Hodgkin's disease five months earlier was referred for FDG PET imaging to evaluate the response to chemotherapy (Figures 6.1.7A and B). Coronal FDG PET images (Figure 6.1.7A) and orthogonal images through the spine (Figure 6.1.7B) are shown. The FDG PET images were acquired with a dedicated PET tomograph (GE Advance) and reconstructed with iterative reconstruction and measured segmented attenuation correction.

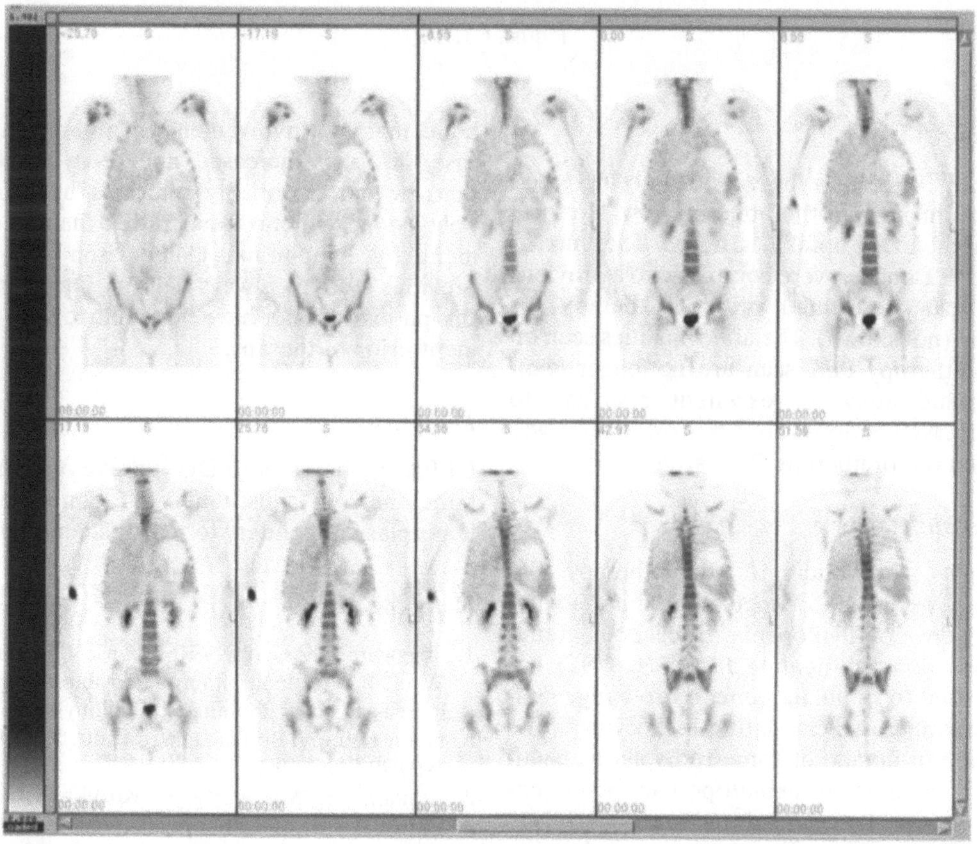

FIGURE 6.1.7A.

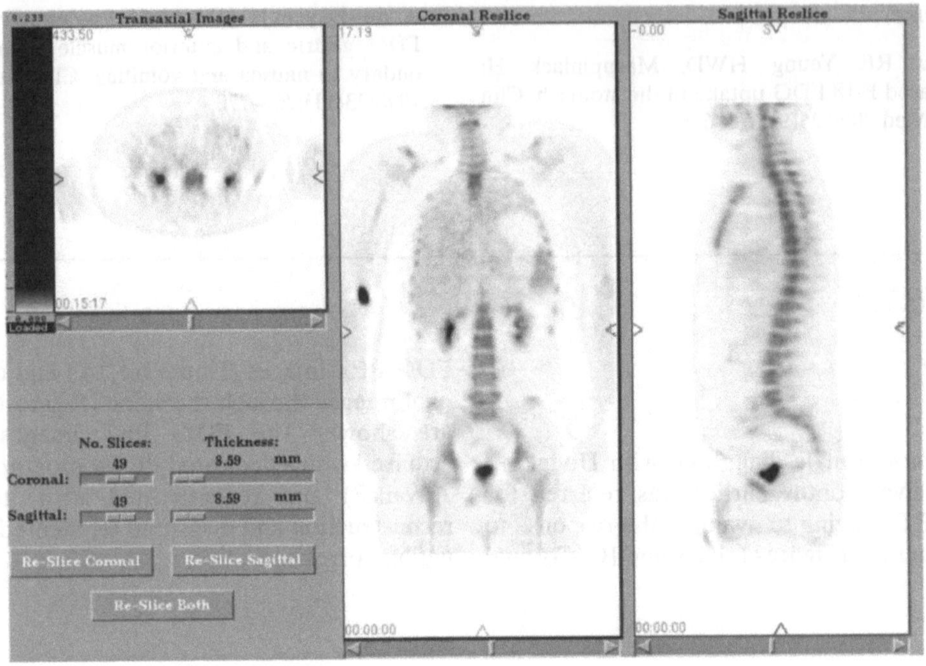

FIGURE 6.1.7B.

Findings

On the FDG images, there is diffusely increased uptake throughout the bone marrow. No focal abnormal FDG uptake is noted. The current FDG PET images were compared to a previous PET scan performed prior to therapy for staging (not shown). The abnormalities seen on the pretherapy PET scan are no longer identified, indicating an excellent response to therapy. No abnormal bone marrow uptake was seen on the pretherapy PET scan.

Discussion

Patients who undergo chemotherapy for primary, recurrent, or metastatic tumors commonly develop leukopenia. Exogenous granulocyte colony-stimulating factor (G-CSF) has been used to stimulate bone marrow regeneration and increase circulating leukocytes.[1,2] The increase in uptake of some radiopharmaceuticals in stimulated hematopoietic tissue has been reported, such as ^{67}gallium[2] and FDG.[1] Homogenous diffuse bone marrow uptake after chemotherapy should not be misinterpreted as bone marrow involvement by tumor. In this case, diffusely increased uptake in the bone marrow most probably indicates hypermetabolic hematopoietic tissue, rather than involvement by lymphoma. Comparison with the previous study is always helpful. For example, this patient did not have bone marrow involvement prior to therapy.

Diagnosis

Diffusely increased FDG uptake within the bone marrow consistent with bone marrow hyperplasia secondary to recent chemotherapy.

References

1. Sugawara Y, Zasadny KR, Kison PV, Baker LH, Wahl RL: Splenic fluorodeoxyglucose uptake increased by granulocyte colony-stimulating factor therapy: PET imaging results. J Nucl Med 1999;40:1456–1462.
2. Kondoh H, Murayama S, Kozuka T, et al.: Enhancement of hematopoietic uptake by granulocyte colony-stimulating factor in Ga-67 scintigraphy. Clin Nucl Med 1995;29(3):250–253.

Case 6.1.8

History

A 45-year-old male was diagnosed with squamous cell carcinoma of the larynx six months earlier and treated with chemotherapy and radiation therapy. He complained of persistent pain and dysphagia, and FDG imaging was performed to assess the presence of residual tumor (Figure 6.1.8). Orthogonal images through the posterior mediastinum are shown. The FDG images were acquired with a dedicated PET tomograph (GE Advance) and reconstructed with iterative reconstruction and measured segmented attenuation correction.

Findings

No abnormal uptake was seen in the region of the neck. However, the FDG images show activity in a linear pattern anterior to the cervical and thoracic spine.

Discussion

The pattern of uptake in this patient is most consistent with diffuse esophageal activity. The gastrointestinal tract can have variable FDG uptake. Uptake along the esophagus is common and is best identified on sagittal images. Activity may often appear more prominent at the gastroesophageal junction. Esophageal diseases such as esophagitis, Barrett's esophagus, and gastroesophageal reflux can demonstrate moderate or even markedly increased uptake of FDG.[1] FDG PET can also be useful in patients with esophageal carcinoma, especially in detecting distant metastasis, although its value in the evaluation of local spread is controversial.[2,3]

Diagnosis

Physiologic uptake in the esophagus.

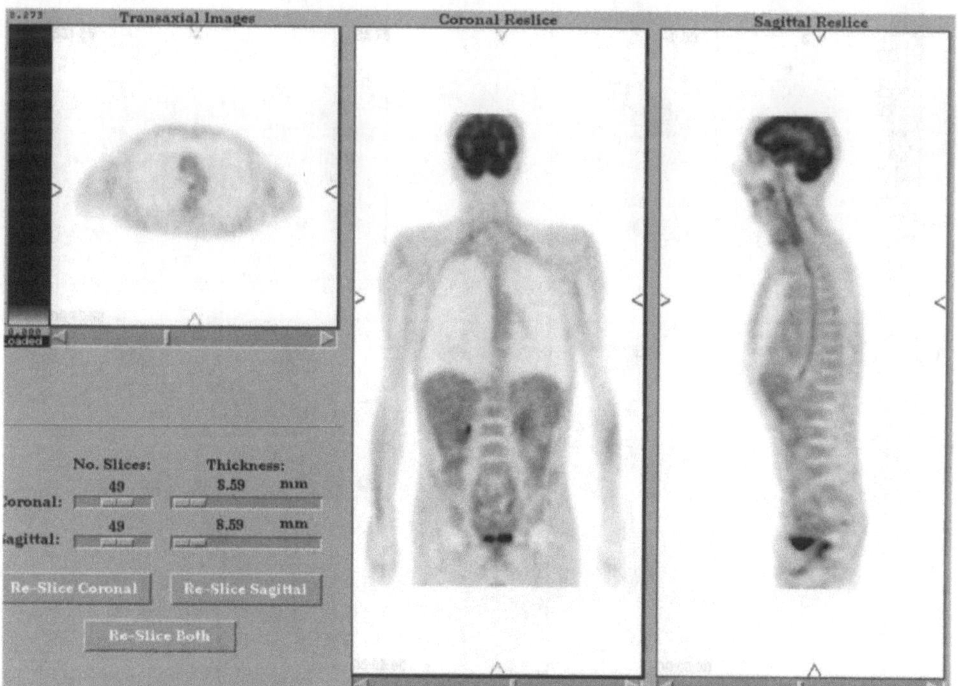

FIGURE 6.1.8.

References

1. Bakheet SM, Amim T, Alia AG, et al.: F-18 FDG uptake in benign esophageal disease. Clin Nucl Med 1999;24:995–997.
2. Flamen P, Lerut A, Van Cutsem E, et al.: Utility of positron emission tomography for the staging of patients with potentially operable esophageal carcinoma. J Clin Oncol 2000;18(18):3202–3210.
3. Skehan SJ, Brown AL, Thompson M, et al.: Imaging features of primary and recurrent esophageal cancer at FDG PET. Radiographics 2000;20(3):713–723.

Case 6.1.9

History

After completing therapy for non-Hodgkin's lymphoma three months earlier, a 36-year-old male presented with a stable right paratracheal node and a new 2 × 3 cm anterior mediastinal mass on CT scan (not shown). He was referred for FDG imaging. Figure 6.1.9A shows coronal FDG PET images acquired with a dedicated PET tomograph (GE Advance) and reconstructed with iterative reconstruction and measured segmented attenuation correction. When the images were displayed, the technologist noted a focus of markedly increased activity on the side of the screen and had to reset the window at a lower level to allow visualization of the outline of the body.

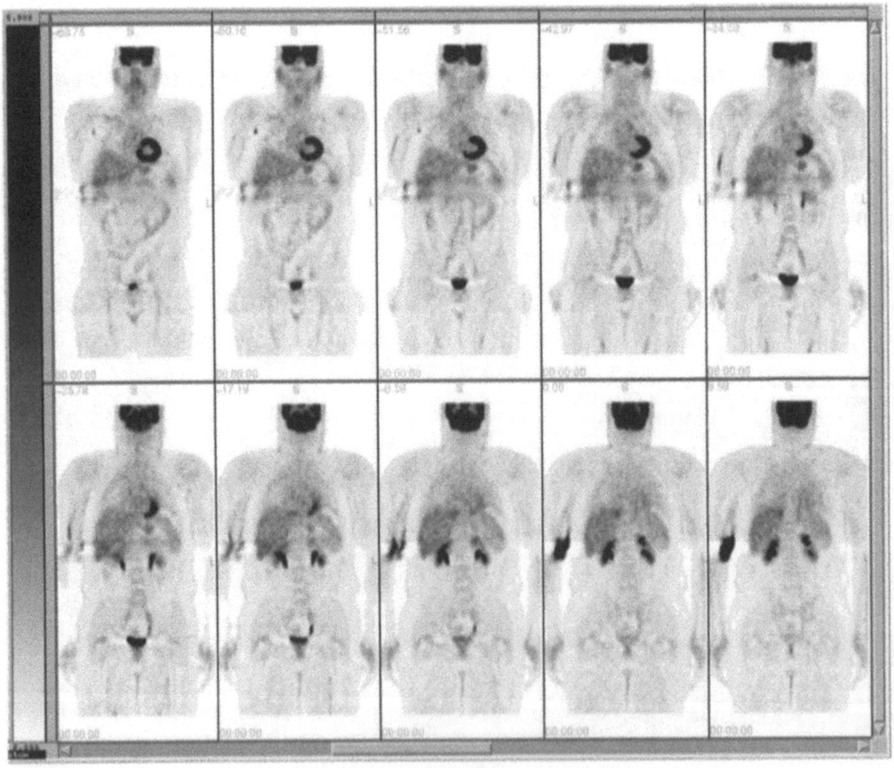

Figure 6.1.9A.

Findings

There is no abnormal uptake in the neck or anterior mediastinum, but there is a focus of markedly increased FDG uptake in the right axilla. Marked physiologic uptake is noted in the myocardium and renal collecting system. The focus of markedly increased activity noted by the technologist is located in the right antecubital fossa at the site of FDG injection.

Discussion

The absence of FDG uptake in the stable right paratracheal lymph node seen on CT indicates a good response to therapy. No FDG uptake corresponding to the new anterior mediastinal mass seen on CT indicates a benign etiology. With the history of recent chemotherapy, rebound thymic hyperplasia is likely (see Case 6.1.1). The uptake in the right antecubital fossa is due to extravasation of FDG into the subcutaneous tissues at the site of injection. There was no adenopathy seen in the right axilla when FDG images were correlated with the CT scan. In the absence of any other evidence of recurrent lymphoma, the uptake in the right axilla is most likely related to lymphatic transport of the extravasated radiopharmaceutical to the sentinel lymph node in the axilla. In addition, uptake is visualized along the vessels of the right upper extremity.

Another case of artifact related to administration of the radiopharmaceutical is illustrated in Figure 6.1.9B. This is a 34-year-old female with a history of recurrent abdominal Hodgkin's disease treated with chemotherapy, radiation therapy, and splenectomy. She was referred for FDG imaging for evaluation of persistent lymphadenopathy at the level of the porta hepatis on CT (not shown). The FDG images demonstrate uptake in these lymph nodes indicating persistent tumor. There is also

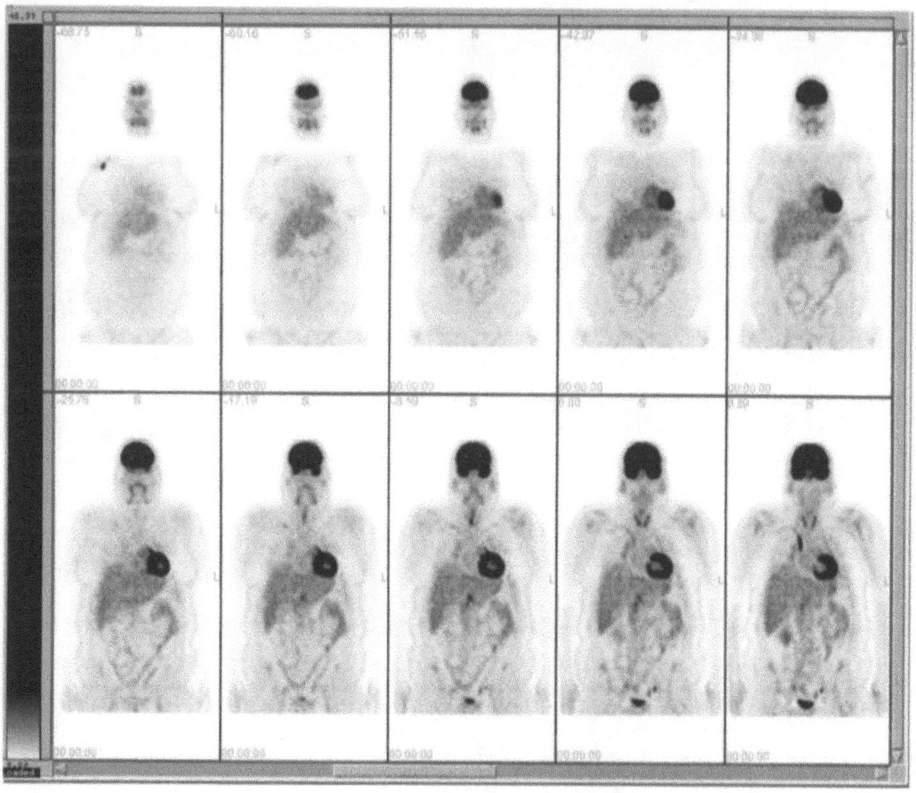

FIGURE 6.1.9B.

uptake in the thyroid gland that can be a normal variant and physiologic myocardial uptake. Another worrisome focus of uptake is noted in the mediastinum in a right paratracheal location, as well as a focus in the right chest wall anteriorly and superiorly. Correlation with the CT scan demonstrates a Portacath in place corresponding to the focus on the chest wall and no adenopathy corresponding to the right paratracheal focus of uptake. Additional history reveals that the FDG was injected through the Portacath because the venous access was difficult. It was concluded that the focus in the mediastinum was probably due to blood pool activity in a central vessel related to administration of the radiopharmaceutical through the Portacath.

Diagnoses

1. Visualization of an axillary sentinel lymph node related to extravasation of the radiopharmaceutical at the injection site.
2. Portacath central venous injection artifact.

6.2 Head and Neck Tumors

Orlin Woodie Hopper, William H. Martin, and Dominique Delbeke

Head and neck cancer represents about 2 to 3% of cancers in the United States, and most of them (90%) are squamous cell carcinomas of the nasopharynx and oropharynx, oral cavity, and larynx.[1] The initial diagnosis is usually obtained with physical and endoscopic examinations. FDG PET may play a role to detect the primary tumor in patients presenting with cervical adenopathy. Evaluation of the extent of the primary tumor, relationship to adjacent organs, and involvement of cervical lymph nodes are performed with CT and MRI. The most common locations for distant metastases are mediastinal lymph nodes, lungs, liver, brain, and occasionally the skeleton. The limitations of anatomical imaging with CT or MRI to monitor therapy or assess residual or recurrent tumors are well recognized. Residual lesions after therapy are common and may be related to scarring or inflammatory changes. There is general agreement in the literature that CT and MRI cannot reliably differentiate these changes from residual or recurrent tumor.

It has been well established that several tumors, including head and neck carcinoma,[2–12] demonstrate increased glucose metabolism both at the primary and metastatic sites. For head and neck carcinoma, there is no correlation between FDG uptake and histological grading.[3,4] Some benign salivary gland tumors, such as pleomorphic adenomas and Warthin's tumors, do accumulate FDG and can be mistaken for metastases.[13–16]

Due to relatively high physiologic FDG uptake in complex structures of the nasopharynx and neck, interpretation of FDG images of the head and neck is challenging, especially in the postsurgical patient. The osseous structures are normally hypometabolic. The maxilla can be identified by its horseshoe shape, and the mandibule can be identified by its typical V-shape. Physiologic FDG uptake is usually seen in the lymphoid tissue of the Waldeyer ring, the palatine and lingual tonsils, and the parotid and other salivary glands. The degree of uptake, however, varies from patient to patient.[17] When some of these metabolically active structures have been surgically resected, the physiologic activity in the contralateral normal paired structure should not be misinterpreted as a metastasis. Detailed correlation with CT is mandatory to avoid errors. Physiologic FDG uptake in activated laryngeal muscle, thyroid, and skeletal muscle are sources of misinterpretation as well.

Detection of Unknown Primary Tumors in Patients with Metastatic Cervical Lymph Nodes

In 20 to 40% of patients presenting with a metastatic cervical lymph node,[18] a primary tumor will be diagnosed in the head and neck during the course of the disease. The primary tumor in these patients may remain undetected during initial evaluation because of its small size, submucosal location, or spontaneous regression.[19,20] Blind biopsy allows detection of the primary tumor in only 10% of these patients, and MRI allows detection in 20%.[1]

The success of FDG PET for identification of the primary tumor varies between 10 percent[1,21] and 47 percent.[18–20,22–24]

Staging Head and Neck Carcinoma

Staging is very important in head and neck carcinoma because the extent of the treatment is determined by the size of the tumor and the presence or absence of metastatic lymph nodes. There is an overlap of sensitivity (range, 67 to 91%) and specificity (range, 88 to 100%) of FDG PET imaging and that of CT/MR imaging (sensitivity of 36 to 82% and specificity of 75 to 97%) in several studies.[1,7–9,11,12,23,24] Therefore, there is still controversy as to whether FDG PET imaging should be included in the routine initial staging of patients with head and neck carcinoma. Some investigators recommend limiting the addition of FDG PET imaging to patients with lesions equivocal by other staging modalities.

Approximately 20% of patients without lymph node involvement detected by conventional staging modalities have micrometastases at surgery. Several studies have demonstrated better sensitivity of FDG PET imaging (78 and 100%) compared to CT imaging (40 to 57% and 88 to 90%, respectively, in two studies).[23,24] The sensitivity of FDG PET to detect lymph node metastases may be better for tumors located in the oral cavity than in the oropharynx or hypopharynx.[24]

When FDG PET imaging detects additional metastases compared to anatomical imaging, the exact anatomical localization of the abnormal PET foci will still require correlation with anatomical imaging. The optimal diagnostic modality may be a fusion image showing the metabolic lesion superimposed onto the anatomical location.

Monitoring Therapy

FDG PET imaging has been used to monitor the response to therapy in patients with a variety of tumors, including head and neck tumors. The vast majority of patients with stage III or IV head and neck carcinoma receive radiation as a component of therapy. Measurements of FDG uptake in the tumors before and during therapy have demonstrated that there is decreased FDG uptake in responding tumors, while FDG uptake persists in nonresponding tumors. Data on a small number of patients suggest that the timing of posttreatment FDG PET may be important.[25–27] For example, Rege et al.[26] reported that FDG uptake in the primary tumor initially increased during the early course of radiation therapy (< 20 GY) but decreased near the end of therapy (> 45 GY), while there is no significant change in uptake in normal structures of the neck six weeks after radiation therapy. Persistent uptake on PET images obtained one month after radiation therapy strongly suggests residual tumor. Studies done too early after completion of therapy may give a false-positive result.

The growth rate and FDG uptake in patients with head and neck carcinoma treated with chemotherapy are highly correlated with clinical response and different regression functions for tumor and lymph node metastases.[28,29] Dalsaso et al.[30] studied 28 patients with stage III and IV head and neck cancer after two or three rounds of chemotherapy and correlated the results of FDG PET and CT (SUV in PET and volume reduction on CT) with posttherapy biopsies. They found a more significant decrease in SUV than decrease in tumor size posttherapy. Lowe et al.[31,32] conducted a trial of 44 patients with stage III or IV head and neck carcinoma who underwent PET imaging as a surveillance tool two and ten months after completing therapy. The results of PET imaging, physical exam, and anatomical imaging with CT were compared. Of the 30 patients who were disease free after therapy, 16 developed residual disease. Recurrence was documented by pathology in 15 of 16 cases. Sensitivity and specificity for each surveillance technique were as follows: 44% and 100% for physical examination, 38% and 85% for CT, and 100% and 93% for PET.

Studies suggest that the degree of pretherapy FDG uptake has prognostic significance.[33–35] In 15 patients with head and neck neoplasms studied before and after intra-arterial chemotherapy and radiotherapy, a relatively low pretreatment uptake of FDG predicts a complete response. PET is useful in predicting the response to treatment, and posttreatment FDG PET can accurately evaluate the presence of residual tumor. Brun et al.[34] showed that low pretherapy FDG uptake predicts local complete response.

Detection of Recurrence

Numerous studies have demonstrated that FDG PET is more accurate than CT in detecting recurrence of head and neck cancer after surgery or irradiation.[36–46] Both the sensitivity and specificity for PET range between 80 and 100%. For CT, the sensitivity ranges from 25 to 80%, and specificity ranges from 31 to 100%. Many investigators have concluded that PET should precede CT or MRI imaging in the search for recurrence because CT and MRI will often be inconclusive.

Summary

In summary, there is a consensus in the literature about the clear advantage of FDG PET imaging over CT or MR imaging in monitoring the effects of therapy and evaluating patients for recurrence of head and neck carcinoma following therapy.

References

1. Keyes JW Jr, Watson NE, Williams DW III, Greven KM, McGuirt WF: FDG-PET in head and neck cancer. Am J Roentgenol 1997;169:1663–1669.
2. Chisin R: Nuclear medicine in head and neck oncology: Reality and perspectives. J Nucl Med 1999;40:91–99.
3. Minn H, Joensuu H, Ahonen A, Klemi P: Fluorodeoxyglucose imaging: A method to assess the proliferative activity in human cancer in vivo—comparison with DNA flow cytometry in head and neck tumors. Cancer 1988;61:1776–1781.
4. Haberkorn U, Strauss LG, Reisser CH, et al.: Glucose uptake, perfusion, and cell proliferation in head and neck tumors: Relation of positron emission tomography to flow cytometry. J Nucl Med 1991;32:1548–1555.
5. Bailet JW, Abermayor E, Jabour BA, Hawkins RA, Ho C, Ward PH: Positron emission tomography: A new, precise imaging modality for detection of primary head and neck tumors and assessment of cervical adenopathy. Laryngoscope 1992;102:281–288.
6. Jabour BA, Choi Y, Hoh CH, et al.: Extracranial head and neck: PET imaging with 2-[F-18]fluoro-2-deoxy-d-glucose and MR imaging correlation. Radiology 1993;186:27–35.
7. Rege S, Maass A, Chaiken L, et al.: Use of positron emission tomography with fluorodeoxyglucose in patients with extracranial head and neck cancers. Cancer 1994;73:3047–3058.
8. Braams JW, Pruim J, Freling NJM, et al.: Detection of lymph nodes metastases of squamous-cell cancer of the head and neck with FDG-PET and MRI. J Nucl Med 1995;36:211–216.
9. McGuirt WF, Williams DW III, Keyes JW Jr, Greven KM, Watson NE Jr, Geisinger KR, et al.: A comparative diagnostic study of head and neck nodal metastases using positron emission tomography. Laryngoscope 1995;105:373–375.
10. Lauenbacher C, Saumweber D, Wagner-Manslau C, et al.: Comparison of fluorine-18-fluorodeoxyglucose PET, MRI and endoscopy for staging head and neck squamous-cell carcinomas. J Nucl Med 1995;36:1747–1757.
11. Benchaou M, Lehmann W, Slosman DO, Becker M, Lemoine R, Rufenacht D, et al.: The role of FDG-PET in the preoperative assessment of N-staging in head and neck cancer. Acta Otolaryngol 1996;116(2):332–335.
12. Adams S, Baum RP, Stuckensen T, Bitter K, Hor G: Prospective comparison of 18F-FDG PET with conventional imaging modalities (CT, MRI, US) in lymph node staging of head and neck cancer. Eur J Nucl Med 1998;25(9):1255–1260.
13. Okamura T, Kawabe J, Koyama K, et al.: Fluorine-18 fluorodeoxyglucose positron emission tomography imaging of parotid mass lesions. Acta Otolaryngol Suppl 1998;538:209–213.
14. Keyes JW Jr, Harkness BA, Greven KM, Williams DW III, Watson NE Jr, McGuirt WF: Salivary gland tumors: Pretherapy evaluation with PET. Radiology 1994;192(1):99–102.
15. Matsuda M, Sakamoto H, Okamura T, Nakai Y, Ohashi Y, Kawabe J, et al.: Positron emission tomography imaging of pleomorphic adenoma in the parotid gland. Acta Otolaryngol Suppl 1998;538:214–220.
16. Horiuchi M, Yasuda S, Shohtsu A, Ide M: Four cases of Wharthin's tumor of the parotid gland detected with FDG PET. Ann Nucl Med 1998; 12:47–50.
17. Jabour BA, Choi Y, Hoh CK, et al.: Extracranial head and neck: PET imaging with 2-[F-18]fluoro-

2-deoxy-D-glucose and MR imaging correlation. Radiology 1993;186(1):27–35.
18. Kole AC, Nieweg OE, Pruim J, et al.: Detection of unknown occult primary tumors using positron emission tomography. Cancer 1998; 82(6):1160–1166.
19. Mukherji SK, Drane WE, Mancuso AA, Parsons JT, Mendenhall WM, Stringer S: Occult primary tumors of the head and neck: Detection with 2-[F-18]fluoro-2-deoxy-D-glucose SPECT. Radiology 1996;199(3):761–766.
20. Assar OS, Fischbein NJ, Caputo GR, et al.: Metastatic head and neck cancer: Role and usefulness of FDG PET in locating occult primary tumors. Radiology 1999;210(1):177–181.
21. Greven KM, Keyes JW Jr, Williams DW III, McGuirt WF, Joyce WT III: Occult primary tumors of the head and neck: Lack of benefit from positron emission tomography imaging with 2-[F-18]fluoro-2-deoxy-D-glucose. Cancer 1999;86(1):114–118.
22. Bohuslavizki KH, Klutmann S, Kroger S, et al.: FDG PET detection of unknown primary tumors. J Nucl Med 2000;41:816–822.
23. Myers LL, Wax MK: Positron emission tomography in the evaluation of the negative neck in patients with oral cavity cancer. J Otolaryngol 1998;27(6):342–347.
24. Myers LL, Wax MK, Nabi H, Simpson GT, Lamonica D: Positron emission tomography in the evaluation of the N0 neck. Laryngoscope 1998;108:232–236.
25. Minn H, Paul R, Ahonen A: Evaluation of treatment response to radiotherapy in head and neck cancer with fluorine-18 fluorodeoxyglucose. J Nucl Med 1988;29(9):1521–1525.
26. Rege SD, Chaiken L, Hoh CK, et al.: Change induced by radiation therapy in FDG uptake in normal and malignant structures of the head and neck: Quantitation with PET. Radiology 1993; 189:807–812.
27. Greven KM, Williams DW, Keyes JW Jr, et al.: Positron emission tomography of patients with head and neck carcinoma before and after high dose irradiation. Cancer 1994;74:1355–1359.
28. Haberkorn U, Stauss LG, Dimitrakopoulou A, et al.: Fluorodeoxyglucose imaging of advanced head and neck cancer after chemotherapy. J Nucl Med 1993;34:12–17.
29. Berlangieri SU, Brizel DM, Scher RL, Schifter T, Hawk TC, Hamblen S: Pilot study of positron emission tomography in patients with advanced head and neck cancer receiving radiotherapy and chemotherapy. Head Neck 1994;16:340–346.
30. Dalsaso TA, Lowe VJ, Dunphy FR, Martin DS, Boyd JH, Stack BC: FDG PET and CT in evaluation of chemotherapy in advanced head and neck cancer. Clin Pos Imag 2000;3:1–5.
31. Lowe VJ, Dunphy FR, Varvares M, et al.: Evaluation of chemotherapy response in patients with advanced head and neck cancer using [F-18]fluorodeoxyglucose positron emission tomography. Head Neck 1997;19:666–674.
32. Lowe VJ, Boyd JH, Dunphy FR, et al.: Surveillance for recurrent head and neck cancer using positron emission tomography. J Clin Oncol 2000;18(3):651–658.
33. Kitagawa Y, Sadato N, Azuma H, Ogazawara T, Yoshida M, Ishii Y, et al.: FDG PET to evaluate combined intra-arterial chemotherapy and radiotherapy of head and neck neoplasms. J Nucl Med 1999;40:1132–1137.
34. Brun E, Ohlsson T, Erlandsson K, et al.: Early prediction of treatment outcome in head and neck cancer with 2-18FDG PET. Acta Oncol 1997;36(7):741–747.
35. Minn H, Lapela M, Klemi PJ, et al.: Prediction of survival with fluorine-18-fluoro-deoxyglucose and PET in head and neck cancer. J Nucl Med 1997;38(12):1907–1911.
36. Chaiken L, Rege S, Hoh C, et al.: Positron emission tomography with fluorodeoxyglucose to evaluate tumor response and control after radiation therapy. Int J Radiat Oncol Biol Phys 1994;29:841–845.
37. Minn H, Paul R, Ahonen A: Evaluation of treatment response to radiotherapy in head and neck cancer with fluorine-18 fluorodeoxyglucose. J Nucl Med 1988;29:1521–1525.
38. Wong WL, Chevretton EB, McGurk M, et al.: A prospective study of PET-FDG imaging for the assessment of head and neck squamous cell carcinoma. Clin Otolaryngol 1997;22:209–214.
39. Keyes JW Jr, Watson NE, Williams DW III, Greven KM, McGuirt WF: FDG-PET in head and neck cancer. AJR Am J Roentgenol 1997; 169:1663–1669.
40. Myers LL, Wax MK, Nabi H, Simpson GT, Lamonica D: Positron emission tomography in the evaluation of the N0 neck. Laryngoscope 1998;108:232–236.
41. Lapela M, Grenman R, Kurki T, et al.: Head and neck cancer: Detection of recurrence with PET and 2-[F-18]fluoro-2-deoxy-D-glucose. Radiology 1995;197:205–211.
42. Hubner KF, Thie JA, Smith GT, Chan AC, Fernandez PS, McCoy JM: Clinical utility of FDG PET in detecting head and neck tumors: A

comparison of diagnostic methods and modalities. Clin Pos Img 2000;3:7–16.
43. Anzai Y, Carroll WR, Quint DJ, et al.: Recurrence of head and neck cancer after surgery or irradiation: Prospective comparison of 2-deoxy-2[F-18]fluoro-D-glucose PET and MR imaging diagnoses. Radiology 1996;200:135–141.
44. Chaiken L, Rege S, Hoh C, et al.: Positron emission tomography with fluorodeoxyglucose to evaluate tumor response and control after radiation therapy. Int J Radiat Oncol Biol Phys 1994;29:841–845.
45. Berlangieri SU, Brizel DM, Scher RL, Schifter T, Hawk TC, Hamblen S: Pilot study of positron emission tomography in patients with advanced head and neck cancer receiving radiotherapy and chemotherapy. Head Neck 1994;16:340–346.
46. Greven KM, Williams DW, Keyes JW Jr, et al.: Distinguishing tumor recurrence from irradiation sequelae with positron emission tomography in patients with advanced head and neck cancer receiving radiotherapy and chemotherapy. Int J Radiat Oncol Biol Phys 1994; 29:841–845.

Case Presentations

Case 6.2.1

History

A 60-year-old male with a history of a large cell neuroendocrine carcinoma of the larynx, who completed both radiation and chemotherapy ten months ago, presented with lung nodules on CT scan (Figure 6.2.1A) and was referred for FDG imaging. FDG images were first acquired using a dedicated full ring PET tomograph (GE Advance) (Figure 6.2.1B) and reconstructed with iterative reconstruction and measured segmented attenuation correction. Then images were obtained using a hybrid gamma camera (VG Millenium) capable of coincidence imaging for FDG imaging (hybrid PET) and CT transmission imaging. CT transmission images provide attenuation maps for attenuation correction and hybrid CT images for image fusion and lesion localization (Figure 6.2.1C, see color plate). Figure 6.2.1B shows coronal FDG PET images with attenuation correction. Figure 6.2.1C shows transaxial images through the chest: hybrid CT (left), hybrid PET (middle), and fusion hybrid CT/hybrid PET (right).

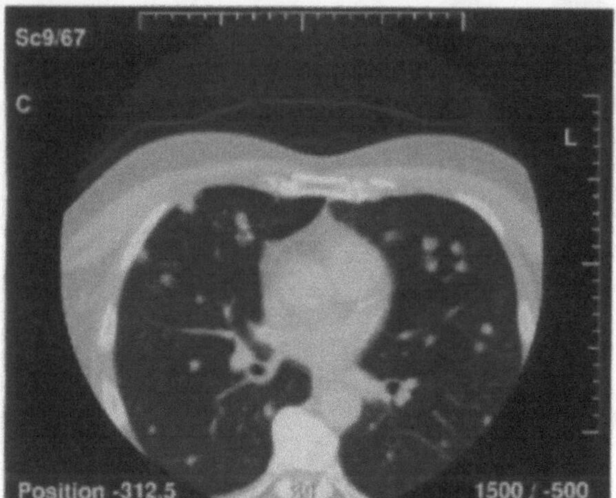

FIGURE 6.2.1A.

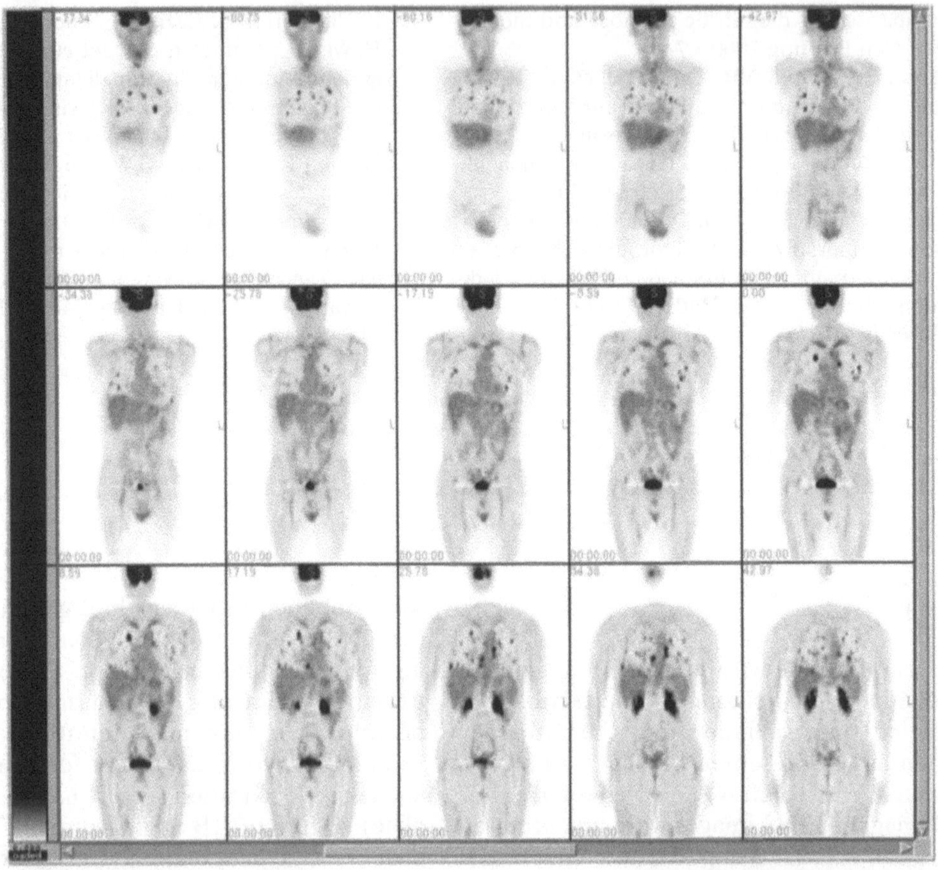

B

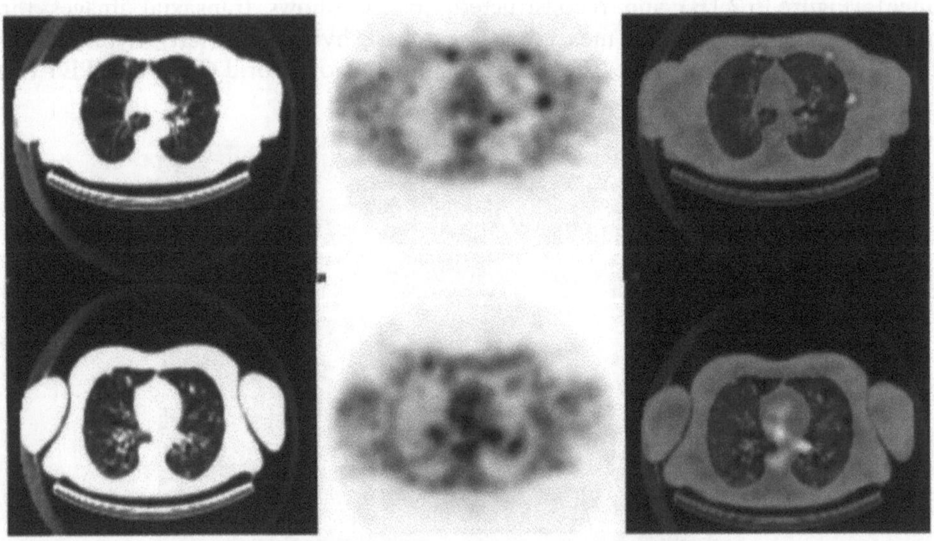

C

FIGURE 6.2.1B,C. (See color plate)

Findings

The chest CT scan and hybrid CT images are remarkable for multiple bilateral lung nodules. The FDG PET and hybrid PET images both demonstrate multiple foci of increased FDG activity throughout both lungs. Many foci of uptake are located peripherally, and the exact location is difficult to assess on functional (FDG) images alone (pleural-based, chest wall, or ribs). Uptake is also seen in the neck at the midline. The fusion hybrid CT/hybrid PET images demonstrate that the peripheral foci of uptake correspond to pleural-based lung nodules, even though the patient moved slightly and the foci of uptake do not superimpose exactly to the anatomical lesion.

Discussion

These findings are consistent with multiple pulmonary metastases. The most common sites of distant spread of head and neck carcinomas are the lungs and the skeleton. This study was undertaken to determine whether the multiple nodules in this patient represented metastatic disease and assess the presence of additional unsuspected metastases. Given the markedly increased FDG activity, the lesions were consistent with pulmonary metastases, although active granulomatous processes can have the same degree of uptake as metastases.

On FDG images, it is sometimes difficult to differentiate lesions within the pulmonary parenchyma from those in adjacent structures such as the chest wall, ribs, and mediastinum. In this patient, many of the nodules were pleural-based, making the exact location of the lesions difficult to ascertain. Attenuation correction can be helpful by providing better anatomical landmarks, but fusion images superimposing functional (FDG) on anatomical (CT) images are superior. In this case, the fusion images demonstrate that each focus of uptake on hybrid PET corresponds to a lung nodule on hybrid CT, making rib metastases unlikely.

The patient had a history of prior tracheostomy. Therefore, the activity in the neck in the midline was most consistent with inflammatory changes related to the prior tracheostomy site. Any process eliciting an inflammatory response such as trauma, granulomatous disease, or osteomyelitis, for example, may demonstrate increased FDG accumulation. For this reason, a brief history and physical examination are often helpful in accounting for otherwise unexplained foci of FDG uptake and thus reducing interpretive errors.

Due to the inherent relative low sensitivity of the imaging system, the hybrid PET images are noisier than those acquired with the dedicated PET system. The accurate attenuation correction and fusion images made possible by the integrated CT system compensated nicely for the limitations of the system, thus facilitating accurate interpretation.

Diagnoses

1. Diffuse bilateral pulmonary metastases.
2. Inflammation secondary to prior tracheostomy.

Case 6.2.2

History

A 53-year-old male with a history of poorly differentiated squamous cell carcinoma of the nasopharynx presented with back pain. Recurrence to a left supraclavicular node was proven by biopsy. He underwent MRI imaging of the spine (Figure 6.2.2A), CT of the chest (Figure 6.2.2B) and abdomen (Figure 6.2.2C), and FDG PET imaging (Figures 6.2.2D and E). Figure 6.2.2A shows T1-weighted sagittal images through the lumbar spine. Figures

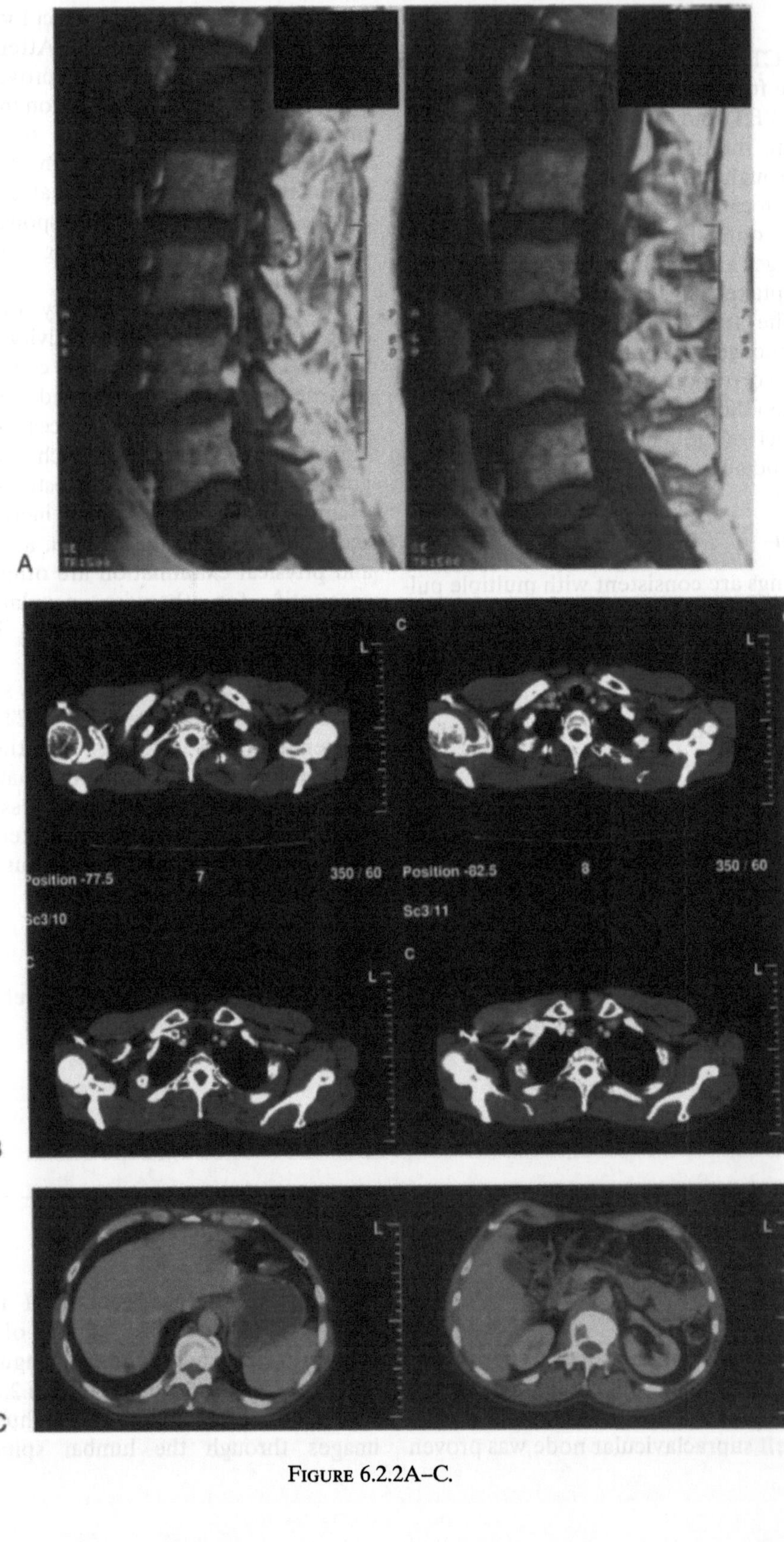

FIGURE 6.2.2A–C.

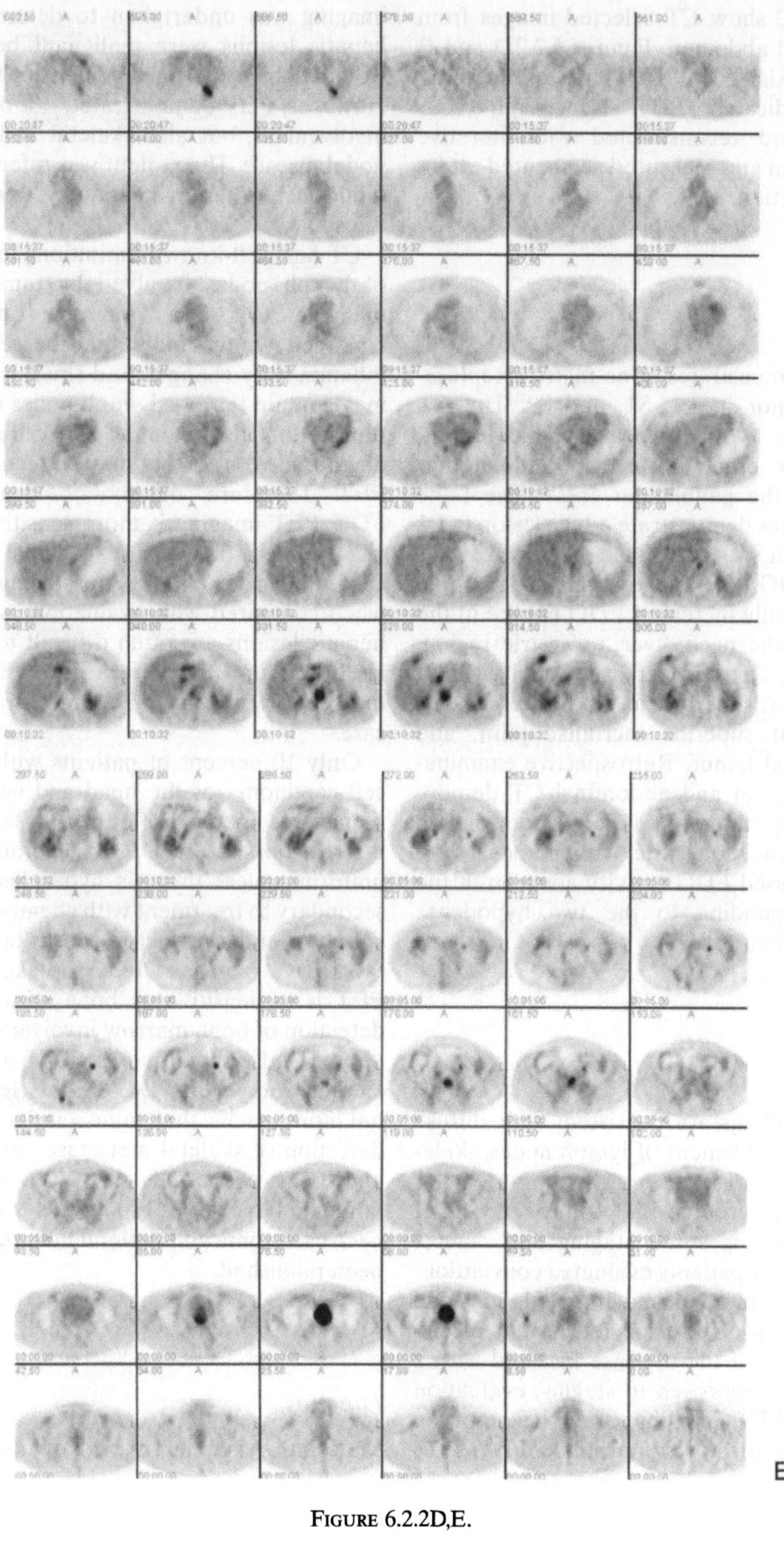

FIGURE 6.2.2D,E.

6.2.2B and C show CT selected images from the chest and abdomen. Figures 6.2.2D and E show transaxial FDG PET images acquired with a dedicated PET tomograph (GE Advance) and reconstructed with iterative reconstruction and measured segmented attenuation correction.

Findings

The MRI demonstrates bone marrow replacement by tumor in L1, S1, and S2. The CT demonstrates two equivocal hepatic lesions, one near the dome posteriorly and another adjacent to the gallbladder fossa. The bone window images demonstrate a lytic lesion in L1 (not well seen with soft tissue windows).

On the FDG PET images, there are multiple foci of markedly increased FDG uptake in the left base of the neck, liver, epigastric region, and skeleton. There is increased activity within a posterior left superior rib, L1 vertebral body, sacrum, right superior sacroiliac joint, and right proximal femur. Retrospective examination of the chest and abdominal CT demonstrates destruction of a left superior rib posteriorly and epigastric lymph nodes. Two foci of increased FDG activity are seen in the liver, corresponding to the two hypodense lesions noted on CT.

Discussion

The PET findings are consistent with diffuse metastatic involvement of lymph nodes, skeleton, and liver.

It is widely accepted that whole-body FDG PET often changes the staging and clinical management of patients evaluated conventionally with CT and other imaging modalities due to its detection of unsuspected distant metastases. Because of the expense incurred with a multimodality approach to staging, evaluation with FDG PET imaging often becomes an economically attractive alternative. FDG PET imaging was undertaken to determine if the hepatic lesions were malignant because that would change the management of the patient. However, PET demonstrated not only hepatic involvement, but also skeletal and additional nodal disease. The patient was referred for systemic chemotherapy in addition to radiation to the spine.

CT has well-known limitations for detection of lymph nodes involved by tumor because malignancy is based on size criteria only. Enlarged lymph nodes may be secondary to inflammatory changes, and small lymph nodes may contain tumors. Lymph nodes involved by tumors that do not meet size criteria are not diagnosed with CT but may be recognized with PET. Therefore, metabolic evaluation with FDG PET imaging is more sensitive and specific than CT for detection of nodal metastases. FDG PET often changes the staging of patients when compared with evaluation by CT. Small hepatic lesions are often difficult to characterize by CT or US, whereas FDG PET imaging may be diagnostic, as is demonstrated in this case.

Only 10 percent of patients with squamous cell carcinoma of the head and neck develop metastases to the skeleton. Physiologic bone marrow uptake of FDG is generally mild and uniform, unless there is hyperplastic marrow secondary to treatment with chemotherapy and colony-stimulating factor. Most skeletal metastases have increased FDG uptake, and FDG PET is as sensitive as bone scintigraphy for detection of bone marrow involvement by lymphoma and skeletal metastases from lung carcinoma. However, FDG PET is less sensitive but more specific than bone scintigraphy for the detection of skeletal metastases from prostate and breast carcinoma. As of yet, a study containing a large series of patients with head and neck carcinoma and skeletal metastases has not been published.

Diagnosis

Metastatic nasopharyngeal carcinoma.

Case 6.2.3

History

A 59-year-old male presented with a history of total laryngectomy for squamous cell carcinoma, followed by multiple subsequent operations for recurrence and treatment with chemotherapy and external beam radiation. A recent biopsy proved recurrence at the site of the stoma. A CT demonstrated nonspecific thickening of deep cervical soft tissue planes anteriorly and esophageal wall thickening (not shown). The CT scan was not able to accurately demonstrate the extent of the recurrence, and the patient was referred for FDG imaging. FDG images were first acquired using a dedicated full ring PET tomograph (GE Advance) (Figures 6.2.3A, B, and C) and reconstructed with iterative reconstruction and measured segmented attenuation correction. Then FDG images were acquired using a hybrid gamma camera (VG Millenium) capable of coincidence imaging for FDG imaging and CT transmission imaging. CT transmission images provide attenuation maps for attenuation correction and hybrid CT images for image fusion and lesion localization (Figure 6.2.3D, see color plate). Figures 6.2.3A, B, and C show coronal (Figure 6.2.3A), transaxial (Figure 6.2.3B), and orthogonal FDG PET images through the neck (Figure 6.2.3C). Figure 6.2.3D shows orthogonal hybrid images through the chest, matching the orthogonal dedicated PET images. Figure 6.2.3E, see color plate, shows transaxial hybrid CT (left), hybrid PET (middle), and fusion hybrid CT/hybrid PET (right), through the stoma site (upper panel) and through the mediastinum (lower panel).

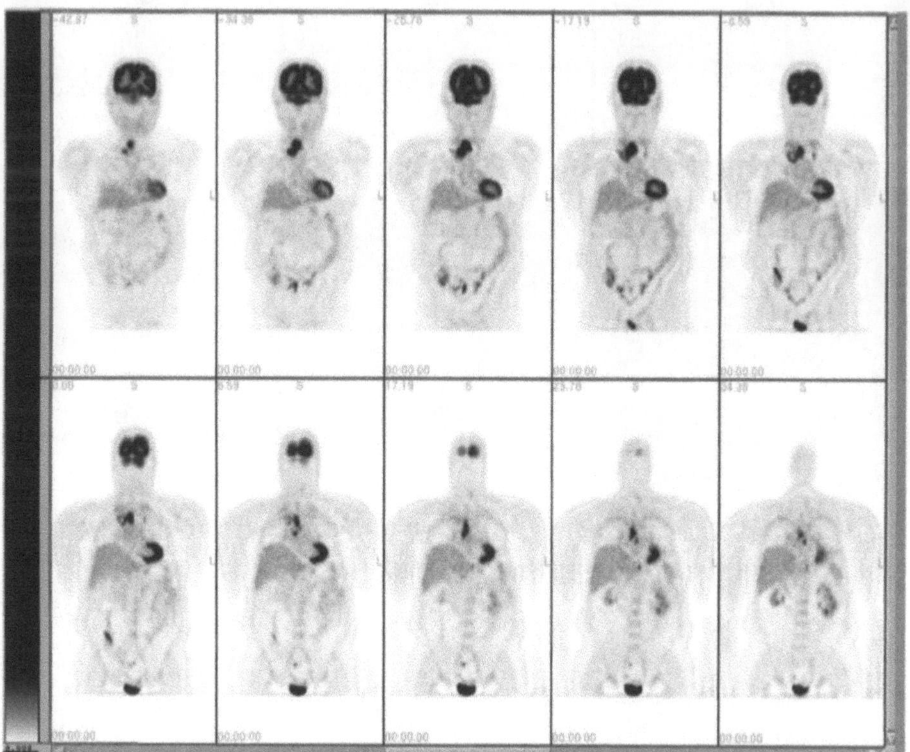

FIGURE 6.2.3A.

B

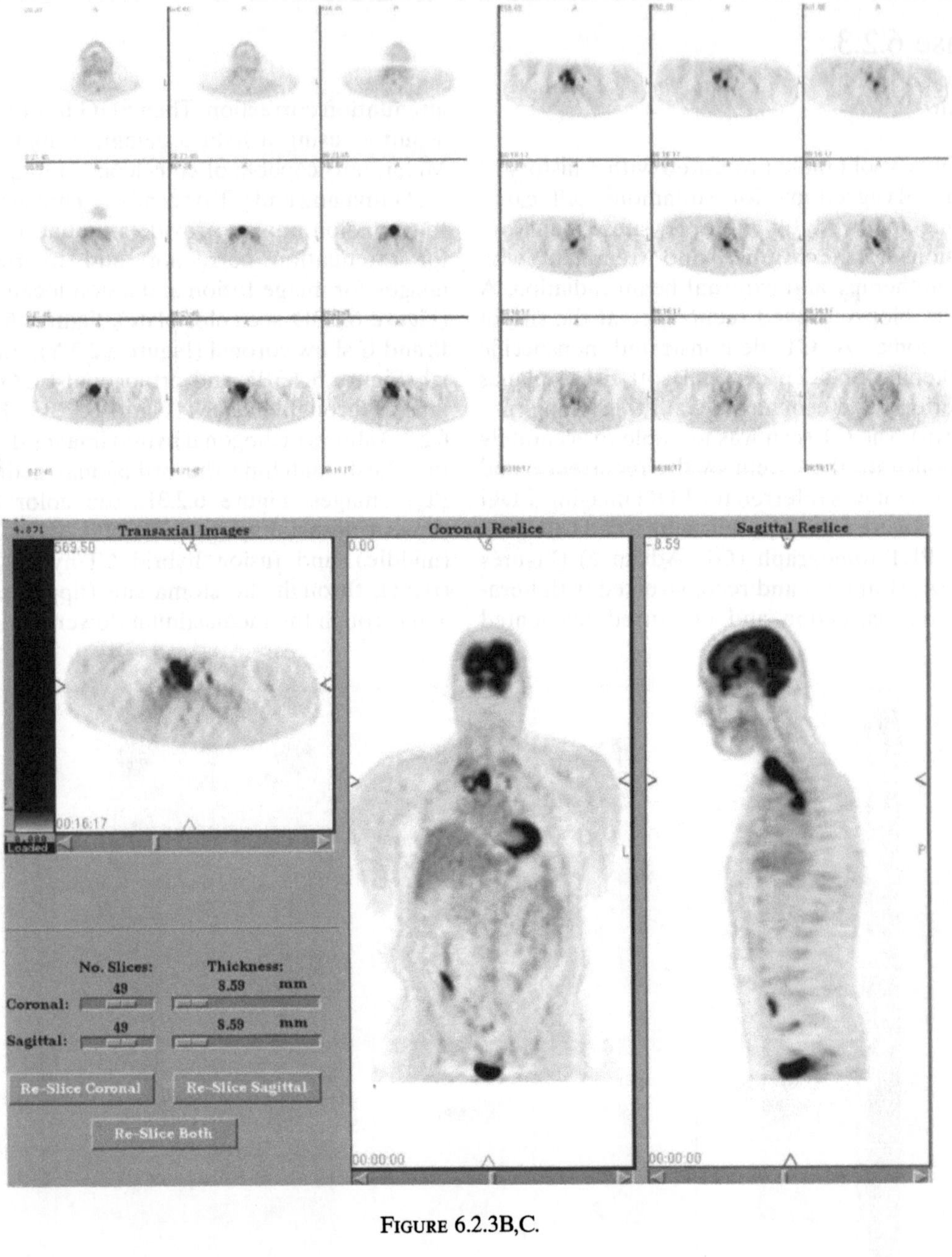

C

FIGURE 6.2.3B,C.

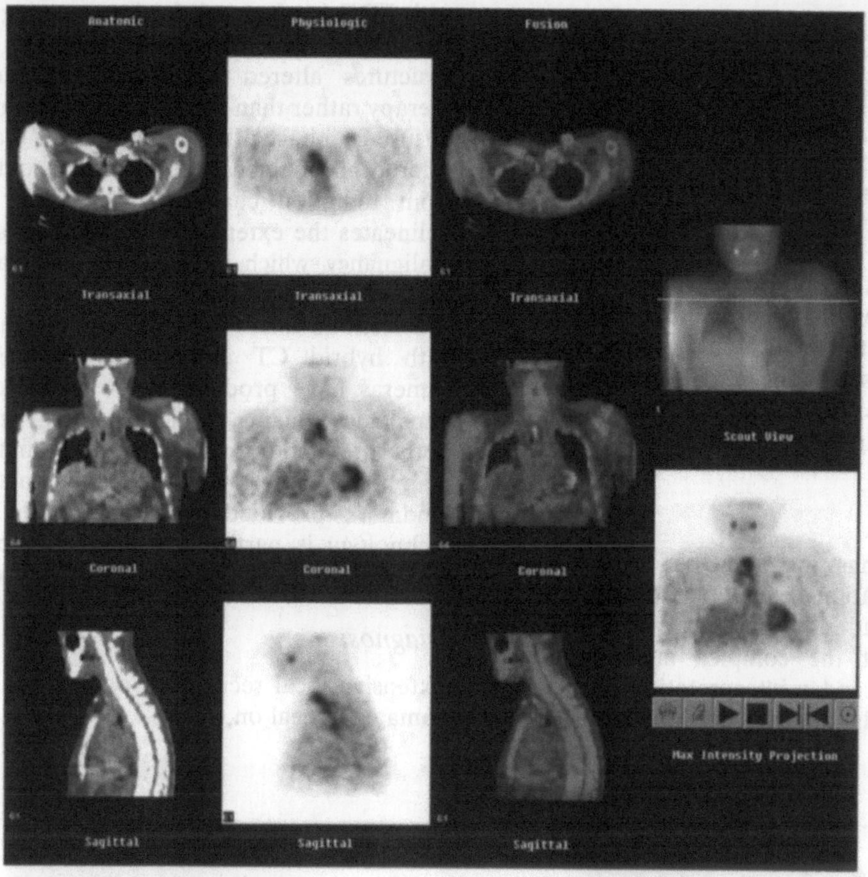

D

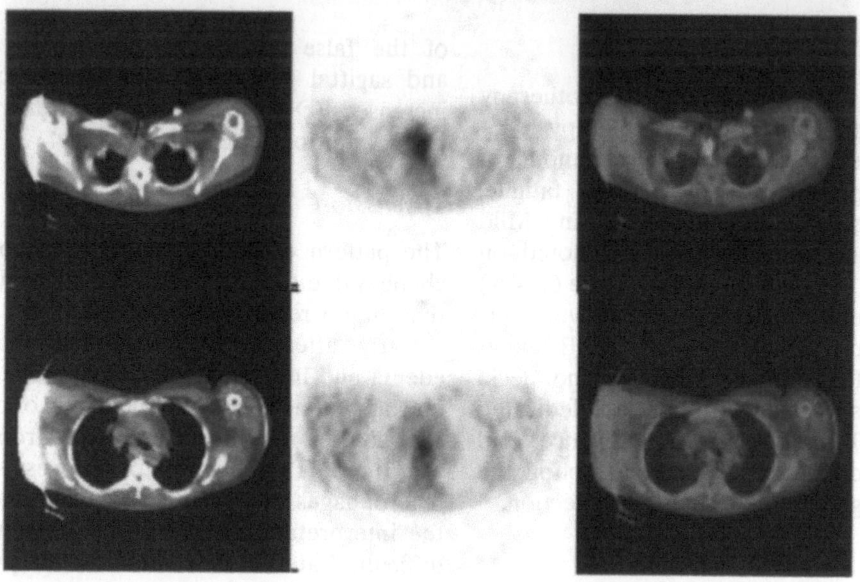

E

FIGURE 6.2.3D,E. (See color plate)

Findings

The FDG PET images demonstrate a large area of markedly increased FDG uptake at the site of the stoma, extending deeply in the neck to the right of midline and inferiorly into the posterior mediastinum along the esophagus to the level of the carina, best seen on the sagittal image.

The selected hybrid CT/hybrid PET and fusion images demonstrate that FDG uptake corresponds to the thickening of the deep cervical soft tissue seen on CT scan and in fact, extends inferiorly into the posterior mediastinum along the esophagus.

Discussion

These findings are diagnostic of extensive tumor infiltration and not posttherapy scarring.

Surgery and radiotherapy involving the neck often distort the complex anatomy of this region and render interpretation of anatomic imaging modalities difficult. Metabolic imaging with FDG is often helpful for assessing recurrence by revealing hypermetabolic foci within structures altered by surgery or radiation therapy rather than by malignancy. In this case, diffuse esophageal thickening on CT was considered an equivocal finding and could result from radiation changes. FDG PET clearly delineates the extent of hypermetabolism and malignancy, which included the esophagus to the level of the carina.

Recent advances in image fusion technology with hybrid CT and hybrid PET gamma cameras have produced a powerful tool for oncologic imaging. This technology permits both attenuation correction and anatomical mapping of hypermetabolic foci on anatomical landmarks provided by the integrated CT. This technology is particularly helpful in patients with distorted anatomy secondary to therapy.

Diagnosis

Extensive local recurrence of laryngeal carcinoma equivocal on CT.

Case 6.2.4

History

Two months after completion of radiotherapy to the neck and systemic chemotherapy, a 45-year-old male with squamous cell carcinoma of the larynx presented with ongoing fatigue, throat soreness, and difficulty swallowing. Mild redness of the anterior neck was noted on examination. A CT of the neck (Figure 6.2.4A) and whole-body FDG PET imaging were performed (Figure 6.2.4B). Figure 6.2.4B shows orthogonal FDG images through the neck. These images were acquired using a dedicated full ring PET tomograph (GE Advance) and reconstructed with iterative reconstruction and measured segmented attenuation correction.

Findings

The CT scan demonstrates mild thickening of the aryepiglottic folds with minimal edema of the false cords. The transaxial, coronal, and sagittal FDG PET images demonstrate increased FDG activity in a linear distribution in the anterior neck at the midline.

Discussion

The pattern of uptake suggests inflammatory changes due to recent radiation therapy rather than tumor recurrence.

Early after radiation therapy, there are edema and inflammatory changes. The edema may appear as abnormal thickening of mucosal surfaces that must be differentiated from recurrent tumor. The inflammatory process includes macrophages that accumulate FDG and make the interpretation of FDG images sometimes difficult. Later after radiation therapy, there is decreased FDG activity because there is decreased vascular patency due to endothelial proliferation and subsequent arteriolar

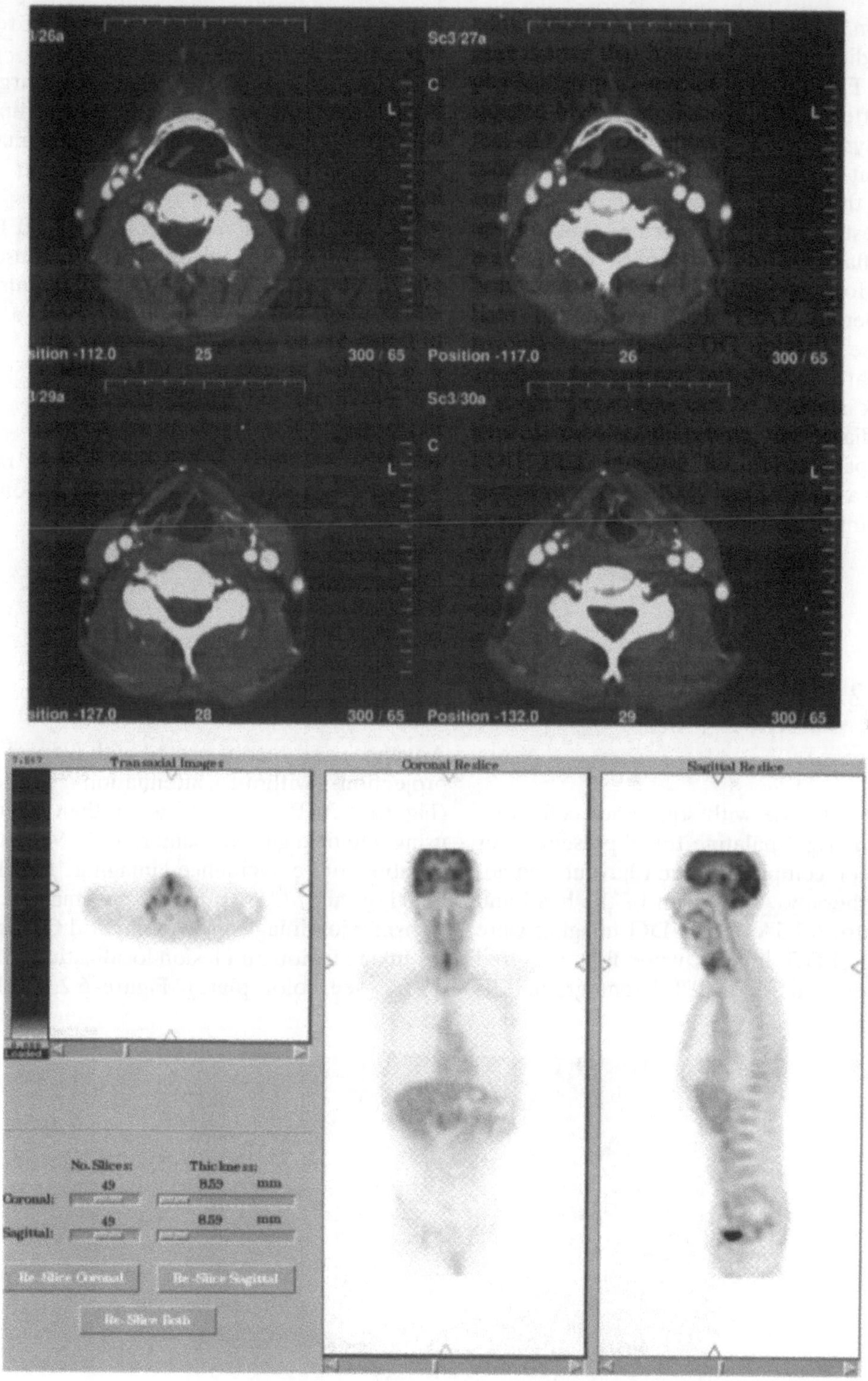

A

B

Figure 6.2.4A,B.

obliteration. At that time, the presence of FDG uptake indicates recurrent tumor. The time course of FDG uptake due to inflammatory changes after radiation therapy has not been studied systematically, but some authors suggest that persistent uptake one month after radiation therapy is worrisome for tumor. Other investigators have suggested that uptake due to inflammation may persist for several months. However, healing time is probably variable between patients, and therefore, the time course of FDG uptake may vary. In this case, the pattern of increased FDG metabolism in the neck in the midline was helpful in the differential diagnosis. Two weeks after the PET scan, the patient presented with acute throat pain and was diagnosed with a fistula. A biopsy revealed inflammatory changes in the soft tissues of the neck with no evidence of recurrent tumor.

Knowledge of the patient's history, a targeted physical examination, and the pattern of uptake allowed correct interpretation of inflammatory reaction to recent radiotherapy rather than underlying tumor.

The symmetrical regions of increased FDG activity in the neck are explained by muscular uptake. This is often seen in tense patients and may be avoided by administration of a mild sedative prior to injection of FDG.

Diagnosis

Inflammatory changes following recent radiotherapy with subsequent fistula formation and chondronecrosis.

Case 6.2.5

History

A 45-year-old male with squamous cell carcinoma of the right palatine tonsil presented for staging after completing neoadjuvant chemoradiation therapy. A CT scan of the head and neck (Figure 6.2.5A) and FDG imaging were performed. FDG images were first acquired using a dedicated full ring PET tomograph (GE Advance) and reconstructed with filtered back projection without attenuation correction (Figure 6.2.5B). Images were then acquired using a hybrid gamma camera (VG Millenium) capable of coincidence imaging for FDG imaging and CT transmission imaging. CT transmission images provide hybrid CT images for image fusion and lesion localization (Figure 6.2.5C, see color plate). Figure 6.2.5B shows

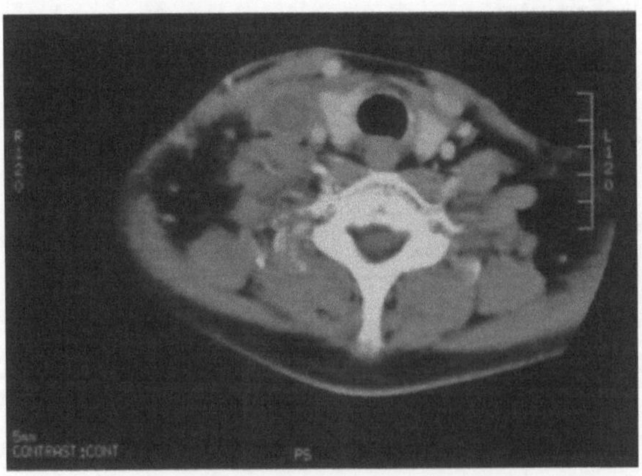

FIGURE 6.2.5A.

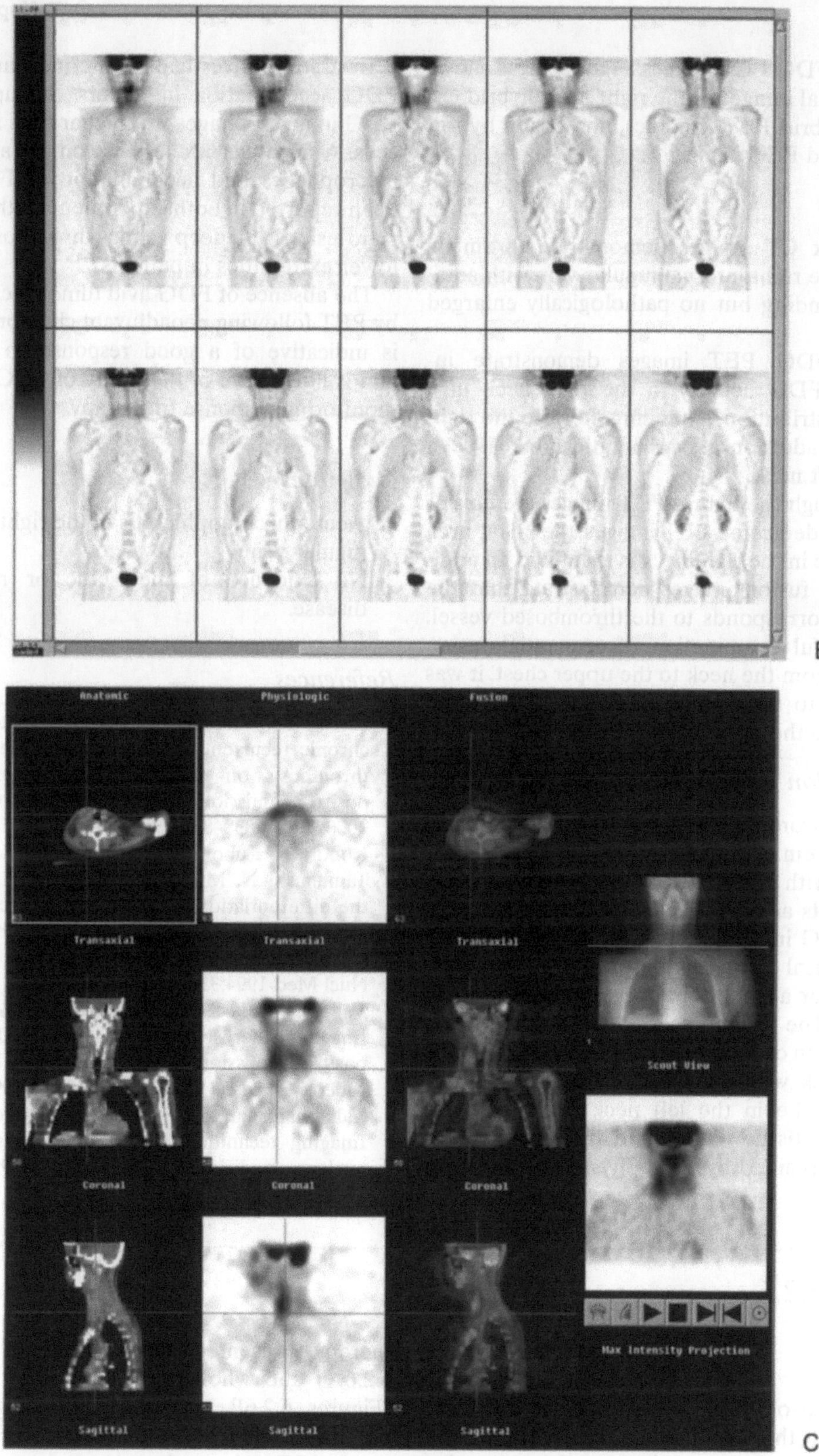

FIGURE 6.2.5B,C. (See color plate)

coronal FDG PET images. Figure 6.2.5C shows orthogonal images of the right neck: hybrid CT (left), hybrid PET (middle), and fusion hybrid CT/hybrid PET (right).

Findings

The neck CT images demonstrate thrombus within the right internal jugular vein with adjacent stranding but no pathologically enlarged nodes.

The FDG PET images demonstrate increased FDG activity in the right neck in a linear distribution, extending down to the right axilla. In addition, a focus of mild uptake is seen in the left neck.

Although the hybrid PET images are noisier than the dedicated PET images, the linear area of uptake in the right neck is identified. In addition, the fusion images demonstrate that the uptake corresponds to the thrombosed vessel. On careful examination of sequential fusion images from the neck to the upper chest, it was possible to trace mild uptake in thrombosed vessels to the right axilla (not shown).

Discussion

Acute thrombophlebitis of the right internal jugular vein was suspected clinically and confirmed with the CT findings. As this process represents active inflammation, it may be seen with FDG imaging. However, correlation with the clinical presentation and CT scan was critical for accurate interpretation of the FDG images. The fusion images demonstrate perfect correlation of the increased FDG activity of the right neck with the CT findings. The focus of mild uptake in the left neck corresponds to muscular tissue on CT and therefore is most likely explained by focal physiologic muscular uptake.

In a study investigating the mechanisms of FDG accumulation in tumors, the uptake of FDG in macrophages was higher than in tumor cells. Atherosclerotic lesions contain abundant macrophages and accumulation of FDG has been reported in both experimental atherosclerotic lesions and deep venous thrombosis of the lower extremities in patients.[1–4]

The absence of FDG avid tumor localization by PET following neoadjuvant chemoradiation is indicative of a good response to therapy and is illustrative of the utility of FDG PET in monitoring response to therapy.

Diagnoses

1. Acute thrombophlebitis of the right internal jugular vein.
2. No evidence of metastatic or recurrent disease.

References

1. Chang KJ, Zhuang H, Alavi A: Detection of chronic recurrent lower extremity deep venous thrombosis on fluorine-18 fluorodeoxyglucose positron emission tomography. Clin Nucl Med 2000;25(10):838–839.
2. Kubota R, Kubota K, Yamada S, Tada M, Ido T, Tamahashi N: Microautoradiographic study for the differentiation of intratumoral macrophages, granulation tissues and cancer cells by the dynamics of fluorine-18-fluorodeoxyglucose uptake. J Nucl Med 1994;35(1):104–112.
3. Vallabhajosula S, Machac J, Knesaurek J, et al.: Imaging atherosclerotic macrophage density by positron emission tomography using F-18-fluorodeoxyglucose (FDG). J Nucl Med 1996;37:38P.
4. Vallabhajosula S, Fuster V: Atherosclerosis: Imaging techniques and the evolving role of nuclear medicine. J Nucl Med 1997;38(11):1788–1796.

Case 6.2.6

History

A 42-year-old male with squamous cell carcinoma of the oropharynx previously treated with chemotherapy and external beam radiotherapy presented for staging CT (Figure 6.2.6A) and whole-body FDG PET imaging (Figures 6.2.6B and C). FDG images were obtained using a dedicated full ring PET tomograph (GE Advance) and reconstructed with

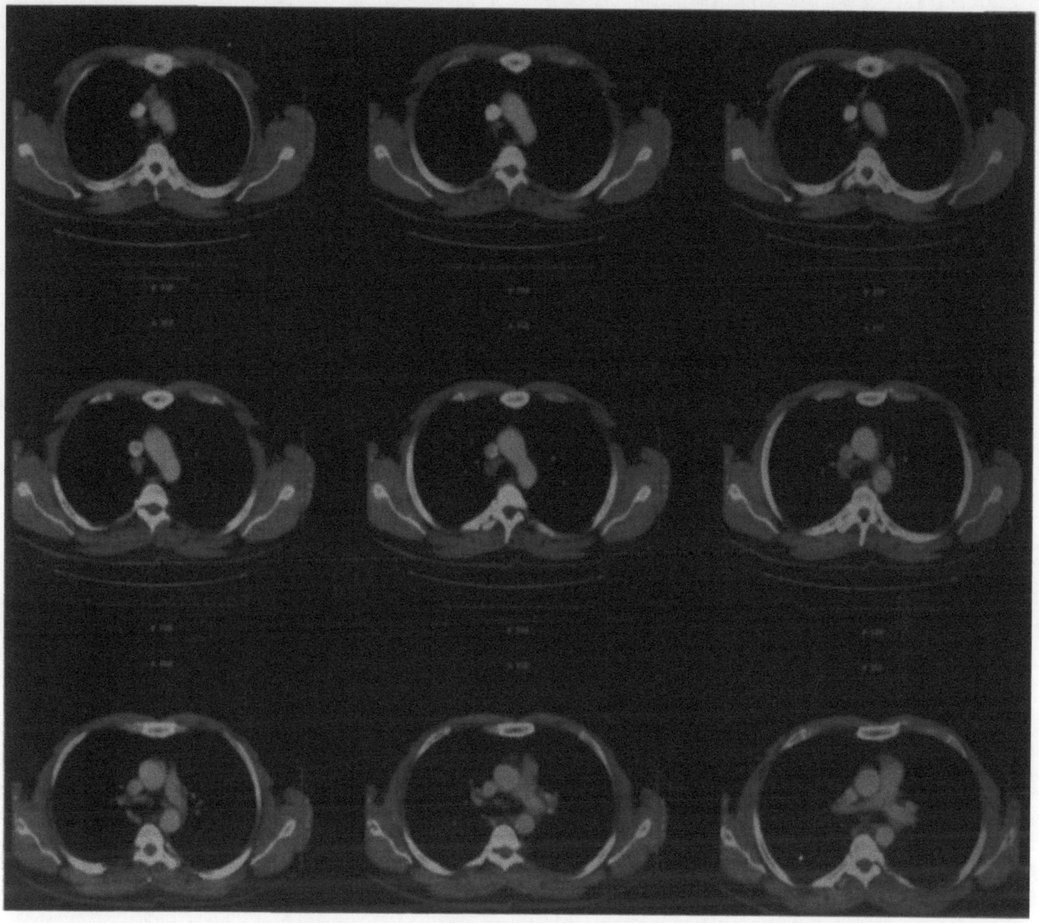

FIGURE 6.2.6A.

iterative reconstruction and measured segmented attenuation correction.

Findings

The CT scan is remarkable for interval decrease in the size of a left jugular node (not shown) and increase in the size of multiple superior mediastinal lymph nodes.

The FDG PET images demonstrate marked activity in the mediastinum extending to the base of the right neck and the left axilla. There are no other foci of abnormal FDG uptake; specifically, the left neck is unremarkable.

Discussion

In a patient with the preceding history, metastatic disease must be a consideration, given the degree of abnormal uptake within the chest and neck. Active granulomatous disease is also a possibility and must be excluded clinically. The referring physician related a history of sarcoidosis, and this was proved with mediastinoscopy.[1–3] The absence of abnormal activity in the region of the persistently enlarged left jugular node is compatible with a favorable response to therapy. However, underlying metastases in the chest cannot be completely excluded.

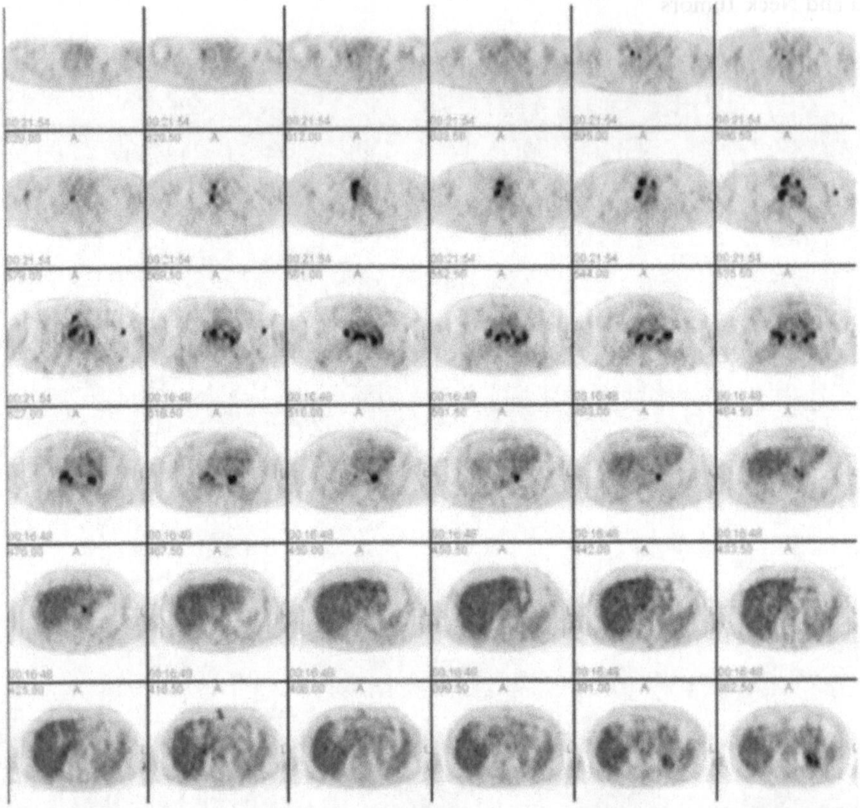
B

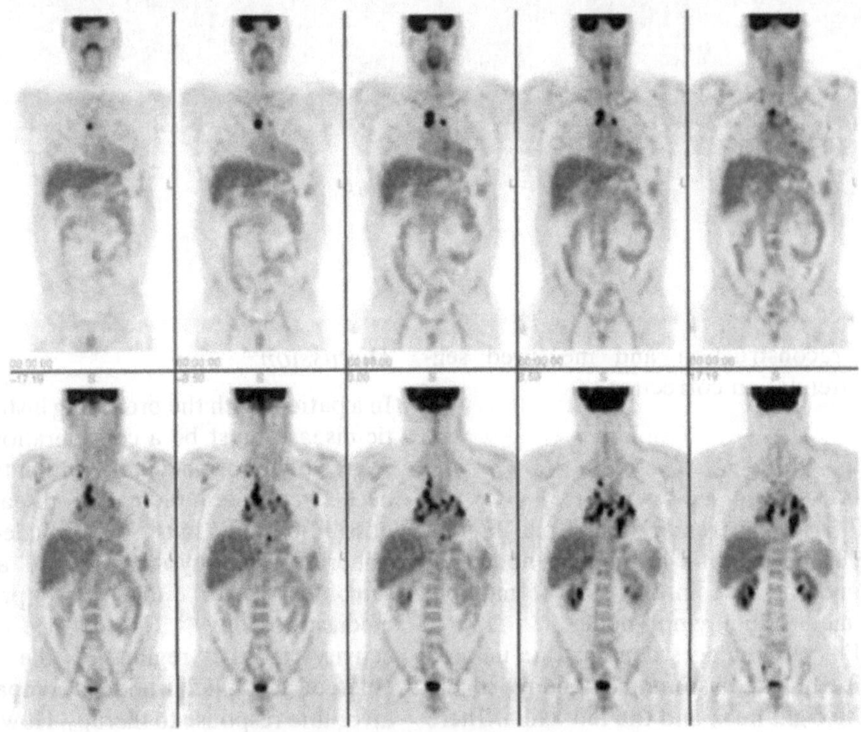
C

FIGURE 6.2.6B,C.

Pulmonary granulomatous disease is endemic in many regions of the United States, especially within the San Joaquin, Mississippi, and Ohio river valleys. This may be problematic, and histologic sampling may be necessary to distinguish malignancy from benign fungal infections, as active lesions may demonstrate prominent uptake of FDG with SUVs sometimes greater than 2.5.

Although FDG PET imaging has not been studied systematically, it may well represent an effective technique for determining the extent of active sarcoidosis, especially in regard to organ (for example, spleen) and skeletal involvement. At present, ^{111}In-octreotide scintigraphy has supplanted ^{67}gallium imaging as the modality of choice for imaging sarcoidosis.

Diagnosis

Sarcoidosis.

References

1. Lewis PJ, Salama A: Uptake of fluorine-18-fluoroglucose in sarcoidosis. J Nucl Med 1994;35: 1647–1649.
2. Kobayashi A, Shinozaki T, Shinjyo Y, Kato K, Oriuchi N, Watanabe H, et al.: FDG PET in the clinical evaluation of sarcoidosis with bone lesions. Ann Nucl Med 2000;14(4):311–313.
3. Lebthahi R, Crestani B, Belmatoug N, et al.: Somatostatin receptors scintigraphy and gallium scintigraphy in patients with sarcoidosis. J Nucl Med 2001;42:21–26.

6.3 Lung Tumors

Mark Kuzucu, William H. Martin, and Dominique Delbeke

Lung cancer is the most common cause of cancer death in both men and women in the United States with approximately 160,000 deaths annually. Only 13% of patients who develop lung cancer survive five years. The classification of the World Health Organization divides these tumors into four major categories: squamous cell carcinoma, 35 to 50%; adenocarcinoma, 15 to 35%; small cell carcinoma, 20 to 25%; and large cell (undifferentiated) carcinoma, 10 to 15%. Squamous cell and small cell carcinomas (SCLC) are predominantly associated with smoking and arise from the proximal bronchial tree. Adenocarcinomas are more often peripherally located in the lung and arise from the alveolar surface epithelium or bronchial mucosal glands. Small cell carcinomas have the poorest prognosis, having usually spread systemically at the time of diagnosis.

Small cell lung carcinoma is not treated surgically. It usually presents with widespread disease, which is initially responsive to combination chemotherapy, although median survival is less than one year despite therapy. In the few patients with disease limited to one hemithorax, external radiation therapy is combined with aggressive chemotherapy. Surgery is the treatment of choice for non–small cell lung cancer (NSCLC) patients with stage I and II disease, although radiation therapy may be administered with curative intent if there are contraindications for surgery. The five-year survival for patients with stage I and II NSCLC is 40% and 20%, respectively. Patients with stage IIIA disease, depending on the clinical circumstances, may be considered for surgery, radiation therapy, chemotherapy, or a combination of these modalities. Five-year survival is 15%. Patients with stage IIIB do not benefit from surgery, having a five-year survival of 5%. Median survival of stage IIIB and IV patients treated with newer combinations of platinum-based regimens is 35 to 45 weeks with a one-year survival of 40%.

Patients who have lung cancer often present with solitary pulmonary nodules (SPN) on chest radiographs performed as preoperative evaluations or part of routine physical examinations.

Diagnosing Lung Carcinoma and Evaluation of Indeterminate Pulmonary Nodules

In the United States, there are 130,000 new pulmonary nodules discovered in patients each year. Only 30 to 50% of these nodules are malignant. Sputum cytology will be positive in 80% of central tumors, but the yield is less than 20% for small, peripheral tumors. Chest radiography and CT imaging have well-known limitations in differentiating benign from malignant nodules, leading to a large number of unnecessary invasive procedures. Transbronchial and transthoracic fine-needle biopsy provide a greater than 90% yield but can suffer from sampling error, and therefore, negative results cannot reliably exclude the presence of a malignant tumor.[1–6] In addition, 2 to 3% of patients who undergo a percutaneous biopsy develop a pneumothorax requiring the placement of a chest tube.[3,6]

FDG PET imaging is used increasingly to differentiate benign from malignant focal pulmonary abnormalities and is gradually replacing some of the invasive modalities previously used. Multiple studies have shown the utility of FDG PET in characterizing pulmonary nodules and opacities that are indeterminate on chest radiography and/or CT scan.[7–22] (Table 6.3.1) The reported performance of FDG PET in these studies to detect a malignant nodule is the following: The sensitivity ranges from 83 to 100%, the specificity is lower due to false-positive inflammatory/granulomatous lesions (62 to 100%), and the accuracy ranges from 86 to 98%. The negative predictive value of 95% is especially reassuring. Active granulomatous processes such as tuberculosis and histoplasmosis and even silicoanthracosis[23] may accumulate FDG and cause false-positive scans in the evaluation of malignancy with PET.[9,11] Other etiologies for false-positives are sarcoidosis, acute radiation pneumonitis, lipoid pneumonia that can be caused by mineral oil ingestion, talc granulomas, and sometimes postobstructive pneumonia. False-negative FDG PET scans can occur for small lesions (< 1 cm) due to partial volume averaging, in patients with elevated serum glucose levels, with bronchial carcinoid, bronchioalveolar carcinoma, and mucinous neoplasms.[24–27] Bronchioalveolar carcinoma represents only 5% of all lung cancers and is a more differentiated subtype of adenocarcinoma occurring in a younger population and with a better prognosis than the other subtypes. Approximately 50 to 80% of bronchioalveolar carcinomas are hypometabolic and therefore undetected by PET.

In our experience,[18] FDG PET is an accurate imaging modality to differentiate malignant from benign pulmonary lesions both in patients with and without a history of prior malignancy. We found, like other studies, that an SUV of 2.5 is the optimal cutoff level to differentiate malignant from benign lesions in the lung. The interpretation is equivalent using as the cutoff level either the standard uptake value (SUV) of 2.5 or the lesion-to-background (L/B) ratio of 5, and the overall accuracy is 88%. Visual analysis without quantitation of activity may be as accurate.

The "Prospective Investigation of PET in Lung Nodules," a multicenter study including 90 patients from five centers, confirmed the findings of the individual studies and led to the following conclusion:[22] Owing to its high sensitivity and negative predictive value for pulmonary lesions greater than 1 cm, FDG PET can exclude the presence of a malignant lesion with great certainty. Because over 50% of solitary pulmonary nodules are benign, no further

TABLE 6.3.1. Evaluation of lung nodules with FDG PET.

Author	Year	No. of patients	Sensitivity (%)	Specificity (%)	Accuracy (%)
Kubota[7]	1990	22	83	90	86
Dewan[9]	1993	30	95	80	90
Patz[10]	1993	51	89	100	92
Lowe[11]	1994	88	97	89	
Dewan[12]	1995	35	100	78	94
Paulus[13]	1995	45	100	93	98
Duhaylongsod[14]	1995	87	97	82	92
Hubner[15]	1995	23	100	67	92
Inoue[16]	1995	39	100	62	87
Gupta[17]	1996	61	93	88	92
Knight[18]	1996	48	100	63	88
Lowe[21]	1997	197	96	77	89
Lowe[22]	1998	89	92	90	91
Total		815	83 to 100	62 to 100	86 to 98

work-up is necessary for patients with a negative FDG PET scan of a mass larger than 1 cm, precluding further use of expensive and invasive procedures. Patients with a positive PET scan require further evaluation by biopsy to establish the tissue diagnosis. The high sensitivity at the expense of lower specificity is acceptable because malignancy will be undiagnosed in few patients. FDG-negative lung masses should be followed with chest CT at six-month intervals for two years.

An analysis of potential cost savings has projected that using the CT plus FDG PET strategy instead of CT alone in the evaluation of patients with solitary pulmonary nodules would result in a cost savings of $91 to $2,200 per patient. This translates into a yearly national savings of $62.7 million by decreasing the need for thoracotomies and transthoracic needle aspirations.[28] A significant reduction in patient morbidity and mortality was also projected.

Staging Non-Small Cell Lung Carcinoma

Lung carcinoma can spread via the lymphatic channels and the vasculature resulting in hematogenous spread of distant metastases. The lymphatic channels follow the bronchioarterial tree to reach the mediastinum. The lower lobes drain primarily to the posterior mediastinum, the right upper lobe drains into the superior mediastinum, and the left upper lobe drains into the anterior and superior mediastinum. Peripheral tumor can spread to pleural lymphatic channels. Staging using the extent of the primary tumor (T), regional lymph nodes (N), and distant metastases (M) is essential in the management of patients with non–small cell bronchogenic carcinoma; the TNM classification has been recently summarized.[29]

For patients with early stage NSCLC, surgical resection is the treatment of choice. The treatment of patients with N2 disease (with ipsilateral lymph node involvement) is still controversial. Patients with minimal N2 disease are potentially curable by surgery, but these represent only 20% of patients with N2 disease. Most of these patients are identified only at thoracotomy. Involvement of contralateral lymph nodes (stage N3), however, is usually a contraindication to surgery.[30] The CT and MRI criteria to detect nodal involvement are based on size and shape of the lymph nodes. These criteria have obvious limitations: Lymph nodes of normal size can be involved by tumors, and inflammatory lymph nodes can be enlarged. In the multi-institutional Radiologic Diagnostic Oncology Group trial sponsored by the National Cancer Institute, CT was 52% sensitive and 69% specific, and MR imaging was 48% sensitive and 64% specific in detecting mediastinal nodal involvement by tumor.[31] As a consequence, mediastinoscopy, which is the most reliable technique to stage the mediastinum, remains an important technique for accurate staging.[31–33]

In contrast to CT and MRI, both of which depend on morphological criteria, the findings on FDG PET imaging depend on the metabolic characteristics of the tissues. It is now well demonstrated that FDG PET imaging is significantly more accurate than CT for noninvasively staging mediastinal disease in patients with NSCLC.[34–52] (Table 6.3.2) In these studies, the sensitivity and specificity of FDG PET imaging ranged from 66 to 100% and 81 to 100%, respectively, and the accuracy ranged from 80 to 100%. The sensitivity and specificity for CT in these studies ranged from 42 to 81% and 44 to 94%, respectively, and the accuracy ranged from 52 to 82%. However, although FDG PET imaging appears more accurate in detecting the extent of mediastinal involvement of NSCLC in preoperative staging, PET may not detect bronchial wall, pleural, and vascular invasion. Therefore, anatomical imaging is also necessary. For this reason, fusion images of CT and PET are probably the best choice for optimizing the strengths of both imaging technologies. A meta-analysis and summary receiver operating curve analysis including 14 studies (514 patients) and 29 studies (2,226 patients) evaluating the performance of PET and CT, respectively, indicated that PET was more accurate than CT for demonstration of nodal metastases. The mean sensitivity and specificity were 79% and 91%, respectively for

TABLE 6.3.2. Mediastinal staging of lung carcinoma with FDG PET.

Authors	Year	No. of patients	No. of LN stations	CT Sensitivity (%)	CT Specificity (%)	CT Accuracy (%)	PET Sensitivity (%)	PET Specificity (%)	PET Accuracy (%)
Wahl[34]	1994	23		64	44	52	82	81	81
Scott[35]	1994	25					83	94	91
Valk[36]	1995	76		63	73	70	83	94	91
Chin[37]	1995	30		56	86	77	78	81	80
Patz[38]	1995	62		42	85	53	83	82	82
Sasaki[39]	1996	29	71	65	87	82	76	98	93
Sazon[40]	1996	32		81	56	69	100	100	100
Scott[41]	1996	27	75	60	93		100	98	
Bury[42]	1996	50		72	81		90	82	
Bury[43]	1997	109					100	94	86
Steinert[44]	1997	47	191	57	94	85	89	99	96
Guhlmann[45]	1997	46		50	75	60	80	100	87
Vansteenkiste[46]	1997	50		67	59	64	67	97	88
Vansteenkiste[47]	1998	68	690	75	63	68	93	95	94*
Total		674		42 to 81	44 to 94	52 to 82	66 to 100	81 to 100	80 to 100

* PET + CT.

PET, and 60% and 77% for CT.[53] A prospective study including 102 patients comparing CT, PET, and histopathology reported a sensitivity of 75% and a specificity of 66% for CT, compared to 91% sensitivity and 86% specificity for PET, supporting the data from the meta-analysis.[54] Because of the high negative predictive value of PET, patients with a negative PET scan can proceed directly to thoracotomy and be spared invasive mediastinal staging. However, because of the false-positive findings due to inflammatory disease, patients with a positive PET scan should be referred for mediastinoscopy.[55]

The cost effectiveness of including PET in staging patients with NSCLC has been demonstrated using decision tree sensitivity analysis.[56] The CT plus PET strategy using the conservative tree showed a savings of $1,154 per patient without a loss of life expectancy, in comparison to the alternate strategy of CT alone.

FDG PET can also provide unique information in the detection of unsuspected distant metastases in patients with pulmonary masses when a whole-body scanning technique is used.[57,58] In a study of 94 patients with stage IIIA disease or less, unexpected extrathoracic metastases were detected using FDG PET imaging in 14% of the patients,[57] thus promoting them to inoperable stage IV. Unsuspected distant metastases were detected in 10% of the patients in the prospective study of Pieterman et al.[54]

Furthermore, semiquantitative FDG PET may provide prognostic information in patients with lung cancer. In a series of 155 patients with NSCLC, a SUV of > 10 provided prognostic information independent of the clinical stage and lesion size, with a survival less than half of that of patients with tumor SUV < 10.[59–61] For lung carcinoma, FDG PET seems to be more sensitive to detect bone metastases than bone scintigraphy.[62,63] A study of 20 patients with osseous lesions demonstrated that using a 2.0 cutoff value for SUV, PET correctly identified 14 of 15 malignant lesions and 4 of 5 benign lesions.[61]

Monitoring Therapy and Detection of Persistent or Recurrent Lung Carcinoma

Another application is the differentiation of recurrent tumor versus scar in patients who have been already treated.[14,16,64,65] Preliminary studies indicate that FDG PET can be useful in predicting and assessing the response to radiation therapy[66–68] and chemotherapy.[69,70] In addition, FDG PET imaging may have a prognostic significance.[71]

Summary

FDG PET imaging is recommended to evaluate indeterminate pulmonary nodules greater in size than the resolution of the system used for imaging (5 to 15 mm). Because of the high negative predictive value of FDG PET, FDG-negative lesions can be followed with imaging studies. FDG-positive lesions should be biopsied because of the relatively high rate of false-positive active granulomatous processes. FDG PET should also be performed for staging NSCLC, because it can detect metastatic lymph nodes that do not meet CT size criteria for malignancy. Because of its whole-body technique, PET imaging is capable of detecting unsuspected distant metastases with a high degree of sensitivity. Unlike CT, FDG PET imaging can differentiate scar tissue from recurrent tumor and therefore has applications for monitoring therapy and the evaluation of recurrent disease.

Common sources of false-positive findings include active granulomatous processes (such as tuberculosis, histoplasmosis, other fungal infections, sarcoidosis, and talc granuloma), postobstructive pneumonia, healing wounds and fractures, postoperative pleural inflammation, and postradiation fibrosis. Cases of FDG-avid lipoid pneumonia have also been described. False-negatives include lesions smaller (< 1 cm) than the resolution of the system used for imaging and bronchioalveolar carcinomas and some carcinoid and mucinous tumors.

References

1. Salathe M, Soler M, Bollinger CT, et al.: Transbronchial needle aspiration in routine fiberoptic bronchoscopy. Respiration 1992;59:5–8.
2. Schenk DA, Bower JH, Bryan CL, et al.: Transbronchial needle aspiration staging of bronchogenic carcinoma. Am Rev Resp Dis 1986; 134:146–148.
3. Wang KP, Kelly SJ, Britt JE: Percutaneous needle aspiration biopsy of chest lesions. New instrument and new technique. Chest 1988;93: 993–997.
4. Polak J, Kubik A: Percutaneous thin needle biopsy of malignant and non-malignant thoracic lesions. Radiologia Diagnostica 1989;30:177–182.
5. Winning AJ, McIvor J, Seed WA, et al.: Interpretation of negative results in fine needle aspiration of discrete pulmonary lesions. Thorax 1986;41:875–879.
6. Williams AJ, Santiago S, Lerhman S, et al.: Trancutaneous needle aspiration of solitary pulmonary masses: How many passes? Am Rev Resp Dis 1987;136:452–454.
7. Kubota K, Matsuzawa T, Fujiwara T, et al.: Differential diagnosis of lung tumor with positron emission tomography: A prospective study. J Nucl Med 1990;31:1927–1933.
8. Gupta NC, Frank AR, Dewan NA, et al.: Solitary pulmonary nodules: Detection of malignancy with PET with 2-[F-18]-fluoro-2-deoxy-D-glucose. Radiology 1992;184:441–444.
9. Dewan NA, Gupta NC, Redepenning LS, et al.: Diagnostic efficacy of PET-FDG imaging in solitary pulmonary nodules: Potential role in evaluation and management. Chest 1993;104: 997–1002.
10. Patz EF, Lowe VJ, Hoffman JM, et al.: Focal pulmonary abnormalities: Evaluation with F-18-fluorodeoxyglucose PET scanning. Radiology 1993;188:487–490.
11. Lowe VJ, Hoffman DM, DeLong DM, Patz EF, Coleman RE: Semiquantitative and visual analysis of FDG-PET images in pulmonary abnormalities. J Nucl Med 1994;35:1771–1776.
12. Dewan NA, Reeb SD, Gupta NC, et al.: PET-FDG imaging and transthoracic needle lung aspiration biopsy in evaluation of pulmonary lesions. A comparative risk-benefit analysis. Chest 1995;108:441–446.
13. Paulus P, Benoit TH, Bury TH, et al.: Positron emission tomography with ^{18}F-fluoro-deoxyglucose in the assessment of solitary pulmonary nodules. Eur J Nucl Med 1995;22:775.
14. Duhaylongsod FG, Lowe VJ, Patz EF, et al.: Detection of primary and recurrent lung cancer by means of F-18 fluorodeoxyglucose positron emission tomography. FDG-PET. J Thorac Cardiovasc Surg 1995;110:130–140.
15. Hubner KF, Buonocore E, Singh SK, et al.: Characterization of chest masses by FDG positron emission tomography. Clin Nucl Med 1995;20: 293–298.
16. Inoue T, Kim EE, Komasi R, et al.: Detecting recurrent or residual lung cancer with FDG-PET. J Nucl Med 1995;36:788–793.

17. Gupta NC, Maloof J, Gunel E: Probability of malignancy in solitary pulmonary nodules using fluorine-18-FDG and PET. J Nucl Med 1996; 37:943–948.
18. Knight SB, Delbeke D, Stewart JR, Sandler MP: Evaluation of pulmonary lesions with FDG-PET: Comparison of findings in patients with and without a history of prior malignancy. Chest 1996;109:982–988.
19. Bury T, Dowlati A, Paulus P, et al.: Evaluation of pulmonary nodules by positron emission tomography. Europ Respiratory J 1996;9:410–414.
20. Dewan NA, Shehan CJ, Reeb SD, Gobar LS, Scott WJ, Ryschon K: Likelihood of malignancy in a solitary pulmonary nodule: Comparison of Bayesian analysis and results of FDG-PET scan. Chest 1997;112:416–422.
21. Lowe VJ, Duhaylongsod FG, Patz EF, et al.: Pulmonary abnormalities and PET data analysis: A retrospective study. Radiology 1997;202:435–446.
22. Lowe VJ, Fletcher JW, Gobar L, et al.: Prospective investigation of PET in lung nodules. J Clin Oncol 1998;16:1075–1084.
23. Pieterman RM, van Putten JWG, Meuzelaar JJ, et al.: Preoperative staging of non-small-cell lung cancer with positron-emission tomography. N Engl J Med 2000;343:254–261.
24. Erasmus JJ, McAdams HP, Patz EF, Coleman RE, Ahuja V, Goodman PC: Evaluation of primary pulmonary carcinoid tumors using FDG PET. Am J Roentgenol 1998;170(5):1369–1373.
25. Kim B, Kim Y, Lee KS, et al.: Localized form of bronchioloalveolar carcinoma: FDG-PET findings. Am J Roentgenol 1998;170:935–939.
26. Yap CS, Schiepers C, Fishbein M, Phelps ME, Czernin J: Metabolic imaging in lung cancer: How sensitive it is for bronchiolo-alveolar carcinoma? J Nucl Med 2001;42:749.
27. Berger KL, Nicholson SA, Dehdashti F, Siegel BA: FDG PET evaluation of mucinous neoplasms: Correlation of FDG uptake with histopathologic features. Am J Roentgenol 2000; 174(4):1005–1008.
28. Gambhir SS, Shepherd JE, Shah BD, et al.: Analytical decision model for the cost-effective management of solitary pulmonary nodules. J Clin Oncol 1998;16:2113–2125.
29. Al-Sugair A, Coleman RE: Applications of PET in lung cancer. Sem Nucl Med 1998;28(4): 303–319.
30. Watanabe Y, Shimizu J, Oda M, et al.: Aggressive surgical intervention in N2 non-small cell cancer of the lung. Ann Thorac Surg 1991;51:253–261.
31. Webb WR, Gatsonis C, Zerhouni EA, et al.: CT and MR imaging in staging non-small cell bronchogenic carcinoma: Report of the Radiologic Diagnostic Oncology Group. Radiology 1991; 178:705–713.
32. McLoud TC, Bourgouin PM, Greenberg RW, et al.: Bronchogenic carcinoma: Analysis of staging in the mediastinum with CT by correlative lymph node mapping and sampling. Radiology 1992;182:319–323.
33. Webb WR, Sarin M, Zerhouini EA, Heelan RT, Glazer GM, Gatsonis C: Interobserver variability in CT and MR staging of lung cancer. J Comput Assist Tomogr 1993;17:841–846.
34. Wahl RL, Quint LE, Greenough RL, Meyer CR, White RI, Orringer MB: Staging of mediastinum non-small cell lung cancer with FDG-PET, CT, and fusion images: Preliminary prospective evaluation. Radiology 1994;191:371–377.
35. Scott WJ, Schwabe JL, Gupta NC, et al.: Positron emission tomography of lung tumors and mediastinal lymph nodes using [^{18}F]fluorodeoxyglucose. Ann Thorac Surg 1994;58:698–703.
36. Valk PE, Poundds TR, Hopkins DM, et al.: Staging non-small cell lung cancer by whole-body positron emission tomographic imaging. Ann Thorac Surg 1995;60:1573–1581.
37. Chin R Jr, Ward R, Keyes JW Jr, et al.: Mediastinal staging of non-small-cell lung cancer with positron emission tomography. Am J Resp Crit Care Med 1995;152:2090–2096.
38. Patz EJ, Lowe VG, Goodman PC, et al.: Thoracic nodal staging with PET imaging with 18FDG in patients with bronchogenic carcinoma. Chest 1995;108:1617–1621.
39. Sasaki M, Ichiya Y, Kuwabara Y, et al.: The usefulness of FDG positron emission tomography for the detection of mediastinal lymph node metastases in patients with non-small cell lung cancer: A comparative study with X-ray computed tomography. Eur J Nucl Med 1996;23; 741–747.
40. Sazon DAD, Santiago SM, Soo GW, et al.: Fluorodeoxyglucose-positron emission tomography in the detection and staging of lung cancer. Am J Respir Crit Care Med 1996;153:417–421.
41. Scott WJ, Gobar LS, Terry JD, et al.: Mediastinal lymph node staging of non-small-cell lung cancer: A prospective comparison of computed tomography and positron emission tomography. J Thorac & Cardiovascul Surg 1996;111:642–648.
42. Bury T, Paulus P, Dowlati A, et al.: Staging of the mediastinum: Value of positron emission tomo-

graphy imaging in non-small cell lung cancer. Eur Respir J 1996;9:2560–2564.
43. Bury T, Dowlate A, Corhay JL, et al.: Whole-body 18-FDG in the staging of non-small cell lung cancer. Eur Respir J 1997;10:2529–2534.
44. Steinert HC, Hauser M, Alleman F, et al.: Non-small cell lung cancer: Nodal staging with FDG-PET versus CT with correlative lymph node mapping and sampling. Radiology 1997;202:441–446.
45. Guhlmann A, Storck M, Kotzerke J, Moog F, Sunder-Plassmann L, Reske SN: Lymph node staging in non-small cell lung cancer: Evaluation by [18F]FDG positron emission tomography (PET). Thorax 1997;52:438–441.
46. Vansteenkiste JF, Stroobants SG, De Lyn PR, et al.: Mediastinal lymph node staging with FDG-PET scan in patients with potentially operable non-small cell lung cancer: A prospective analysis of 50 cases. Leuven Lung Cancer Group. Chest 1997;112:1480–1486.
47. Vansteenkiste JF, Stroobants SG, De Lyn PR, et al.: Lymph node staging in non-small cell lung cancer with FDG-PET scan: A prospective study on 690 lymph node stations from 68 patients. J Clin Oncol 1998;16:2142–2149.
48. Weder W, Schmid RA, Brushhaus H, Hillinger S, von Schulthess GK, Steinert HC: Detection of extrathoracic metastases by positron emission tomography in lung cancer. Ann Thorac Surg 1998;66:892–893.
49. Gupta CG, Graeber GM, Rogers JS, Bishop HA: Comparative efficacy of positron emission tomography with FDG and computed tomographic scanning in preoperative staging of non-small cell lung cancer. Annals of Surgery 1999;229(2):286–291.
50. Kernstine KH, Stanford W, Mullan BF, et al.: PET, CT, and MRI with Combidex for mediastinal staging in non-small cell lung carcinoma. Ann Thoracic Surg 1999;68(3):1022–1028.
51. Farrell MA, McAdams HP, Herndon JE, Patz EF: Non-small cell lung cancer: FDG PET for nodal staging in patients with stage I disease. Radiology 2000;215:886–890.
52. Saunders CA, Dussek JE, O'Doherty MJ, Maisey MN: Evaluation of fluorine-18-fluorodeoxyglucose whole body positron emission tomography imaging in the staging of lung cancer. Ann Thorac Surg 1999;67(3):790–797.
53. Dwamena BA, Sonnad SS, Angobaldo JO, Wahl RL: Metastases from non-small cell lung cancer: Mediastinal staging in the 1990s—Meta-analytic comparison of PET and CT. Radiology 1999; 213:530–536.
54. Pieterman RM, van Putten JWG, Meuzelaar JJ, et al.: Preoperative staging of non-small-cell cancer with positron emission tomography. N Engl J Med 2000;343:254–261.
55. Berlangieri SU, Scott AM: Metabolic staging of lung cancer. N Engl J Med 2000;34:290–292.
56. Gambhir SS, Hoh CK, Phelps ME, Madar I, Maddahi J: Decision tree sensitivity analysis for cost-effectiveness of FDG-PET in the staging and management of non-small-cell lung carcinoma. J Nucl Med 1996;37:1428–1436.
57. Rege SD, Hoh CK, Glaspy JA, et al.: Imaging of pulmonary mass lesions with whole body positron emission tomography and fluorodeoxyglucose. Cancer 1993;72:82–90.
58. Weder W, Schmid RA, Bruchhaus H, Hillinger S, son Schulthess GK, Steinert HC: Detection of extrathoracic metastases by positron emission tomography in lung cancer. Ann Thorac Surg 1998;66:886–892.
59. Ahuja V, Coleman RE, Herndon J, Patz EF: The prognostic significance of fluorodeoxyglucose positron emission tomography imaging for patients with non-small-cell lung carcinoma. Cancer 1998;83:918–924.
60. Shreve PD, Grossman HB, Gross MD, Wahl RL: Metastatic prostate cancer: Initial findings of PET with 2-deoxy-2-[F18]fluoro-D-glucose. Radiology 1996;199:751–756.
61. Dehdashti F, Siegel BA, Griffeth LK, et al.: Benign versus malignant intraosseous lesions: Discrimination by means of PET with 2-[F18] fluoro-2-deoxy-D-glucose. Radiology 1996;200: 243–247.
62. Bury T, Barreto A, Daenen F, Barthelemy N, Ghaye B, Rigo P: Fluorine-18 deoxyglucose positron emission tomography for the detection of bone metastases in patients with non-small cell lung cancer. Eur J Nucl Med 1998;9:1244–1247.
63. Cook GJ, Houston S, Rubens R, Maisey MN, Fogelman I: Detection of bone metastases in breast cancer by 18FDG PET: Differing metabolic activity in osteoblastic and osteolytic lesions. J Clin Oncol 1998;10:3375–3379.
64. Patz E, Lowe VJ, Hoffman JM, et al.: Persistent or recurrent bronchogenic carcinoma using 18F-2-deoxy-D-glucose and positron emission tomography (PET) imaging. Radiology 1994; 191:379–384.
65. Bury T, Cordhay JL, Duysinx B, et al.: Value of FDG PET in detecting residual or recurrent

non-small cell cancer. Eur Respir J 1999;14(6): 1376–1380.
66. Hebert M, Lowe V, Hoffman J, et al.: Positron emission tomography in the pretreatment, evaluation, and follow-up of non-small-cell lung cancer patients treated with radiotherapy. Am J Clin Oncol 1996;19:416–421.
67. Ichija Y, Kuwabara Y, Sasaki M, et al.: A clinical evaluation of FDG-PET to assess the response in radiation therapy for bronchogenic carcinoma. Ann Nucl Med 1996;10:193.
68. Nestle U, Walter K, Schmidt S, et al.: 18F-deoxyglucose positron emission tomography (FDG-PET) for the planning of radiotherapy in lung cancer: High impact in patients with atelectasis. Int J Radiat Oncol Biol Phys 1999;44(3): 593–597.
69. Patz EF, Connolly J, Herndon J: Prognostic value of thoracic FDG PET imaging after treatment for non-small cell lung cancer. Am J Roentgenol 2000;174:769–777.
70. Vansteenkiste JF, Stroobants SG, De Leyn PR, et al.: Potential use of FDG-PET scan after induction chemotherapy in surgically staged IIIa-N2 non-small-cell lung cancer: A prospective pilot study. The Leuven Lung Cancer Group. Ann Oncol 1998;9:1193–1198.
71. Ahuja V, Coleman RE, Herndon J, Patz EF Jr: The prognostic significance of fluorodeoxyglucose positron emission tomography imaging for patients with non-small cell lung carcinoma. Cancer 1998;83(5):918–924.

Case Presentations

Case 6.3.1

History

A 79-year-old man presented with hemoptysis. During the patient's evaluation, a chest radiograph demonstrated a possible right upper lobe soft tissue mass. A CT of the chest and upper abdomen (Figure 6.3.1A) and FDG PET imaging (Figure 6.3.1B, top left, transaxial; bottom, coronal; top right, sagittal) were then performed. The FDG images were acquired with a dedicated PET tomograph (Siemens ECAT 933) and reconstructed using filtered back projection without attenuation correction. FDG images were then obtained with a hybrid dual-head gamma camera (VG Millenium) operating in the coincidence mode (Figure 6.3.1C, see color plate). The hybrid FDG PET images were reconstructed using an iterative

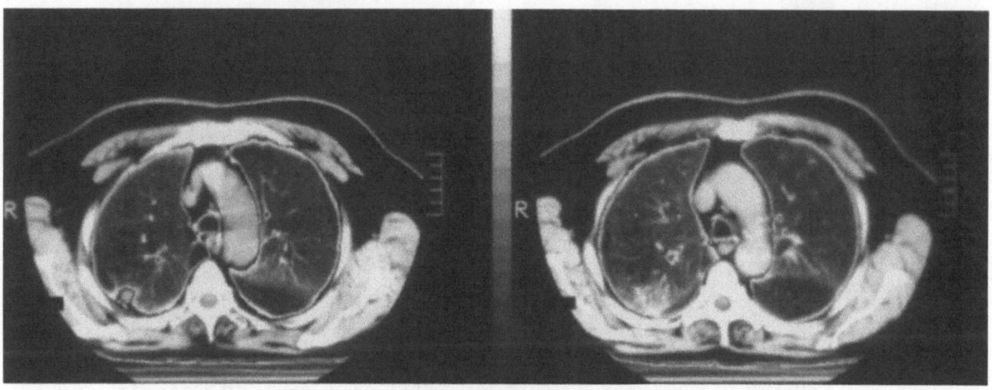

FIGURE 6.3.1A.

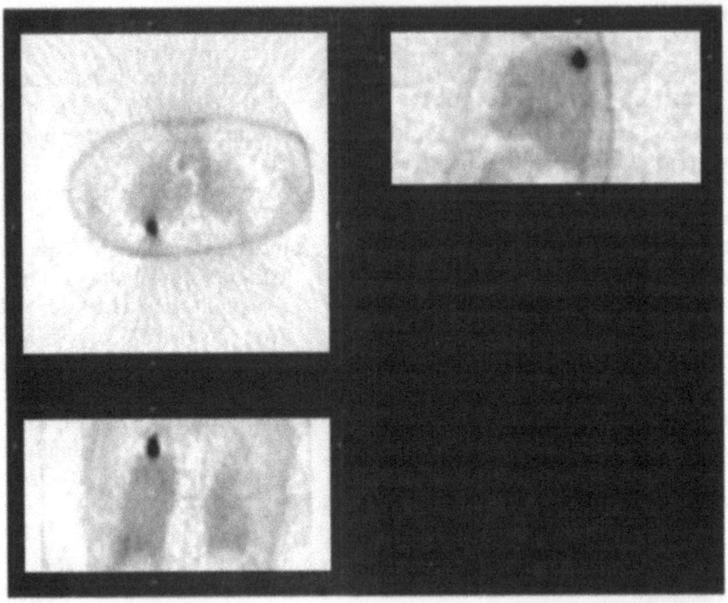

B

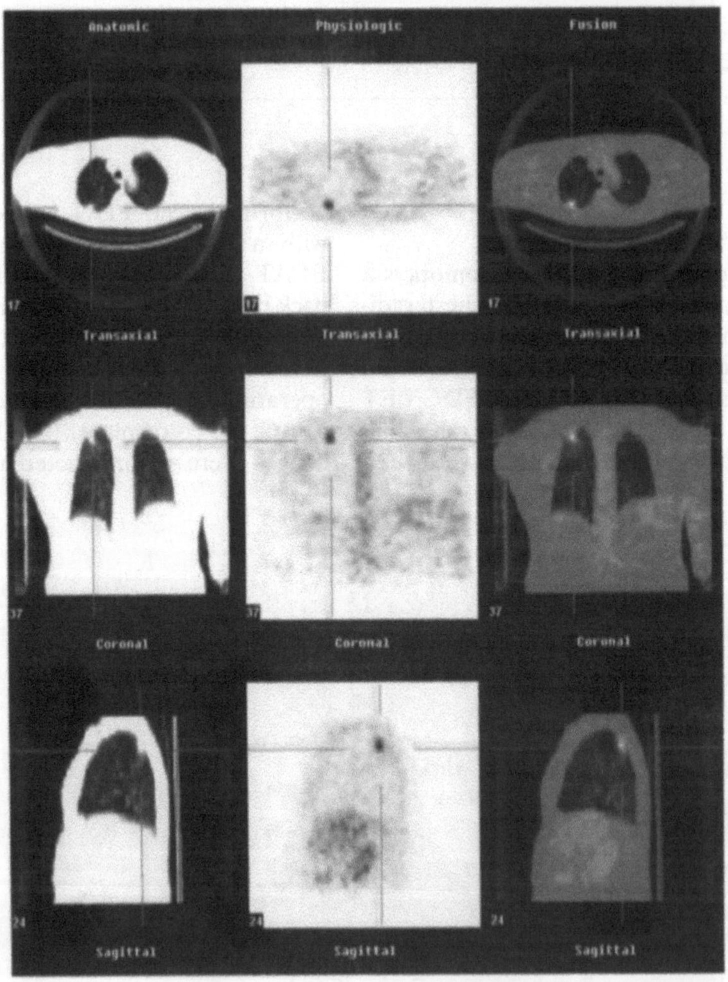

C

FIGURE 6.3.1B,C. (See color plate)

reconstruction algorithm and corrected for attenuation using attenuation maps obtained with a X-ray tube and array of detectors mounted on the gantry of the camera and functioning basically as a third-generation CT scanner. These attenuation maps also provide hybrid CT images for image fusion and anatomical mapping. Figure 6.3.1C shows orthogonal images of the hybrid CT (left), hybrid PET (middle), and fusion image (right).

Findings

The CT of the chest and upper abdomen confirmed a 1 cm area of indeterminate nodularity and scarring within the posterior segment of the right upper lobe, abutting the posterior pleural surface. There was no rib destruction, pleural effusion, adenopathy, adrenal mass, nor other pulmonary parenchymal abnormalities with the exception of emphysematous changes.

The dedicated PET images demonstrate a focus of markedly increased uptake within the posterior right lung apex congruent with the CT abnormality.

The hybrid PET images show a focus of FDG uptake in the same location as the dedicated PET images, although the images are noisier. The hybrid CT image demonstrates the same nodule as the dedicated CT scan, although the resolution of the images is limited compared to the dedicated CT scan. The fusion image demonstrates that the metabolic focus superimposes to the nodule.

Discussion

Intense FDG uptake within a solitary pulmonary nodule is most consistent with malignancy. However, benign inflammatory lesions such as granulomatous infection from tuberculosis, histoplasmosis, or other fungal infections can also show increased activity, although the degree of activity is often less than that seen with malignancy. Therefore, biopsy is necessary for confirmation of malignancy. In this case, the patient refused invasive procedures. Subsequent radiographic and CT evaluation performed over the next year demonstrated progressive enlargement of this lesion.

Although hybrid PET has limitations for lesion detectability compared to dedicated PET (15 to 20 mm versus 5 to 10 mm), this 1 cm lesion was easily detected by both techniques because of the high tumor-to-background ratio present in most pulmonary malignancies.

The dedicated PET images shown have not been corrected for attenuation because that particular model of PET tomograph required acquisition of the transmission scan before FDG administration, involving repositioning of the patient in the scanner gantry between transmission and emission scanning. This can lead to errors in the registration of the transmission and emission data resulting in poor quality images, as was the case in this patient. Without attenuation correction, the lungs typically show higher uptake than the chest wall and mediastinum despite the fact that they contain less metabolically active tissue per volume. This is because the pulmonary parenchyma is filled with air (a low density compound), resulting in less photon attenuation. With the model of hybrid gamma camera used, the CT transmission and FDG emission scans are performed sequentially in time without repositioning of the patient on the scanner bed, and good quality images are more often obtained. On images with attenuation correction, the lungs appear hypometabolic compared to chest wall and mediastinum. The fusion images do not improve sensitivity but do enhance accurate localization of the lesion.

Diagnosis

Malignant solitary pulmonary nodule.

Case 6.3.2

History

A 46-year-old man presented with pleuritic chest pain and dyspnea without fever or constitutional symptoms. A chest radiograph demonstrated a new 1.5 cm focal mass/infiltrate inferior to a large right apical bulla. CT imaging confirmed this finding and showed no addi-

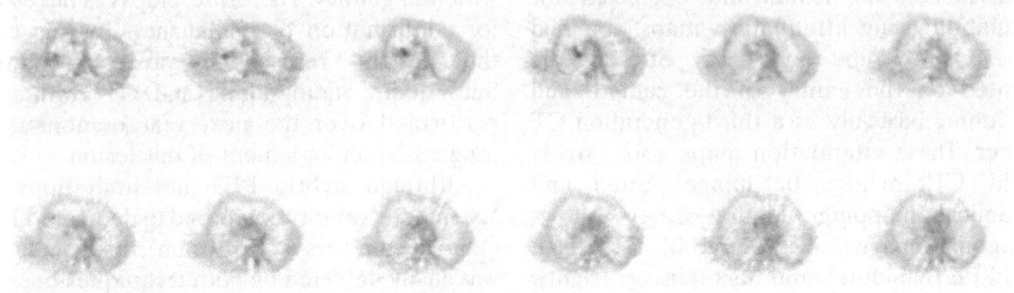

FIGURE 6.3.2A.

tional parenchymal lesions nor evidence of lymphadenopathy. Transbronchial biopsy was nondiagnostic. The patient then underwent FDG imaging with a dedicated PET tomograph (Siemens ECAT 933) with full rings of BGO detectors and with a hybrid PET gamma camera (VG Millenium). Figure 6.3.2A shows transaxial FDG PET images reconstructed using filtered back projection and attenuation correction. The hybrid PET FDG images were reconstructed using an iterative algorithm and corrected for attenuation using attenuation maps obtained with an X-ray tube and array of detectors mounted on the gantry of the camera and functioning basically as a third-generation CT. These attenuation maps also provide hybrid CT images for image fusion and anatomical mapping (Figure 6.3.2B, see color plate). Figure 6.3.2B shows transaxial images of the hybrid CT (left), hybrid PET (middle), and fusion image (right).

Findings

The dedicated PET images demonstrate three small, discrete foci of increased FDG uptake within the right upper lobe, one of which corresponds to the focal abnormality present on the CT scan. The second focus is located just lateral and superior to the focus described preceding. The third one is located just inferior, lateral, and anterior to the other two lesions. The hybrid PET images demonstrate two of these three foci of increased uptake (Figure 6.3.2B, upper and middle panel); the third lesion is not seen (Figure 6.3.2B, lower panel).

Discussion

The patient's initial CT scan demonstrated an ill-defined focus of infiltrate/nodularity within the right upper lobe. However, the PET images demonstrated three discrete foci in this location. The first lesion had the highest SUV (2.6) of the three foci. SUV of 2.5 has been reported to be a defining cutoff value for differentiating benign from malignant lesions within the lung. Because infectious processes can also have FDG uptake approaching this level, biopsy is often necessary to exclude malignancy. The patient underwent subsequent right upper lobectomy. The pathology results were negative for malignancy but did demonstrate the presence of acid-fast bacilli, most consistent with an atypical mycobacterium infection.

The most common cause for a false-positive pulmonary nodule seen with FDG imaging is acute granulomatous infection, including tuberculosis, atypical mycobacteria, histoplasmosis, other fungal infections, and sarcoidosis. Although other inflammatory processes, such as bacterial pneumonia, can demonstrate increased FDG uptake, it is typically a more diffuse low-grade process. FDG PET imaging identified two satellite foci of uptake adjacent to the main one. Although satellite lesions can be seen with malignancy, this finding is atypical and should heighten suspicion for a granulomatous process. Tuberculoma typically appears as a relatively discrete mass with smooth borders and of less than 3cm in diameter, although lesions as large as 5cm have been reported, and irregular edges and spiculation are not uncommon. Satellite lesions are seen in up to 80% of cases. Calcification is seen in 20

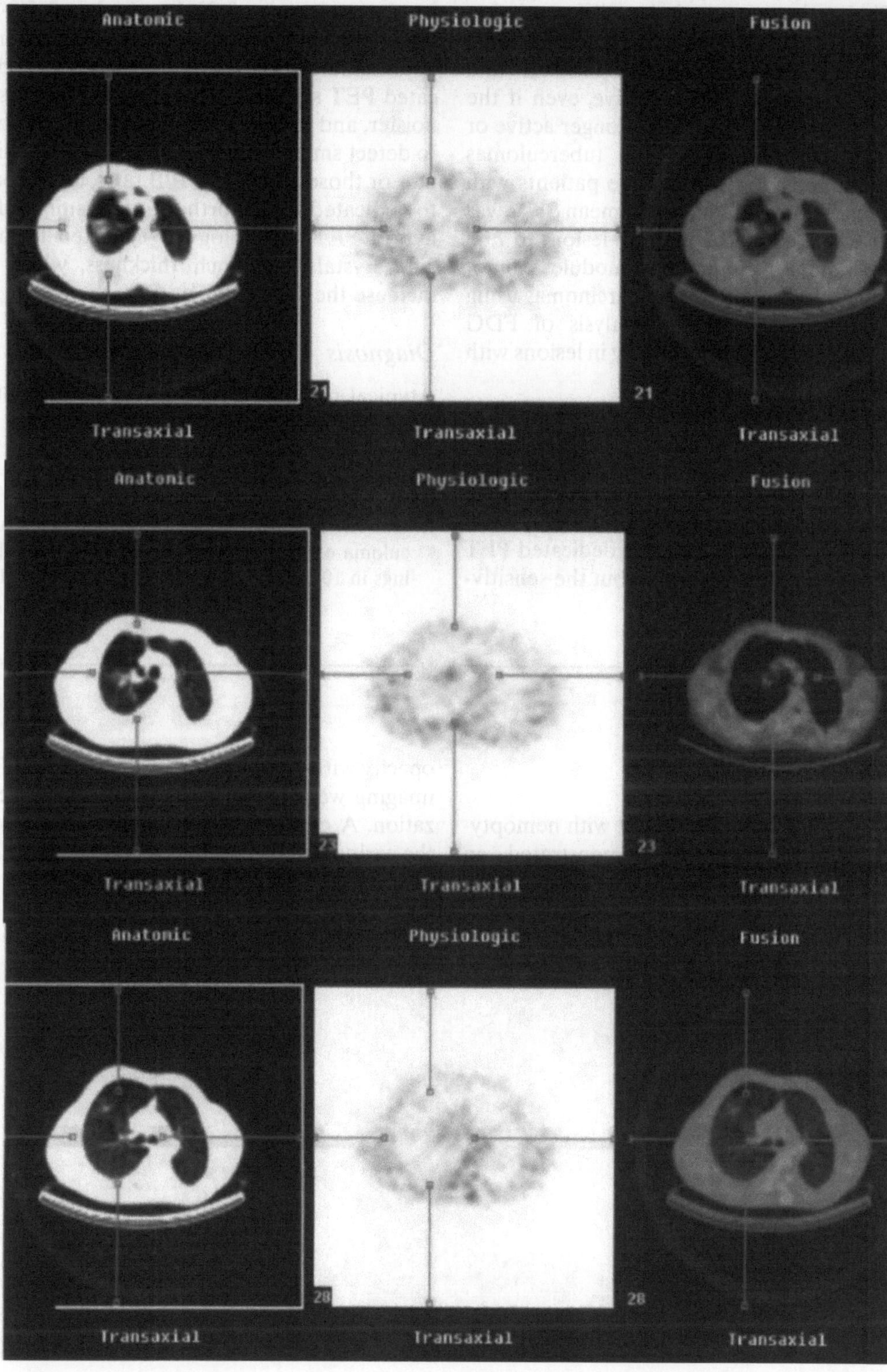

FIGURE 6.3.2B. (See color plate)

to 30%, but in the remainder, differentiation from carcinoma is difficult using conventional radiography. Inflammatory mediastinal and hilar nodes may be FDG-positive, even if the primary pulmonary focus is no longer active or FDG-avid. In a series of ten tuberculomas detected among 150 consecutive patients with solitary pulmonary nodules, the mean SUV was 4.2 with a range of 0 (in an 8 mm lesion) to 7.0.[1] Thus, inflammatory pulmonary nodules cannot always be differentiated from carcinomas using visual or semiquantitative analysis of FDG PET images, necessitating biopsy in lesions with high uptake.

This case illustrates the limitations of hybrid PET compared to dedicated PET for detection of small lesions or lesions with a relatively low SUV or L/B ratio. Gamma cameras operating in the coincidence mode (hybrid PET) have resolution in the same range as dedicated PET scanners, approximately 5 mm, but the sensitivity (count rate) of NaI crystals of 5/8-inch thickness for detection of 511 keV photons is approximately ten times less than that of dedicated PET scanners. Therefore, the images are noisier, and hybrid PET is limited in its ability to detect small lesions less than 1.5 cm in diameter or those with a low L/B ratio, as compared to dedicated PET. Further improvement of the hybrid PET technology is expected by using NaI crystals of 1-inch thickness, which will increase the sensitivity by 50%.

Diagnosis

Atypical mycobacteria infection with multiple small pulmonary nodules.

Reference

1. Goo JM, Im J-G, Do K-H, et al.: Pulmonary tuberculoma evaluated by means of FDG PET: Findings in 10 cases. Radiology 2000;216:117–121.

Case 6.3.3

History

A 72-year-old female presented with hemoptysis. A chest radiograph demonstrated an opacity within the left upper lobe. CT and FDG imaging were performed for lesion characterization. A contrasted CT image at the level of the carina is shown in Figure 6.3.3A. FDG PET

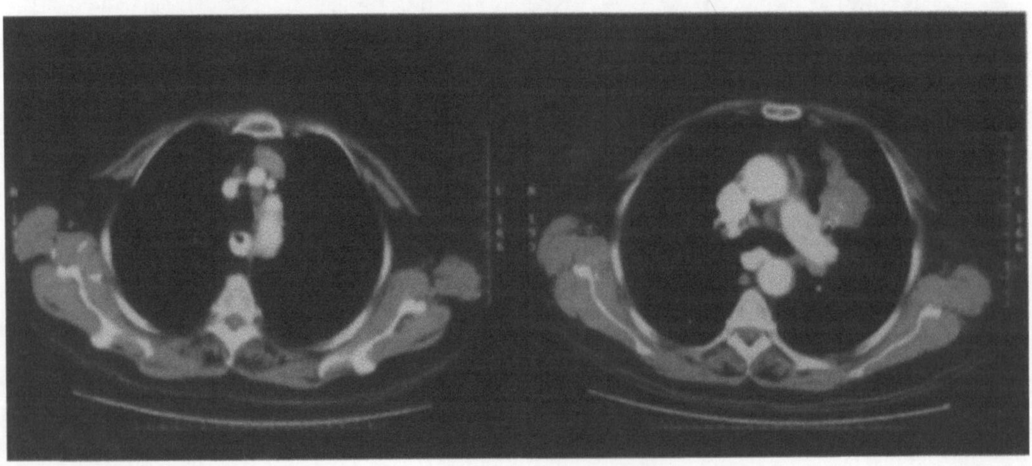

FIGURE 6.3.3A.

images acquired with a dedicated PET tomograph (GE Advance) and reconstructed with iterative reconstruction and measured segmented attenuation correction are shown in Figures 6.3.3B and C. Transaxial images are shown in Figure 6.3.3B, and orthogonal images through the upper mediastinum are shown in Figure 6.3.3C.

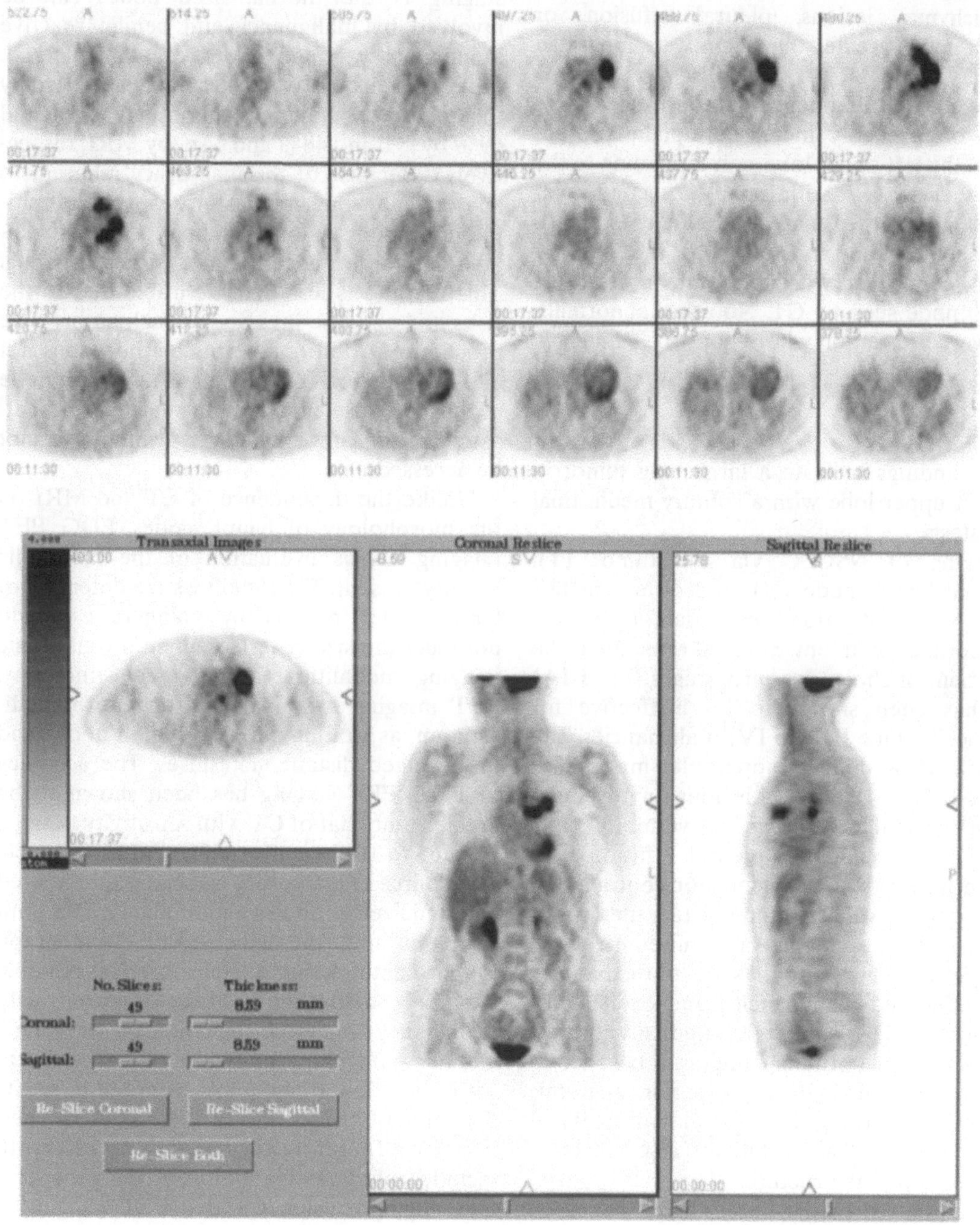

B

C

FIGURE 6.3.3B,C.

Findings

The CT image shows an irregular 4 cm spiculated mass adjacent to the main pulmonary artery extending to the anterior mediastinum. An 8 mm soft tissue density mass is also seen on this image just anterior to the carina. No other parenchymal lesions, pleural effusion, or lymph nodes greater than 1 cm were identified by CT.

The FDG PET images demonstrate a large focus of markedly increased uptake present within the left upper lobe, corresponding to the mass seen by CT. Additionally, a second separate small focus of increased activity is identified superior and posterior to the primary lesion, congruent with the 8 mm pretracheal lymph node seen by CT. No other abnormalities were present on whole-body PET imaging.

Discussion

These findings indicate a large lung tumor in the left upper lobe with a solitary mediastinal metastasis.

Staging of NSCLC via the tumor (T), regional lymph node (N), and distant metastases (M) classification is essential for planning appropriate treatment. Surgical resection is the treatment of choice for early stages (I to IIIA) but has been shown to be ineffective for advanced (stage IIIB to IV) malignancies. The criteria that define inoperable malignancy (stage IIIB or IV) are T4 lesions (involvement of mediastinal organs, carina, vertebral body invasion, or malignant pleural effusion), N3 lymph nodes (supraclavicular or contralateral hilar or mediastinal), or any distant metastases (M1). Accurate staging is required to avoid unnecessary thoracotomies on those patients with advanced malignancies and overstaging, which could deny patients a potentially curative resection. The T (tumor) staging is best evaluated by CT due to its superior anatomic resolution, allowing accurate measurement of tumor size as well as its ability to assess involvement of adjacent structures.

Traditionally, mediastinal staging has been dependent on anatomical imaging with CT or MRI, as well as invasive mediastinoscopy and transbronchial biopsy. The anatomical imaging criterion used to identify nodal metastasis is based purely on the size of the visualized lymph nodes, with a short axis diameter of greater than 1 cm typically used for mediastinal nodes. The obvious limitation of this method of staging is that normal-sized nodes can be involved by malignancy and benign reactive inflammatory lymph nodes can be enlarged. Thus, the sensitivity and specificity achieved by this method of staging is suboptimal (52% and 69% by CT and 48% and 64% by MRI, respectively). Because of the inaccuracy inherent to anatomic imaging, mediastinoscopy with multiple node biopsies has remained the most reliable method for accurate preoperative staging. This method is less than desirable due to the risks and expense involved in such an invasive procedure. Additionally, this method does not allow evaluation of all mediastinal lymph node groups because nodes in the posterior mediastinum and aortopulmonary window cannot be accessed.

Unlike the dependence of CT and MRI on the morphology of lymph nodes, FDG PET imaging allows evaluation of the metabolic activity present. Thus, it allows the detection of lymph nodes involved by malignancy that do not meet the size criteria defined for anatomic imaging modalities. Unlike mediastinoscopy, PET imaging can evaluate the entire mediastinum, as well as the hilar lymph nodes and unsuspected distant metastases. The accuracy of FDG PET staging has been shown to be greater than that of CT, with sensitivity ranging from 66 to 100% and specificity of 81 to 100%.

A source of inaccuracy is the inherent limited anatomic resolution of the modality. The limit of resolution of the dedicated PET tomograph is approximately 5 mm. Therefore, it is possible for very small lymph nodes involved with malignancy to escape detection by both PET and CT imaging. Another potential problem with the limited anatomic resolution is the detection of bronchial wall, pleural, or vascular invasion. Therefore, it remains necessary to include anatomic evaluation in the preoperative staging. Fusion CT and PET imaging is likely the best method to optimize the strengths of both techniques. Mediastinoscopy will exclude from thoracotomy 30 to 40% of patients initially thought to have surgically resectable disease.

Another source of inaccuracy in PET evaluation is the potential false-positive findings caused by inflammatory processes. It is well known that benign reactive lymph nodes can demonstrate increased FDG uptake. The level of activity is often but not always less than that seen with malignancy. Granulomatous infection by tuberculosis or fungal organisms is a potential cause of a false-positive study. Increased uptake due to inflammation has also been identified in the presence of postobstructive pneumonitis. Because of the high negative predictive value of PET, patients with a negative PET scan can proceed directly to thoracotomy and be spared invasive mediastinal staging. However, because of the false-positive findings due to inflammatory disease, patients with a positive PET scan should be referred for mediastinoscopy.

A less common cause of FDG PET inaccuracy that is seen in all indications for FDG imaging is the poor uptake present in individuals with hyperglycemia. Therefore, it is necessary to have the patient in a fasting state and measure serum glucose prior to FDG administration.

In the case described, PET imaging not only detected the primary lung mass and characterized it as malignant, but PET imaging also detected a pretracheal lymph node deemed benign by CT criteria. Mediastinoscopy confirmed mediastinal metastases, including contralateral lymph node involvement (N_3). The patient was upstaged from stage I to IIIB. The patient was treated with chemotherapy and radiation, and an unnecessary surgical resection with its associated morbidity was avoided based on the results of the PET study.

Diagnosis

Squamous cell carcinoma of the left upper lobe with an FDG-positive subcentimeter lymph node metastasis in the pretracheal region, representing a stage IIIB nonsurgical malignancy.

Case 6.3.4

History

A 21-year-old male college student presented with progressive dyspnea and a low-grade fever. A chest radiograph demonstrated a large left-sided pleural effusion. Following two weeks of empiric antibiotic therapy, a follow-up chest X-ray showed interval progression of the pleural effusion. Thoracentesis produced 5 liters of bloody fluid with cytology suspicious for malignancy. Chest CT demonstrated a large multiloculated cystic lesion occupying over 90% of the left hemithorax. The right lung and upper abdomen appeared normal, and no lymphadenopathy was identified. Subsequent bronchoscopy was negative, and thoracoscopy revealed numerous pleural-based implants on the chest wall, diaphragm, and pericardium. The pathology was consistent with adenocarcinoma, with mesothelioma considered a less likely possibility. Chemotherapy was started for stage IIIB malignancy.

One month after chemotherapy was initiated, the patient complained of left-sided rib pain, and a chest CT showed interval progression of the lesion. Bone scintigraphy was negative. Staging FDG PET imaging was acquired with a dedicated PET tomograph (GE Advance) and reconstructed with iterative reconstruction and measured segmented attenuation correction. Coronal FDG PET images are shown in Figures 6.3.4A and B, and orthogonal FDG PET images through an upper thoracic vertebral body are shown in Figure 6.3.4C.

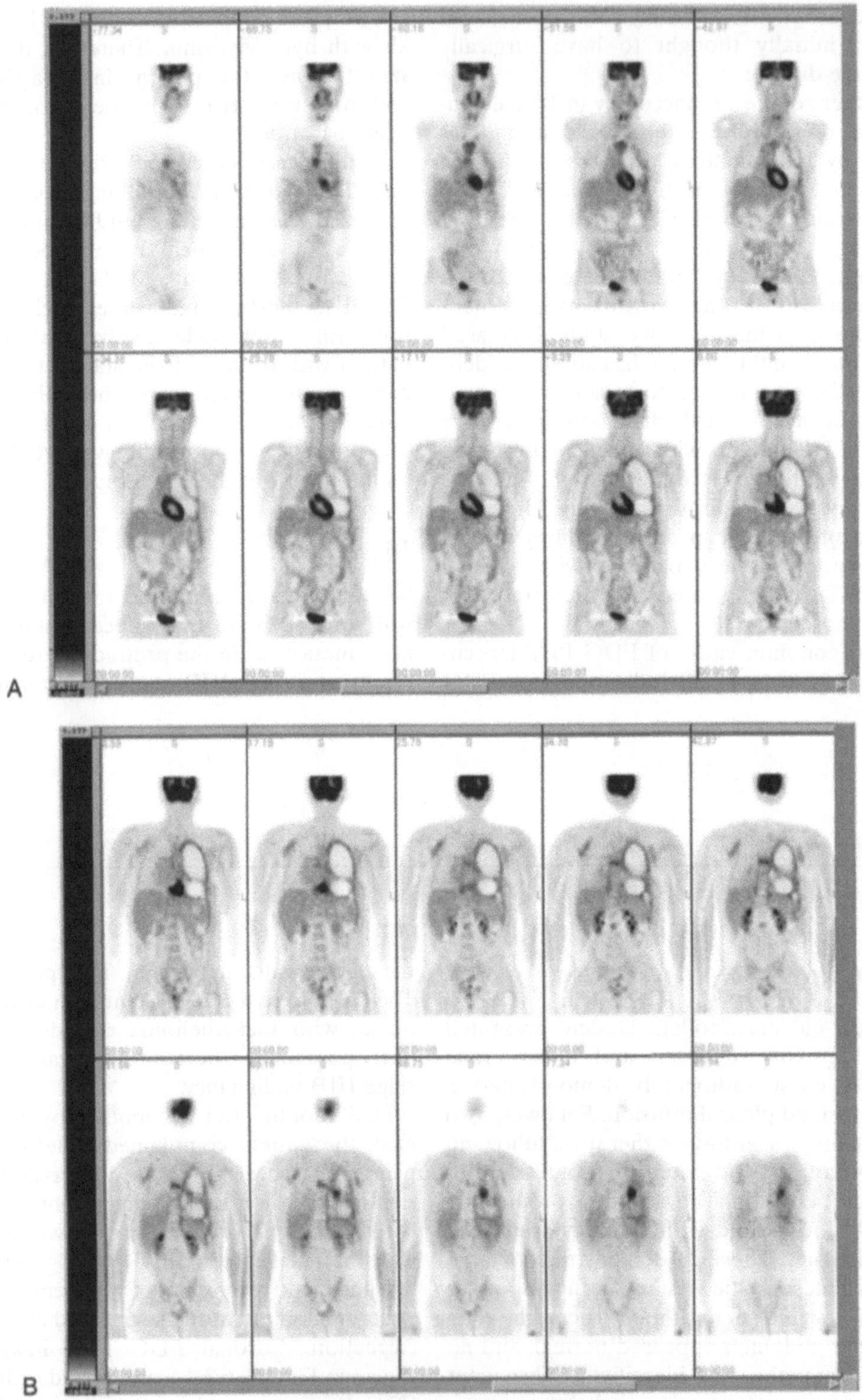

FIGURE 6.3.4A,B.

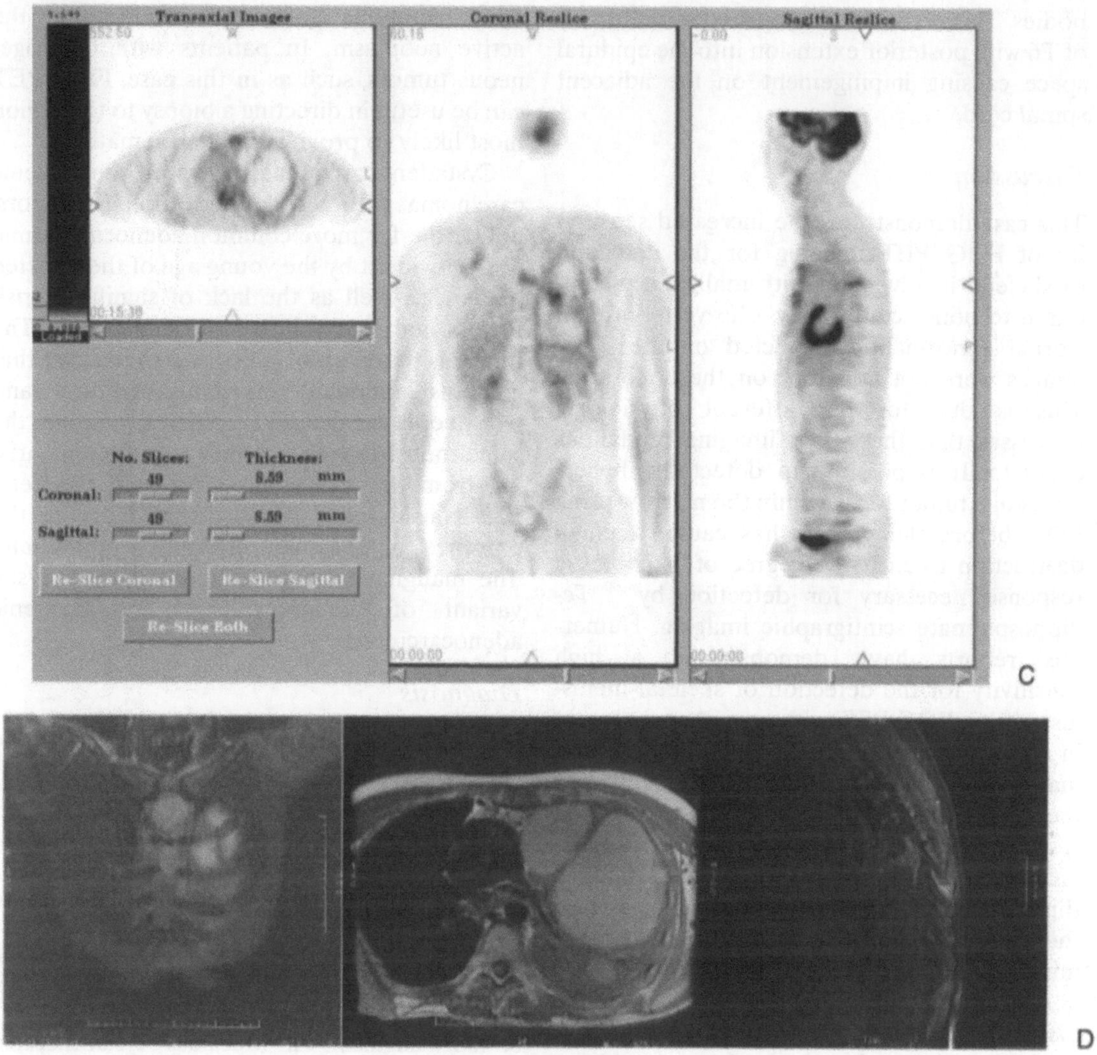

FIGURE 6.3.4C,D.

Findings

The FDG PET images demonstrate near total replacement of the left hemithorax with a predominately nonhypermetabolic cystic mass. However, the periphery of the mass, as well as the thick-walled septa within the mass, exhibit increased FDG uptake. Furthermore, there is a large focus of increased FDG activity present posteriorly just below the level of the carina, which correlates with a focal soft tissue mass present on CT. The right lung displays normal activity, and no hypermetabolic mediastinal or hilar lymphadenopathy is apparent. No abnormalities are seen within the abdomen or pelvis. However, focal increased activity is present within the sternum and a mid-thoracic vertebral body. These foci are suspicious for skeletal involvement by either direct extension or metastatic involvement.

Subsequent MR images (Figure 6.3.4D, coronal T2-weighted, left; transaxial T2-weighted, middle; sagittal gadolinium-enhanced T1-weighted, right) demonstrate abnormal decreased T1 (not shown) and increased T2 signal and contrast enhancement within the manubrium and superior sternum, as well as within the T6 and T9 (not in FOV) vertebral bodies. There is also a compression deformity of T6 with posterior extension into the epidural space causing impingement on the adjacent spinal cord.

Discussion

This case demonstrates the increased sensitivity of FDG PET imaging for the detection of skeletal involvement with malignancy compared to bone scintigraphy. The vertebral and sternal abnormalities detected on the FDG images were not apparent on the bone scan. This is due to the different physiologic processes that these two imaging modalities evaluate. It is possible to detect the hypermetabolic tumor focus within the marrow using FDG before the process has caused enough destruction to elicit the degree of osteoblastic response necessary for detection by ^{99m}Tc-diphosphonate scintigraphic imaging. Numerous reports have demonstrated a high sensitivity for the detection of skeletal metastases using FDG PET with some improvement in sensitivity over bone scintigraphy and marked improvement in specificity. However, the demonstration of osteoblastic metastases, such as with prostate carcinoma, is less satisfactory.[1] The presence of skeletal metastases in this patient, confirmed by MR imaging, altered the patient's staging from stage IIIB (determined by the CT and bone scan) to stage IV.

Also evident from this example is that the cystic (or hemorrhagic/necrotic) portion of a cystic neoplasm does not demonstrate increased metabolic activity. The solid, viable region demonstrates a focus of hypermetabolism, and this includes the walls and septa of the lesion. The cystic material, however, is merely a nonmetabolic by-product produced by the active neoplasm. In patients with heterogeneous tumors, such as in this case, FDG PET can be useful in directing a biopsy to the region most likely to provide diagnostic material.

Cystadenocarcinoma is a rare bronchogenic carcinoma with few known etiologic factors, unlike the far more common adenocarcinoma. This is evident by the young age of the affected patient, as well as the lack of significant risk factors and family history of malignancy. The tumor is made up of a fibrous-walled cyst that contains abundant mucinous material and few neoplastic cells. Pathologically, it has the same morphology as cystadenocarcinoma arising from the ovary, appendix, and pancreas. It is considered a primary tumor due to the presence of reactive respiratory epithelium. The malignancy is considered to be a cystic variant of mucin-producing bronchogenic adenocarcinoma.[2–4]

Diagnosis

Cystadenocarcinoma with metastases to the sternum and spine.

References

1. Cook GJ, Fogelman: The role of positron emission tomography in the management of bone metastases. Cancer 2000;88(S12):2927–2933.
2. Gaeta M: Mucinous cystadenocarcinoma of the lung: CT-pathologic correlation in three cases. J Comput Assist Tomogr 1999;23(4):641–643.
3. Tangthangtham A: Mucinous cystadenocarcinoma of the lung. J Med Assoc Thai 1998;81(10): 794–798.
4. Papla B: Pulmonary mucinous cystadenoma of borderline malignancy: A report of two cases. Pol J Pathol 1996;47(2):87–90.

Case 6.3.5

History

A 51-year-old female referred for FDG PET imaging had a history of right mastectomy for breast carcinoma eight years ago. Two of thirteen lymph nodes were positive for malignancy, so she received postoperative chemotherapy. At the time of breast reconstruction two years later, two metastatic lung nodules detected by CT were resected. Follow-up CT examinations showed no evidence of additional metastatic disease until the most recent study (Figure

6.3.5A). Figure 6.3.5B shows transaxial FDG images through the chest acquired with a dedicated PET tomograph (GE Advance) and reconstructed with iterative reconstruction and measured segmented attenuation correction.

Findings

The CT image shows a 2 cm pleural-based soft tissue density nodule within the posterior right mid-lung. The margins are smooth, without evi-

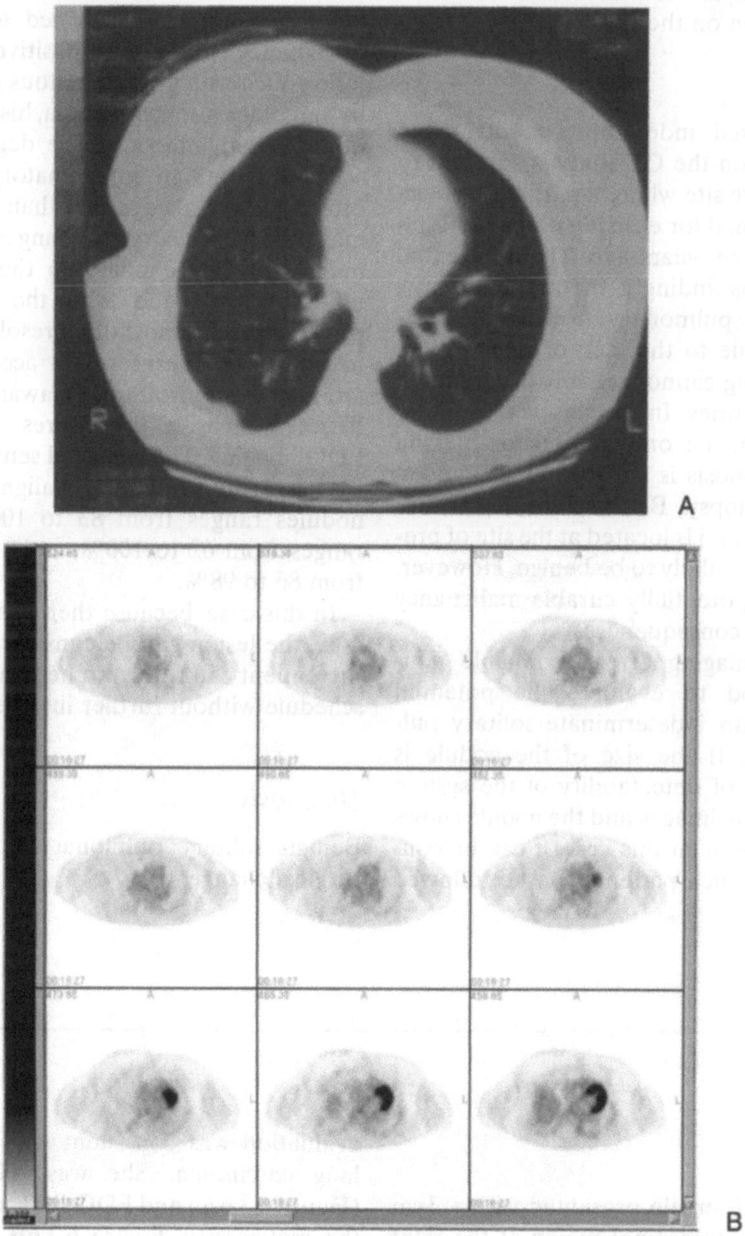

FIGURE 6.3.5A,B.

dence of spiculation. There is no calcification present within the lesion. No other evidence of metastatic nodules, pathologic lymphadenopathy, nor pleural effusion was apparent on this study.

The FDG PET images demonstrate physiologic distribution of activity within the myocardium, but no abnormal uptake is present within the lung parenchyma or pleura in the location of the lesion seen on the CT.

Discussion

The pleural-based indeterminate soft tissue nodule present on the CT study is adjacent to the postoperative site where a partial rib resection was performed for excision of the metastatic lung nodule six years ago. The differential diagnosis for this finding is metastatic disease, benign solitary pulmonary nodule, or post-surgical scar. Due to the lack of calcification, anatomic imaging cannot reliably differentiate among these entities. In the absence of metabolic evaluation, the only option for making this crucial diagnosis is an open or CT-guided percutaneous biopsy. Because the lesion has smooth margins and is located at the site of previous surgery, it is likely to be benign. However, follow-up of a potentially curable malignancy could have dire consequences.

FDG PET imaging offers a reliable non-invasive method to evaluate the potential malignancy of an indeterminate solitary pulmonary nodule. If the size of the nodule is above the limit of detectability of the system used to obtain the images and the nodule shows no FDG uptake, as in this case, it can be considered benign; such patients can be followed using CT without biopsy. False-negative results can occur with small lesions; the limit of detectability is in the 5 to 10 mm range for dedicated PET systems and in the 15 to 20 mm range with hybrid PET gamma cameras. False-negative results can also be seen in patients with hyperglycemia and with bronchioalveolar, carcinoid, and mucinous tumors. If, however, a lesion demonstrates increased FDG uptake, biopsy should be performed to differentiate malignancy from a false-positive inflammatory lesion such as a granulomatous process caused by sarcoidosis, mycobacteria, histoplasmosis, or other fungal infection. The degree of uptake seen with benign inflammatory processes is often, but not always, less than that seen with malignancy. Postsurgical changes can also accumulate FDG secondary to the inflammatory infiltrate associated with the acute healing process, but this most often resolves within four to six weeks. Therefore, for accurate interpretation, it is important to be aware of the timing between invasive procedures or trauma and FDG imaging. The reported sensitivity of FDG PET imaging to identify malignant pulmonary nodules ranges from 83 to 100%; specificity ranges from 62 to 100%; and accuracy ranges from 86 to 98%.

In this case, because there was no FDG uptake, the lesion can be considered benign, and the patient can return to her routine follow-up schedule without further intervention.

Diagnosis

Benign solitary pulmonary nodule or post-surgical change.

Case 6.3.6

History

This 71-year-old female presented with a 3 cm mass within the paraspinal region of the right lower lobe. Subsequent fine-needle aspiration evaluation was consistent with non-small cell lung carcinoma. She was referred for CT (Figure 6.3.6A) and FDG PET imaging to stage the malignancy. Figure 6.3.6B shows coronal FDG PET images acquired with a dedicated

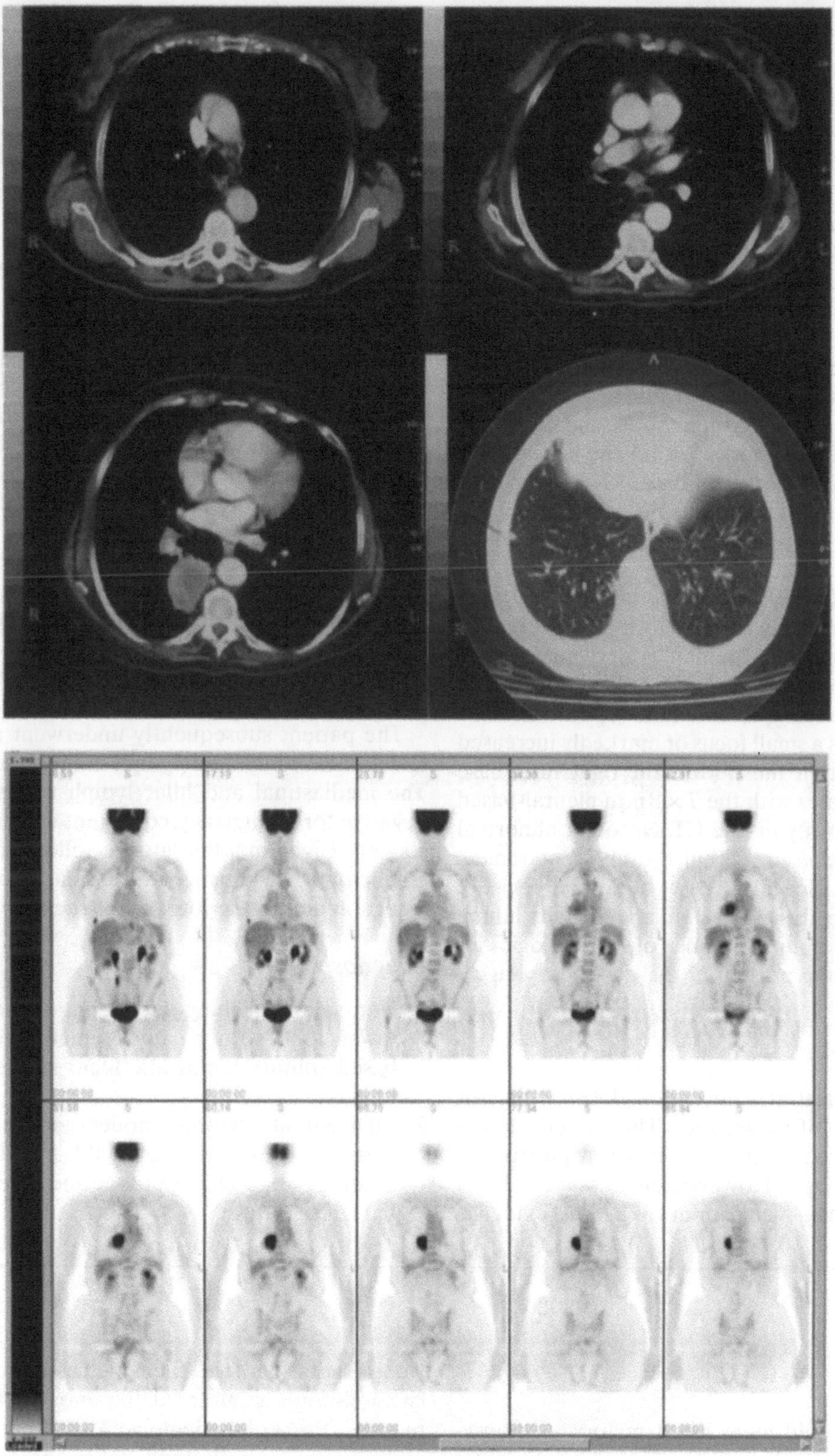

FIGURE 6.3.6A,B.

PET tomograph (GE Advance) and reconstructed using iterative reconstruction and measured segmented attenuation correction.

Findings

The CT image demonstrates a 3 × 4cm mass of soft tissue density located in the right paraspinal region at the level of the left atrium. It abuts the adjacent pleural surface, but no definite invasion or pleural effusion is apparent. Also present are at least two 8mm lymph nodes in the aortopulmonary window, as well as a 14mm subcarinal lymph node and a 10mm right hilar lymph node. Within the lateral right lower lobe is a pleural-based 7 × 8mm soft tissue density that exhibits no calcification and is difficult to characterize further due to its small size.

The FDG PET images demonstrate a large focus of markedly increased uptake present in the right paraspinal region, congruent with the soft tissue mass seen on the CT and proven to be malignant by fine-needle aspiration. Also identified is a small focus of markedly increased activity within the peripheral right lung base that correlates with the 7 × 8mm pleural-based nodular density on the CT. No other abnormal activity is present within the chest, abdomen, and pelvis. Specifically, no abnormal foci are seen within the mediastinum and right hilum. Incidental note is made of physiologic increase uptake present at the gastroesophageal junction.

Discussion

This case illustrates the use of FDG imaging for the staging of malignancy. The primary lesion known to be malignant is obviously positive on the PET images. However, the absence of FDG uptake in the mediastinum is strong evidence against malignant involvement of the lymph nodes seen on the CT scan, even though they reach borderline size criteria for malignancy by CT. They may be enlarged due to a benign reactive phenomenon. According to current literature, no further evaluation of these lymph nodes is necessary, and they can be considered benign for staging purposes. Thus, the stage is T2N2 with CT and T2N0 with FDG.

However, the small pleural-based nodule present by CT demonstrates markedly increased activity. Although too small to characterize by CT, the FDG uptake demonstrated in the face of known malignancy is highly suggestive of a metastasis. Unfortunately, an active granuloma could demonstrate similar uptake, and the diagnosis of metastatic disease is not definitive. Therefore, biopsy should be considered for further staging purposes. However, if this nodule did not demonstrate FDG uptake, it could be considered benign, and the malignancy would then be isolated to the primary focus (T2N0).

The patient subsequently underwent a right lower lobectomy and lymph node resection. The mediastinal and hilar lymph nodes were negative for malignancy, consistent with a T2N0 staging. Eight months later, a follow-up PET scan showed recurrence at the hilar margin of resection and in the low lateral chest wall.

Diagnoses

1. Non-small cell lung carcinoma in the right lower lobe with a subcentimeter pleural-based solitary metastatic focus in the same lobe.
2. Mediastinal lymph nodes approaching pathologic size criteria by CT but demonstrating no FDG uptake and therefore benign in nature.

Case 6.3.7

History

An 81-year-old male has a history of biopsy-proven large cell carcinoma of the right lower lobe with mediastinal involvement. He underwent radiation to the mediastinum and chemotherapy completed five months ago. A recent CT scan has demonstrated a persistent infiltrate within both upper lobes and a persistent mass in the location of the primary tumor

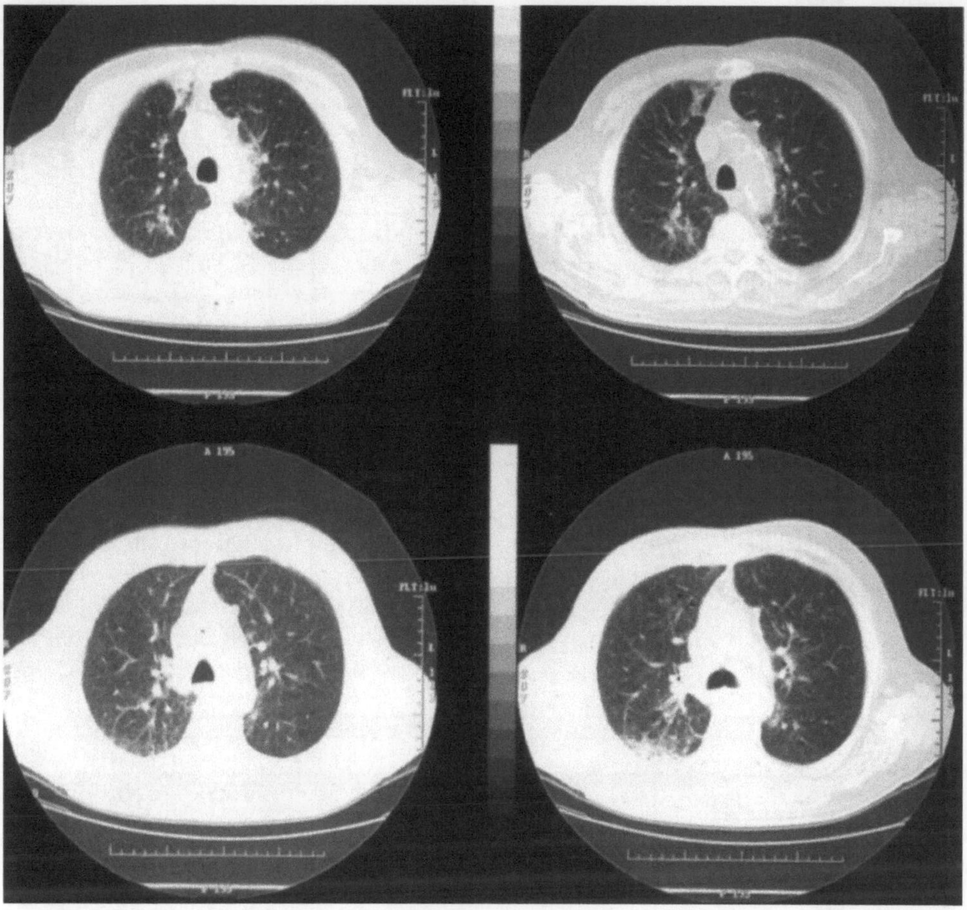

FIGURE 6.3.7A.

in the right lower lobe (Figure 6.3.7A). The patient was referred for FDG PET evaluation. Figures 6.3.7B and C show transaxial and coronal FDG images acquired with a dedicated PET tomograph (GE Advance) and reconstructed with iterative reconstruction and measured segmented attenuation correction.

Findings

The CT study demonstrates patchy areas of increased density within both upper lobes, greater on the right side. No focal lesion is present, and these findings have developed since the previous study. The study also shows a soft tissue mass within the right lower lobe in the location of the primary malignancy (not shown).

The FDG PET images demonstrate markedly increased uptake within both medial upper lobes, also greater on the right side and correlating with the CT findings. There is also markedly increased uptake present within the superior portion of the right lower lobe, seen on the coronal images (not in the field of view of the FDG transaxial images shown).

Discussion

These findings indicate residual or recurrent viable tumor in the primary lesion in the right

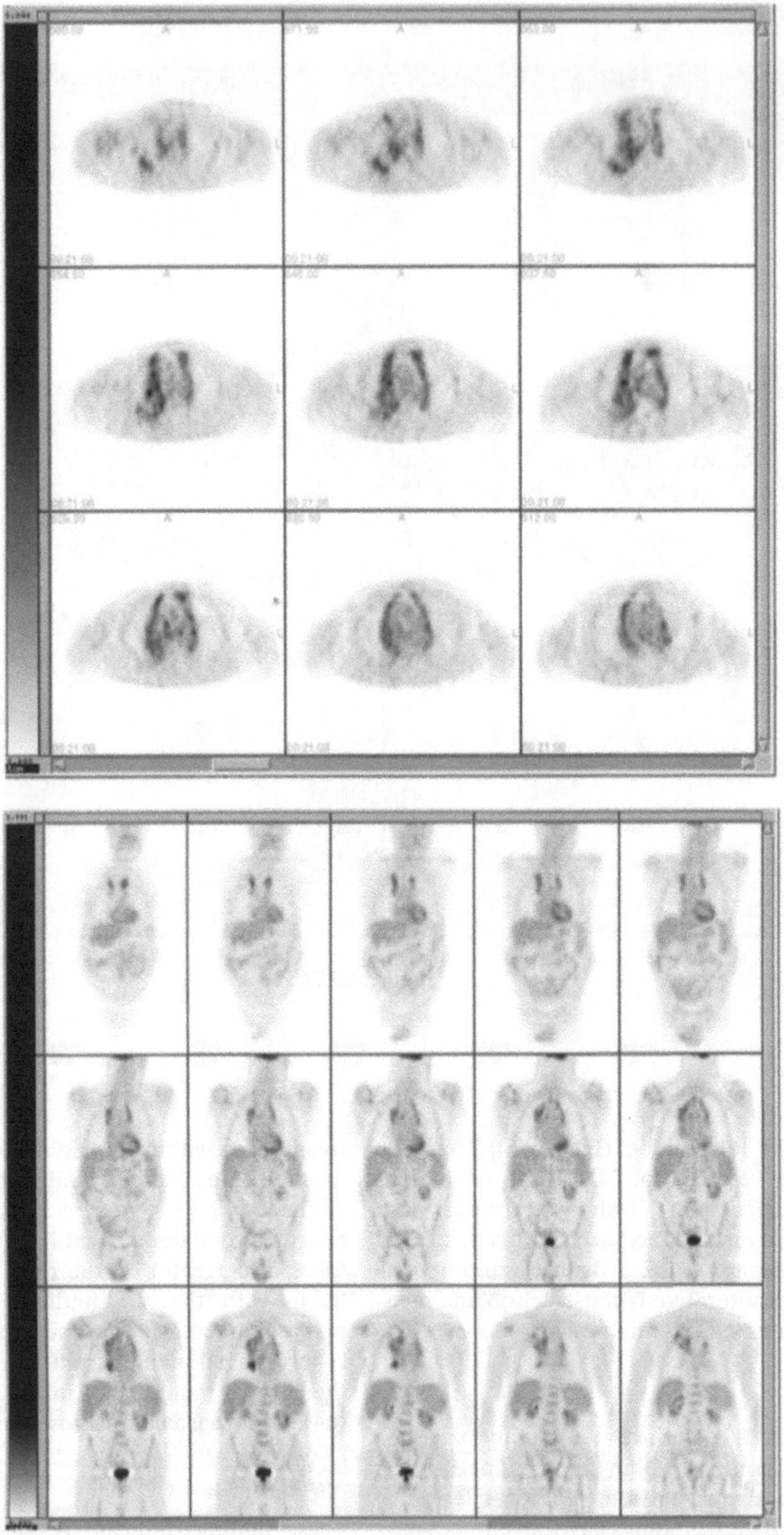

B

C

FIGURE 6.3.7B,C.

lower lobe and postradiation pneumonitis in both upper lobes.

The differential diagnosis for the CT findings of new patchy densities within both upper lobes includes postradiation pneumonitis or fibrosis, superimposed infectious pneumonia, post-obstructive atelectasis, active tuberculosis or fungal infection, and metastatic disease. With FDG PET imaging, infectious and malignant processes would be expected to demonstrate increased uptake. This excludes the possibilities of atelectasis and fibrosis. Infectious pneumonia and tuberculosis should be apparent clinically. Therefore, the differential diagnosis is narrowed to postradiation pneumonitis or malignancy.

The degree of damage to the lungs caused by postradiation pneumonitis depends on several factors including the volume of lung irradiated, the radiation dose, the dose fractionation, and concurrent chemotherapy. Pathologically, there are three phases: the exudative phase, characterized by edema fluid and hyaline membranes six to eight weeks after exposure due to depletion of surfactant and desquamation of alveolar and bronchial cells; the organizing phase; and the fibrotic phase, characterized by interstitial fibrosis seen six to twelve months following therapy. The findings are confined to the radiation port and usually have sharp lateral margins. There are patchy consolidation and signs of volume loss within the paramediastinal upper lobes. Dilated air bronchograms are often seen as a result of traction bronchiectasis. Pleural thickening is an associated finding, and pericardial effusions can be seen occasionally. In the early stages, the patient can be treated with steroid administration for the symptoms of insidious onset of dyspnea, nonproductive cough, and weakness, but the majority of patients are asymptomatic. The fibrotic changes that occur later in the disease process are irreversible.

Because of the inflammatory reaction incited by the radiation-induced damage to the lung, increased FDG uptake is expected due to the increased metabolism. Histological examination of biopsy specimen of these regions has demonstrated infiltration of macrophages, which are believed to be responsible for the increased FDG uptake. Once this has resolved late in the fibrotic phase, the increased FDG activity also resolves. The time course of FDG uptake in postradiation pneumonitis has not been studied systematically.

In this case, because the CT and FDG PET findings are limited to the typical radiation port and because of the timing of the study five months after treatment, postradiation pneumonitis prior to end stage fibrosis is the most likely diagnosis.

Diagnoses

1. Postradiation pneumonitis of both upper lobes.
2. Residual or recurrent carcinoma in the right lower lobe.

Case 6.3.8

History

An 81-year-old male was referred for FDG evaluation due to multiple pulmonary nodules detected on CT (Figure 6.3.8A). The patient had a previous history of smoking, and his occupation was mining. Figure 6.3.8B shows transaxial FDG PET images acquired with a dedicated PET tomograph (GE Advance) and reconstructed using iterative reconstruction and measured segmented attenuation correction.

Findings

On CT, the largest nodule is seen within the apical segment of the right upper lobe, measuring 2.5 cm. It is lobulated and spiculated in contour and contains eccentric calcifications. A 1 cm soft tissue nodule with central calcification is seen within the anterior segment of the right upper lobe. There are several subpleural satellite nodules measuring up to 1 cm adjacent to the mass. The left upper lobe also demonstrates several nodules measuring up to 1.2 cm, many

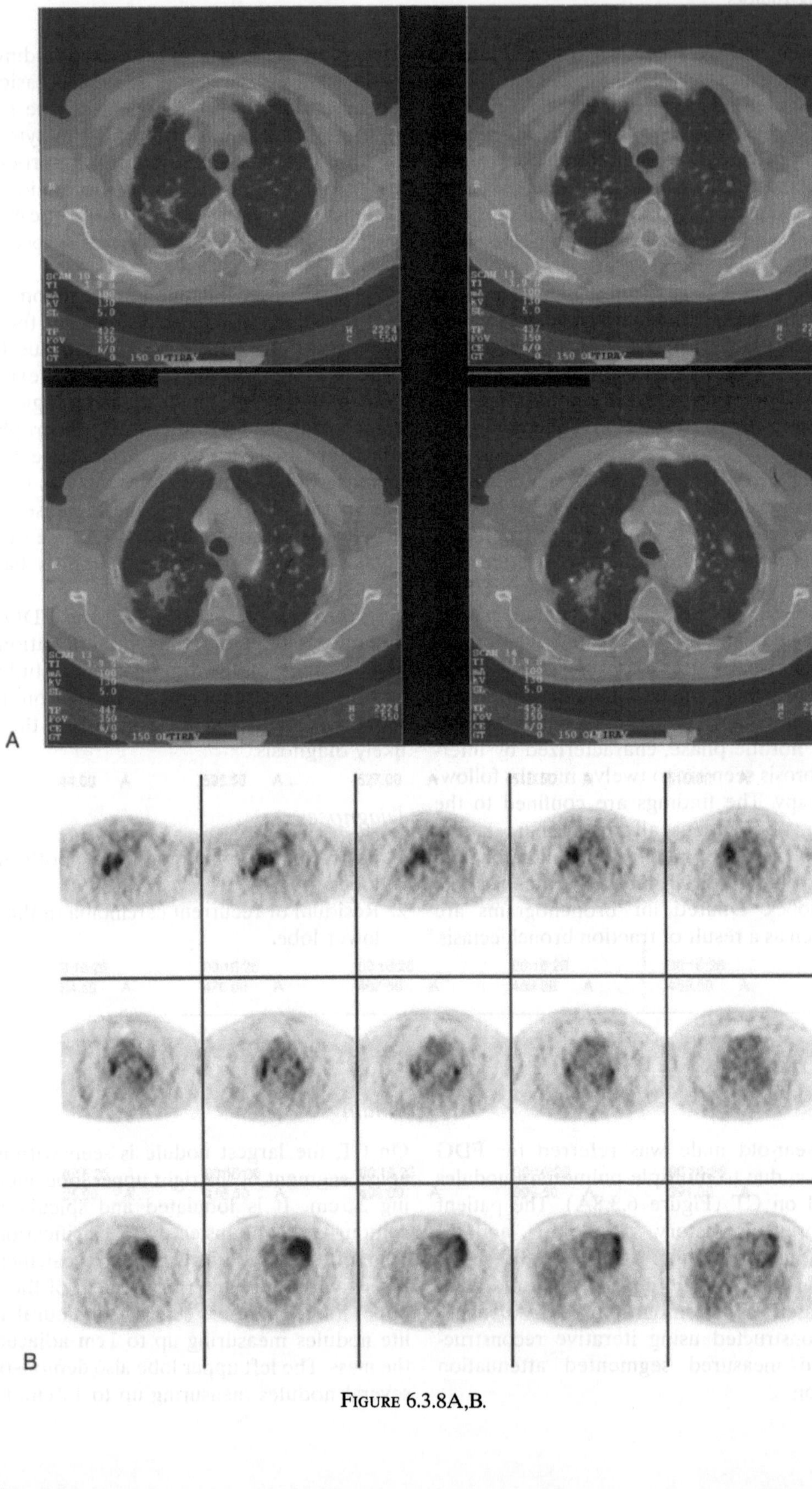

FIGURE 6.3.8A,B.

of which contain faint central calcification. Calcified hilar and mediastinal lymph nodes are also identified (not shown).

The FDG PET images demonstrate marked uptake present within the large lesion of the right upper lobe, as well as within the multiple small adjacent nodules described. Within the left upper lobe, there is mildly increased activity present within several foci correlating with the nodular densities on the CT. There are also several small foci of considerable FDG uptake present within the mediastinum and both hilar regions. Incidental note is made of physiologic uptake present within the myocardium. No abnormal activity is present within the abdomen, pelvis, or skeleton.

Discussion

The degree of uptake present within these lung lesions is worrisome for malignancy. The patient was referred for subsequent mediastinoscopy, right upper lobe wedge resection, and pulmonary needle biopsy. Histologic examination of the specimens revealed a benign right hilar lymph node demonstrating hyperplasia, as well as lung tissue with inflammation and fibrosis. The specimens contained extensive anthracotic pigment. There was no evidence of malignancy.

Given the patient's history of mining, as well as the multiple calcifications present on the CT study, a granulomatous process must be considered as the etiology for these nodules. The size and distribution of the nodules is consistent with a pneumoconiosis. An active granulomatous process can demonstrate nodular increased FDG uptake. Although the level is often less than that seen with malignancy (SUV < 2.5), this is unfortunately not always the case. Therefore, biopsy is necessary to exclude malignancy. If no abnormal FDG uptake was present on the study, the nodules could be considered benign, and the patient could be followed clinically and radiographically.

Diagnosis

Pneumoconiosis with multiple FDG-avid granulomas.

Case 6.3.9

History

A 65-year-old man presented with several months of neck pain. He had no significant neurological symptoms or past medical history. Radiographs of the cervical spine showed degenerative changes at the C4 through C7 levels. He was treated with anti-inflammatory medicines but later returned with persistent pain. A chest radiograph demonstrated a 3 cm mass within the right lower lobe. He was referred for chest CT (Figure 6.3.9A, axial image at the level of the right hilum), bone scintigraphy (Figure 6.3.9B, anterior and posterior whole-body images), cervical spine MRI (Figure 6.3.9C, sagittal postcontrast fat saturated T1-weighted image), and FDG PET (Figures 6.3.9D and E, transaxial images and orthogonal images through the neck). The FDG images were acquired with a dedicated PET tomograph (GE Advance) and reconstructed with iterative reconstruction and measured segmented attenuation correction.

Findings

The chest CT demonstrates a 3 cm lesion within the posterior portion of the superior segment of the right lower lobe, which does not appear to invade the adjacent chest wall. Also noted is a 2 cm lesion in the right hilum worrisome for metastatic adenopathy. There is no pleural effusion or other pathologic mediastinal, hilar, or axillary lymphadenopathy. CT of the abdomen

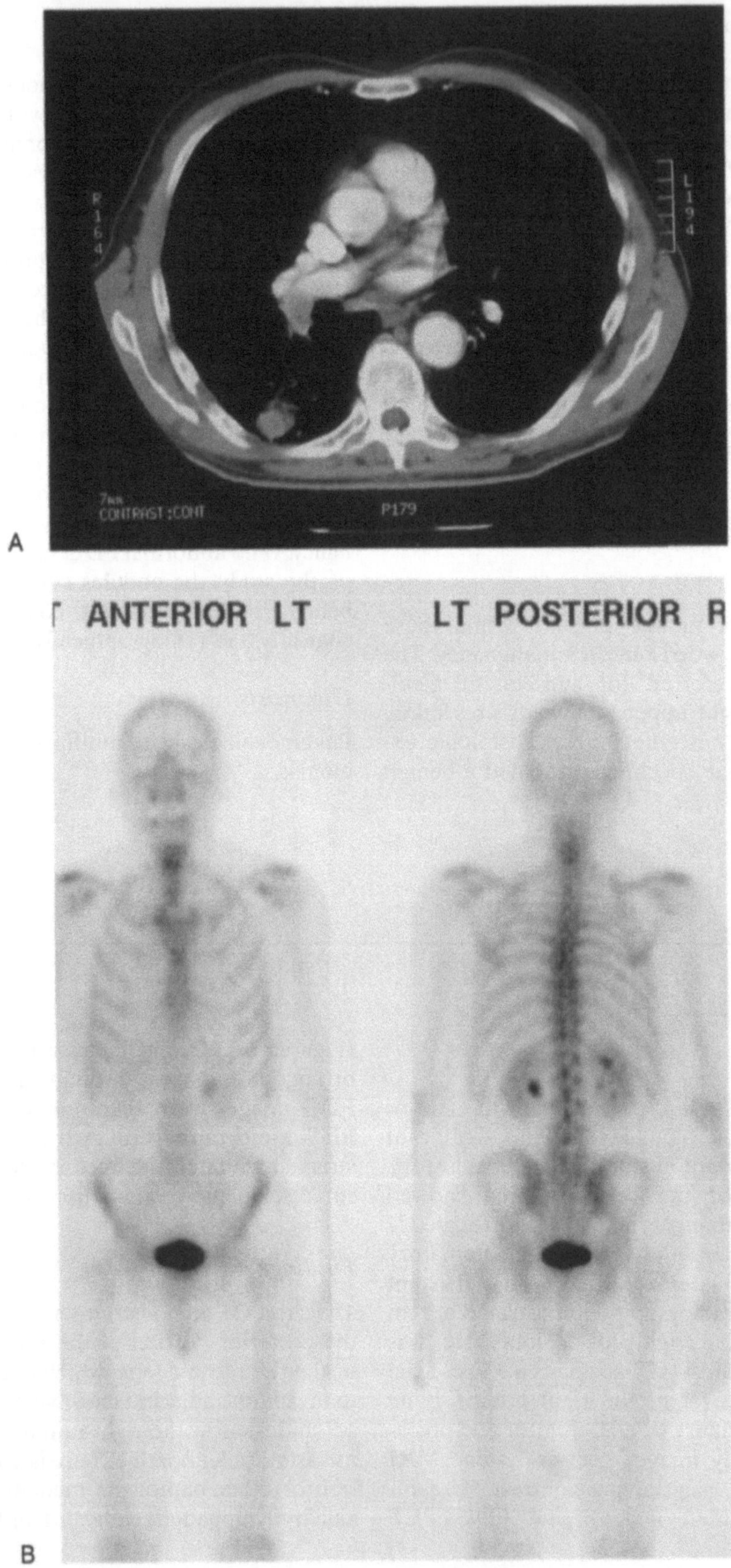

FIGURE 6.3.9A,B.

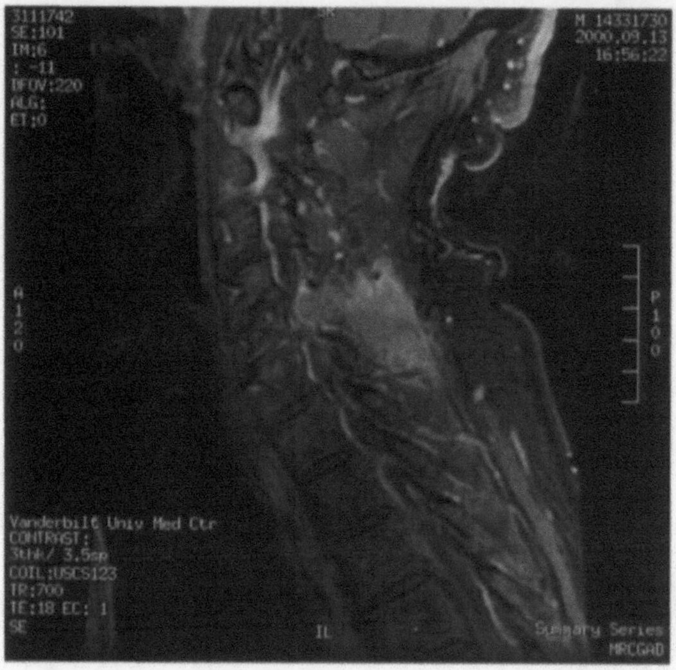

C

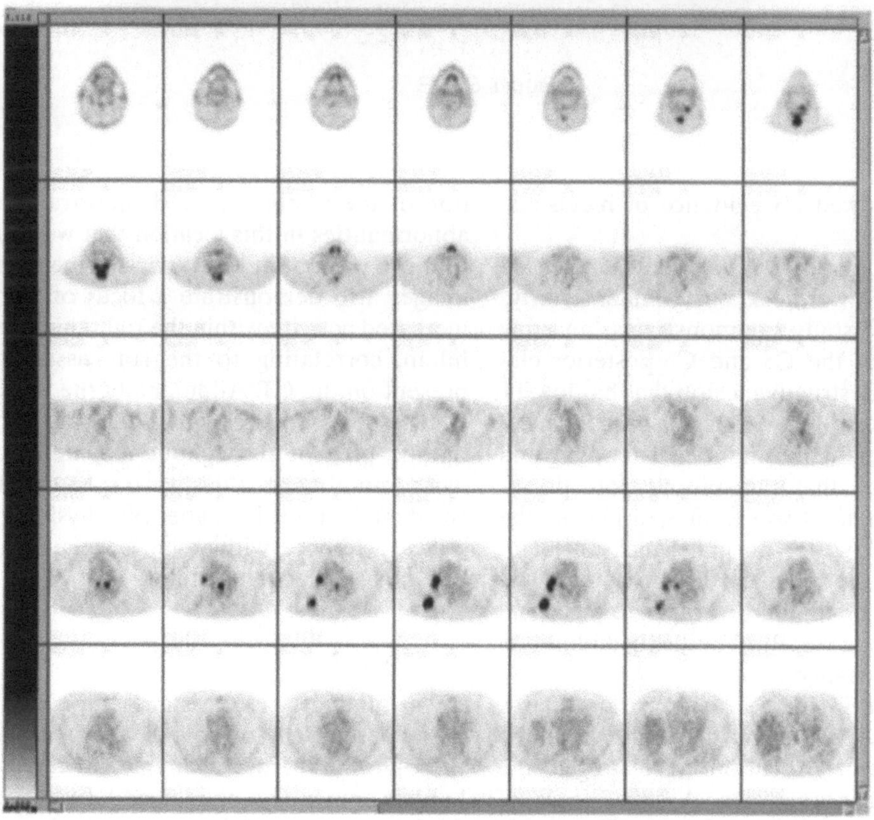

D

FIGURE 6.3.9C,D.

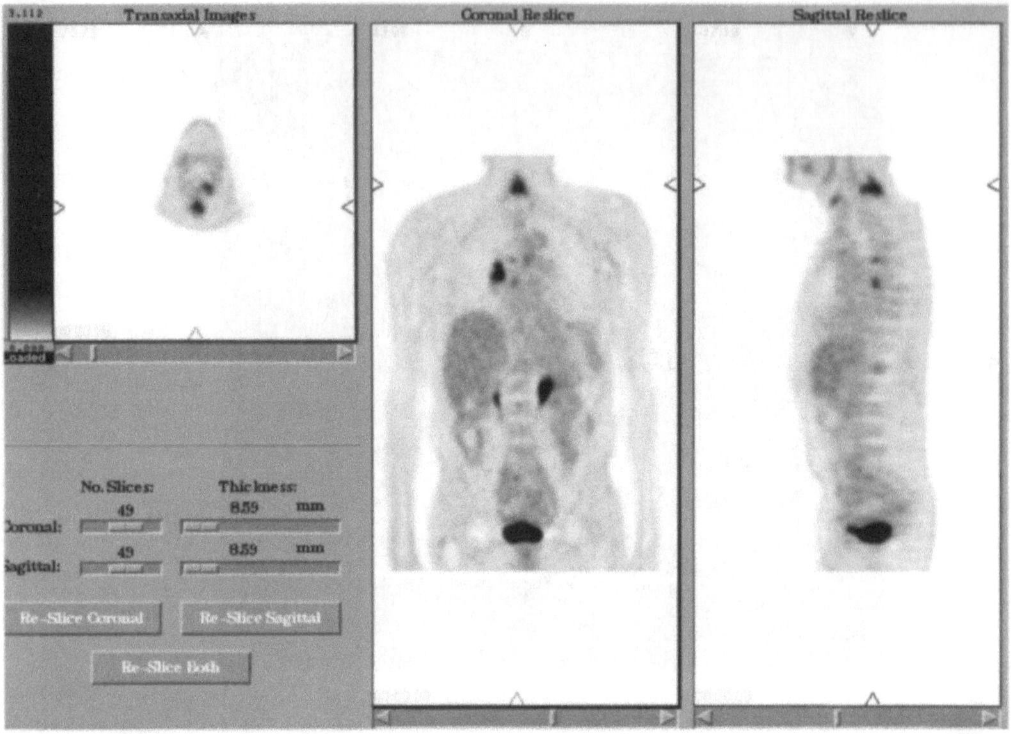

Figure 6.3.9E.

and pelvis showed no evidence of metastatic disease.

Bone scintigraphy reveals mild increased uptake in the lower neck, best seen anteriorly.

The MRI study demonstrates marrow replacement of the C5 and C6 posterior elements with a destructive lesion that has low T1 and high T2 signal, as well as contrast enhancement. The signal abnormalities extend beyond the bone into the paraspinous soft tissues and lateral epidural soft tissues, displacing the spinal cord. However, normal signal was maintained within the spinal cord. Also notable was a generalized mottled appearance to the signal of the remaining vertebral bodies in addition to degenerative changes.

The FDG PET images demonstrate a large focus of markedly increased activity within the cervical spine in a location correlating to the MRI signal abnormalities. A small focus of increased uptake was also noted in the L1 vertebral body, and a subsequent MRI examination of the lumbar spine demonstrated signal abnormalities in this location that were similar to those present in the cervical spine. The PET images also demonstrate a focus of markedly increased activity within the right mid-lung and hilum, correlating to the soft tissue masses present on the CT. Additionally, the FDG PET study shows several small foci of increased uptake present throughout the mediastinum, where no abnormalities were seen on the CT. Incidental note is made of physiologic increased activity within the laryngeal muscles and renal collecting system.

Discussion

These findings are consistent with a lung carcinoma in the right lower lobe with metastases to the right hilum, mediastinum, and cervical and lumbar spine. The patient underwent cervical laminectomy and fusion with resection of the paraspinal muscles and extradural tumor. Histologic examination of the specimen revealed a large cell neuroendocrine carcinoma as the primary tumor.

This case illustrates the high sensitivity of FDG PET imaging for detection of skeletal metastases from lung carcinoma compared to bone scintigraphy, as previously discussed in Case 6.3.4. In this case, FDG imaging demonstrated an obvious metastasis in the cervical spine and an additional metastasis within the L1 vertebral body that were inconspicuous or not apparent on bone scintigraphy. FDG imaging is also more specific than bone scintigraphy and, for example, does not demonstrate increased activity in locations with degenerative changes. This case also illustrates how easily bone scintigraphy findings can be misinterpreted. Because of the typical location and low level of increased activity present at the base of the cervical spine, it is easy to discount such findings as being due to degenerative change and calcifications in the thyroid cartilage, particularly if degenerative changes are present in that location on a correlative radiographic study.

As expected, increased uptake was also noted within the right lower lobe and right hilum, confirming the malignant nature of these abnormalities present on CT. In addition, numerous small foci of increased FDG activity were present throughout the mediastinum, whereas there were no lymphadenopathies on CT. This illustrates the role of FDG PET imaging for mediastinal staging, as described in Case 6.3.3.

Diagnosis

Large cell lung carcinoma with metastases to the right hilum, mediastinum, C5, C6, and L1.

Case 6.3.10

History

A 71-year-old female diagnosed with lung carcinoma one year ago and treated with surgery and chemotherapy presented with back pain. Bone scintigraphy was performed (Figure 6.3.10A, whole-body planar images in the anterior and posterior projections) and followed by a contrast enhanced MRI examination. Figure 6.3.10B shows T1-weighted (left) and T2-weighted (right) sagittal images from this study. FDG PET imaging was requested for evaluation of metastatic disease. FDG images were acquired with a dedicated PET tomograph (GE Advance) and reconstructed with filtered back projection without attenuation correction. Figure 6.3.10C shows transaxial images, and Figure 6.3.10D shows orthogonal images through the spine.

Findings

The bone scan demonstrates mild diffusely increased activity within the T12 vertebral body. A radiograph showed a compression deformity at this level, and therefore, it was considered a relatively acute injury. Otherwise, there are no additional foci of abnormal activity to suggest metastatic disease.

MRI examination was then performed to determine if the compression deformity represented a pathologic fracture or was merely due to osteopenia. The MRI images reveal increased T_2-signal within this vertebral body, a finding that is often seen in an acute or subacute compression fracture. Additionally, there is a small focus of contrast enhancement within this vertebral body (not shown), but this did not extend outside the vertebral body nor was focal contrast enhancement apparent within other levels. Although somewhat atypical, mild enhancement can be seen with an acute compression fracture. Otherwise, the study demonstrates heterogeneous bone marrow signal with mild patchy enhancement, another nonspecific finding that can be seen with diffuse metastases or hematopoietic marrow changes. Therefore, the MRI is not diagnostic for metastatic disease.

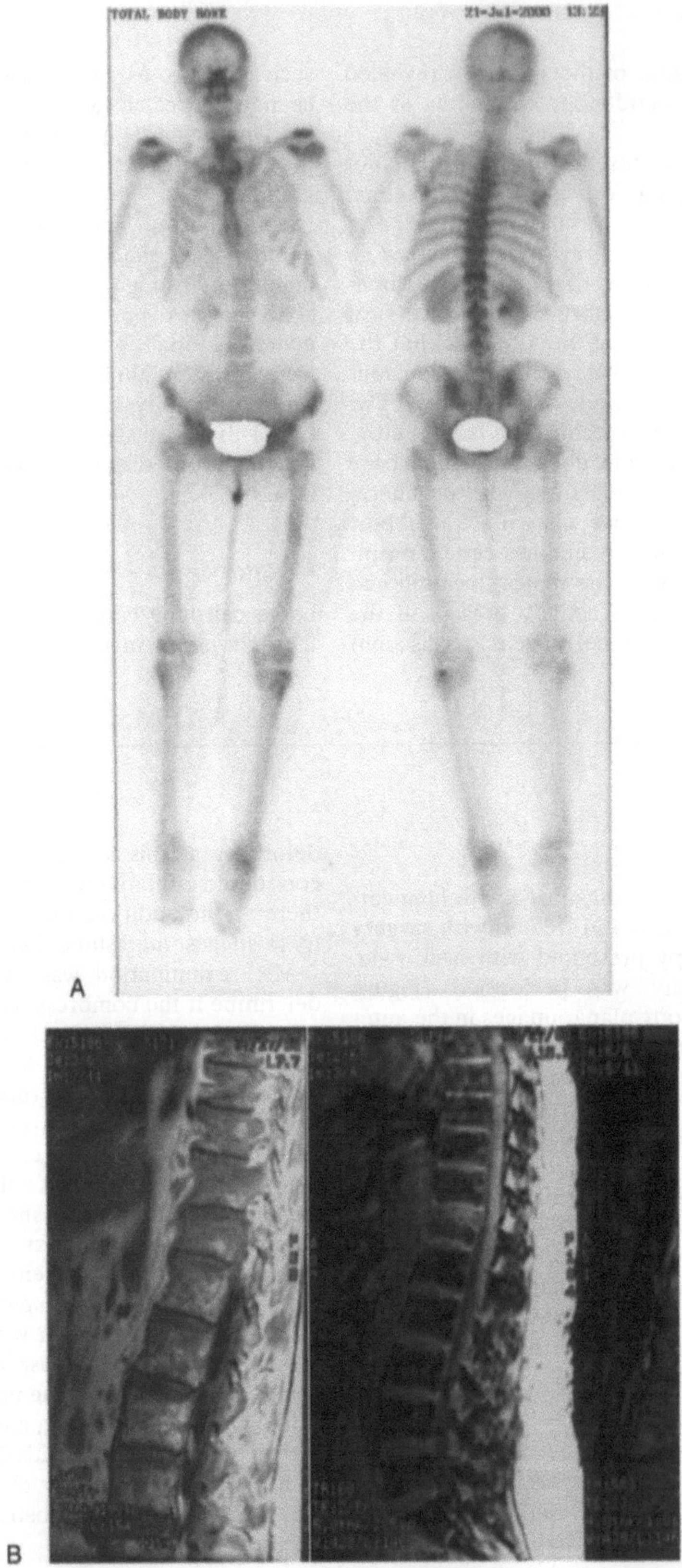

FIGURE 6.3.10A,B.

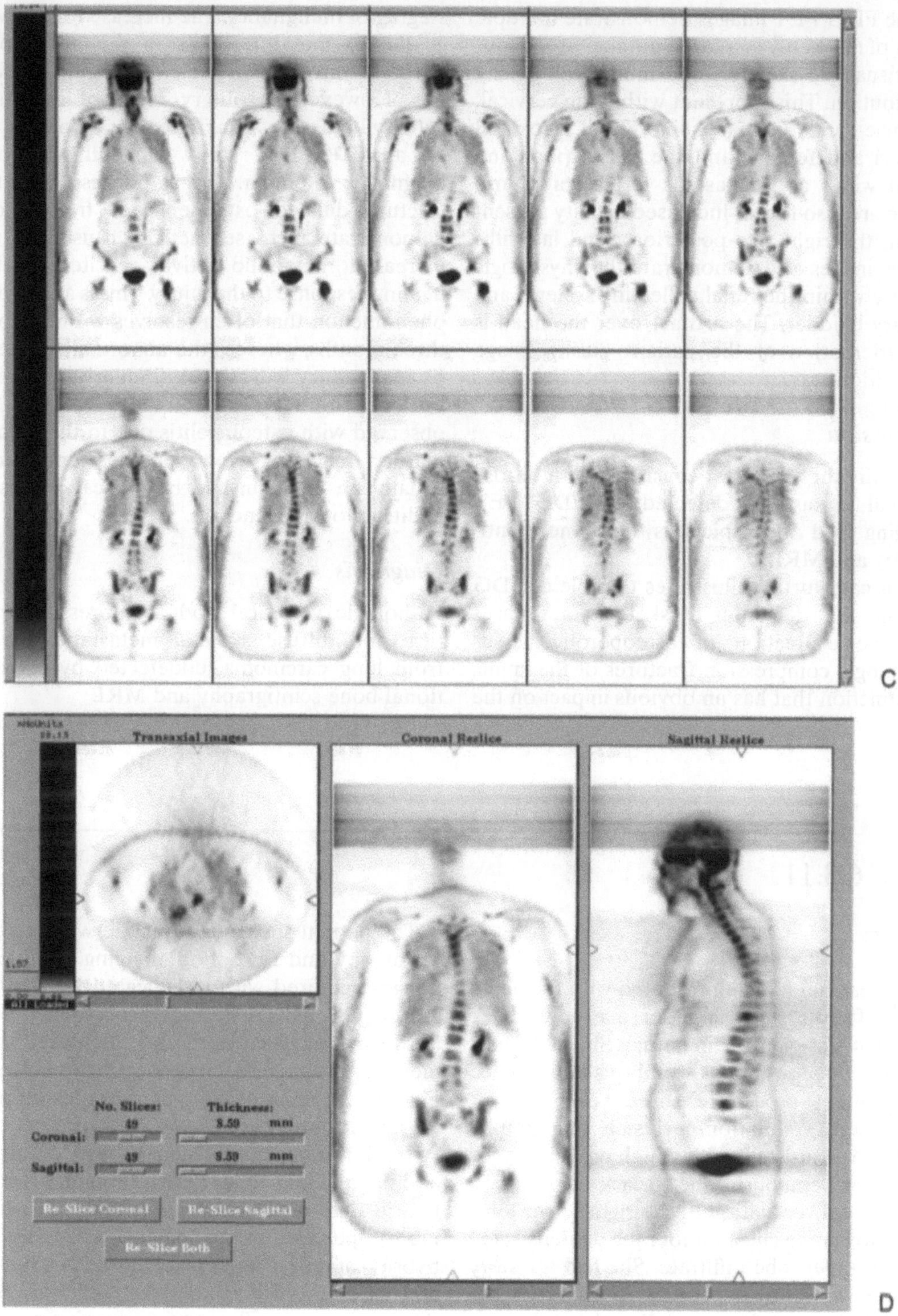

FIGURE 6.3.10C,D.

The FDG PET images demonstrate multiple areas of markedly increased uptake throughout the visualized skeleton in a multifocal, patchy distribution. This is present within the cervical, thoracic, and lumbar spine, both proximal humeri and femurs, and the pelvis (iliac and sacral wings as well as the left acetabulum). There are also foci of increased activity present within the right ribs posteriorly and laterally. These images also demonstrate the physiologic activity within the renal collecting systems and urinary bladder. The artifact over the head is due to motion of the patient during image acquisition.

Discussion

These findings are most consistent with diffuse skeletal metastases detected on FDG PET imaging and inconspicuous on bone scintigraphy and MRI.

This case further illustrates the role of FDG imaging for detection of skeletal metastases and the evaluation of osteoporotic versus pathologic compression fractures of the spine, a distinction that has an obvious impact on the staging of malignancy. The increased sensitivity is due to the differences in the physiologic processes involved in the two imaging modalities. However, a solitary focus of increased activity limited to a single vertebral body noted on an FDG PET study can still present a diagnostic dilemma. This is because an acute fracture due to osteopenia or trauma can demonstrate increased activity caused by the increased metabolic activity elicited by the healing response to the injury. This is a transient phenomenon that often resolves within two to three months, whereas the abnormality caused by malignancy will persist. Similarly, increased activity within a vertebral body can also be observed with osteomyelitis due to the inflammatory reaction. However, this entity can usually be distinguished by clinical means in addition to MRI findings.

Diagnosis

Pathologic vertebral body compression fracture and diffuse skeletal metastatic disease from lung carcinoma, undetected by conventional bone scintigraphy and MRI.

Case 6.3.11

History

A 31-year-old female presented with the acute onset of right chest, shoulder, and upper back pain that was pleuritic in nature. She had a past history of deep venous thrombosis after a knee replacement procedure three years ago. A subsequent ventilation-perfusion scintigraphy study was consistent with a high probability for pulmonary embolism due to lack of perfusion and normal ventilation to the right upper lobe. The correlating chest radiograph demonstrated a right upper lobe infiltrate. She had a history of smoking up to two packs of cigarettes per day for the past 15 years. Therefore, she was referred for a chest CT (Figure 6.3.11A). Sputum cytology was suspicious for squamous cell carcinoma.

The patient subsequently underwent mediastinoscopy and FDG PET imaging. Transaxial images acquired with a dedicated PET tomograph (GE Advance) and reconstructed with iterative reconstruction and measured segmented attenuation correction are shown in Figure 6.3.11B, and orthogonal images through the mediastinum are shown in Figure 6.3.11C. After the dedicated PET images were obtained, additional FDG images were obtained with a hybrid dual-head gamma camera (VG Millenium) operating in the coincidence mode. The hybrid camera is equipped with an X-ray tube and an array of detectors that functions as a third-generation CT scanner, allowing acquisition of attenuation maps for attenuation correction and anatomical mapping. Figure 6.3.11D shows transaxial hybrid PET images corresponding to the dedicated PET images. Figure 6.3.11E, see color plate, shows transaxial images of the hybrid CT (left), hybrid PET (middle), and fusion (right) at the level of the upper mediastinum (upper panel) and lung mass (lower panel).

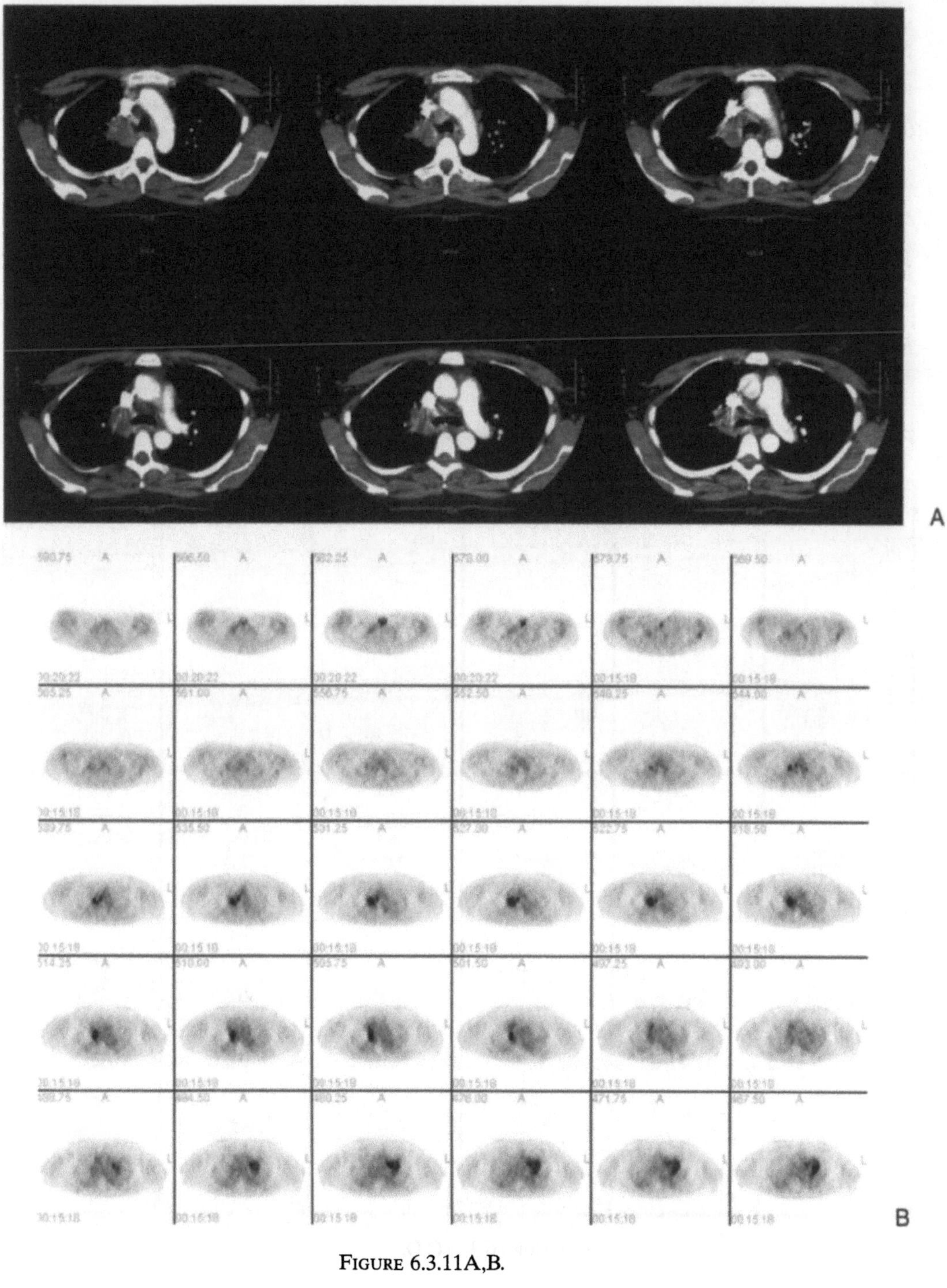

FIGURE 6.3.11A,B.

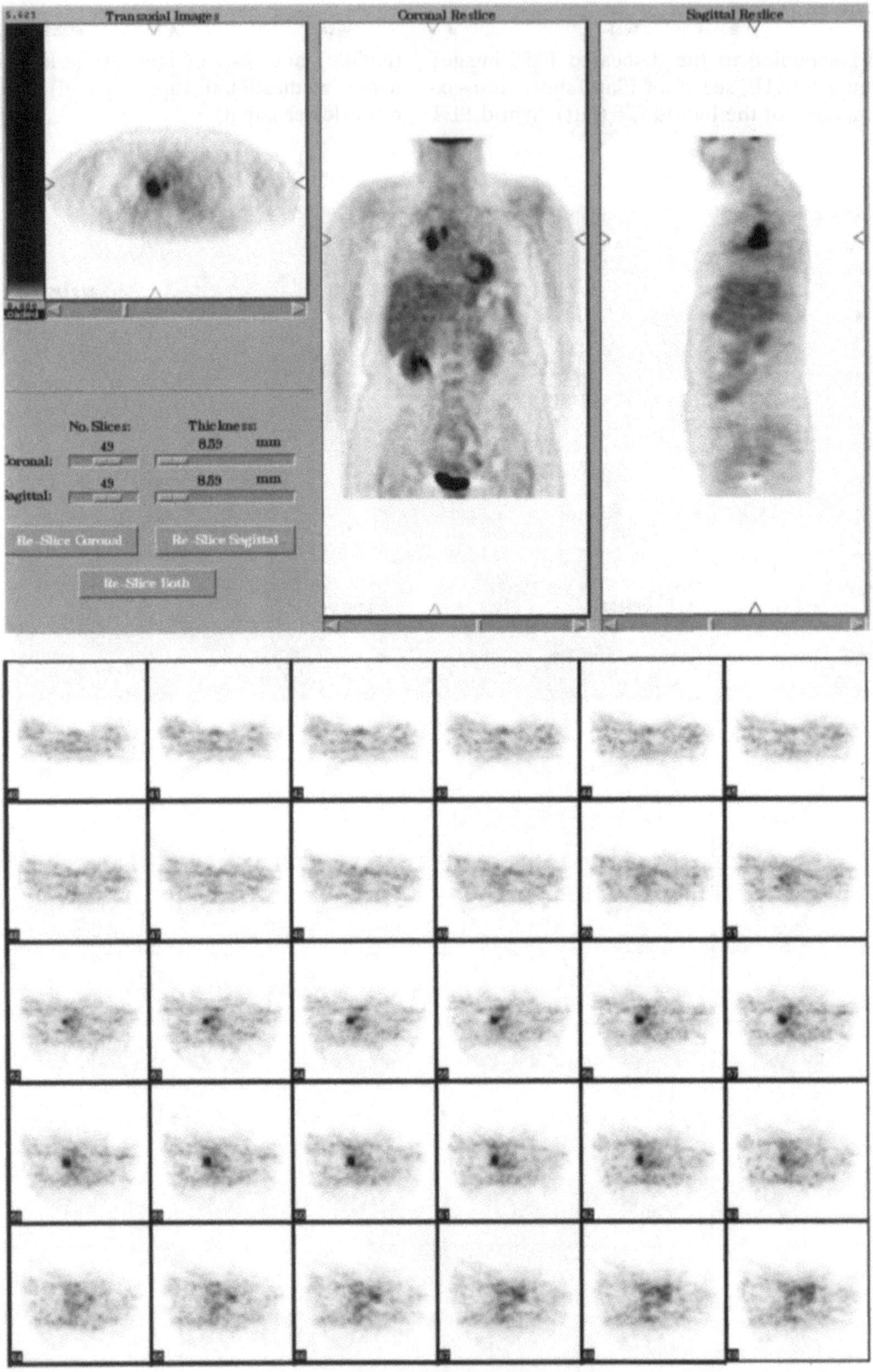

C

D

FIGURE 6.3.11C,D.

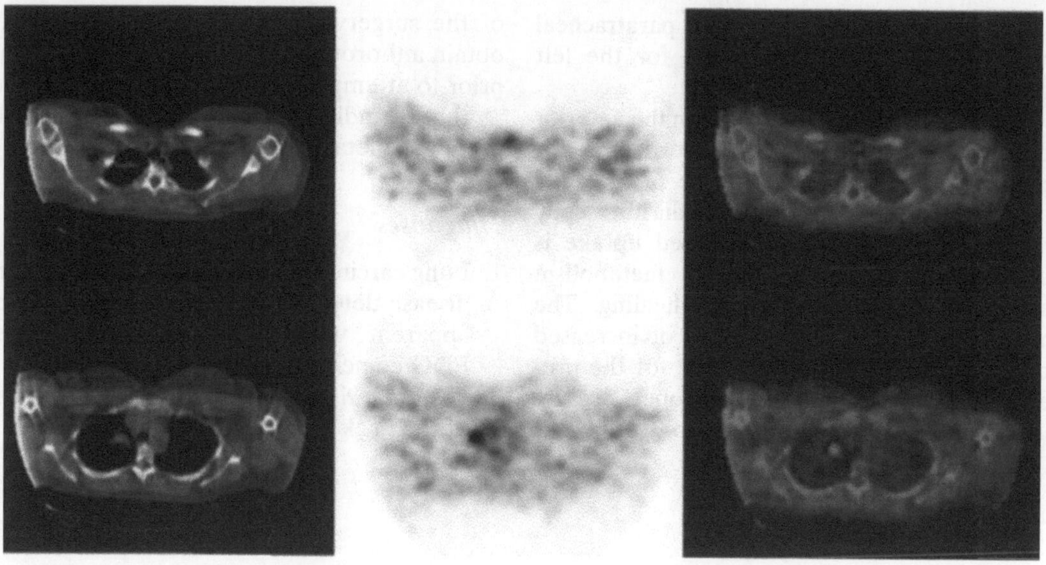

FIGURE 6.3.11E. (See color plate)

Findings

The chest CT reveals a soft tissue density mass within the right upper lobe in a paratracheal location. It surrounded the right main stem bronchus and pulmonary artery and extended into the pretracheal, hilar, and subcarinal regions. Infiltrate was present distally within the right apex, presumably representing post-obstructive pneumonia.

The dedicated FDG PET images demonstrate a large focus of markedly increased activity present within the medial right upper lobe, correlating with the soft tissue mass seen on CT. A small focus of increased activity is also seen in the mediastinum. In addition, there is moderately increased uptake at the base of the neck in the midline. Physiologic activity is present within the myocardium.

As with the dedicated PET images, the hybrid PET images show increased activity present within the right upper lobe, and the fusion image definitively localizes this to the CT abnormality. The hybrid PET images also show the increased activity present at the base of the neck. The fusion image localizes this to the anterior chest wall, but no CT abnormality is identified in this location. The small focus of uptake in the mediastinum can only be identified retrospectively on the hybrid PET images.

Discussion

These findings are consistent with a primary lung carcinoma metastatic to the mediastinum. The uptake in the upper anterior chest wall is due to inflammatory changes related to recent mediastinoscopy.

This case further demonstrates the differences of limits of lesion detectability between dedicated PET camera images as compared to those obtained with dual-head coincidence cameras (hybrid PET). Dedicated PET allows detection of lesions of approximately 5 mm in diameter, whereas the size limit is 15 to 20 mm with hybrid PET. This can have a drastic effect on mediastinal staging of malignancy. The small focus of increased activity seen on dedicated PET is equivocal on hybrid PET. However, the fusion hybrid CT/hybrid PET image reveals that the equivocal focus of uptake corresponds to a pretracheal lymph node. The histological examination from the specimens from the mediastinoscopy were consistent with metastatic involvement of the right paratracheal lymph nodes but were negative for the left paratracheal lymph nodes.

The increased activity present on the anterior chest wall superiorly is also worrisome for metastatic disease. However, the FDG study was obtained shortly after the mediastinoscopy was performed, and this increased uptake is consistent with the increased metabolism caused by postsurgical wound healing. The fusion image localizes this focus of increased activity to the typical incision site for the procedure. Increased uptake at a postoperative site is a common finding within one to two months of the surgery. Therefore, it is imperative to obtain a thorough history of recent procedures prior to attempting to interpret an FDG study, so that a finding such as this is not misinterpreted as metastatic disease.

Diagnoses

1. Lung carcinoma with metastatic mediastinal disease detected by dedicated PET, but not apparent with dual-head hybrid camera FDG coincidence imaging (hybrid PET).
2. Postoperative increased uptake at the base of the neck from recent mediastinoscopy.

6.4 Breast Carcinoma

LeAnn Simmons-Stokes, William H. Martin, and Dominique Delbeke

Breast carcinoma is the most common malignancy in women in North America. If diagnosed early, it is a curable disease. The estimated incidence of breast carcinoma is about 180,000 cases per year. One in nine women will develop breast carcinoma in their lifetime, and about one-third of these patients will die from their disease.[1]

Detection of Breast Carcinoma

The initial diagnosis of breast cancer is usually made by physical examination or mammography and confirmed by biopsy. Mammography is difficult to interpret in women who have dense breasts, who have had mammoplasties, and in whom prior biopsies have been performed. Despite the high sensitivity of mammography for the detection of breast cancer, its specificity is less than 30%, leading to a large number of biopsies for benign lesions.

FDG PET allows accurate detection of breast carcinoma with sensitivity and specificity both ranging from 80% to 100%.[2–12] As with other types of tumors, false-negative results can occur when lesions are less than 1 cm in size or when the tumor is well-differentiated, such as tubular carcinoma and carcinoma in situ. A high rate of false-negative findings has been reported in lobular carcinomas[13] as well. False-positive results occur in patients with inflammatory processes in the breast or early after biopsy or surgery. Benign breast tumors usually have low FDG uptake;[14] only about 10% of fibroadenomas accumulate FDG. Technically, examination of the breast in the prone position is preferable to differentiate breast lesions from lesions in the chest wall. However, this requires a special imaging table.

FDG PET imaging is particularly useful in patients with small lesions, nonpalpable lesions, equivocal mammographic findings, and fibrocystic disease in which fine-needle biopsy is less reliable. FDG PET imaging can also be useful in women with dense breasts or after augmentation mammoplasty; mammographic detection of cancer in these women is challenging, owing to the radiodensity of the implant.[15]

Staging Breast Carcinoma

Since the presence of nodal metastases is the most important prognostic factor in patients with breast carcinoma,[16] axillary lymph node dissection is usually performed as a diagnostic procedure for staging purposes. Although several studies have demonstrated the ability of PET to detect axillary lymph node metastases with relatively high sensitivities and specificities,[17–20] FDG PET cannot delineate the number of lymph nodes involved, which is an important prognostic factor. Patients with a positive PET scan should undergo axillary dissection to confirm the presence and number of lymph nodes involved. The anticipated limitation of this approach is that 5% of women with microscopic lymph node metastases not detected by PET would be understaged. Therefore, for staging early breast carcinoma, identification and sampling of the sentinel lymph node may be the technique of choice.

The advantages of FDG PET imaging are the detection of unsuspected distant metastases[21] and the capability of detecting internal mammary lymph node metastases that are not routinely sampled with the current standard of care.

Monitoring Therapy of Breast Carcinoma

Preliminary reports indicate that FDG PET may be able to differentiate responders from nonresponders as early as after the first course of chemotherapy.[22–25] If these data are confirmed, predicting the tumor responsiveness to therapy would avoid unnecessary toxicity and expenses in nonresponsive patients.

Detection of Recurrent or Metastatic Breast Carcinoma

In a study of 75 patients, Bender et al.[26] found that FDG PET detected six local recurrences and eight nodal and seven bone metastases not seen on CT/MRI. In another study of 57 patients, the sensitivity and specificity of FDG PET to detect recurrence was 93% and 79%, respectively.[27] False-negative results were mostly bone metastases. Cook et al.[28] compared FDG PET and bone scintigraphy in 23 patients with skeletal metastases from breast cancer. They concluded that FDG PET was superior to bone scintigraphy to detect osteolytic metastases that had a poorer prognosis. Osteoblastic metastases had lower FDG uptake and were frequently undetectable by FDG PET.

Summary

Because of the limitations of FDG PET imaging to detect small tumors, FDG PET is not recommended for routine evaluation of primary breast tumors. However, it is useful in selected difficult cases, such as patients with fibrocystic disease, dense breasts, equivocal mammographic or MRI findings, and patients with mammoplasties or prior biopsies. In early stage disease, FDG PET is limited by detection of micrometastases, and therefore, the axillary node status is better predicted by sentinel lymph node identification, resection, and histopathological examination. In patients with advanced disease, FDG PET is helpful to stage loco-regional lymph nodes and distant metastases. In addition, FDG PET seems to be very accurate to monitor therapy and detect recurrent disease.

References

1. Parker SL, Tong T, Bolden S, Wingo PA: Cancer statistics, 1997. CA Cancer J Clin 1997;1:5–27.
2. Kubota K, Matsuzawa T, Amemiya A, et al.: Imaging of breast cancer with [18F]fluorodeoxyglucose and positron emission tomography. J Comput Assist Tomogr 1989;13:1097–1098.
3. Wahl RL, Cody R, Hutchins GD, Mudgett E: Primary and metastatic breast carcinoma: Initial clinical evaluation with PET with the radiolabeled glucose analog 2-[F-18]-fluorodeoxy-2-D-glucose (FDG). Radiology 1991;179:765–770.
4. Tse NY, Hoh CK, Hawkins RA, et al.: The application of positron emission tomographic imaging with fluorodeoxyglucose to the evaluation of breast disease. Ann Surg 1992;216:27–34.
5. Nieweg OE, Kim EE, Wong WH, et al.: Positron emission tomography with fluorine-18-deoxyglucose in the detection and staging of breast cancer. Cancer 1993;71:3920–3925.
6. Adler LP, Crowe JP, al-Kaisi NK, Sunshine JL: Evaluation of breast masses and axillary lymph nodes with [F-18]2-deoxy-2-fluoro-D-glucose PET. Radiology 1993;187:743–750.
7. Hoh K, Hawkins RA, Glaspy JA, et al.: Cancer detection with whole-body PET using [F-18]fluoro-2-deoxy-D-glucose. J Comput Assist Tomogr 1993;17:582–589.
8. Dehdashti F, Mortimer JE, Siegel BA, et al.: Positron tomographic assessment of estrogen receptors in breast cancer. Comparison with FDG-PET and in vitro receptor assays. J Nucl Med 1995;36:1766–1774.
9. Avril N, Dose J, Janicke F, et al.: Metabolic characterization of breast tumors with positron emission tomography using F-18 fluorodeoxyglucose. J Clin Oncol 1996;14:1848–1857.
10. Schiedhauer K, Scharl A, Pietrzyk U, Wagner R, Gohring UJ, Schomaker K, Schica H: Qualitative [18F]FDG positron emission tomography in

primary breast cancer: Clinical relevance and practicability. Eur J Nucl Med 1996;23:618–623.
11. Palmedo H, Bender H, Grunwald F, et al.: Comparison of fluorine-18-fluorodeoxyglucose positron emission tomography and technetium-99m methoxyisobutylisonitrile scintimammography in the detection of breast tumors. Eur J Nucl Med 1997;24:1138–1145.
12. Noh DY, Yun IJ, Kim JS, et al.: Diagnostic value of positron emission tomography for detecting breast cancer. World J Surg 1998;22:223–227.
13. Crippa F, Seregni E, Agresti R, et al.: Association between [18F]fluorodeoxyglucose uptake and postoperative histopathology, hormone receptor status, thymidine labeling index and p53 in primary breast cancer: A preliminary observation. Eur J Nucl Med 1998;10:1429–1434.
14. Avril N, Schelling M, Dose J, et al.: Utility of PET in breast cancer. Clin Pos Imag 1999;2:261–271.
15. Wahl RL, Helve MA, Chang AE, Andersson I: Detection of breast cancer in women after augmentation mammoplasty using fluorine-18-fluorodeoxyglucose-PET. J Nucl Med 1994;35:872–875.
16. Wilking N, Rutqvist LE, Cartensen J, Mattson A, Skoog L: Prognostic significance of axillary nodal status in primary breast cancer in relation to the number of resected nodes. Acta Oncol 1992;31:29–35.
17. Utech CI, Young CS, Winter PF: Prospective evaluation of fluorine-18 fluorodeoxyglucose positron emission tomography in breast cancer for staging of the axilla related to surgery and immunocytochemistry. Eur J Nucl Med 1996;23:1588–1593.
18. Adler LP, Faulhaber PF, Schnur KC, Al-Kasi NC, Shenk RR: Axillary lymph node metastases: Screening with [F-18]2-deoxy-2-fluoro-D-glucose (FDG) PET. Radiology 1997;203:323–327.
19. Crippa F, Agresti R, Seregni E, et al.: Prospective evaluation of fluorine-18-FDG-PET in presurgical staging of the axilla in breast cancer. J Nucl Med 1998;39:4–8.
20. Smith IC, Ogston KN, Whitford P, et al.: Staging of the axilla in breast cancer: An accurate in vivo assessment using positron emission tomography with 2-(fluorine-18)-fluoro-2-deoxy-D-glucose. Ann Surg 1998;228:220–227.
21. Avril N, Dose J, Janicke F, et al.: Assessment of axillary lymph node involvement in breast cancer patients with positron emission tomography using radiolabeled 2-(fluorine-18)-fluoro-2-deoxy-D-glucose. J Natl Cancer Inst 1996;88(17):1204–1209.
22. Wahl RL, Zasadny K, Helvie M, et al.: Metabolic monitoring of breast cancer chemohormonotherapy using positron emission tomography: Initial evaluation. J Clin Oncol 1993;11:2101–2111.
23. Jansson T, Westlin JE, Ahlstrom H, Lilja A, Langstrom B, Bergh J: Positron emission tomography studies in patients with locally advanced and/or metastatic breast cancer: A method for early therapy evaluation? J Clin Oncol 1995;13:1470–1477.
24. Bassa P, Kim EE, Inoue T, et al.: Evaluation of preoperative chemotherapy using PET with fluorine-18-fluorodeoxyglucose in breast cancer. J Nucl Med 1996;37(6):931–938.
25. Schelling M, Avril N, Nahrig J, et al.: Positron emission tomography using [(18)F]fluorodeoxyglucose for monitoring primary chemotherapy in breast cancer. J Clin Oncol 2000;18(8):1689–1695.
26. Bender H, Kirst J, Palmedo H, et al.: Value of 18fluoro-deoxyglucose positron emission tomography in the staging of recurrent breast carcinoma. Anticancer Res 1997;17:1687–1692.
27. Moon DP, Maddahi J, Silverman DHS, et al.: Accuracy of whole-body fluorine-18-FDG-PET for the detection of recurrent or metastatic breast carcinoma. J Nucl Med 1998;39:431–435.
28. Cook GJ, Houston S, Rubens R, Maisey MN, Fogelman I: Detection of bone metastases in breast cancer with FDG-PET: Differing metabolic activity in osteoblastic and osteolytic lesions. J Clin Oncol 1998;16:3375–3379.

Case Presentations

Case 6.4.1

History

A 68-year-old female presented with a one-year history of rising tumor markers. Seven years earlier she had undergone a left breast lumpectomy followed by radiation and chemotherapy. Coronal FDG images (Figure 6.4.1A, chest and Figure 6.4.1B, abdomen and pelvis) were acquired with a dedicated full ring PET (Siemens ECAT 933) and reconstructed using filtered back projection without attenuation correction.

Findings

No abnormal uptake is seen in the chest. A focus of increased FDG activity is seen in the

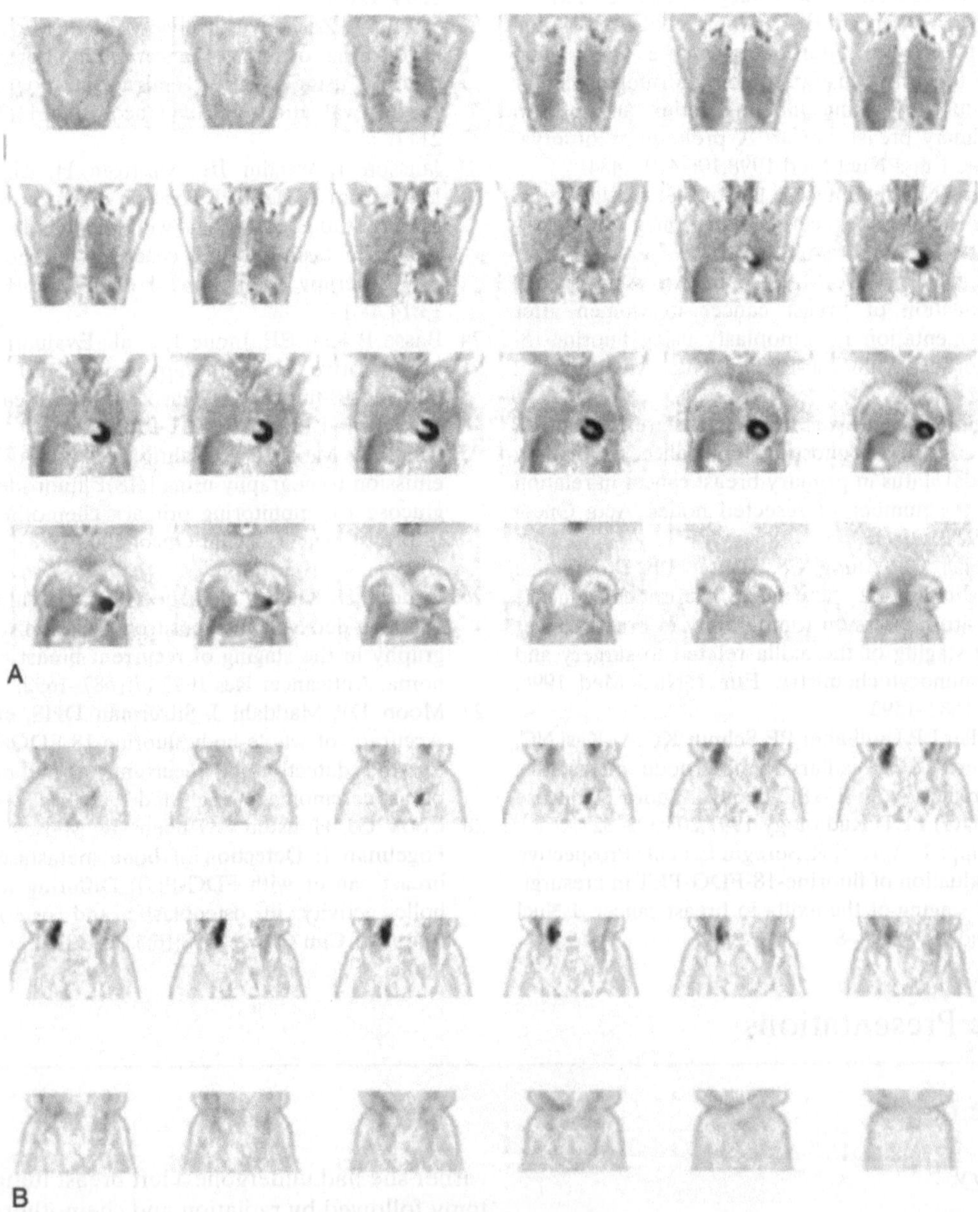

FIGURE 6.4.1A,B.

region of the left sacroiliac joint. Intense activity is also noted in the collecting system of the right kidney on these images.

Discussion

As with other nuclear medicine techniques, the increased activity in the collecting system of the right kidney should be correlated with ultrasound and/or CT to exclude ureteral obstruction. The focus of increased activity in the pelvis is consistent with a solitary metastatic skeletal lesion. Both FDG PET and conventional diphosphonate bone scintigraphy may be used to detect skeletal metastases in cancer patients. Because the agents utilized in these studies have different characteristics and different mechanisms of uptake, there may be different indications for and applications of these techniques. The ^{99m}Tc-diphosphonate radiopharmaceutical used in conventional bone scintigraphy is chemically adsorbed onto the bone surface, its uptake dependent on local blood flow, osteoblastic activity, and capillary permeability. Since most metastatic skeletal lesions are associated with an osteoblastic reaction in the surrounding bone as well as increased vascularity, there is focal accumulation of the radiopharmaceutical in and around the metastasis. Purely lytic lesions, unaccompanied by osteoblastic activity, may demonstrate poor or absent activity.

However, FDG accumulates in viable neoplastic tissues, including skeletal metastases, that have a higher glycolytic rate than the surrounding tissues and is not dependant on other factors such as a surrounding osteoblastic reaction to the predominantly medullary tumor. FDG PET imaging has both advantages and disadvantages when compared with bone scintigraphy. Whole-body FDG PET imaging can demonstrate not only skeletal metastases, but also any other metastatic lesions as well as local recurrences. Since FDG accumulates in viable tumor cells and PET allows for the measurement of standard uptake values within specific lesions, FDG PET has the potential to characterize and grade lesions and monitor response to therapy. Furthermore, due to its mechanism of uptake, the specificity of FDG for malignant neoplasm is much higher than that of the diphosphonates. The main advantage of bone scintigraphy over FDG PET imaging is that scintigraphy is more sensitive in the detection of sclerotic bone lesions.

Diagnosis

Breast carcinoma with unsuspected metastasis to the sacrum.

Case 6.4.2

History

A 43-year-old female underwent right mastectomy followed by chemotherapy one year ago for breast cancer. She now presents with elevated serum tumor markers (CEA and CA125) as well as a CT scan (Figure 6.4.2A) demonstrating a new lesion in the liver. Coronal FDG images (Figure 6.4.2B) acquired on a dedicated full ring PET tomograph (GE Advance) and reconstructed using an iterative algorithm and measured segmented attenuation correction as well as orthogonal (Figure 6.4.2C) slices through the liver are displayed.

Findings

The CT image shows a 2 cm lesion in segment VIII of the liver. A 1.5 cm low attenuation lesion is also seen in segment VI. The axial, coronal, and sagittal FDG PET images demonstrate a focus of increased activity in the lateral right lobe of the liver near the dome that corresponds with the lesion seen in segment VIII on CT. A second focus of increased uptake is not seen in the region of segment VI on the FDG PET scan. Symmetrically increased activity present in the upper chest on the coronal images is due to contraction of skeletal muscu-

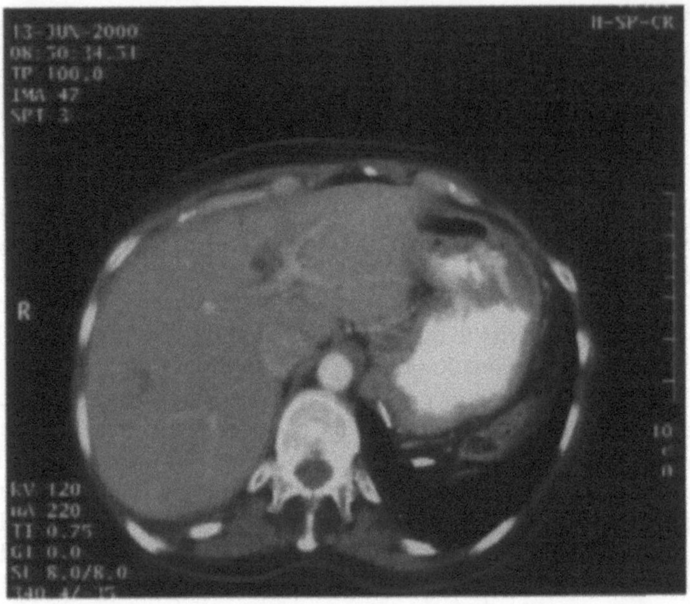

A

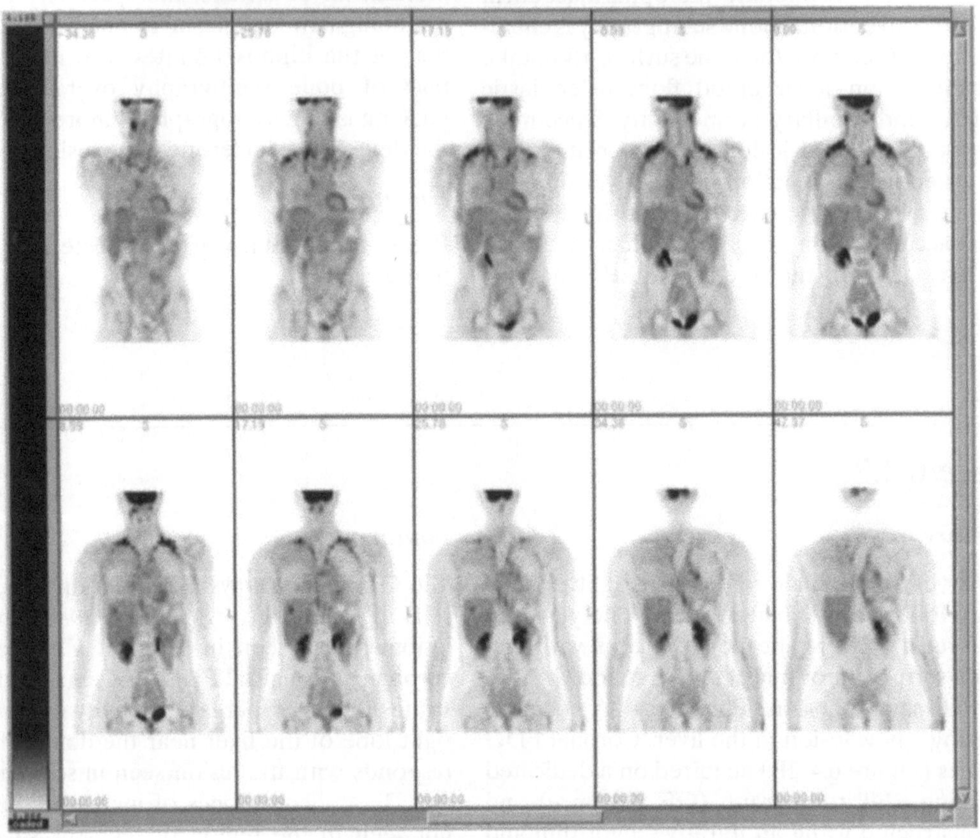

B

FIGURE 6.4.2A,B.

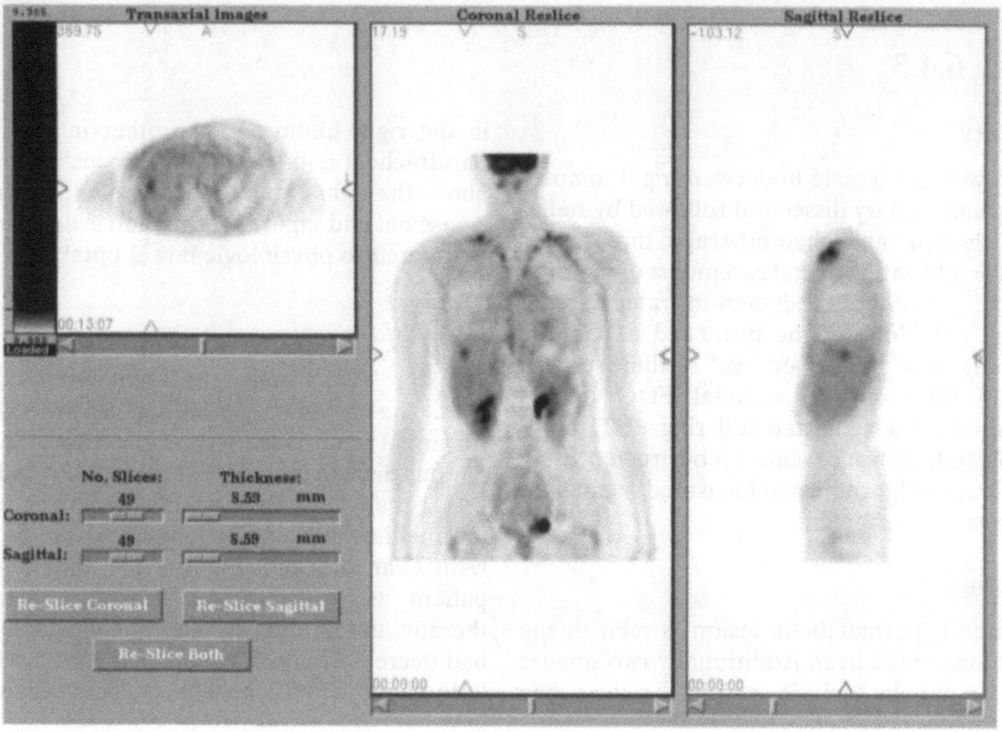

FIGURE 6.4.2C.

lature during FDG distribution and is often seen in anxious or tense individuals.

Discussion

The FDG PET images indicate the presence of a single metastatic lesion in the liver. This lesion was later biopsied and histologically proven to be metastatic breast carcinoma. The second liver lesion seen on the CT scan did not demonstrate increased uptake and was therefore felt to represent a benign lesion, probably a simple hepatic cyst. The information added by FDG PET changed the patient's therapy. Since only a single hepatic metastasis was identified, the patient underwent radiofrequency ablation of the lesion in segment VIII. A later postprocedural CT scan demonstrated a nonenhancing lesion in segment VIII of the liver with no evidence of residual tumor. The lesion in segment VI that was felt to represent a cyst was stable in size and appearance on the repeat CT.

Although not performed in this case, functional imaging with FDG PET imaging following therapy is felt to be superior to anatomical imaging with CT; this has been shown to be true in a variety of neoplasms following surgery, radiation, chemotherapy, and local procedures such as chemoembolization, ethanol instillation, and radiofrequency ablation. In patients with residual masses after therapy, functional imaging can distinguish viable tumor from scar or nonviable tumor mass. Therefore, FDG PET imaging may identify nonresponders earlier, allowing for a more timely change in therapy if indicated.[1]

Diagnoses

1. Breast carcinoma with a solitary hepatic metastasis.
2. Benign hepatic lesion in segment VI.

Reference

1. Smith IC, Welch AE, Hutcheon AW, et al.: Positron emission tomography using [(18)F]-fluorodeoxy-D-glucose to predict the pathologic response of breast cancer to primary chemotherapy. J Clin Oncol 2000;18(8):1676–1688.

Case 6.4.3

History

A 56-year-old female underwent right lumpectomy and axillary dissection followed by radiation therapy and chemotherapy three years ago for infiltrating ductal carcinoma of the right breast. A recent CT scan demonstrated a lesion in the right lobe of the liver, and FDG PET imaging was performed for further staging. Figure 6.4.3 displays coronal FDG images acquired on a dedicated full ring PET tomograph (GE Advance) and reconstructed using an iterative algorithm and measured segmented attenuation correction.

Findings

A large hypermetabolic lesion is seen in the right lobe of the liver. Additionally, two smaller hypermetabolic foci are seen in the chest, one in the right hilum and the other in the right paratracheal region. The small focus of uptake above the right kidney had a tubular pattern on transaxial and sagittal images and is believed to be related to physiologic bowel uptake.

Discussion

The large liver lesion is consistent with a metastasis. The two thoracic lesions are worrisome for nodal metastases, although active granulomatous disease may appear similarly. A follow-up CT scan demonstrated small lymph nodes in the mediastinum corresponding to the foci of right hilar and right paratracheal uptake. The patient was treated with aggressive chemotherapy, and six months later the hepatic lesion had decreased in size, whereas the mediastinal lesions remained unchanged. These findings

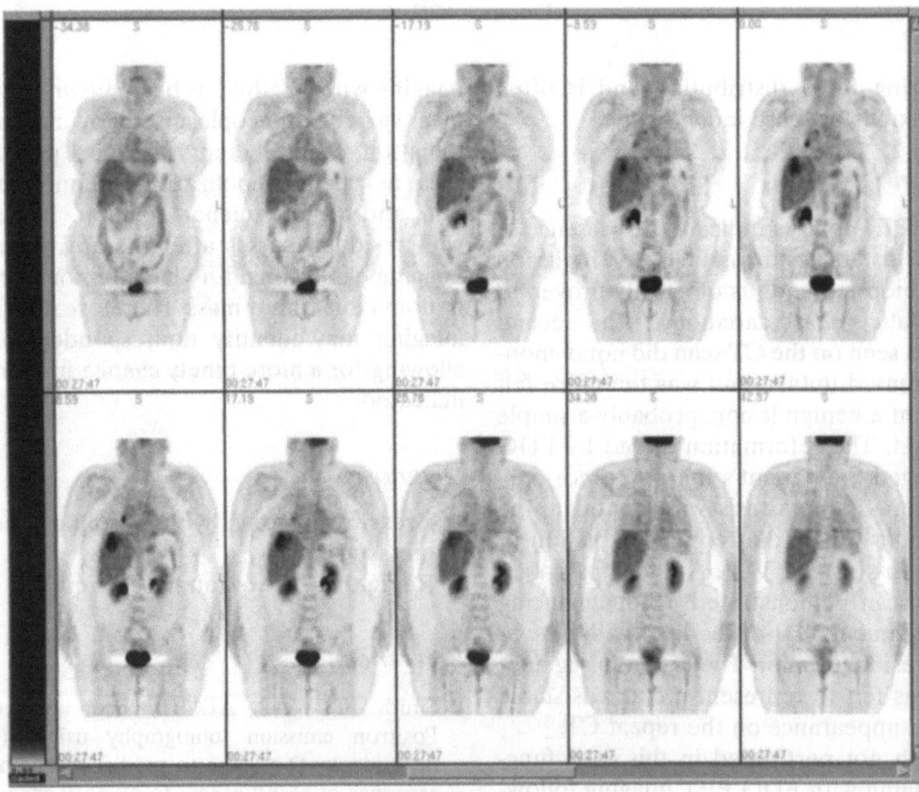

FIGURE 6.4.3.

suggest that the hepatic lesion was a metastasis and the mediastinal lesions were due to a benign inflammatory process. There was no new lesion above the right kidney.

FDG PET has been shown to be the most accurate method available for restaging breast cancer patients.[1] FDG PET imaging is particularly advantageous because whole-body imaging can demonstrate the complete extent of metastatic disease. The finding of distant metastases signifies stage IV disease and changes the patient's prognosis and treatment. Stage IV disease is associated with only an 18% five-year survival,[2] and the treatment is generally palliative, although more aggressive therapies are under investigation.

FDG PET imaging may prove to be even more powerful as a tool for monitoring response to therapy. In a study of 22 patients with locally advanced breast cancer, significant differences in tracer uptake between nonresponding and responding tumors were observed as early as after the first course of chemotherapy. A decrease in the standard uptake value of the tumor to below 55% of the baseline scan identified responders with 100% specificity and 85% sensitivity. Using the same criterion, histologic response was predicted with an accuracy of 88% and 91% after the first and second courses of chemotherapy, respectively.[3]

Diagnosis

Breast carcinoma with a solitary hepatic metastasis.

References

1. Boerner AR, et al.: Optimal scan time for fluorine-18 fluorodeoxyglucose positron emission tomography in breast cancer. Eur J Nucl Med 1999;26(3):226–230.
2. Sainsbury JR, et al.: ABC of breast diseases: Breast cancer. BMJ 2000;321:745–750.
3. Schelling M, et al.: Positron emission tomography using [18F]fluorodeoxyglucose for monitoring primary chemotherapy in breast cancer. J Clin Oncol 2000;18(8):1689–1695.

Case 6.4.4

History

Two years earlier, a 40-year-old female underwent a left mastectomy followed by chemotherapy for breast cancer. The patient is now referred for FDG PET imaging because of elevated serum tumor markers with a CT scan interpreted as negative for recurrence (Figure 6.4.4A). Coronal (Figure 6.4.4B) and transaxial (Figure 6.4.4C) FDG images through the upper

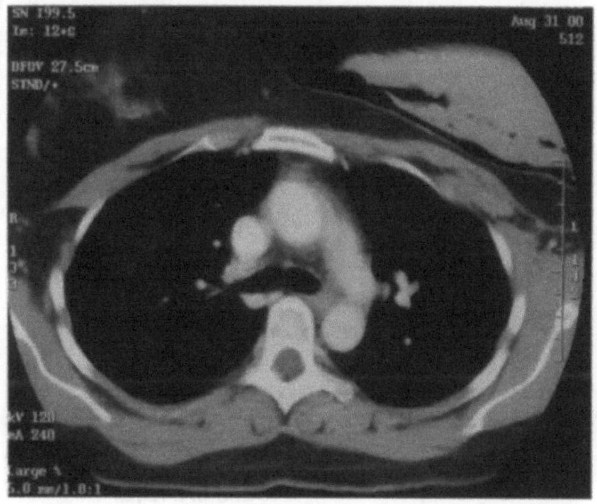

FIGURE 6.4.4A.

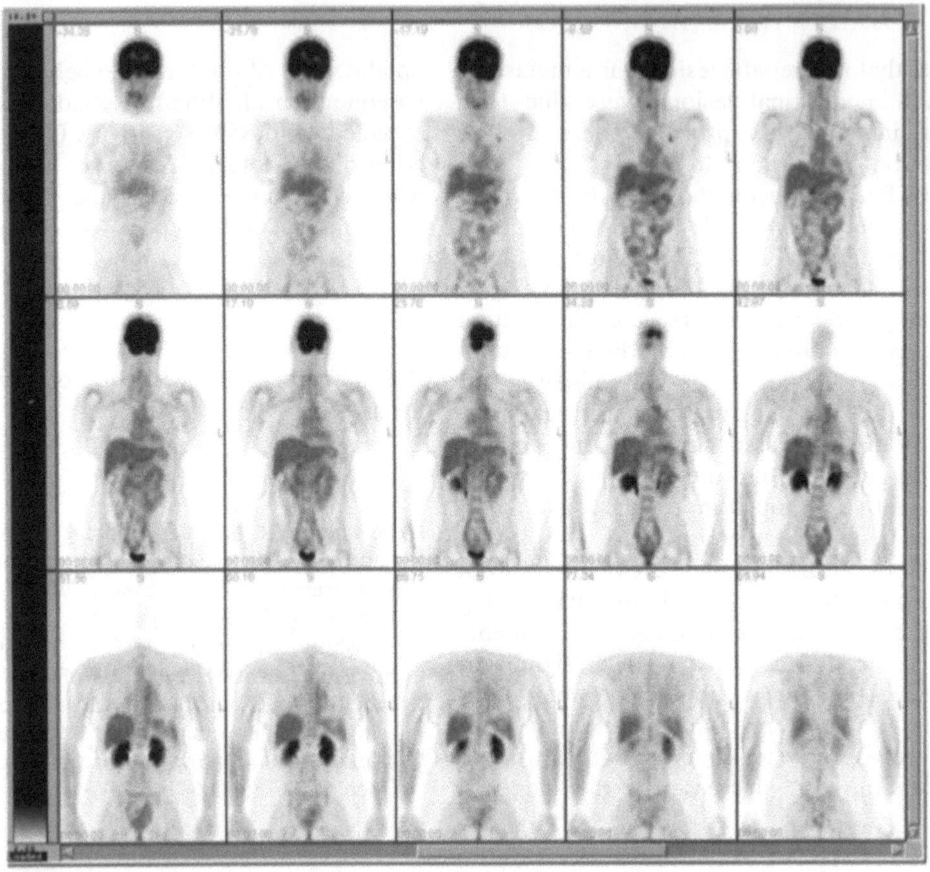

B

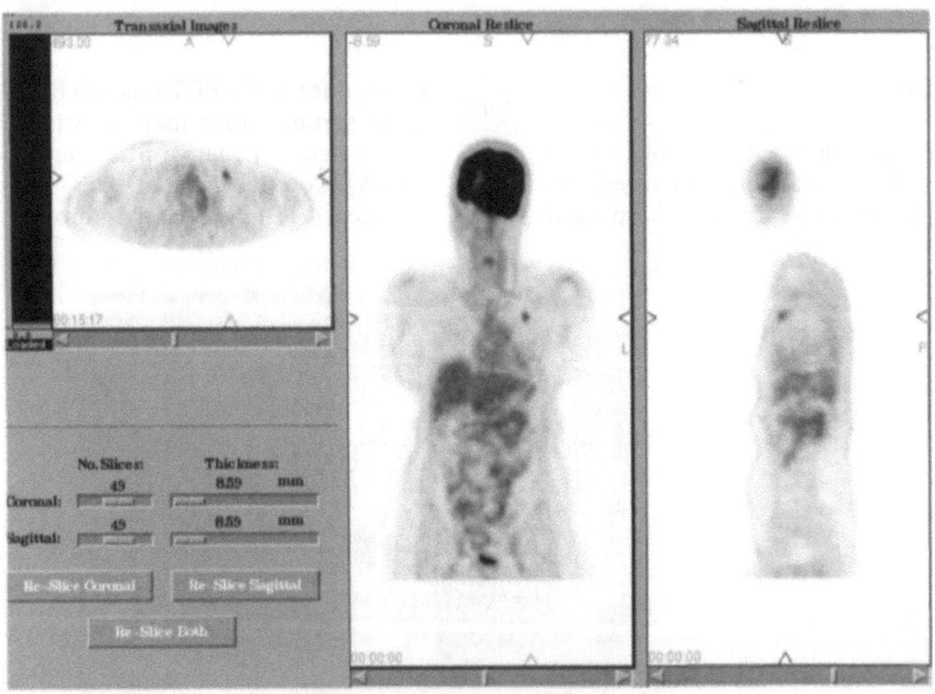

C

FIGURE 6.4.4B,C.

chest acquired on a dedicated full ring PET tomograph (GE Advance) and reconstructed using an iterative algorithm and measured segmented attenuation correction are displayed.

Findings

The FDG images demonstrate a focus of increased metabolism in the left chest wall. In retrospect, a small, enhancing nodule can be seen in the same area on the CT scan.

Discussion

The focus of increased activity in the left chest wall seen on the FDG PET images is consistent with local recurrence of breast cancer. Although the CT scan of the chest was initially interpreted as negative, review of the CT in light of the FDG PET findings revealed a small, enhancing nodule in the left chest wall.

In a retrospective study aimed at evaluating the diagnostic value of PET in primary, recurrent, or metastatic breast cancer, histologic findings in 105 patients who had undergone PET plus X-ray or CT of the chest, ultrasound or CT of the liver, and bone scintigraphy were reviewed. The sensitivity, specificity, and accuracy of the PET scan were calculated for the diagnosis of both tumor and lymph node involvement. In patients with metastatic disease, the accuracy of PET was compared with other imaging modalities. The PET scan was 89% and 91% accurate in diagnosing the tumor and lymph node status, respectively. In the 86 patients in this study who also had a mammogram, PET accurately diagnosed the tumor in 90%, while only 72% of tumors were identified with mammography. In the 19 patients who had metastatic disease, the PET findings were consistent with those of the other imaging modalities in 100% of cases.[1]

While PET was 100% consistent with the findings made using other modalities, the correlate is not always true. Although no results specific to breast cancer have been reported, studies comparing the use of PET and CT for the assessment of other malignancies such as lung and colon cancer consistently report higher sensitivity and specificity of PET over CT.[2] In this case, the CT identified the abnormality only in retrospect; the finding was much more easily made with FDG PET imaging.

Diagnosis

Breast carcinoma with local recurrence to the chest wall.

References

1. Rostom AY, et al.: Positron emission tomography in breast cancer: A clinicopathological correlation of results. Br J Radiol 1999;72:1064–1068.
2. Mascaro F, et al.: Assessment of intrathoracic metastatic lung cancer using FDG-PET and CT of the thorax. Clin Positron Imaging 2000;3(4): 163.

Case 6.4.5

History

A 46-year-old female with a history of comedocarcinoma of the left breast diagnosed ten years earlier was referred for FDG PET imaging due to the finding of foci of increased activity on bone scintigraphy (Figures 6.4.5A and B). She had experienced two prior recurrences. The first involved several internal mammary nodes treated with surgical resection, chemotherapy, and radiation therapy. The second was a local chest wall recurrence. Figure 6.4.5C displays coronal FDG images acquired with a dedicated full ring PET tomograph (GE Advance) and reconstructed using an iterative algorithm and measured segmented attenuation correction.

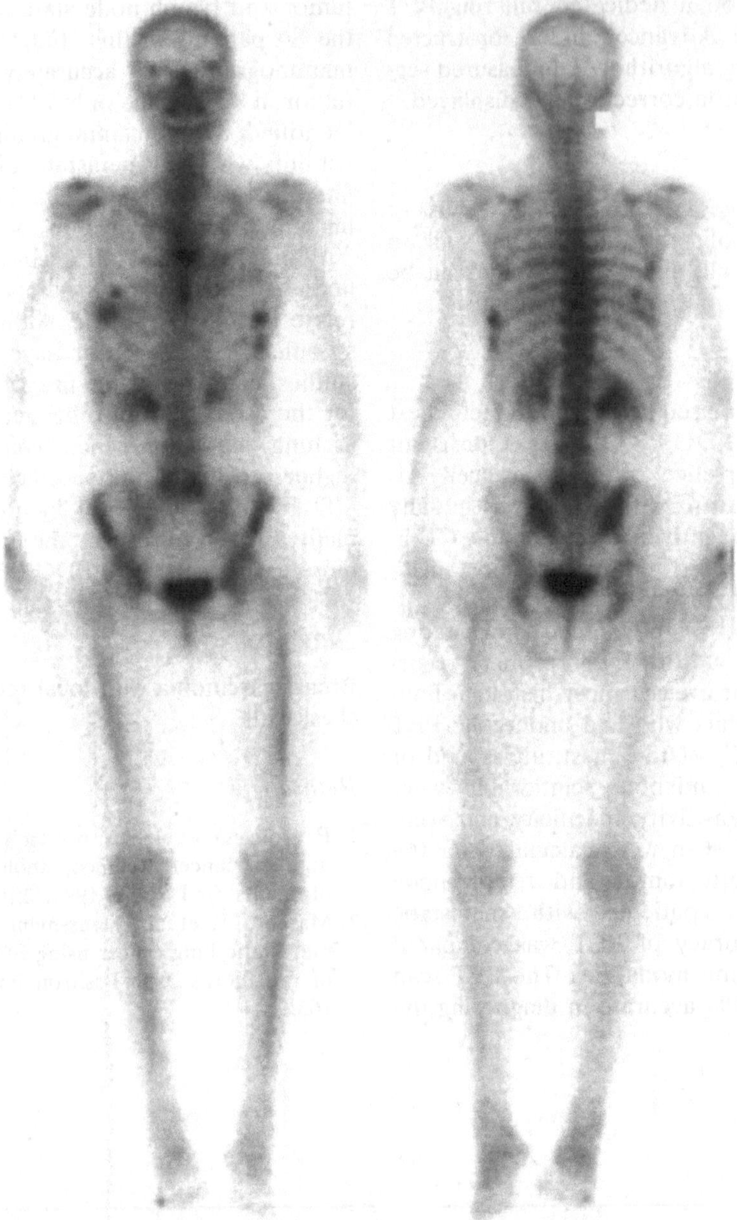

FIGURE 6.4.5A.

Findings

Bone scintigraphy demonstrate foci of increased uptake in the sternum, bilateral ribs laterally, L5, and subtle left anterior iliac wing. Although the pattern of uptake in L5 suggests degenerative disease, the other foci are worrisome for bone metastases.

The FDG images demonstrate no abnormal activity in the chest, abdomen, or pelvis.

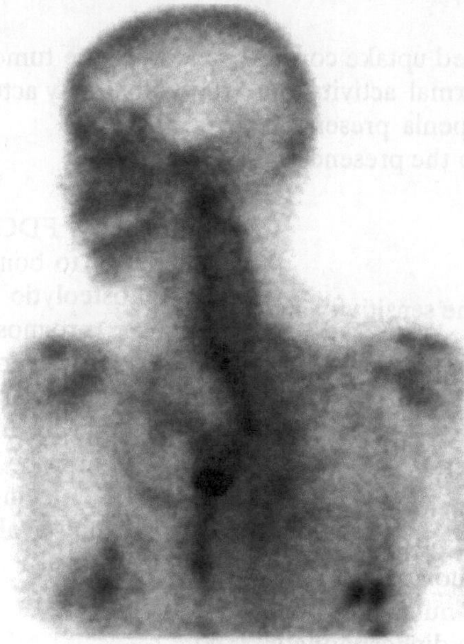

LAO B

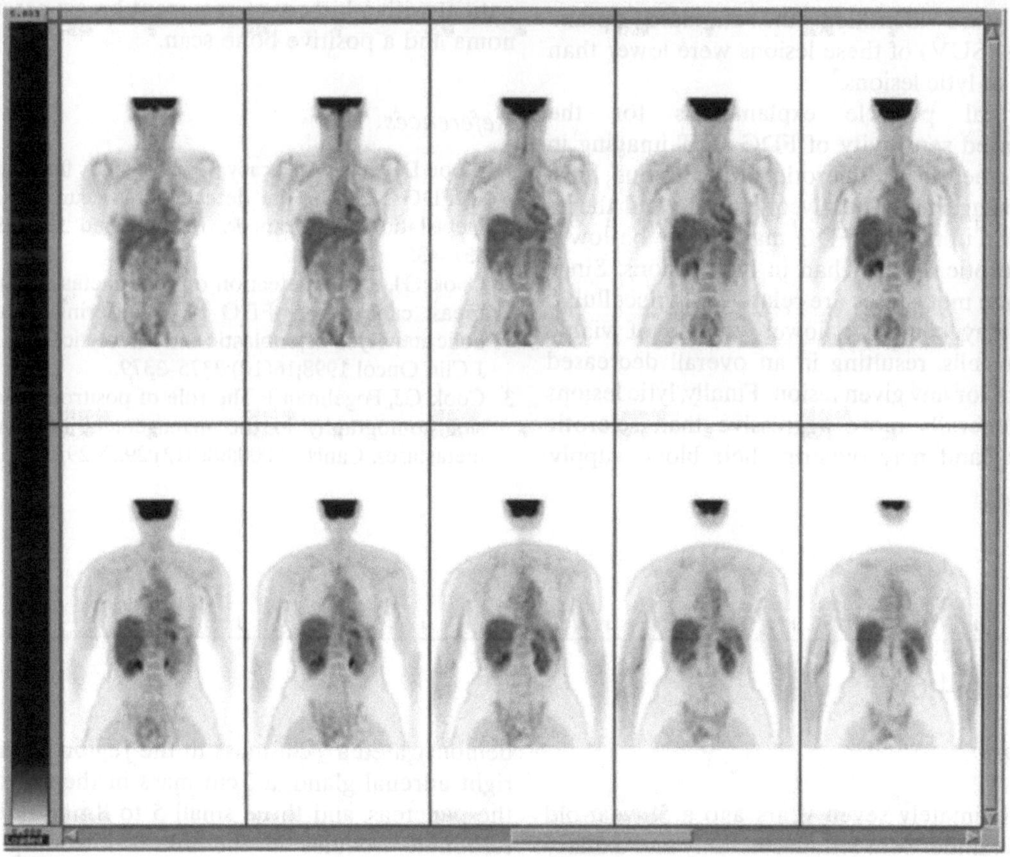

C

FIGURE 6.4.5B,C.

Specifically, there is no increased uptake corresponding to the foci of abnormal activity on bone scintigraphy. The photopenia present in the left anterior chest is due to the presence of a breast prosthesis.

Discussion

In a study that demonstrated the sensitivity and specificity of FDG PET for detecting breast cancer recurrence to be 93% and 79%, respectively, the most common cause of false-negative results was failure to detect bone metastases.[1] A more recent study comparing FDG PET imaging with ^{99m}Tc-diphosphonate images for the evaluation of progressive bone metastases in patients with breast cancer showed that FDG detected a significantly greater number of bone metastases overall than ^{99m}Tc-diphosphonate; however, FDG was less sensitive for detecting sclerotic bone lesions. When sclerotic metastases were identified, the standard uptake values (SUV) of these lesions were lower than those of lytic lesions.[2]

Several possible explanations for the decreased sensitivity of FDG PET imaging in the detection of sclerotic bone lesions have been suggested. The glycolytic rate and therefore the uptake of FDG may simply be lower in sclerotic lesions than in lytic lesions. Since sclerotic metastases are relatively hypocellular, they may contain a lower volume of viable tumor cells, resulting in an overall decreased uptake for any given lesion. Finally, lytic lesions are generally more aggressive than sclerotic lesions and may outstrip their blood supply, rendering the tumor relatively hypoxic, a condition that may actually increase FDG uptake.[3]

Summary

In summary, FDG PET has been shown to be superior to bone scintigraphy in the detection of osteolytic metastases, which do have a poorer prognosis than osteoblastic bone lesions. However, osteoblastic metastases demonstrate lower FDG uptake and are often undetectable by FDG PET imaging. For this reason, it may be necessary to perform both FDG PET imaging and bone scintigraphy in order to fully evaluate patients with sclerotic bone metastases.

Diagnosis

Probable false-negative FDG PET images in a patient with a history of recurrent breast carcinoma and a positive bone scan.

References

1. Moon DP, et al.: Accuracy of whole-body fluorine-18-FDG PET for the detection of recurrent or metastatic breast cancer. J Nucl Med 1998;39:431–435.
2. Cook GJ, et al.: Detection of bone metastases in breast cancer by 18FDG PET: Differing metabolic activity in osteoblastic and osteolytic lesions. J Clin Oncol 1998;16(10):3375–3379.
3. Cook GJ, Fogelman I: The role of positron emission tomography in the management of bone metastases. Cancer 2000;88(S12):2927–2933.

Case 6.4.6

History

Approximately seven years ago a 58-year-old female underwent left mastectomy and axillary dissection for breast cancer. A CT performed recently because of abdominal pain reportedly demonstrated a 7 cm mass in the region of the right adrenal gland, a 3 cm mass in the tail of the pancreas, and three small 5 to 8 mm indeterminate nodules in the mid-to-lower right lung field. A biopsy of the right adrenal gland was nondiagnostic. Figures 6.4.6A and B

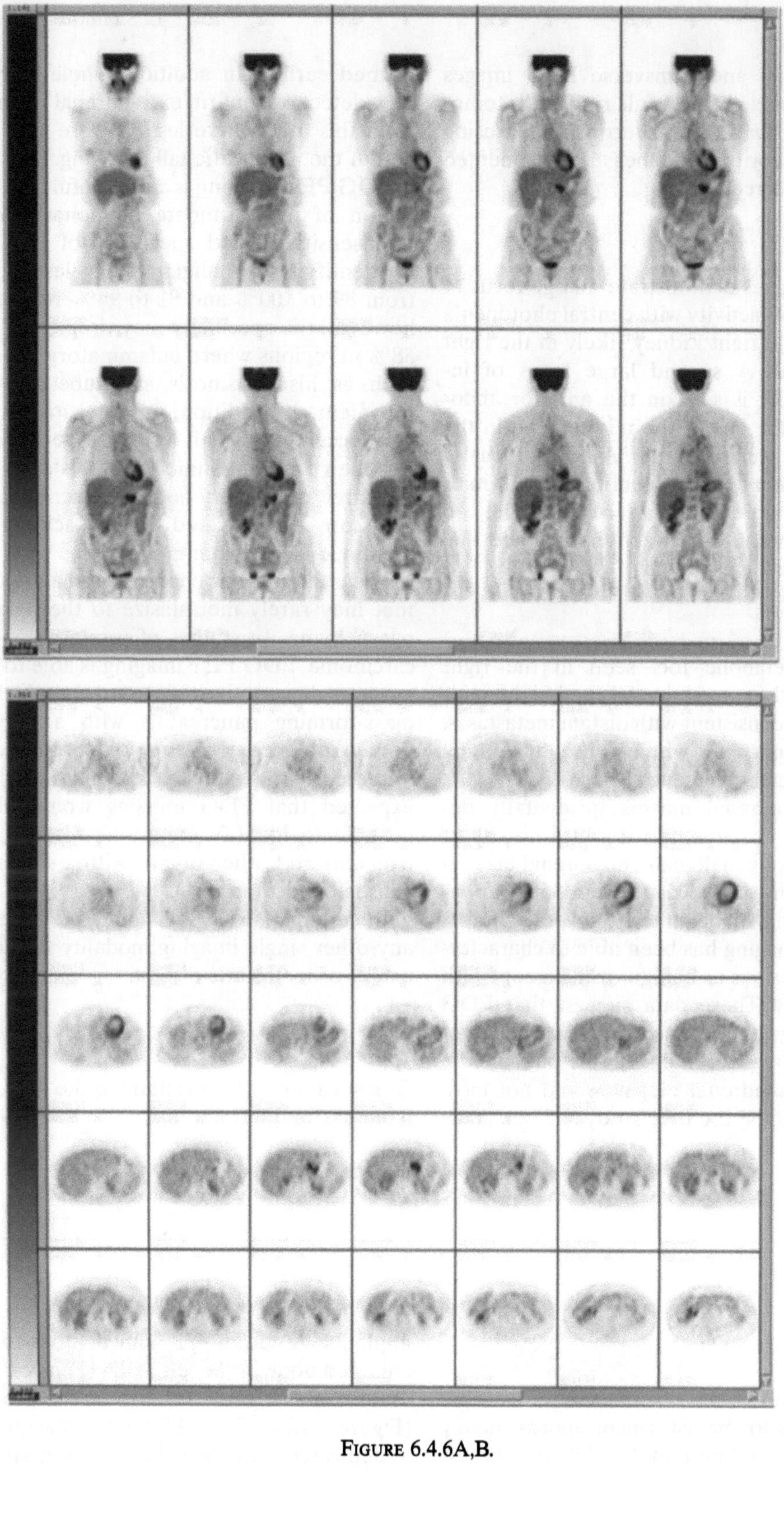

A

B

FIGURE 6.4.6A,B.

display coronal and transverse FDG images acquired on a dedicated full ring PET tomograph (GE Advance) and reconstructed using an iterative algorithm and measured segmented attenuation correction.

Findings

The FDG images demonstrate a large focus of increased FDG activity with central photopenia superior to the right kidney, likely in the right adrenal gland. A second large focus of increased activity is seen in the anterior abdomen, just to the left of the midline and in the region of the pancreatic tail. A subtle focus of increased activity is also seen in the right mid-lung field (Figure 6.4.6A, second image, top row). Asymmetric breast activity is noted due to the prior left mastectomy.

Discussion

The hypermetabolic foci seen in the right adrenal gland, pancreatic tail, and right mid-lung field are consistent with distant metastases. The photopenia seen within the right adrenal lesion is indicative of central necrosis.

Although adrenal masses incidentally detected by CT in patients without a history of cancer are rarely malignant, an adrenal mass in a patient with cancer has up to a 36% probability of being malignant. In several studies, FDG PET imaging has been able to characterize adrenal lesions as benign or malignant with high accuracy. These data suggest that FDG PET imaging may be used to avoid biopsy of adrenal lesions. Certainly in this patient, the nondiagnostic adrenal biopsy would not have been attempted if the PET study had been performed earlier. In addition, whole-body PET may detect or confirm extraadrenal metastases, as in this case where lesions were also identified in the pancreatic tail and lung.

FDG PET imaging is also helpful in the evaluation of indeterminate pulmonary nodules. The sensitivity and specificity of FDG PET in identifying a malignant lung lesion ranges from 89 to 100% and 81 to 94%, respectively; however, the specificity may drop to as low as 58% in regions where inflammatory conditions such as histoplasmosis and tuberculosis are prevalent. In addition, false-negative findings may occur with small lesions, especially those less than 5 mm in diameter. In this case, one of the three pulmonary nodules described on the CT scan demonstrated enough activity to be identified as malignant.

Breast, lung, and renal carcinoma are tumors that may rarely metastasize to the pancreatic parenchyma. In studies of primary pancreatic carcinoma, FDG PET imaging is able to distinguish malignant lesions from chronic benign mass-forming pancreatitis with a very high degree of accuracy, superior to that of CT. Although not studied systematically, it is expected that FDG imaging would likewise be able to identify metastatic disease to the pancreas and other organs with a similar high degree of accuracy.

In summary, FDG PET may be better than any other single imaging modality for defining extent of metastatic disease.

Diagnosis

Breast carcinoma metastatic to the lung, tail of pancreas, and left adrenal.

Case 6.4.7

History

A 53-year-old female underwent bilateral mastectomies for breast cancer approximately seven years ago. She now has bilateral breast implants. A recent CT scan demonstrated an enlarged node in the left axilla (Figure 6.4.7A). Transaxial (Figure 6.4.7B) and orthogonal (Figure 6.4.7C) FDG PET images acquired on a dedicated full ring PET tomograph (GE

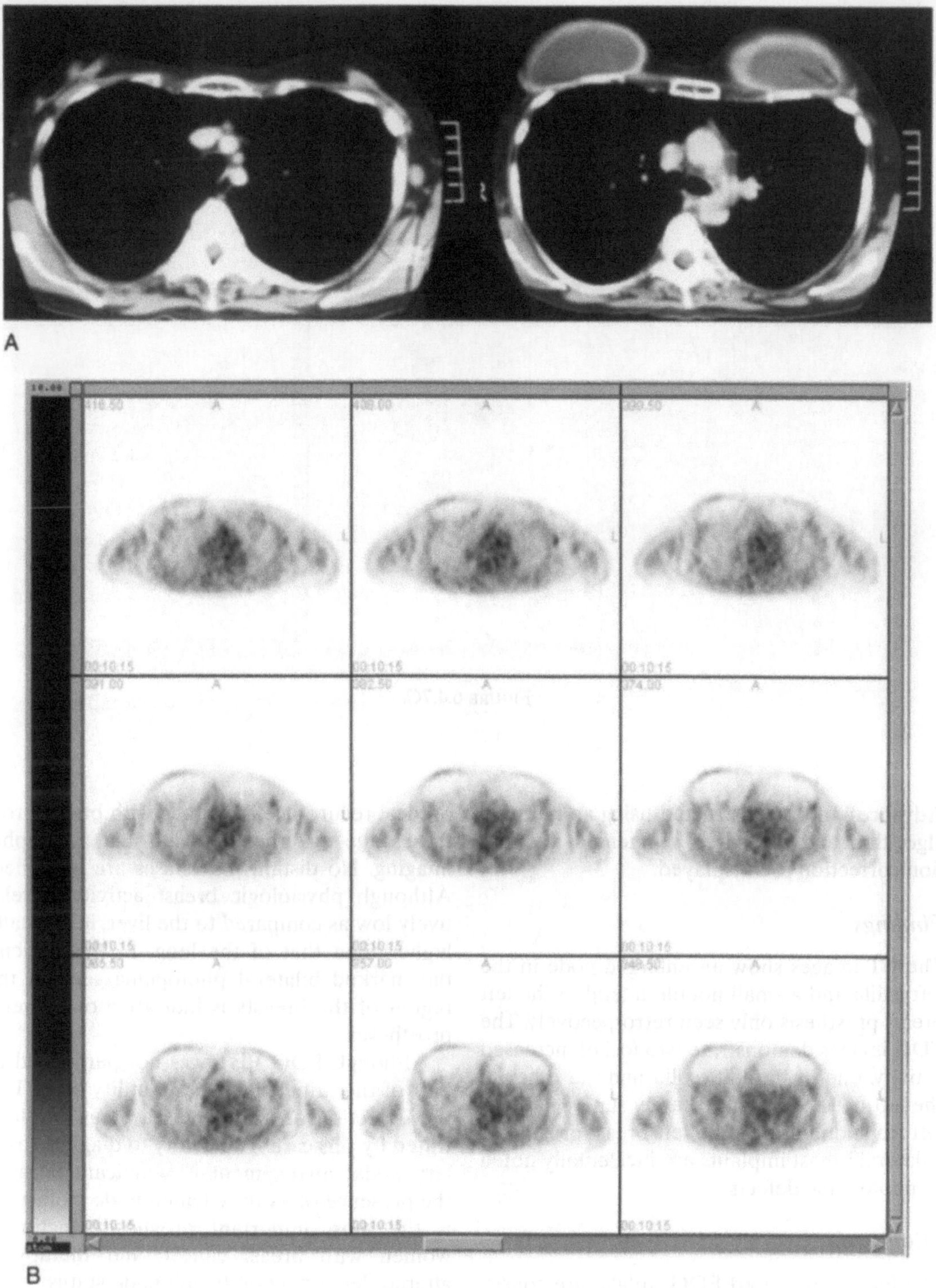

FIGURE 6.4.7A,B.

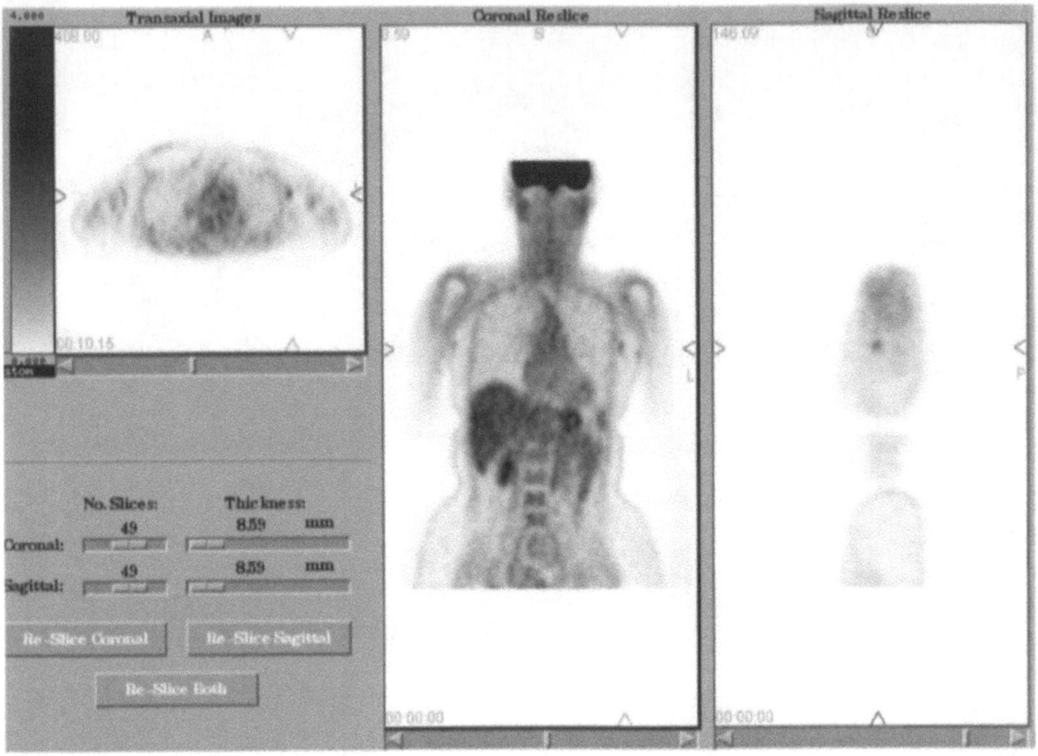

FIGURE 6.4.7C.

Advance) and reconstructed using an iterative algorithm and measured segmented attenuation correction are displayed.

Findings

The CT images show an enlarged node in the left axilla and a small nodule lateral to the left breast prosthesis only seen retrospectively. The FDG images demonstrate two foci of increased activity, one in the left axilla and the other in the left chest wall immediately superficial to a left rib and lateral to the left breast prosthesis. Bilateral breast implants are incidentally noted as photopenic defects.

Discussion

The foci of increased FDG uptake are consistent with local recurrence of breast cancer in both the left axilla and left chest wall. FDG imaging may be especially useful in detection of local recurrence in women with breast prostheses due to difficulties with mammographic imaging. No distant metastases are identified. Although physiologic breast activity is relatively low as compared to the liver, it is usually higher than that of the lung. In this patient, the marked bilateral photopenia seen in the region of the breasts is indicative of bilateral prostheses.

Although FDG PET was not performed as part of the initial staging, the utility of PET in the detection of axillary disease can be illustrated by this case. The ability to diagnose axillary nodal involvement is significant because the presence of axillary lymph node metastasis is the most important prognostic factor in women with breast cancer, and therapy is altered depending on lymph node status.

Several studies have shown the ability of PET to stage the axilla with high sensitivity and specificity. In one study of 27 patients with histologically proven axillary metastases, PET had a detection accuracy of 96% as compared with 74% for physical examination and 60% for mammography. In this same study, PET was even able to accurately predict the number of nodes involved if fewer than three axillary nodes were positive.[1] In another study of 50 patients with either histologically positive or negative axillary nodes, the overall sensitivity of PET was 90%, and the specificity was 97%. In the subset of patients with locally advanced disease, PET had a sensitivity of 93% and a specificity of 100%. The positive predictive value of PET for staging the axilla was over 90%.[2] In a third study of 124 women who underwent PET followed by axillary dissection, PET demonstrated 100% sensitivity in the detection of axillary metastases.[3]

These studies taken together suggest that PET shows promise as an accurate and reliable noninvasive method of determining axillary lymph node status in patients with breast cancer. However, PET is unable to delineate the exact number of positive nodes, which is an important prognostic indicator. In addition, PET will never detect micrometastases, resulting in understaging of approximately 5% of women with breast cancer. In a detailed study of melanoma patients, FDG PET had high sensitivity only for metastases with more than 50% lymph node involvement or capsular infiltration and nodes larger than 0.5 cm in diameter.[4] For these reasons, sentinel node mapping with axillary dissection may remain the technique of choice for the initial staging of breast carcinoma, while PET may be most useful in restaging patients with possible recurrence of disease.

Diagnoses

1. Local recurrence of breast cancer involving the left axilla and left chest wall.
2. Bilateral breast prostheses.

References

1. Noh DY, et al.: Diagnostic value of positron emission tomography for detecting breast cancer. World J S 1998;22:223–227.
2. Smith IC, et al.: Staging of the axilla in breast cancer: An accurate in vivo assessment using positron emission tomography with 2-(fluorine-18)-fluoro-1-deoxy-D-glucose. Annals of Surgery 1998;228:220–227.
3. Pisano, Parham CA: Breast imaging: Digital mammography, sestamibi breast scintigraphy and positron emission tomography breast imaging. Radiologic Clinics of North America 2000;38(4): 861–869.
4. Crippa F, Leutner M, Belli F, et al.: Which kinds of lymph node metastases can FDG PET detect? J Nucl Med 2000;41:1491–1494.

Case 6.4.8

History

A 74-year-old female with a history of breast cancer was referred for FDG PET imaging due to the detection a 5 cm hypodense mass within the left lobe of the liver by CT scan (not shown). Figure 6.4.8A shows coronal FDG images acquired with a dedicated full ring PET tomograph (GE Advance) and reconstructed using an iterative algorithm with measured segmented attenuation correction.

Findings

On the FDG PET images there is markedly increased activity within the left lobe of the liver congruent with the hypodense lesion seen on CT (not shown). There is no evidence of abdominal or axillary hypermetabolic lymphadenopathy. There is a linear focus of increased uptake at the base of the neck on the right.

Discussion

The marked uptake of FDG within the known hepatic mass is consistent with a malignant process. Although active inflammation must always be a consideration when increased FDG activity is noted, the CT does not support a diagnosis of such a process. A cavernous hemangioma and other benign lesions of the

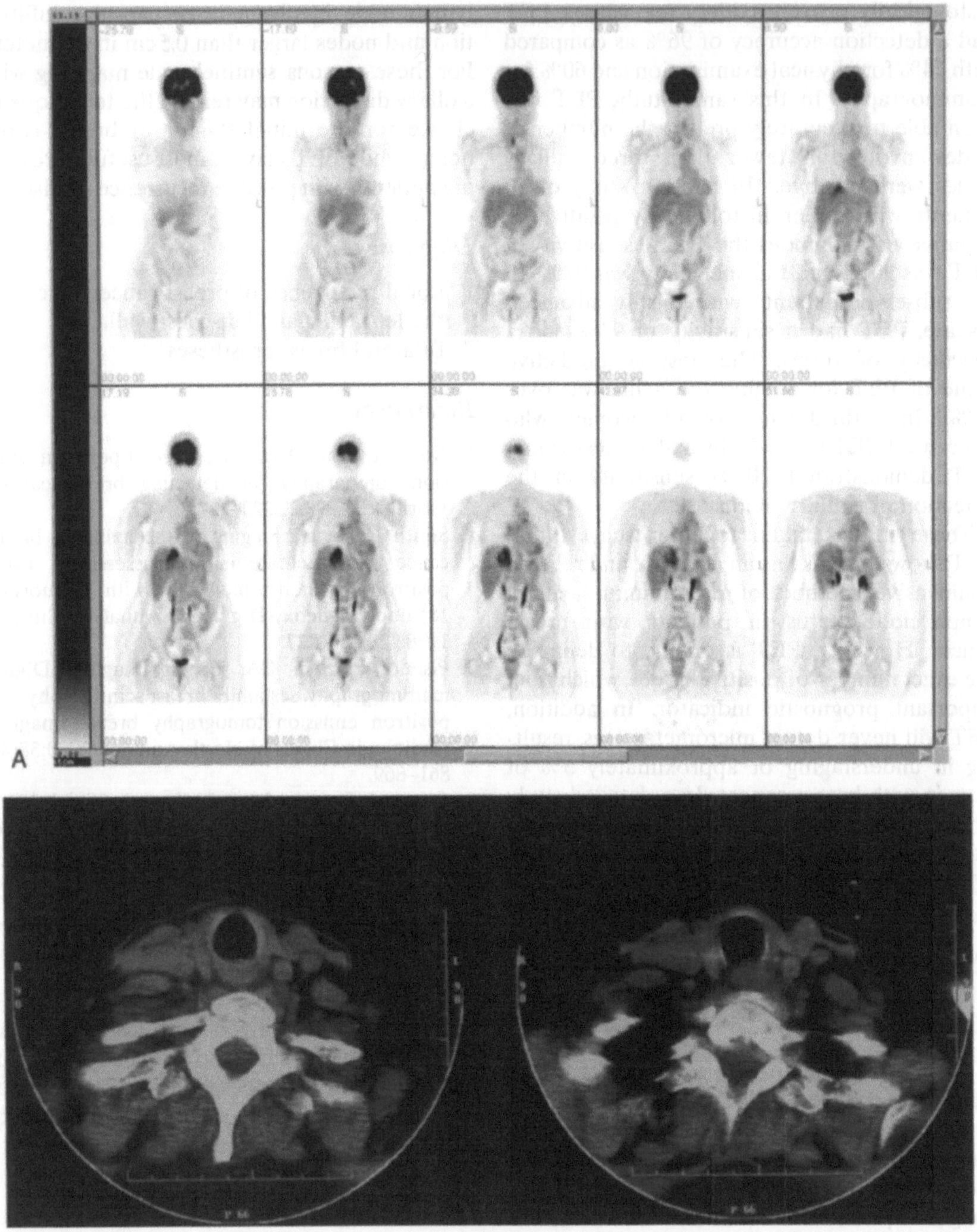

FIGURE 6.4.8A,B.

liver can be easily excluded, as these entities do not demonstrate increased FDG activity.

Any discrete focus of asymmetrically increased FDG activity in a patient with an underlying malignancy should be viewed with suspicion. In this case, the focus at the base of the right neck is worrisome for a metastasis. On questioning the patient, however, a history of a left thyroid lobectomy was obtained and confirmed by CT (Figure 6.4.8B).

FDG PET imaging has established applications for imaging anaplastic or dedifferentiated thyroid tumors that no longer accumulate ^{131}I. In addition, some benign thyroid neoplasms, especially autonomous adenomas, may accumulate FDG. Furthermore, diffuse thyroid disorders including Graves' disease, diffuse toxic goiter, chronic autoimmune thyroiditis, and adenomatous goiter may be visualized on FDG PET studies.[1] In patients with an incidental finding of diffusely increased FDG uptake within the thyroid, it has been suggested that this often represents the presence of chronic thyroiditis with or without hypothyroidism. Yasuda et al.[2] in a review of patients without known thyroid pathology, but with diffusely increased FDG activity, demonstrated chronic thyroiditis in 34 of 36 total patients. Several investigators have reported that the normal thyroid gland is not visualized on whole-body FDG images. In this patient, the additional history of prior thyroid lobectomy, most likely performed for chronic goitrous thyroiditis or adenomatous goiter, facilitated the correct interpretation of benign lobar diffuse thyroid FDG activity rather than extrahepatic metastasis.

On the anterior coronal images, asymmetrically absent soft tissue activity in the left thorax is consistent with the patient's prior left mastectomy.

Diagnoses

1. Breast cancer metastatic to the left lobe of the liver.
2. Hemithyroidectomy.

References

1. Borner AR, Voth E, Wienhard K, Wagner R, Schicha H: F-18-FDG PET in autonomous goiter. Nuclearmedizin 1999;38:1–6.
2. Yasuda S, Shohtsu A, Ide M, et al.: Chronic thyroiditis: Diffuse uptake of FDG at PET. Radiology 1998;207:775–778.

6.5
Colorectal Carcinoma

Dominique Delbeke, Tsuyoshi Komori, and William H. Martin

Colorectal carcinoma is the third most common noncutaneous malignancy in the United States, representing 13% of all malignancies. There are over 133,000 new cases detected annually with almost 55,000 annual deaths.

Preoperative Diagnosis

Only a small number of studies have been performed with FDG PET in the preoperative diagnosis of colorectal carcinoma.[1,2] False-positives include abscesses, fistulas, diverticulitis, and occasionally adenomas. Although the sensitivity of FDG PET for the detection of a primary colon carcinoma is high, it presently plays no role in the preoperative diagnosis or initial staging except on occasion to define or identify hepatic or distant extrahepatic metastases.

Detection and Staging of Recurrent Colorectal Carcinoma

Approximately 14,000 patients per year present with isolated liver metastases as their first recurrence, and 20% of these patients die with metastases exclusive to the liver. Hepatic resection may result in a cure in up to 25% of these patients, but the size and number of hepatic metastases and the presence of extrahepatic metastases all adversely affect prognosis. The presence of extrahepatic metastases is thought to represent a contraindication to hepatic resection.

Serial serum carcinoembryonic antigen (CEA) determinations are used to monitor patients for recurrences with a sensitivity of 59% and a specificity of 84%, and CT has been the conventional imaging modality used to localize recurrence. However, CT fails to demonstrate hepatic metastases in up to 7% of patients and underestimates the number of lobes involved in up to 33% of cases.[3] Extrahepatic abdominal metastases are commonly missed on CT, and the differentiation of postsurgical changes from tumor recurrence is problematic. Superior mesenteric arterial CT portography is more sensitive than CT for detection of hepatic metastases but has a high rate of false-positive findings, lowering the positive predictive value.

Numerous studies have demonstrated a strong role for FDG PET in identifying recurrences of colorectal carcinoma (see Table 6.5.1).[4–20] For detection of recurrent colon carcinoma, FDG PET has been found to be more sensitive than CT at all anatomic sites except the lung, where the two modalities are equivalent. One-third of PET-positive metastases in the extrahepatic abdomen and pelvis are CT-negative. Whole-body PET is especially useful for detecting distant metastatic disease, including abdominal nodal disease and pulmonary metastases (indeterminate lung nodules), and differentiating postsurgical scarring from recurrent disease, all of which are problematic for CT.[21] For differentiation of posttherapy scar from local recurrence, PET is clearly more accurate (90 to 100%) than CT (48 to 65%),

TABLE 6.5.1. Comparison of PET and CT for staging recurrent colorectal carcinoma.

Author	Year	No. of patients	CT Sensitivity (%)	CT Specificity (%)	CT Accuracy (%)	PET Sensitivity (%)	PET Specificity (%)	PET Accuracy (%)
Yonekura[4]	1982	3				100	100	100
Strauss[5]	1989	29				100	100	100
Ito[6]	1992	15				100	100	100
Gupta[7]	1993	16	60	100	65	90	66	87
Falk[8]	1994	16	47	100	56	87	67	83
Schiepers[9]	1995	76			65 to 93			95 to 98
Vitola[10]	1996	24	86	100	76	90	100	93
Ogunbiyi[22]	1997	58			66			95
Delbeke[11]	1997	61	79	58	76	93	89	92
Ruhlmann[13]	1997	59				100	67	
Valk[12]	1999	155	69	96		93	98	
Imbriaco[18]	2000	40	75	90		94	98	
Staib[20]	2000	100	91	72	82	98	90	95
Total		652	47 to 91	58 to 100	56 to 93	87 to 100	66 to 100	83 to 100

and CT is often equivocal.[5,6,8,9,22,23] For hepatic metastases, FDG PET has a higher accuracy (92%) than CT (78%) and CT portography (80%) despite the slightly higher sensitivity of CT portography.[10] A meta-analysis of the literature including 11 reports and encompassing 281 patients evaluated FDG PET for detection of recurrent colorectal carcinoma and determined that the overall sensitivity and specificity were 97% and 76% respectively.[24]

In two small studies of patients with unexplained CEA elevation and no abnormal findings on conventional evaluation, including CT, the sensitivity of PET for the detection of recurrent disease was 93 to 100%; PET correctly demonstrated tumors in two-thirds of patients with an unexplained carcinoembryonic antigen elevation.[12,25]

In a cumulative population of 532 patients, FDG PET imaging led to a change in management in 36% of the patients (see Table 6.5.2). At Vanderbilt University Medical Center, surgical management was altered by PET in 28% of patients, in one-third by initiating surgery and in two-thirds by avoiding hepatectomy. The meta-analysis of the literature determined that overall FDG PET changed the management in 102 out of 349 (29%) patients.[24]

TABLE 6.5.2. Clinical impact of FDG PET in patients with colorectal carcinoma.

Author	Year	No. of patients	Accuracy PET (%)	Detection of unsuspected metastases (%)	Clinical impact (%)
Beets[23]	1994	35			40 (14/35)
Schiepers[9]	1995	76	95 to 98	13 (10/76)	
Lai[21]	1996	34		32 (11/34)	29 (10/34)
Delbeke[11]	1997	61	92	28 (17/61)	28 (17/61)
Valk[12]	1999	155		36 (35/96)	34 (17/73)
Imdahl[19]	2000	71		20.8 (16/71)	20.8 (16/71)
Staib[20]	2000	100	95		61 (61/100)
Total		532		26.3 (89/338)	36.1 (135/374)

Including FDG PET in the evaluation of patients with recurrent colorectal carcinoma was shown to be cost-effective in studies using both a retrospective review of costs[12] and decision tree sensitivity analysis.[26]

False-negative lesions can be due to partial volume averaging, leading to underestimation of the uptake in small lesions (<1 cm) or in necrotic lesions with a thin viable rim, classifying these lesions as benign instead of malignant. The sensitivity of FDG PET for detection of mucinous adenocarcinoma is lower than for nonmucinous adenocarcinoma (41% to 58% versus 92%), probably because of the relative hypocellularity of these tumors.[27,28]

Some inflammatory lesions, especially granulomatous lesions, can accumulate significant FDG due to uptake by activated macrophages and can be mistaken for malignancies. FDG activity normally present in the gastrointestinal tract can sometimes be difficult to distinguish from a malignant lesion.

Based on these data, patients referred for evaluation of potentially resectable recurrent colorectal carcinoma should undergo FDG PET imaging preoperatively. If limited hepatic metastases are seen, CT portography should be performed to evaluate their resectability and the possible presence of small metastases that are below PET resolution. If extrahepatic foci of uptake are present on the PET images (with or without liver metastases), a CT of the corresponding region of the body should be performed for anatomical correlation. This approach allows more accurate selection of the patients who will benefit from surgery and, more importantly, patients who will not benefit from laparotomy and liver resection because of unsuspected or unrecognized extrahepatic recurrence.

Monitoring Therapy of Colorectal Carcinoma

Two studies have shown that FDG PET can differentiate local recurrence from scarring after radiation therapy.[5,6] However, increased FDG uptake immediately following radiation may be due to inflammatory changes and is not always associated with residual tumor. The time course of postirradiation FDG activity has not been studied systematically. However, it is generally accepted that FDG activity present six months after completion of radiation therapy most likely represents tumor recurrence. There are preliminary reports suggesting that the response to chemotherapy in patients with hepatic metastases can be predicted with PET. Responders may be discriminated from nonresponders after four to five weeks of chemotherapy with fluorouracil by measuring FDG uptake before and during therapy.[29] Regional therapy to the liver by chemoembolization can also be monitored with FDG PET imaging. FDG uptake decreases in responding lesions. The presence of residual uptake in some lesions can help in guiding further regional therapy.[30] A pilot study of 15 patients with primary rectal carcinoma in place demonstrated that FDG PET imaging adds incremental information for assessing the response to preoperative radiation and 5-fluorouracil-based chemotherapy.[31]

Summary

At present, the indications for FDG PET whole-body imaging in patients with suspected recurrent or metastatic colorectal carcinoma are as follows: (1) when there is a rising serum CEA level in the absence of a known source, (2) to increase the specificity of structural imaging when an equivocal lesion is detected, (3) as a screening method for the entire body in the preoperative staging before curative resection of recurrent disease, (4) to differentiate posttherapy changes versus persistent/recurrent viable tumor, and (5) possibly to monitor response to therapy.

References

1. Gupta NC, Falk PM, Frank AL, Thorson AM, Frick MP, Bowman B: Preoperative staging of colorectal carcinoma using positron emission tomography. Nebr Med J 1993;78(2):30–35.
2. Abdel-Nabi H, Doerr RJ, Lamonica DM, et al.: Staging of primary colorectal carcinomas with fluorine-18 fluorodeoxyglucose whole-body

PET: correlation with histopathologic and CT findings. Radiology 1998;206(3):755–760.
3. Steele G Jr, Bleday R, Mayer R, Lindblad A, Petrelli N, Weaver D: A prospective evaluation of hepatic resection for colorectal carcinoma metastases to the liver: Gastrointestinal Tumor Study Group protocol 6584. J Clin Oncol 1991; 9:1105–1112.
4. Yonekura Y, Benua RS, Brill AB, et al.: Increased accumulation of 2-deoxy-2[^{18}F]fluoro-D-glucose in liver metastases from colon carcinoma. J Nucl Med 1982;23:1133–1137.
5. Strauss LG, Clorius JH, Schlag P, et al.: Recurrence of colorectal tumors: PET evaluation. Radiology 1989;170:329–332.
6. Ito K, Kato T, Tadokoro M, et al.: Recurrent rectal cancer and scar: Differentiation with PET and MR imaging. Radiology 1992;182:549–552.
7. Gupta NC, Falk PM, Frank AL, Thorson AM, Firck MP, Bowman B: Preoperative staging of colorectal carcinoma using positron emission tomography. Nebr Med J 1993;78:30–35.
8. Falk PM, Gupta NC, Thorson AG, et al.: Positron emission tomography for preoperative staging of colorectal carcinoma. Dis Colon Rectum 1994; 37:153–156.
9. Schiepers C, Penninckx F, De Vadder N, et al.: Contribution of PET in the diagnosis of recurrent colorectal cancer: Comparison with conventional imaging. Eur J Surg Oncol 1995;21: 517–522.
10. Vitola JV, Delbeke D, Sandler MP, et al.: Positron emission tomography to stage metastatic colorectal carcinoma to the liver. Am J Surg 1996;171:21–26.
11. Delbeke D, Vitola J, Sandler MP, et al.: Staging recurrent metastatic colorectal carcinoma with PET. J Nucl Med 1997;38:1196–1201.
12. Valk PE, Abella-Columna E, Haseman MK, et al.: Whole-body PET imaging with F-18-fluorodeoxyglucose in management of recurrent colorectal cancer. Arch Surg 1999;134:503–511.
13. Ruhlmann J, Schomburg A, Bender H, et al.: Fluorodeoxyglucose whole-body positron emission tomography in colorectal cancer patients studied in routine daily practice. Dis Colon Rectum 1997;40:1195–1204.
14. Flamen P, Stroobants S, Van Cutsem E, et al.: Additional value of whole-body positron emission tomography with fluorine-18-2-fluoro-2-deoxy-D-glucose in recurrent colorectal cancer. J Clin Oncol 1999;17(3):894–901.
15. Akhurst T, Larson SM: Positron emission tomography imaging of colorectal cancer. Semin Oncol 1999;26(5):577–583.
16. Kim EE, Chung SK, Haynie TP, et al.: Differentiation of residual or recurrent tumors from post-treatment changes with F-18 FDG PET. Radiographics 1992;12:269–279.
17. Vogel SB, Drane WE, Ros PR, Kerns SR, Bland KI: Prediction of surgical resectability in patients with hepatic colorectal metastases. Ann Surg 1994;219:508–516.
18. Imbriaco M, Akhurst T, Hilton S, et al.: Whole-body FDG-PET in patients with recurrent colorectal carcinoma. A comparative study with CT. Clin Positron Imaging 2000;3(3):107–114.
19. Imdahl A, Reinhardt MJ, Nitzsche EU, et al.: Impact of 18F-FDG-positron emission tomography for decision making in colorectal cancer recurrences. Arch Surg 2000;385(2):129–134.
20. Staib L, Schirrmeister H, Reske SN, Beger HG: Is (18)F-fluorodeoxyglucose positron emission tomography in recurrent colorectal cancer a contribution to surgical decision making? Am J Surg 2000;180(1):1–5.
21. Lai DT, Fulham M, Stephen MS, et al.: The role of whole-body positron emission tomography with [18F]fluorodeoxyglucose in identifying operable colorectal cancer. Arch Surg 1996;131:703–707.
22. Ogunbiyi OA, Flanagan FL, Dehdashti F, et al.: Detection of recurrent and metastatic colorectal cancer: Comparison of positron emission tomography and computed tomography. Ann Surg Oncol 1997;4:613–620.
23. Beets G, Penninckx F, Schiepers C, et al.: Clinical value of whole-body positron emission tomography with [18F]fluorodeoxyglucose in recurrent colorectal cancer. Br J Surg 1994;81:1666–1670.
24. Huebner RH, Park KC, Shepherd JE, et al.: A meta-analysis of the literature for whole-body FDG PET detection of colorectal cancer. J Nucl Med 2000;41:1177–1189.
25. Flanagan FL, Dehdashti F, Ogunbiyi OA, Siegel BA: Utility of FDG PET for investigating unexplained plasma CEA elevation in patients with colorectal cancer. Annals of Surgery 1998;227(3): 319–323.
26. Gambhir SS, Valk P, Shepherd J, Hoh C, Allen M, Phelps ME: Cost effective analysis modeling of the role of FDG PET in the management of patients with recurrent colorectal cancer. J Nucl Med 1997;38:90P.
27. Whiteford MH, Whiteford HM, Yee LF, et al.: Usefulness of FDG-PET scan in the assessment

of suspected metastatic or recurrent adenocarcinoma of the colon and rectum. Dis Colon Rectum 2000;43(6):759–767; discussion 767–770.
28. Berger KL, Nicholson SA, Dehadashti F, Siegel BA: FDG PET evaluation of mucinous neoplasms: Correlation of FDG uptake with histopathologic features. Am J Roentgenol 2000; 174(4):1005–1008.
29. Findlay M, Young H, Cunningham D, et al.: Noninvasive monitoring of tumor metabolism using fluorodeoxyglucose and positron emission tomography in colorectal cancer liver metastases: Correlation with tumor response to fluorouracil. J Clin Oncol 1996;14:700–708.
30. Vitola JV, Delbeke D, Meranze SG, Mazer MJ, Pinson CW: Positron emission tomography with F-18-fluorodeoxyglucose to evaluate the results of hepatic chemoembolization. Cancer 1996;78: 2216–2222.
31. Guillem J, Calle J, Akhurst T, et al.: Prospective assessment of primary rectal cancer response to preoperative radiation and chemotherapy using 18-fluorodeoxyglucose positron emission tomography. Dis Colon Rectum 2000;43:18–24.

Case Presentations

Case 6.5.1

History

A 62-year-old man with a history of colectomy for colon carcinoma presented with a rising serum CEA level and an indeterminate solitary pulmonary nodule (1.5 cm) in the right lower lobe on chest CT (not shown). FDG PET images were acquired with a dedicated PET tomograph (GE Advance) and reconstructed using an iterative algorithm and measured segmented attenuation correction. Coronal images are shown in Figure 6.5.1A, and orthogonal images through the abdomen are shown in Figure 6.5.1B.

Findings

The FDG images show abnormal increased uptake corresponding to the lung nodule seen on CT. In addition, there is an abnormal focus of increased activity in the abdomen lying immediately superior and anterior to the upper pole of the right kidney; the orthogonal images help locate it to the expected location of the right adrenal gland. Retrospective review of the CT images demonstrated equivocal enlargement but normal contour of the right adrenal gland (not shown).

Discussion

These findings indicate a pulmonary metastasis and a metastasis to the right adrenal gland, whereas the CT was nondiagnostic.

Anatomical imaging with CT demonstrated an indeterminate pulmonary nodule, suspicious for a metastasis in a patient with a rising CEA level. Metabolic imaging with FDG demonstrates increased glucose metabolism most consistent with a metastasis, although an active granuloma is a less likely possibility. In addition, FDG PET was able to detect the adrenal metastasis before any significant morphological changes had occurred. Detectable hypermetabolism often precedes anatomical changes, and therefore, metabolic imaging can detect metastases before the shape and size of structures are altered.

FDG PET imaging can accurately differentiate benign from malignant pulmonary nodules in patients with and without a known primary malignant tumor. Pulmonary nodules greater than 1 cm in diameter that do not accumulate FDG can be considered benign and followed by sequential CT imaging. Pulmonary nodules accumulating FDG require biopsy because of the possibility of false-positive granulomatous processes. FDG PET imaging is also highly accurate in differentiating benign from malignant adrenal lesions and may obviate the need for percutaneous adrenal biopsy.

When whole-body PET is performed, FDG imaging detects unsuspected metastases in up to one-third of patients with suspected recurrent or metastatic colorectal carcinoma, and in most of these cases, the management of the

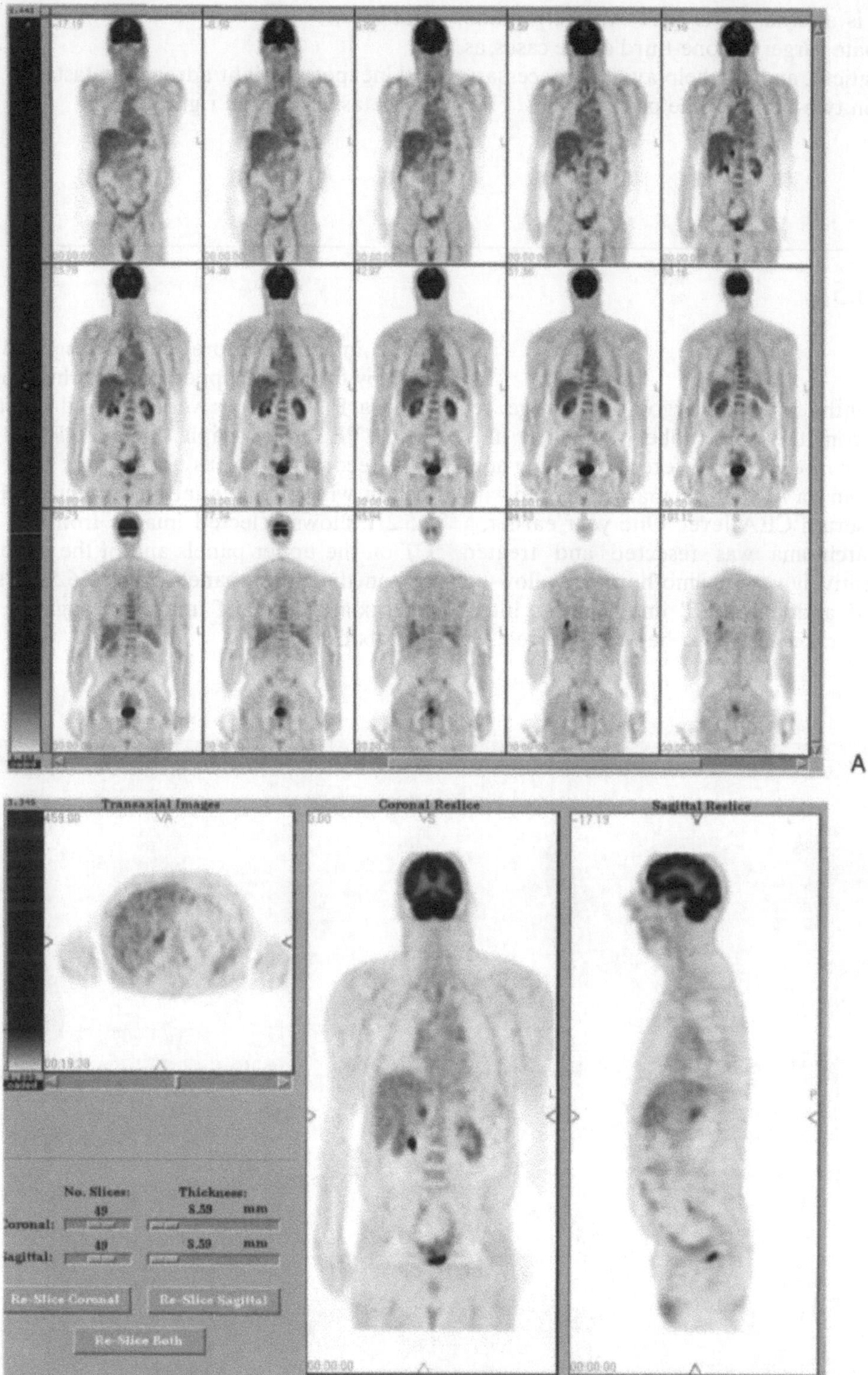

FIGURE 6.5.1A,B.

patients is altered. FDG PET will help guide appropriate surgery in one-third of the cases, as in this patient, and will help avoid unnecessary surgery in two-thirds of the patients.

Diagnoses

1. Unexpected right adrenal metastasis.
2. Metastasis to the right lung.

Case 6.5.2

History

Four months after undergoing a wedge resection from the upper lobe of the left lung revealing a moderately differentiated lung adenocarcinoma, a 70-year-old man presented with a rising serum CEA level. One year earlier, a colon carcinoma was resected and treated postoperatively with chemotherapy. Follow-up chest and abdominal CT imaging was interpreted as inconclusive, so he was referred for FDG imaging before considering radiation therapy to the left upper chest for his lung carcinoma. FDG images were acquired with a dedicated PET tomograph (Siemens ECAT 933) and reconstructed using filtered back projection without attenuation correction. Figure 6.5.2A shows selected images from the chest CT on the upper panels and of the abdominal CT on the lower panels. Figure 6.5.2B shows transaxial FDG PET images through the chest and abdomen.

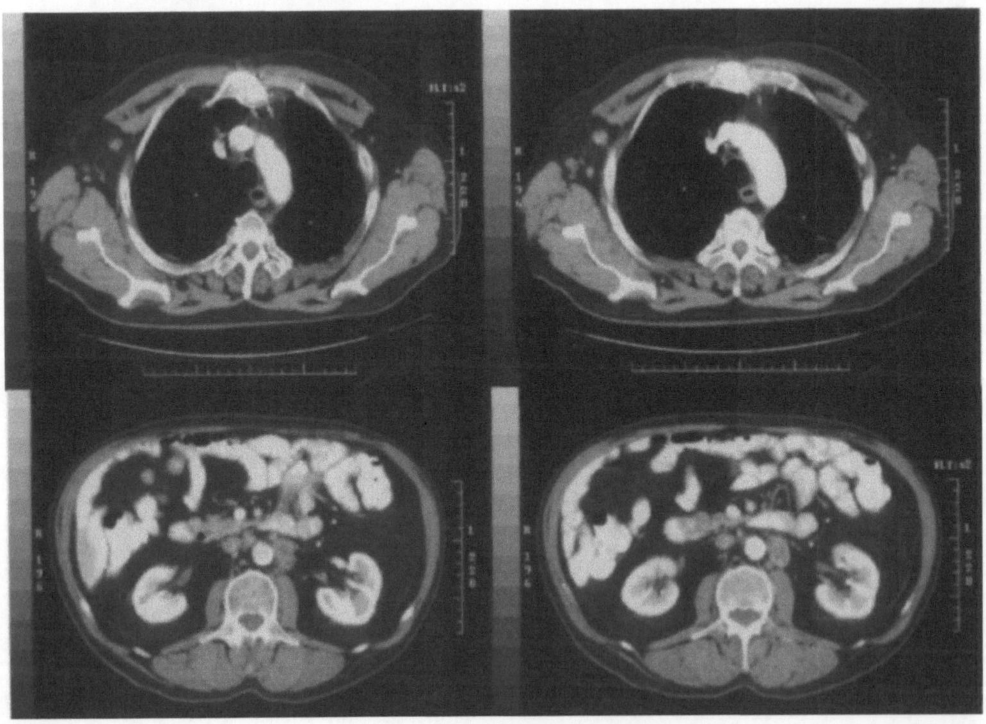

FIGURE 6.5.2A.

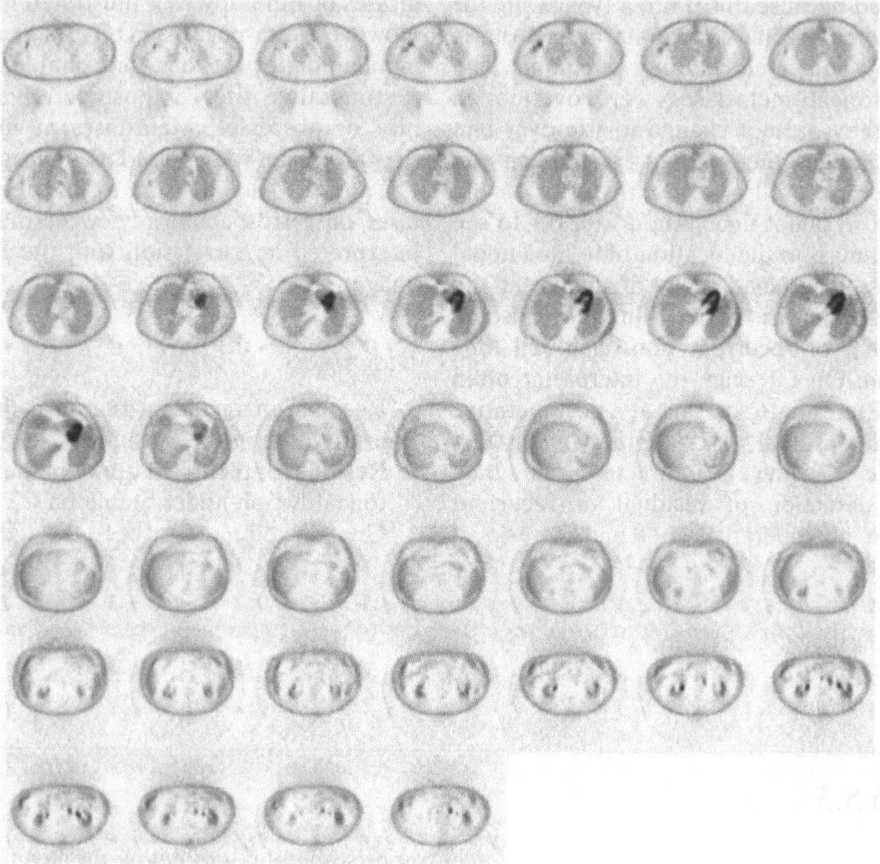

FIGURE 6.5.2B.

Findings

Initially the abdominal CT scan was interpreted as showing stable retroperitoneal lymphadenopathy; one of the enlarged retroperitoneal lymph nodes in Figure 6.5.2A has central necrosis. The FDG images demonstrate multiple foci of abnormal increased FDG activity in the right axilla. These correspond to lymph nodes seen in retrospect on the CT scan (Figure 6.5.2A, upper panels) that were overlooked when the CT was first interpreted. There are also multiple foci of increased activity in the abdomen corresponding to the stable retroperitoneal nodes seen on CT (Figure 6.5.2A, lower panels). In addition, there is a small focus of increased FDG activity in the left upper lung field corresponding to an area of scarring seen on CT (not shown).

Discussion

These findings indicate unsuspected metastases in the right axilla and residual or recurrent metastases in the stable retroperitoneal lymph nodes. The uptake in the left lung field indicates probable residual or recurrent lung carcinoma.

This case demonstrates the utility of FDG PET in (1) characterization of solitary pulmonary nodules, (2) detection of unsuspected distant (axillary) metastases, and (3) differentiation of posttherapy changes (in the lung and abdomen) versus persistent/recurrent viable tumor. Rising serum CEA levels can be seen in patients with recurrent colorectal carcinoma and in patients with recurrent bronchogenic carcinoma. Although there were abnormal findings on the CT scan, they were nondiagnostic. The right axillary lymph nodes were overlooked because this is not a typical site for metastatic colorectal carcinoma or metastasis from a left non-small cell lung carcinoma. The retroperitoneal metastases were overlooked because they did not change in size over one year, although the patient had been on chemotherapy until two months prior to the PET scan. It is not uncommon with CT to see a residual mass in the location of treated nodal metastases. The small focus of uptake at the site of resection in the left lung is worrisome for residual or recurrent non-small cell lung carcinoma. On CT scan, the interpreter often cannot differentiate scarring at a postoperative site from residual or recurrent metastasis. Metabolic imaging is more accurate than CT for detection of residual or recurrent disease at postoperative sites and in residual masses posttherapy, as is illustrated in this case. However, false-positive FDG uptake may occur in inflammatory lesions, for example, at healing postoperative sites or postoperative granulomas or abscesses. Metastases at unexpected sites are easier to see on FDG images than with CT, and it is not unusual to find these metastases on retrospective review of the CT scan interpreted in correlation with the FDG PET images.

Diagnoses

1. Residual or recurrent tumor at the postoperative site in the left lung.
2. Residual or recurrent tumor in the retroperitoneal lymph nodes, stable on CT.
3. Unexpected metastases to the right axilla.

Case 6.5.3

History

A 66-year-old female was diagnosed with carcinoma of the left colon and a large hepatic metastasis. She was referred for preoperative staging with FDG PET imaging. The FDG images were acquired with a dedicated PET tomograph (Siemens ECAT 933) and reconstructed using filtered back projection without attenuation correction. Transaxial images are shown in Figure 6.5.3A, and orthogonal images through the abdomen are shown in Figure 6.5.3B.

Findings

The FDG images reveal a large area of increased uptake with a photopenic center in the right lobe of the liver. A focus of moderate uptake is also noted in the left upper quadrant, approximately 4cm above the upper pole of the left kidney. Another focus of marked uptake is seen in the midline of the abdomen anteriorly, approximately 3cm below the level of the left kidney. This focus is seen on the orthogonal images but is difficult to localize.

Discussion

The large focus of uptake in the liver is consistent with the known hepatic metastasis, and the photopenic center indicates central necrosis. By history, the patient has the primary colon carcinoma in place, and it is located at the splenic flexure of the left colon. Therefore, the focus of uptake in the left upper quadrant at the splenic flexure likely represents the primary carcinoma rather than physiologic bowel uptake. The focus of uptake in the abdomen on the midline below the level of the left kidney was initially interpreted as a metastatic retroperitoneal lymph node. The CT scan was not available for correlation at the time of the interpretation. When the CT scan became available, visual correlation revealed that this focus of uptake corresponded to the right renal pelvis, which was

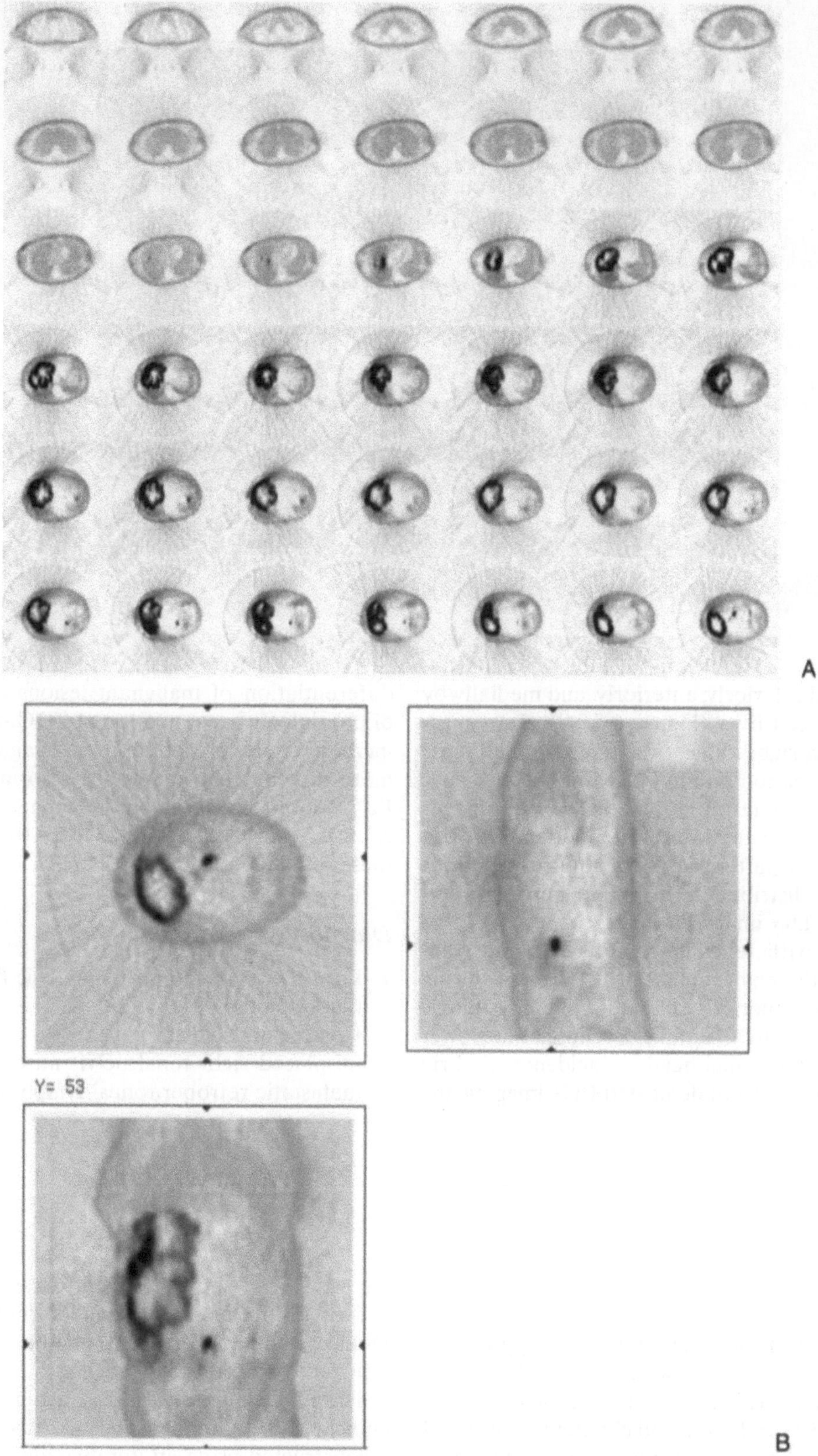

FIGURE 6.5.3A,B.

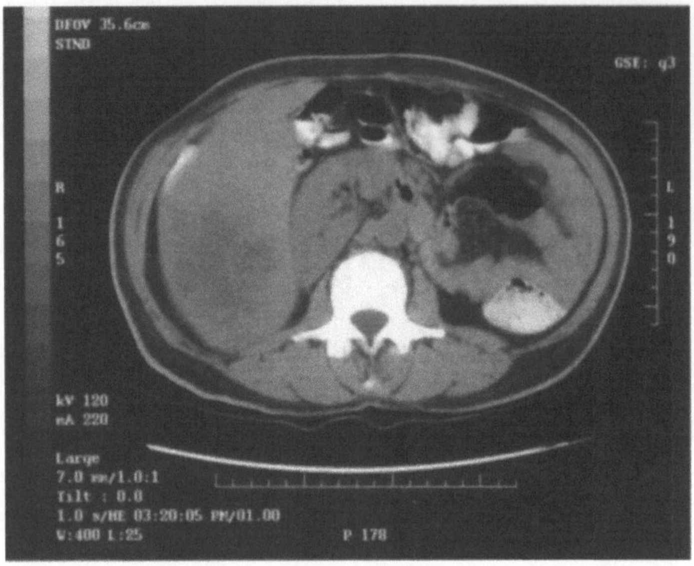

FIGURE 6.5.3C.

displaced inferiorly, anteriorly, and medially by the enlarged liver (Figure 6.5.3C). Retrospectively, the right kidney was not identified in its normal location on the FDG images.

Accurate interpretation of FDG PET images demands that the interpreter be familiar with the normal pattern and physiologic variations of FDG distribution. To avoid misinterpretation of FDG images, it is also important to be familiar with relevant clinical data and standardize the environment of the patient during the uptake period so as to limit physiologic variations in FDG uptake. Because of the lower sensitivity of dual-head coincidence (hybrid PET) compared to dedicated PET imaging, the differentiation of malignant lesions from foci of physiologic accumulation of FDG or merely increased noise present in these images may be more difficult than it would be normally with PET. Close correlation of FDG images with the clinical history and CT scans helps to minimize these difficulties.

Diagnoses

1. Primary carcinoma at the splenic flexure of the left colon.
2. Hepatic metastasis.
3. Displaced right renal pelvis mistaken for a metastatic retroperitoneal lymph node.

Case 6.5.4

History

A 62-year-old woman with a history of rectal carcinoma presented with a rising CEA level. Three years ago she had undergone colectomy followed by radiation and chemotherapy. A CT scan (not shown) performed two months before the PET scan showed a 5 cm presacral mass, a liver lesion, and a 1 cm indeterminate pulmonary nodule at the right lung base. She was referred for FDG PET imaging.

The FDG images were first acquired with a dedicated PET tomograph (GE Advance) and reconstructed using an iterative algorithm and

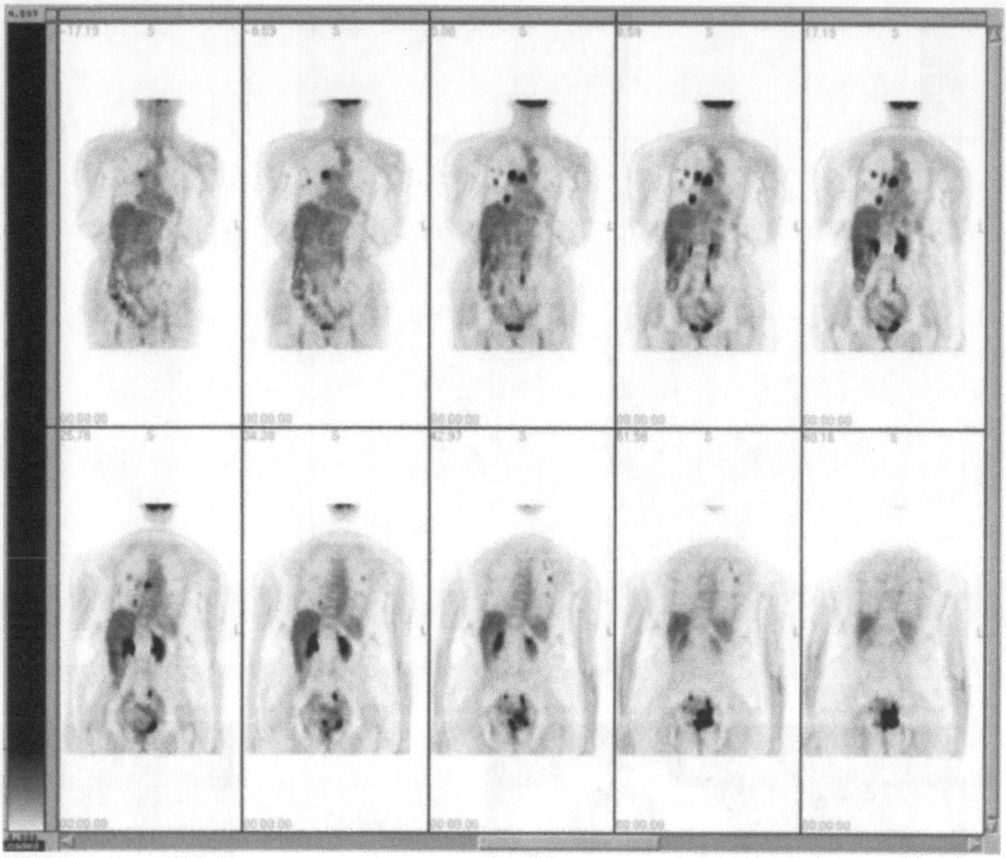

FIGURE 6.5.4A.

measured segmented attenuation correction. Coronal images are shown in Figure 6.5.4A, and orthogonal images through the chest are shown in Figure 6.5.4B. FDG images were then obtained with a hybrid dual-head gamma camera operating in the coincidence mode (Figure 6.5.4C, see color plate) (VG Millenium). The hybrid FDG PET images were reconstructed using an iterative algorithm and corrected for attenuation using attenuation maps obtained with a X-ray tube and array of detectors mounted on the gantry of the camera and functioning basically as a third-generation CT scanner. These attenuation maps also provide hybrid CT images for image fusion and anatomical mapping. Figure 6.5.4C shows a transaxial image of the study on the hybrid system corresponding to the transaxial dedicated PET image seen in Figure 6.5.4B: hybrid CT (left with soft tissue window, middle left with lung window), hybrid PET (middle right), and fusion image (right).

Findings

There is a large area of increased metabolic activity in the presacral region on the left corresponding to the presacral mass on CT, best seen on the sagittal image in Figure 6.5.4B. This may involve the sacrum as well. The FDG PET images demonstrate multiple foci of markedly increased FDG metabolism in the lungs bilaterally and in the mediastinum. The largest are seen in the right hilum and medial right lung base. There is no abnormal increased activity in the liver. The uptake in the right abdomen has a tubular pattern, best seen on the coronal

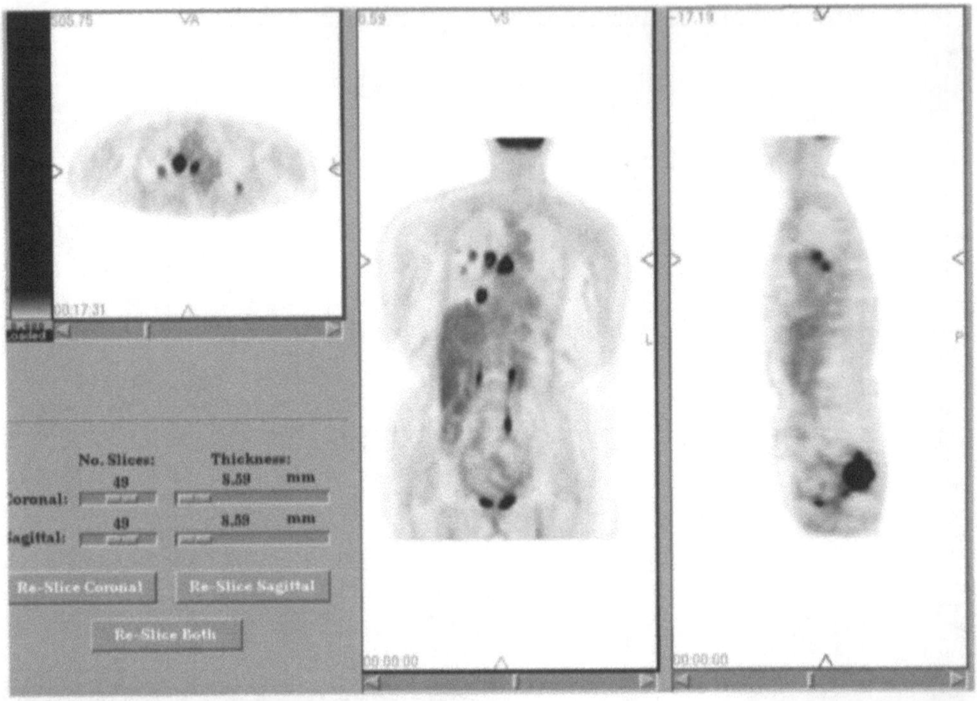

B

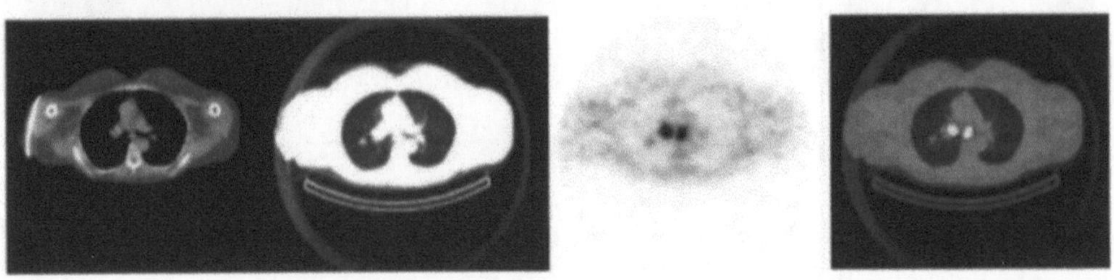

C

FIGURE 6.5.4B,C. (*Continued*) (See color plate)

images. Uptake is also noted at a superficial location in the left lower quadrant congruent with the patient's colostomy site. Retention of activity is seen along the course of both ureters.

With the hybrid system, the images were acquired over the chest and upper abdomen. The fusion images demonstrate superimposition of the abnormal foci of uptake over parenchymal lung nodules and mediastinal soft tissue densities.

Discussion

These findings are consistent with the known large presacral recurrence and unsuspected multiple lung and mediastinal metastases. The FDG PET images suggest involvement of the sacrum that was later confirmed on a repeat CT scan. The multiple pulmonary and mediastinal metastases were confirmed with a follow-up chest CT scan. The demonstration of extensive metastases by FDG PET imaging spared this patient unnecessary pelvic surgery. She was referred for chemotherapy.

The absence of abnormal FDG uptake in the region of the liver lesion seen on CT is indicative of a benign process. This lesion was biopsied during the original rectal resection, and histological examination of the specimen revealed focal nodular hyperplasia. Other similar benign hepatic processes, such as cysts and hemangiomas, do not accumulate FDG.

The tubular pattern of uptake in the right abdomen is consistent with physiologic uptake in the right colon. Uptake in the right colon and cecum is commonly seen probably due to the abundant lymphoid tissue in the wall of the cecum, although other mechanisms such as smooth muscle uptake occurring during peristalsis and even secretion into the lumen have been suggested. Usually, the tubular pattern of uptake allows identification of physiologic bowel accumulation, but when the uptake is focal, it cannot be differentiated from a malignant neoplasm. Correlation with a CT scan is sometimes helpful if a corresponding lesion can be identified. Uptake at the colostomy site is almost always seen. Uptake along the course of the ureters should not be confused with nodal metastases on transaxial images; correlation with coronal images usually clarifies the issue.

One of the advantages of whole-body PET imaging is the evaluation of the chest in addition to the abdomen, pelvis, and skeleton. As illustrated in this case, findings on FDG PET imaging allow identification of metastatic disease in the chest, abdomen, or pelvis, guiding subsequent CT examination of these regions to evaluate the exact anatomic location and potential resectability of any extrahepatic lesions. Outside the liver, FDG PET is especially helpful in detecting nodal involvement, differentiating local recurrence from postsurgical changes, and evaluating the malignancy of indeterminate pulmonary nodules, indications for which CT has known limitations. In the study of 61 patients performed at Vanderbilt University, PET changed the surgical management of 28% of patients, either by identifying a resectable metastasis or demonstrating unresectable extrahepatic disease that was unsuspected clinically and negative or equivocal on CT. PET changed the management by initiating surgery in one-third of the patients and avoiding surgery in two-thirds of the patients.[1]

Diagnoses

1. Local recurrence of colorectal carcinoma in the presacral region involving the sacrum.
2. Multiple metastases to the lungs and mediastinum.
3. Focal nodular hyperplasia.

References

1. Gupta NC, Falk PM, Frank AL, Thorson AM, Frick MP, Bowman B: Preoperative staging of colorectal carcinoma using positron emission tomography. Nebr Med J 1993;78(2):30–35.

Case 6.5.5

History

A 52-year-old woman with a history of sigmoid colectomy two years ago followed by chemotherapy and radiation therapy presented with palpable inguinal lymphadenopathy. A recent colonoscopy revealed local recurrence at the anastomotic site. Her CEA levels have always been normal. An outside CT scan performed one month before was reported as normal. She was referred for FDG imaging. Figures 6.5.5A and B show coronal and orthogonal FDG images through the pelvis acquired with a dedicated PET tomograph (GE Advance) and reconstructed with iterative reconstruction and measured segmented attenuation correction.

Findings

There is markedly increased FDG uptake posteriorly in the pelvis, just superior and posterior to the bladder in the midline. In addition, there are two foci of markedly increased uptake in the groin on the right, as well as a focus of increased FDG uptake in the groin on the left. No other foci of abnormal activity are identified. Physiologic uptake is seen in myocardium and at the colostomy site in the left upper quadrant.

Discussion

These findings are consistent with the known local recurrence of colorectal carcinoma and

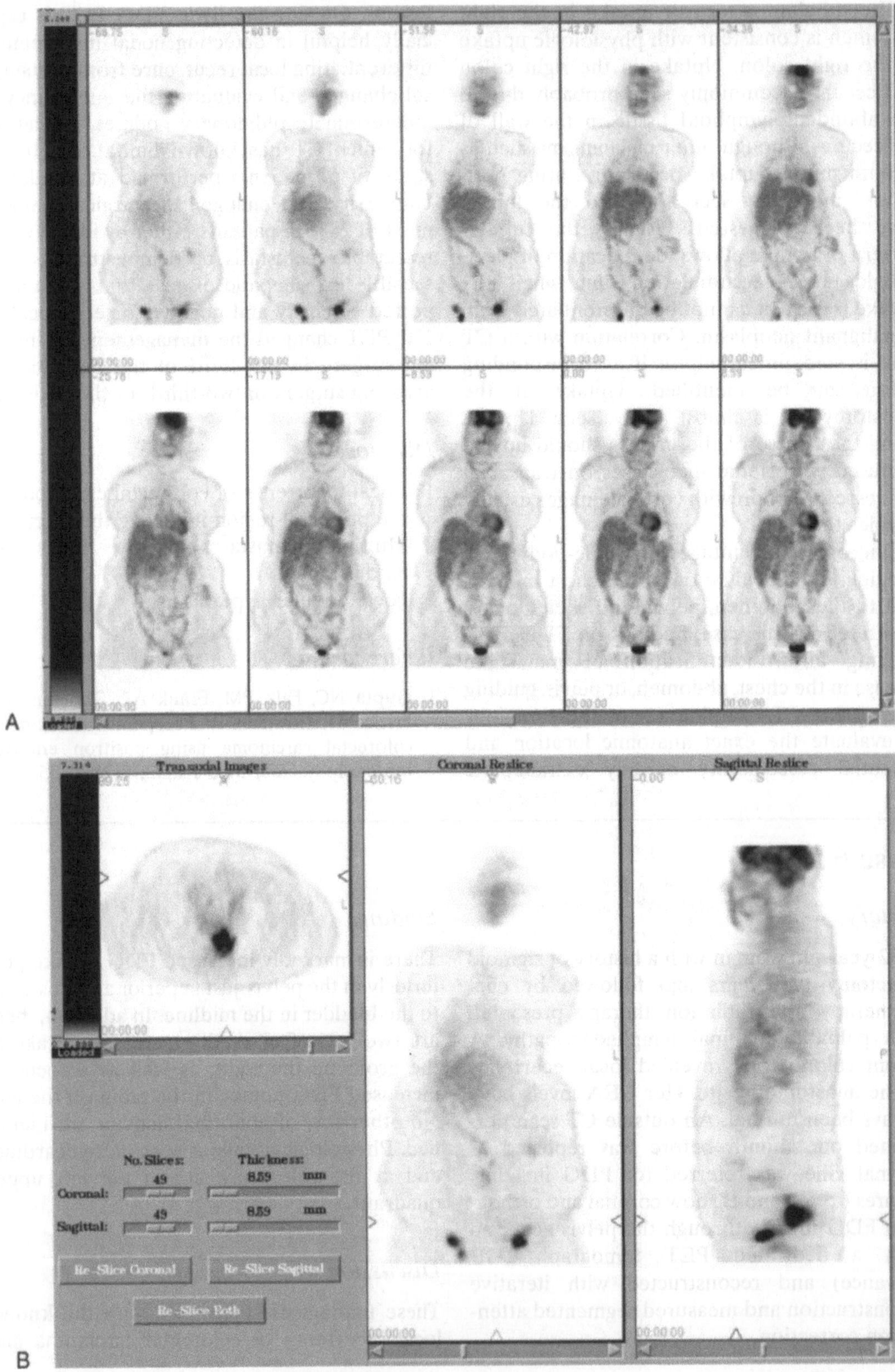

FIGURE 6.5.5A,B.

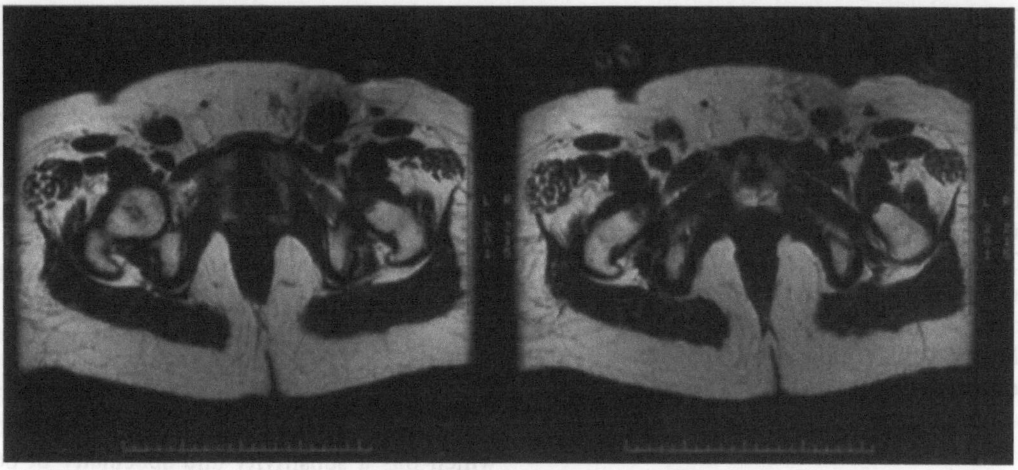

FIGURE 6.5.5C.

unsuspected metastases in multiple inguinal lymph nodes bilaterally. Enlarged inguinal lymph nodes were seen on an MRI performed to evaluate resectability of the pelvic tumor (Figure 6.5.5C, T2-weighted images). A fine-needle biopsy of these lymph nodes confirmed involvement by metastatic colon carcinoma. Pelvic wall involvement demonstrated by MRI in addition to the metastatic inguinal lymph nodes precluded surgical cure, so she was referred for chemotherapy.

For detection of recurrent colon carcinoma, FDG PET has been found to be more sensitive than CT at all anatomic sites except the lung, where the two modalities are equivalent. One-third of PET-positive metastases in the extrahepatic abdomen and pelvis are CT-negative. Although in this case the local recurrence was known, it was not identified on CT. Several studies have compared FDG PET imaging and CT to differentiate scar from local recurrence[1–6] and demonstrated that FDG PET is clearly more accurate (range 90 to 100%) than CT (range 48 to 65%), and CT is often interpreted as equivocal in these cases.

This case also illustrates the ability of FDG PET findings to efficiently guide the performance of other procedures, leading to a change in therapy. This patient was spared the morbidity of an unnecessary pelvic exenteration.

Diagnoses

1. Local recurrence at the anastomotic site.
2. Metastases to bilateral inguinal lymph nodes.

References

1. Strauss LG, Clorius JH, Schlag P, et al.: Recurrence of colorectal tumors: PET evaluation. Radiology 1989;170:329–332.
2. Ito K, Kato T, Tadokoro M, et al.: Recurrent rectal cancer and scar: Differentiation with PET and MR imaging. Radiology 1992;182:549–552.
3. Falk PM, Gupta NC, Thorson AG, et al.: Positron emission tomography for preoperative staging of colorectal carcinoma. Dis Colon Rectum 1994; 37:153–156.
4. Schiepers C, Penninckx F, De Vadder N, et al.: Contribution of PET in the diagnosis of recurrent colorectal cancer: Comparison with conventional imaging. Eur J Surg Oncol 1995;21:517–522.
5. Ogunbiyi OA, Flanagan FL, Dehdashti F, et al.: Detection of recurrent and metastatic colorectal cancer: Comparison of positron emission tomography and computed tomography. Annals of Surgical Oncology 1997;4:613–620.
6. Beets G, Penninckx F, Schiepers C, et al.: Clinical value of whole-body positron emission tomography with [18F]fluorodeoxyglucose in recurrent colorectal cancer. Br J Surg 1994;81:1666–1670.

Case 6.5.6

History

A 48-year-old female diagnosed with colon cancer three years earlier presented with a rising serum CEA level. She was referred for a CT scan (Figure 6.5.6A) and FDG PET imaging. Figures 6.5.6B and C show coronal and transverse FDG PET images acquired with a dedicated PET tomograph (GE Advance) and reconstructed with iterative reconstruction and measured segmented attenuation correction.

Findings

The CT images show several peripheral lesions in the liver. The FDG images demonstrate physiologic distribution of FDG in the gastrointestinal and genitourinary tracts. No areas of focal abnormal uptake are seen corresponding to the abnormalities seen on the CT scan.

Discussion

The abnormalities seen on the CT scan are greater than a centimeter and well within the resolution of FDG PET, though not seen on FDG PET imaging. This is most likely related to the histologic diagnosis of the primary tumor of this patient as mucinous adenocarcinoma. She underwent a segmental resection of the transverse colon, right salpingo-oophorectomy, and wedge biopsy of the liver revealing metastatic mucinous adenocarcinoma.

A meta-analysis of 11 clinical reports determined that the sensitivity and specificity for FDG PET detecting recurrent colorectal cancer are 97% (95% confidence level, 95 to 99%) and 76% (95% confidence level, 64 to 88%), respectively. These values are superior to CT, which has a sensitivity and specificity of 86% and 58% for detecting extrahepatic recurrence.[1] However, false-negative FDG PET findings have been reported with mucinous adenocarcinoma. Whiteford et al.[2] reported that the sensitivity of FDG PET imaging for detection of mucinous adenocarcinoma ($n = 16$) is significantly lower than nonmucinous adenocarcinoma ($n = 93$), 58% and 92% respectively ($p = 0.005$). They reported that FDG PET detected 60% (15 of 25) of patients with mucinous carcinoma (11 colorectal, 8 gastroesophageal, 2 pancreatic, 3 lung, and 1 breast). They suspect that the low sensitivity of FDG PET for detection of mucinous adenocarcinoma is due to the relative hypocellularity of

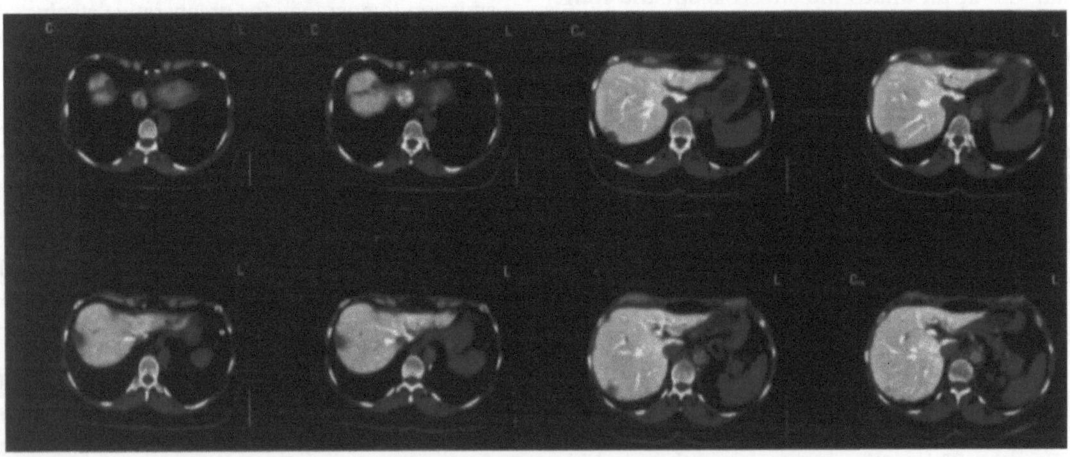

FIGURE 6.5.6A.

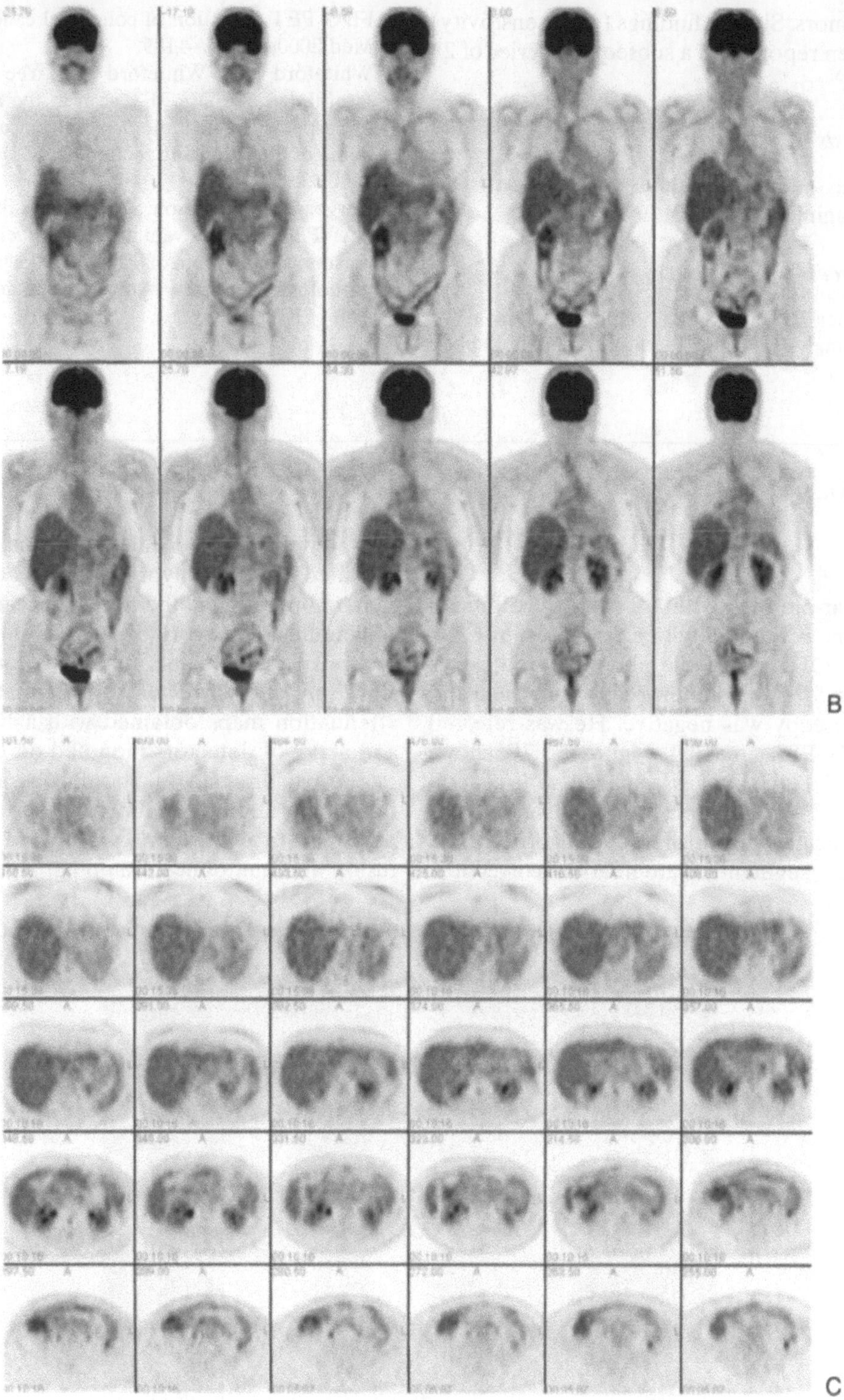

FIGURE 6.5.6B,C.

these tumors. Similar findings (41% sensitivity) have been reported in a subsequent series of 22 patients.[3]

Diagnosis

Mucinous adenocarcinoma, not seen on FDG PET imaging.

References

1. Huebner RH, Park KC, Shepherd JE, et al.: A meta-analysis of the literature for whole-body FDG PET detection of colorectal cancer. J Nucl Med 2000;41:1177–1189.
2. Whiteford MH, Whiteford HM, Yee-LF, et al.: Usefulness of FDG-PET scan in the assessment of suspected metastatic or recurrent adenocarcinoma of the colon and rectum. Dis Colon Rectum 2000;43:759–770.
3. Berger KL, Nicholson SA, Dehadashti F, Siegel BA: FDG PET evaluation of mucinous neoplasms: Correlation of FDG uptake with histopathologic features. Am J Roentgenol 2000; 174(4):1005–1008.

Case 6.5.7

History

A 44-year-old man with a history of colorectal carcinoma presented with a rising serum CEA level. A CT scan of the abdomen and pelvis (Figure 6.5.7A) was interpreted as normal, and a colonoscopy was negative. He was referred for FDG PET imaging. Figure 6.5.7B shows transaxial FDG images acquired with a dedicated PET tomograph (GE Advance) and reconstructed with an iterative algorithm and measured segmented attenuation correction. Two days later, repeat FDG images were obtained with a hybrid dual-head gamma camera operating in the coincidence mode (VG Millenium). The hybrid FDG PET images were reconstructed using an iterative reconstruction algorithm and corrected for attenuation using attenuation maps obtained with a X-ray tube and array of detectors mounted on the gantry of the camera and functioning basically as a third-generation CT scanner. These attenuation maps also provide hybrid CT images for image fusion and anatomical mapping. Figure 6.5.7C

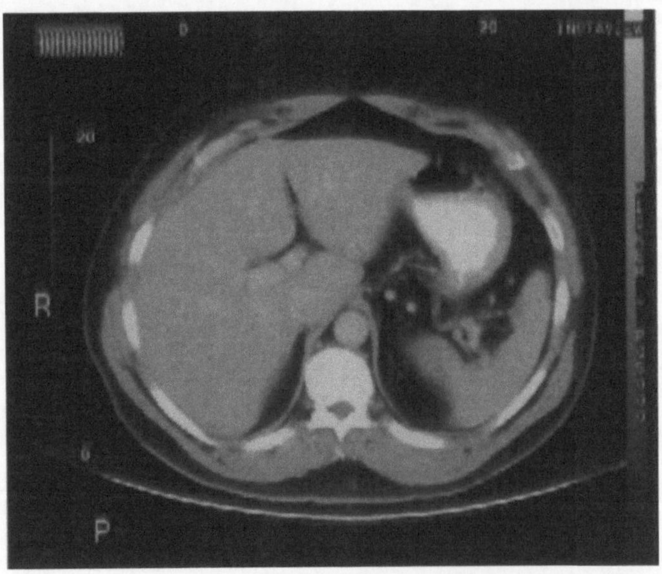

FIGURE 6.5.7A.

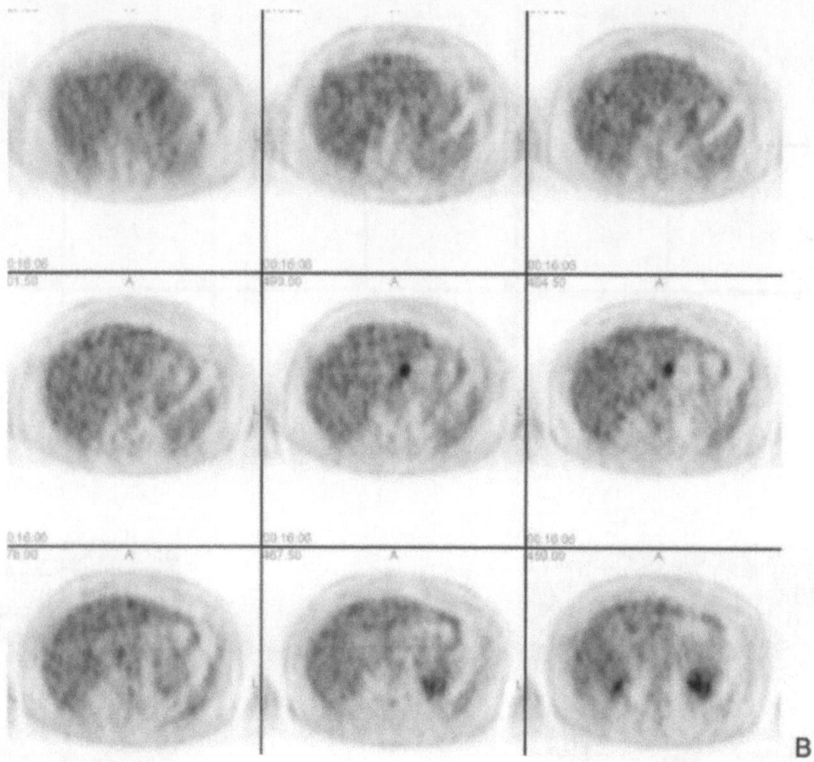

FIGURE 6.5.7B.

shows a series of transaxial hybrid PET images, and Figure 6.5.7D, see color plate, shows a selected transaxial image of the hybrid CT (left), hybrid PET (middle), and fusion image (right).

Findings

The FDG PET images demonstrate one focus of marked uptake that seems to be located in the left lobe of the liver, posteriorly on the midline near the edge. Although on the coronal images this seems to be located along a loop of bowel, this is still highly suspicious for metastasis in the left lobe of the liver or a hilar lymph node. No definite corresponding abnormality is seen on the CT scan, so the possibility that this focus represents physiological uptake in the bowel cannot be excluded. No other foci of abnormal uptake are seen.

Two days later after another administration of FDG, images were acquired using the dual-head gamma camera equipped with an integrated X-ray tube on the gantry. Figure 6.5.7C demonstrates a small focus of uptake (images #20 and #21 on the second row) in the same location as the dedicated PET images, although more difficult to identify because the images are noisier. Mild myocardial uptake can be seen on the top row images as a landmark. Figure 6.5.7D shows enlargement of image #20 (from Figure 6.5.7C); the fusion image on the right demonstrates that this uptake is most certainly located in the left lobe of the liver rather than within adjacent bowel.

Discussion

These findings are consistent with a metastasis in the left lobe of the liver. A subsequent abdominal MRI (Figure 6.5.7E, T2-weighted image) confirmed the hepatic metastasis, and the patient underwent a successful left hepatectomy. Even in retrospect, the metastasis was isointense on precontrasted and postcontrasted CT images.

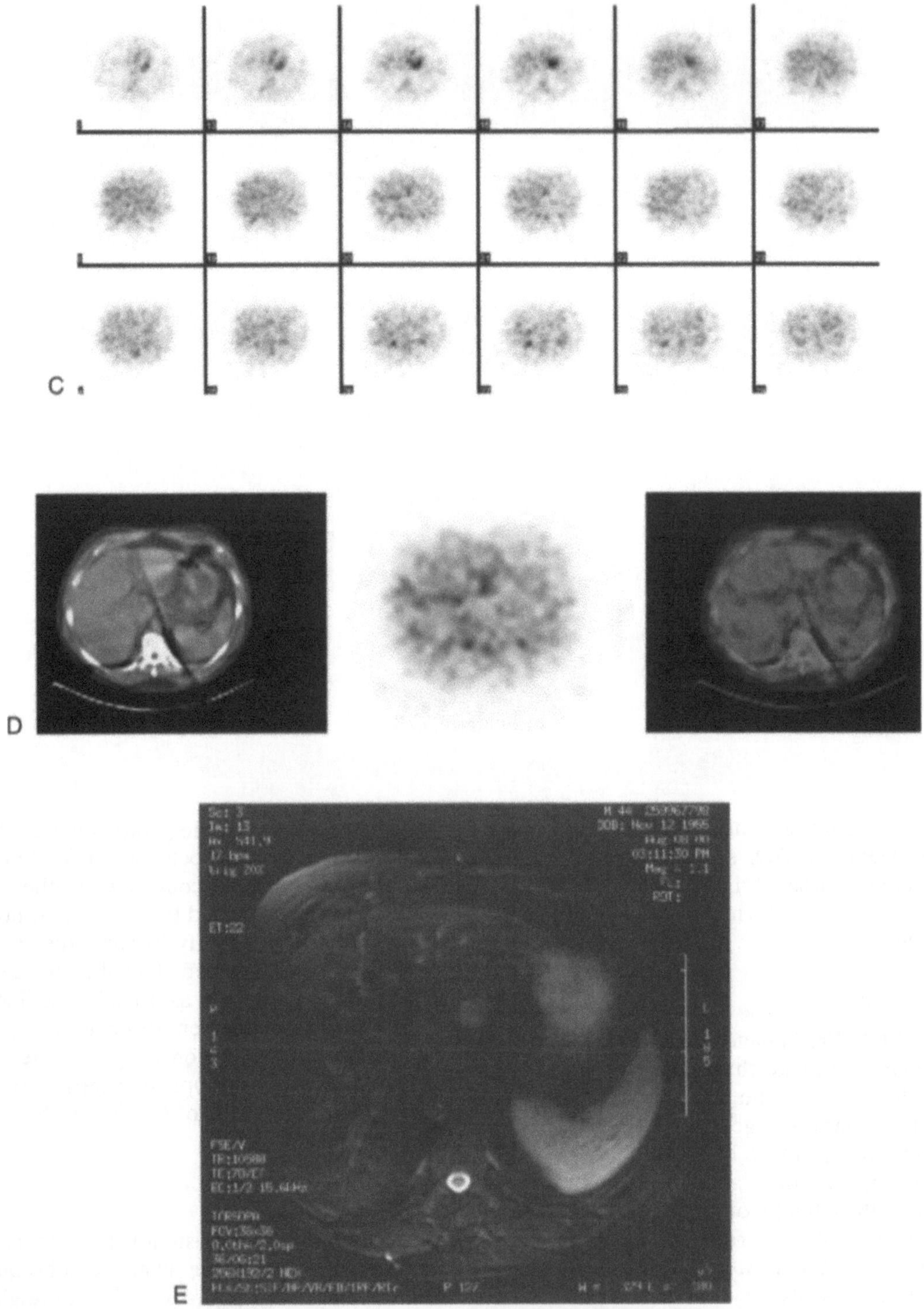

FIGURE 6.5.7C–E. (See color plate)

This case illustrates the power of PET for detection of metastases occult on CT. Flanagan et al.[1] reported the use of FDG PET in 22 patients with unexplained elevation of serum CEA level after resection of colorectal carcinoma and no abnormal findings on conventional work-up, including CT. Sensitivity and specificity of PET for tumor recurrence were 100% and 71% respectively. Valk et al.[2] reported sensitivity of 93% and specificity of 92% in a similar group of 18 patients. In both studies, PET correctly demonstrated tumors in two-thirds of patients with rising CEA levels and negative CT scans. Therefore, one of the first oncologic indications of FDG PET imaging approved by the Health Care Financing Administration (HCFA) for reimbursement was unexplained rising CEA level in patients with a history of colorectal carcinoma.

The localization of the focus of FDG uptake was equivocal on the dedicated FDG PET images, even when images with attenuation correction were reviewed and correlated with CT images. The images from the hybrid system were critical in localizing the focus of uptake in the liver. This system provides hybrid PET images limited by a lesion detectability of 15 mm or greater, but this lesion was greater than 15 mm and seen on the hybrid PET images, although faintly. The X-ray tube and array of detectors mounted on the dual-head camera gantry allow acquisition of attenuation maps for attenuation correction and hybrid CT images for lesion localization. The fusion hybrid PET on hybrid CT image was helpful for localization of the lesion in this patient. The major advantage of fusion of metabolic and anatomic images is improved localization of PET-detected abnormal foci.

Diagnosis

Hepatic metastasis, isodense on CT.

References

1. Flanagan FL, Dehdashti F, Ogunbiyi OA, Siegel BA: Utility of FDG PET for investigating unexplained plasma CEA elevation in patients with colorectal cancer. Annals of Surgery 1998;227(3): 319–323.
2. Valk PE, Abella-Columna E, Haseman MK, et al.: Whole-body PET imaging with F-18-fluorodeoxyglucose in management of recurrent colorectal cancer. Arch Surg 1999;134:503–511.

Case 6.5.8

History

A 43-year-old-female recently diagnosed with colon cancer presented for staging after two months of neoadjuvant chemotherapy and radiation therapy. CT (Figure 6.5.8A) and FDG PET imaging were performed. Figures 6.5.8B and C show coronal and transaxial FDG PET images acquired with a dedicated PET tomograph (GE Advance) and reconstructed with iterative reconstruction and measured segmented attenuation correction.

Findings

The CT shows multiple lesions in the liver, three in the right lobe and one in the left lobe. In the right lobe, one is located in the anterior segment and one is located in the posterior segment, both measuring 2 cm, and a third is located more inferiorly, measuring 1 cm. There was also thickening at the rectosigmoid junction (not shown).

The FDG PET images demonstrate two foci of markedly increased activity within the right lobe of the liver, corresponding to the lesion in the posterior segment and the one more inferiorly. The two other lesions do not accumulate FDG. There is an additional focus of increased activity within the right iliac wing near the sacroiliac joint. There is moderate uptake along the sigmoid colon and rectum, seen on the coronal images.

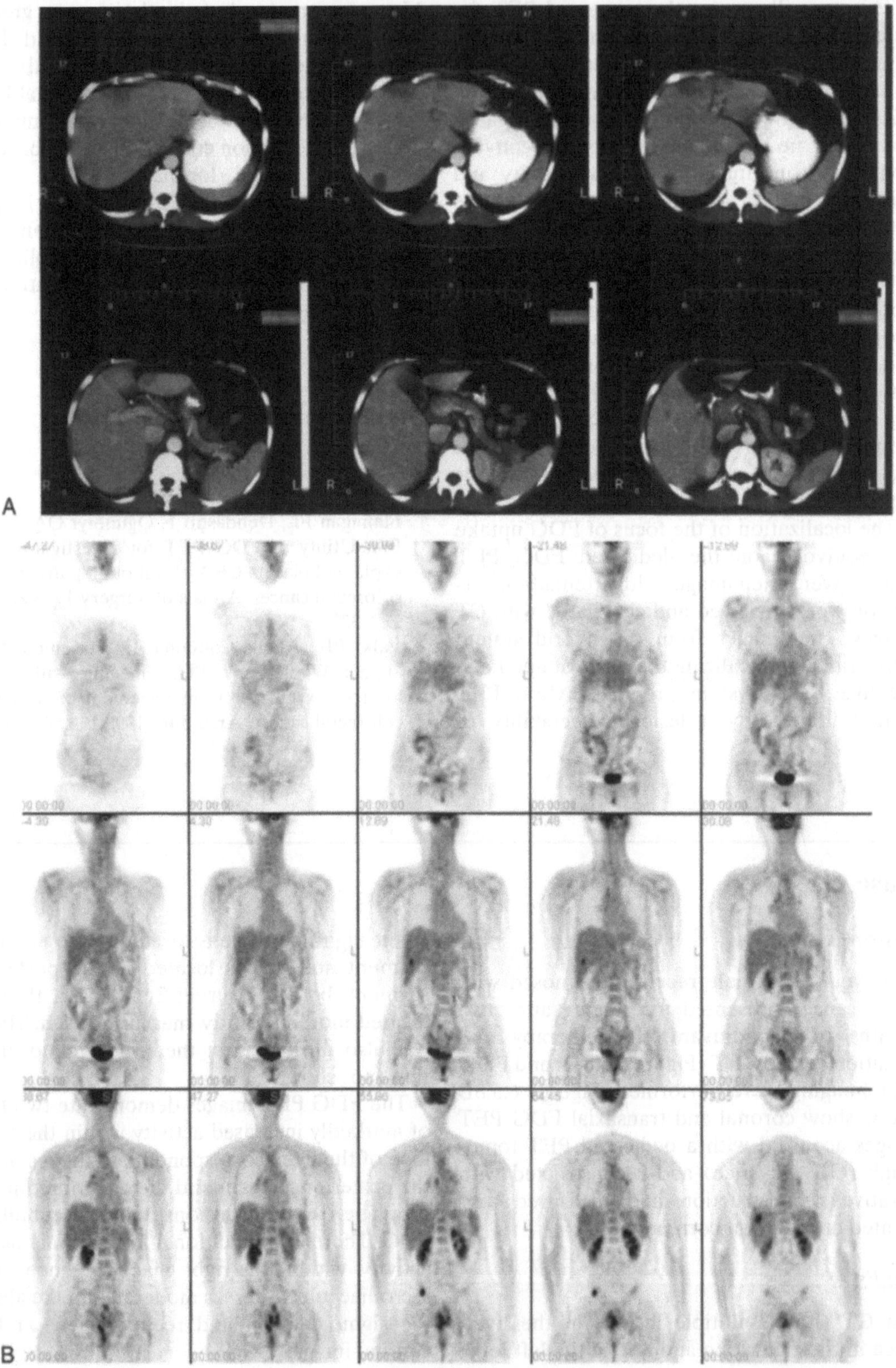

FIGURE 6.5.8A,B.

Discussion

These findings are consistent with two hepatic metastases seen on CT. The two hepatic lesions that do not accumulate FDG are probably benign. This is supported by the findings on an abdominal MRI demonstrating the two lesions accumulating FDG, but not the two other lesions (Figure 6.5.8D, T1-weighted image). In addition, FDG PET imaging detected an unsuspected skeletal metastasis adjacent to the right sacroiliac joint that could be identified retrospectively on the pelvic CT scan (Figure 6.5.8E, upper panel, middle image). The uptake in the sigmoid colon and rectum is nonspecific and may represent physiologic bowel uptake, uptake related to recent radiation therapy, or residual tumor.

Several studies have compared the accuracy of PET and CT for detection of liver metastases. Overall, PET was more accurate than CT.[1–5] However, most of these studies suffered from a major limitation: PET was performed prospectively while CT was reviewed retrospectively and performed at various institutions, resulting in variable quality. Vitola et al.[2] and Delbeke et al.[3] reported comparison of FDG with CT and CT portography for detecting both hepatic and extrahepatic metastases. CT portography, which is more invasive and more costly than PET or CT alone, is regarded as the most effective means of determining resectability of hepatic metastasis. PET had a higher accuracy (92%) than CT (78%) and CT portography (80%) in detecting liver metastases, and although the sensitivity of FDG PET

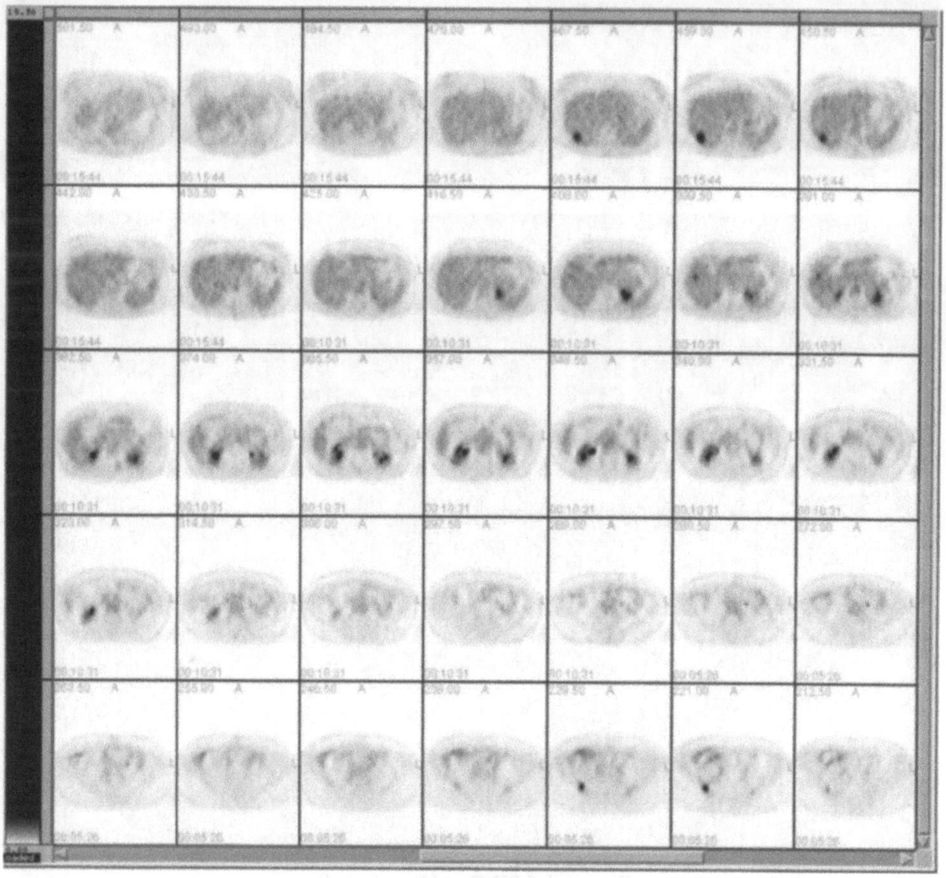

FIGURE 6.5.8C.

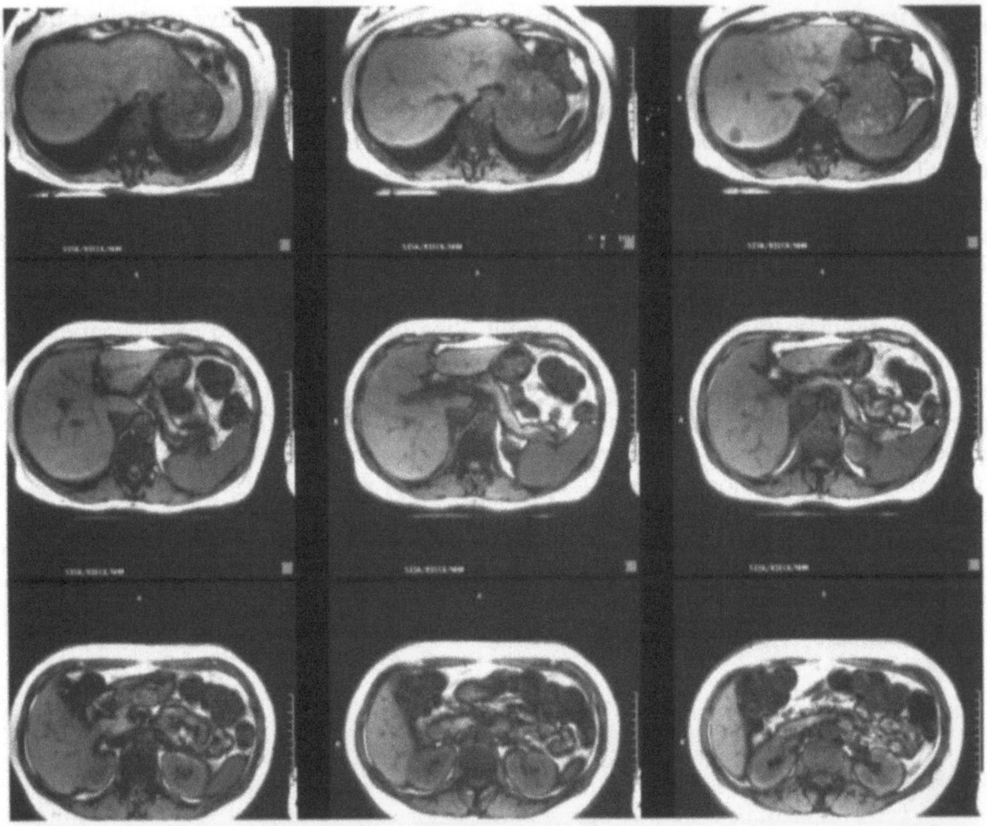

D

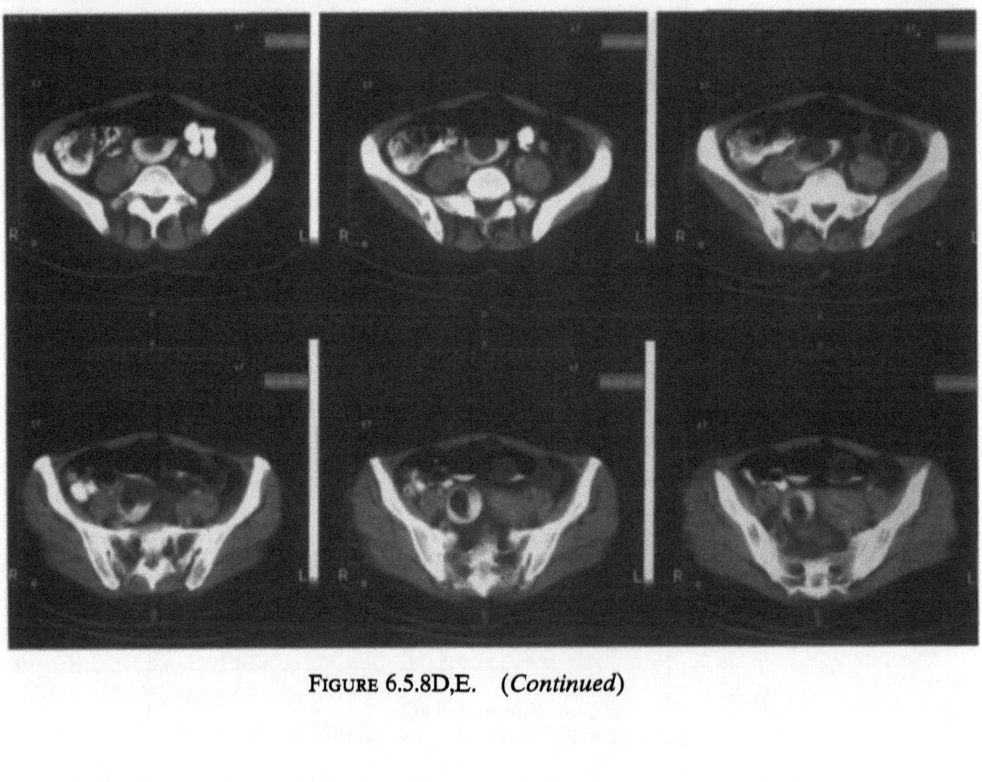

E

FIGURE 6.5.8D,E. (*Continued*)

(91%) was lower than CT portography (97%), the specificity was much higher, particularly at postsurgical sites.

There are numerous reports about the role of PET for detection of bone metastases.[6–12] FDG PET has high sensitivity for the detection of osteolytic skeletal metastasis, but the demonstration of osteoblastic metastases, such as with prostate carcinoma, is less satisfactory. Kao et al.[6] reported FDG PET has a better specificity but a lower sensitivity for detecting malignant bone metastases when compared with diphosphonate skeletal scintigraphy. Yeh et al.[10] reported that only 18% (24 of 131 sites) of bony lesions apparent on the conventional bone scans of patients with prostate carcinoma have corresponding foci of increased FDG uptake. They suggest that other metabolic processes are more important than glycolysis for providing prostate cancer with a source of energy and nutrients. However, Moog et al.[9] demonstrated that in a population of 56 patients with lymphoma, FDG PET is suitable for identifying osseous involvement with a high positive predictive value and is thereby more sensitive and specific than bone scintigraphy. Franzius et al.[8] reported that the sensitivity, specificity, and accuracy of FDG PET in the detection of osseous metastases from Ewing's sarcomas are superior to those of bone scintigraphy but not in the detection of osseous metastases from osteosarcoma. Although there is no series of patients with colon carcinoma and bone metastases that have been studied with FDG PET, bone metastases from colon carcinoma tend to be osteolytic, and therefore, it is expected that they will be FDG-avid.

Diagnoses

1. Primary rectosigmoid carcinoma post–neoadjuvant chemotherapy and radiation therapy.
2. Two metastatic lesions and two benign lesions in the liver.
3. Unsuspected skeletal metastasis adjacent to the right sacroiliac joint.

References

1. Schiepers C, Penninckx F, De Vadder N, et al.: Contribution of PET in the diagnosis of recurrent colorectal cancer: Comparison with conventional imaging. Eur J Surg Oncol 1995;21:517–522.
2. Vitola JV, Delbeke D, Sandler MP, et al.: Positron emission tomography to stage metastatic colorectal carcinoma to the liver. Am J Surg 1996; 171:21–26.
3. Delbeke D, Vitola JV, Sandler MP, et al.: Staging recurrent metastatic colorectal carcinoma with PET. J Nucl Med 1997;38:1196–1201.
4. Ogunbiyi OA, Flanagan FL, Dehdashti F, et al.: Detection of recurrent and metastatic colorectal cancer: Comparison of positron emission tomography and computed tomography. Annals of Surgical Oncology 1997;4:613–620.
5. Valk PE, Abella-Columna E, Haseman MK, et al.: Whole-body PET imaging with F-18-fluorodeoxyglucose in management of recurrent colorectal cancer. Arch Surg 1999;134:503–511.
6. Kao CH, Hsieh JF, Tsai SC, Ho YJ, Yen RF: Comparison and discrepancy of 18F-2-deoxyglucose positron emission tomography and Tc-99m MDP bone scan to detect bone metastases. Anticancer Research 2000;20:2189–2192.
7. Cook GJR, Fogelman I: The role of positron emission tomography in the management of bone metastases. Cancer 2000;88(S12):2927–2933.
8. Franzius C, Sciuk J, Daldrup-Link HE, et al.: FDG-PET for detection of osseous metastases from malignant primary bone tumors: Comparison with bone scintigraphy. Eur J Nucl Med 2000;27:1305–1311.
9. Moog F, Kotzerke J, Reske SN: FDG PET can replace bone scintigraphy in primary staging of malignant lymphoma. J Nucl Med 1999;40:1407–1413.
10. Yeh SD, Imbriaco M, Larson SM, et al.: Detection of bony metastases of androgen-independent prostate cancer by PET-FDG. Nucl Med Biol 1996;23:693–697.
11. Shreve PD, Grossman HB, Gross MD, Wahl RL: Metastatic prostate cancer: Initial findings of PET with 2-deoxy-2-(F-18)fluoro-D-Glucose. Radiology 1996;199:751–756.
12. Bury T, Barreto A, Daenen F, et al.: Fluorine-18 deoxyglucose positron emission tomography for the detection of bone metastases in patients with non-small cell lung cancer. Eur J Nucl Med 1998;25:1244–1247.

6.6 Other Gastrointestinal Tumors

Darrin L. Johnson, William H. Martin, and Dominique Delbeke

Esophageal and Gastric Carcinomas

Approximately one-third of the patients undergoing surgery for esophageal and gastric carcinoma are found to have occult metastases. The published experience with esophageal and gastric carcinomas suggests that FDG PET is highly sensitive to detect both the primary tumors and hepatic and distant metastases.[1–15] The sensitivity of both PET and CT appears limited for the detection of local lymph node involvement, probably due to the proximity of the primary tumor. Peritoneal spread is also difficult to identify using CT or FDG PET. Because patients usually present more often with distant metastases at the time of recurrence than at the time of initial diagnosis, FDG PET may be most helpful in staging patients when they present with recurrence.[16] For example, in the study of Flanagan et al.,[1] PET detected the primary esophageal tumor in all 36 patients and detected distant metastases in 5 patients. CT failed to detect any of the distant metastases. Among the 29 patients who underwent surgery, the extent of nodal disease was revealed in 76% by PET and in 45% by CT. In the study of Block et al.,[2] PET detected 53 out of 58 primary tumors and distant metastases in 17 patients as compared to 5 patients with CT. Of the 21 patients with lymph node involvement found at surgery, 52% were detected with FDG PET, and 28% with CT were detected. In a report of 35 patients,[3] the sensitivity, specificity, and accuracy of FDG PET were 88%, 93%, and 91%, respectively, for distant metastases and 45%, 100%, and 48% for locoregional nodal metastases. In a prospective study of staging 74 patients with esophageal carcinoma, FDG PET had a higher accuracy than the combination of CT and endoscopic ultrasound for diagnosing stage IV disease (82% versus 64%).[11] Endoscopic ultrasound was more sensitive than FDG PET for local lymph node staging (81% versus 33%), but the specificity of FDG PET was superior to CT and endoscopic ultrasound combined for staging local and distant lymph nodes. FDG PET changed the stage in 16 out of 74 (22%) patients, by upstaging two-thirds of the patients and downstaging one-third of the patients. For gastric carcinomas, the sensitivity, specificity, and accuracy of PET for the detection of the primary tumor, locoregional metastases, and distant metastases is in the same range as for esophageal carcinomas.[5] In patients who had a PET scan before and after chemotherapy, FDG uptake appears to decrease in patients who respond to treatment but does not decrease in nonresponders.[4]

In summary, FDG PET, by virtue of its whole-body technique, is more effective than CT or ultrasound in the detection of distant metastases from esophageal and gastric carcinomas. On that basis, PET may change the staging of up to 25% of these patients. Locoregional nodal metastases are detected better with FDG PET than CT but not as well as compared to endoscopic ultrasound. The utility of FDG PET may be more important in the evaluation of patients with recurrence or suspected recurrence and assessing the response to therapy.

Pancreatic Carcinoma

Pancreatic ductal adenocarcinoma is the fourth leading cause of death in the United States and is increasing in incidence. The preoperative diagnosis, staging, and treatment of pancreatic cancer remain challenging.

The suspicion for pancreatic cancer is often raised by US or CT findings, including the presence of a low-attenuation pancreatic mass and dilatation of the pancreatic duct and/or biliary tree. CT is the most common diagnostic imaging modality utilized in the preoperative diagnosis of pancreatic cancer. CT is also important to assess vascular involvement and invasion of adjacent organs. In a multicenter trial,[17] the diagnostic accuracy of CT for staging and resectability was 73%, with a positive predictive value for nonresectability of 90%, but more recent studies have reported accuracies of 85 to 95%, likely related to improvements in CT technology.[18,19] Unfortunately, interpretation of the CT scan is sometimes difficult in the setting of mass-forming pancreatitis or questionable findings such as enlargement of the pancreatic head without definite signs of malignancy or discrete mass.[20,21] The diagnosis of locoregional lymph node metastases is also difficult with CT, because they often are small. In addition, small hepatic metastases (< 1 cm) cannot reliably be differentiated from cysts.[22] Therefore, the reported negative predictive value for nonresectability is less than 30%. Despite recent technical improvements in MRI, including MR cholangiopancreatography (MRCP), the diagnostic performance of MRI remains similar to CT.[23–26] Endoscopic ultrasound offers the possibility of tissue diagnosis with fine-needle biopsy, but the field of view is limited.[27–29] The accuracy of endoscopic retrograde cholangiopancreatography (ERCP) is 80 to 90% to differentiate benign from malignant pancreatic mass, including differentiation of tumor from chronic pancreatitis because of the high degree of resolution of ductal structures. The limitations include false-negative findings when the tumor does not originate from the main duct, a 10% rate of technical failure, and up to 8% morbidity due to iatrogenic pancreatitis. The main advantages are the possibilities of fine-needle aspiration biopsy and interventional procedures. Although fine-needle biopsy may provide a tissue diagnosis with a high degree of accuracy, this technique suffers from significant sampling error,[30,31] with a false-negative incidence of 8 to 17%.

The difficulty in making a preoperative diagnosis is associated with two types of adverse outcomes. First, less aggressive surgeons may abort attempted resection due to a lack of tissue diagnosis. This is borne out by the significant rate of "reoperative" pancreaticoduodenectomy performed at major referral centers.[32–34] A second type of adverse outcome generated by failure to obtain a preoperative diagnosis occurs when more aggressive surgeons inadvertently resect benign disease. This is particularly notable in those patients who present with suspected malignancy without an associated mass on CT scan. This has been reported to occur in up to 55% of patients in some series.[35]

Role of FDG PET in the Preoperative Diagnosis of Pancreatic Carcinoma

In order to avoid these adverse outcomes, metabolic imaging with FDG PET may improve the accuracy of the preoperative diagnosis of pancreatic carcinoma. Most malignancies, including pancreatic carcinoma, demonstrate increased glucose utilization due to an increased number of glucose transporter proteins and increased hexokinase and phosphofructokinase activity.[36,37] There is recent evidence that the over-expression of glucose transporters by malignant pancreatic cells contributes to the increased uptake of FDG by these neoplasms.[38,39] In 11 studies,[40–50] the overall performance of PET to differentiate benign from malignant lesions is: sensitivity, 85 to 100%; specificity, 67 to 99%; and accuracy, 85 to 93%. The majority suggest improved accuracy compared to CT. These results are similar to the findings in our series with a sensitivity of 92% and a specificity of 85% for FDG PET as compared to 65% and 62%, respectively, for CT scanning.[50] In addition, the sensitivity of CT imaging improves with the size of the lesion, but the sensitivity of FDG PET is not as dependent on size.[51] However, these studies suffer from biases. For example, the acquisition of the CT data is often not performed prospectively, and the quality of the CT images may be variable among different institutions. Together, these series support the conclusion that FDG PET imaging may represent a useful adjunctive study in the evaluation of patients with suspected pancreatic cancer.

As with any imaging modality, FDG PET has limitations in the evaluation of pancreatic cancer. The high incidence of glucose intolerance and diabetes exhibited by patients with pancreatic pathology represents a potential limitation of this modality in the diagnosis of pancreatic cancer. Elevated serum glucose levels result in decreased FDG uptake in tumors due to competitive inhibition; low SUV values with false-negative FDG PET scans have been noted in hyperglycemic patients. This has led some investigators to suggest that the SUV be corrected according to serum glucose level.[52–55] The true impact of serum glucose levels on the accuracy of FDG PET in pancreatic cancer and other neoplasms remains controversial. Several studies have demonstrated a lower sensitivity in hyperglycemic as compared to euglycemic patients.[43,47,50] For example, in a study of 106 patients with a disease prevalence of 70%,[47] FDG PET had a sensitivity of 98%, specificity of 84%, and accuracy of 93% in a subgroup of euglycemic patients as compared to 63%, 86%, and 68%, respectively, in a subgroup of hyperglycemic patients. Other investigators[45,46] noted no variation in the accuracy of FDG PET based on serum glucose levels. In the studies of Delbeke et al.[50] and Diederichs et al.,[55] the presence of elevated serum glucose levels and/or diabetes mellitus may have contributed to false-negative interpretations, but correction of the SUV for serum glucose level has not significantly improved the accuracy of FDG PET in the diagnosis of pancreatic carcinoma. False-negative studies may also occur when the tumor diameter is < 1 cm (that is, small ampullary carcinoma). Ampullary carcinomas arise from the ampulla of Vater and have a better prognosis than pancreatic carcinoma because they cause biliary obstruction and are diagnosed earlier in the course of the disease. The detection rate with FDG imaging is only 70 to 80%, probably because of their smaller size at the time of clinical presentation.

Both glucose and FDG are substrates for cellular mediators of inflammation. Some benign inflammatory lesions, including chronic and acute pancreatitis with or without abscess formation, can accumulate FDG and give false-positive interpretations on PET images.[43,46,56,57] In addition, poststenotic pancreatitis can obscure FDG uptake in the tumor itself. Other reported false-positive images include serous cystadenoma and retroperitoneal fibrosis. False-positive studies are more frequent in patients with elevated C-reactive protein and/or acute pancreatitis with a specificity as low as 50%.[57,58] Therefore, screening for acute inflammatory disease with serum C-reactive protein has been recommended.

Preliminary reports suggest that the degree of FDG uptake has a prognostic value. Nakata et al.[59] noted a correlation between SUV and survival in 14 patients with pancreatic adenocarcinoma. Patients with an SUV > 3.0 had a mean survival of five months as compared to 14 months in those with an SUV < 3.0. Zimny et al.[60] performed a multivariate analysis on 52 patients, including SUV and accepted factors of prognosis, to determine the prognostic value of FDG PET. The median survival of 26 patients with SUV > 6.1 was five months as compared to nine months for 26 patients with SUV < 6.1. SUV and the serum level of the tumor marker Ca 19-9 were independent prognostic factors.

In summary, FDG PET imaging is complementary to CT in the evaluation of patients with pancreatic masses or in whom the diagnosis of pancreatic carcinoma is suspected. In view of the probable decreased sensitivity seen in patients with hyperglycemia, acquisition should be performed under controlled metabolic conditions and in the absence of acute inflammatory abdominal disease.

Role of FDG PET in Staging Pancreatic Carcinoma

Stage II disease is characterized by extrapancreatic extension (T stage), stage III is characterized by lymph node involvement (N stage), and stage IV is characterized by distant metastases (M stage). T-staging can only be evaluated with anatomical imaging modalities, which demonstrate best the relationship between the tumor, adjacent organs, and vascular structures. Functional imaging modalities can obviously not replace anatomical imaging in the assessment of local tumor resectability.

As for other neoplasms, FDG imaging has not been superior to helical CT for N staging but is more accurate than CT for M staging. In the study of Delbeke et al.,[50] metastases were diagnosed both on CT and PET in 10 out of 21 patients with stage IV disease, but PET demonstrated hepatic metastases not identified or equivocal on CT and/or distant metastases unsuspected clinically in seven additional patients. In four patients, neither CT nor PET imaging showed evidence of metastases, but surgical exploration revealed carcinomatosis in three patients and a small liver metastasis in one patient. FDG PET is sensitive for detection of hepatic metastases, but false-positive findings have been reported in the liver of patients with dilated bile ducts and formation of inflammatory granulomas.[61]

Impact of FDG PET on the Management of Patients with Pancreatic Carcinoma

The rate with which FDG PET results may lead to alterations in clinical management clearly depends on the specific therapeutic philosophy employed by an evaluating surgeon. In our center, we advocate pancreaticoduodenectomy only for those patients with potentially curable pancreatic cancer and take an aggressive approach to resection including en bloc retroperitoneal lymphadenectomy and selective resection of the superior mesenteric-portal vein confluence when necessary. While certain patients with chronic pancreatitis may also benefit from pancreaticoduodenectomy, the majority of patients with nonmalignant biliary strictures are optimally managed without resection. In a series of 65 patients, the application of FDG PET imaging in addition to CT altered the surgical management in 41% of the patients, 27% by detecting CT-occult pancreatic carcinoma and 14% by identifying unsuspected distant metastases or clarifying the benign nature of lesions equivocal on CT.[50] In this regard, FDG PET may allow selection of the optimal surgical approach in patients with pancreatic carcinoma.

The Role of FDG PET in Monitoring Therapy of Pancreatic Carcinoma

The potentially significant morbidity associated with pancreaticoduodenectomy, which can compromise the delivery of postoperative adjuvant chemoradiation, has led to the development of preoperative adjuvant (neoadjuvant) chemoradiation in these patients. In addition, preliminary studies suggest that neoadjuvant chemoradiation improves the resectability rate and survival of patients with pancreatic carcinoma.[62,63] A recent report from Vanderbilt University determined that FDG PET imaging may be useful for the assessment of tumor response to neoadjuvant therapy and the evaluation of suspected recurrent disease following resection.[51] Nine patients underwent FDG PET imaging before and after neoadjuvant chemoradiation therapy. FDG PET successfully predicted histological evidence of chemoradiation-induced tumor necrosis in all four patients who demonstrated at least a 50% reduction in tumor SUV following chemoradiation. Among these patients, none showed a measurable reduction in tumor diameter as assessed by CT. Three patients showed stable FDG uptake, and two patients showed increasing FDG uptake indicative of tumor progression. Among the two patients with progressive disease demonstrated by FDG PET, one patient showed tumor progression on CT, and the other patient demonstrated stable disease. The four patients who had FDG PET evidence of tumor response went on to successful resection, all showing 20 to 80% tumor necrosis in the resected specimen. Among the five patients who showed no response by FDG PET, the disease could be subsequently resected in only two patients, and only one patient who underwent resection showed evidence of chemoradiation-induced necrosis in the resected specimen. Another pilot study suggests that the absence of FDG uptake at one month following chemotherapy is an indicator of improved survival.[64] Definitive conclusions regarding the role of FDG PET in assessing treatment response will obviously require evaluation in a larger population of patients. However, given the poor track record of CT in assessing histological response to neoadjuvant chemoradiation, the potential utility of FDG PET in this capacity deserves further investigation.

The majority of reports concerning the clinical utilization of FDG PET scanning for pancreatic malignancy have emphasized the identification of recurrent nodal or distant metastatic disease. In a preliminary study,[51] eight patients were evaluated for possible recurrence because of either indeterminate CT findings or a rise in serum tumor marker levels. All were noted to have significant new regions of FDG uptake, four in the surgical bed and four in new hepatic metastases. In all patients, metastasis or local recurrence was confirmed pathologically or clinically. Another study of 19 patients concluded that FDG PET added important incremental information in 50% of the patients, resulting in a change of therapeutic procedure.[65] This included patients with elevated serum tumor marker levels but no findings on anatomical imaging. Therefore, FDG PET may be particularly useful (1) when CT identifies an indistinct region of change in the bed of the resected pancreas that is difficult to differentiate from postoperative or postradiation fibrosis, (2) for the evaluation of new hepatic lesions that may be too small to biopsy, and (3) in patients with rising serum tumor marker levels and a negative conventional work-up.

Summary

Overall, FDG PET imaging appears to be a sensitive and specific adjunct to CT when applied to the preoperative diagnosis of pancreatic adenocarcinoma. This imaging modality is of particular use in patients with suspected pancreatic cancer in whom CT fails to identify a discrete tumor mass. By providing preoperative documentation of pancreatic malignancy in these patients, laparotomy may be undertaken with a curative intent, and the risk of aborting resection due to diagnostic uncertainty is minimized. FDG PET imaging would also appear to be useful in the clarification of CT-occult metastatic disease, allowing nontherapeutic resection to be avoided altogether in this group of patients.

Hepatobiliary Tumors

Metastases to the liver from various primary neoplasms occur 20 times more often than primary hepatic carcinoma and are often multifocal. Although many tumors may metastasize to the liver, the most common primaries producing liver metastases are colorectal, gastric, pancreatic, lung, and breast carcinoma. Ninety percent of malignant primary liver tumors are tumors from epithelial origin: hepatocellular carcinoma and cholangiocarcinoma.

Hepatocellular carcinoma (92% of epithelial tumors) arise from the malignant transformation of hepatocytes and are common in the setting of chronic liver disease such as viral hepatitis, cirrhosis, or in patients exposed to carcinogens. Hepatocellular carcinoma most frequently metastasizes to regional lymph nodes, the lung, and the skeleton.

Cholangiocarcinomas arise from biliary cells and represent only 10% of the epithelial tumors. About 20% of the patients who develop cholangiocarcinomas have predisposing conditions, including sclerosing cholangitis, ulcerative colitis, Caroli's disease, choledocal cyst, infestation by the fluke Clonorchis sinensis, cholelithiasis, or exposure to Thorotrast among others. Approximately 50% of cholangiocarcinomas occur in the liver, and the other 50% are extrahepatic. These tumors are often unresectable at the time of diagnosis and have a poor prognosis. Intrahepatic cholangiocarcinomas can be further subdivided in two categories: the peripheral type arising from the interlobular biliary duct and the hilar type (Klatskin's tumor) arising from the main hepatic duct or its bifurcation. In addition, they can develop in three different morphological types: infiltrating sclerosing lesions (most common), exophytic lesions, and polypoid intraluminal masses. Malignant tumors arising along the extrahepatic bile ducts are usually diagnosed early because they cause biliary obstruction. Tumors arising near the hilum of the liver have a worse prognosis because of their direct extension into the liver. Distant metastases occur late in the disease and most often affect the lungs.

Mesenchymal tumors such as angiosarcomas, epithelioid angioendothelioma, and primary lymphoma are relatively rare malignant tumors that can affect the liver.

Gallbladder carcinoma is uncommon and is associated with cholelithiasis in 75% of the cases. These tumors are insidious, not suspected clinically, and often discovered at surgery or incidentally in the surgical specimen. They frequently spread to the liver and can perforate the wall of the gallbladder, metastasizing to the abdomen. Distant metastases may occur in the lungs, pleura, and diaphragm.

The diagnostic issues of conventional imaging include early detection of these tumors, differentiation from cirrhosis and other benign liver tumor, and assessment of the response to therapy. Screening for hepatic lesions is commonly performed with transabdominal ultrasound. Ultrasound can detect lesions as small as 1 cm in diameter but is operator-dependent, inherently two-dimensional, and suffers from poor specificity. Hepatic metastases can be hypoechoic, hyperechoic, cystic, or have mixed echogenicity. Isoechoic metastases are undetected. CT is the conventional method for screening the liver at many institutions. Metastases may be better seen during the arterial or portal venous phase after contrast injection, depending on the vascularity of the tumor. The development of the helical technique has resulted in a sensitivity comparable to that of MRI, although CT portography remains the most sensitive technique for detection of small lesions.

As hepatocellular carcinoma is often associated with elevated serum levels of alpha-fetoprotein, serum alpha-fetoprotein measurements and ultrasound are conventional methods for screening patients at risk for hepatocellular carcinoma. Differentiation of low-grade hepatocellular carcinomas from hepatic adenoma can be difficult even on core biopsy. Although a capsule is often present in small hepatocellular carcinoma, it is seldom seen in large ones. Invasion of the portal vein is often present, especially with large hepatocellular carcinomas. Hepatocellular carcinoma can undergo hemorrhage and necrosis or demonstrate fatty metamorphosis. The presence of these characteristics on imaging studies is suggestive of hepatocellular carcinoma but requires high-resolution techniques for successful detection. Dynamic multiphase gadolinium-enhanced MRI may be superior to dual-phase spiral CT to characterize hepatocellular carcinoma.[66] Although large lesions (> 3 cm) may be visualized by CT and US with a sensitivity in the 80 to 90% range, smaller lesions may be difficult to distinguish from the surrounding hepatic parenchyma, especially in patients with cirrhosis and regenerating nodules; sensitivity for small hepatocellular carcinomas is in the range of 50%. CT portography is the most sensitive technique for detection of lesions less than 1 cm in size. ^{67}Gallium or ^{201}thallium scintigraphy may be helpful to identify hepatocellular carcinoma if the findings on other imaging modalities are equivocal. Seventy to 90% of hepatocellular carcinoma have ^{67}gallium or ^{201}thallium uptake greater than the liver, and ^{67}gallium scintigraphy has been used in conjunction with a sulfur colloid scan to differentiate hepatocellular carcinoma from regenerating nodules in cirrhotic patients.[67] Fibrolamellar carcinoma, a low-grade malignant tumor representing 6 to 25% of hepatocellular carcinoma, occurs in a younger population of patients without underlying cirrhosis. An avascular scar that may contain calcifications is characteristic. In contrast, focal nodular hyperplasia, is characterized by a vascular scar without calcifications. MRI and SPECT scintigraphy with radiolabeled red blood cells, ^{99m}Tc-sulfur colloid, or ^{99m}Tc-HIDA agents can help to further characterize some lesions (hemangioma, focal nodular hyperplasia, and adenoma).

Cholangiocarcinomas are often not seen on CT because they are small and isodense. When this is the case (most hilar tumors and 25% of peripheral tumors), the level of biliary ductal dilatation infers the location of the tumor.

When the tumor is visible on CT, it most often appears as a nonspecific hypodense mass. Delayed retention of contrast material is characteristic and must be differentiated from cavernous hemangioma. A central scar or calcification is seen in 25 to 30% of the cases. On MRI, these tumors are usually hypointense on T1-weighted images and hyperintense on T2-weighted images. The central scar is best seen as a hypointense structure on the T2-weighted images. After gadolinium administration, there is early peripheral enhancement with progressive concentric enhancement, as with CT. MRI may demonstrate tumors not seen on CT and should be utilized as a problem solving tool.[66] For example, MR cholangiopancreatography used as an adjunct to conventional MRI may provide additional information regarding the extension of hilar cholangiocarcinoma. If MR cholangiopancreatography can establish the resectability of the tumor, the patient may undergo immediate surgery and be spared a percutaneous cholangiography and biliary drainage procedure. Percutaneous cholangiography and/or endoscopic retrograde cholangiopancreatography are usually not indicated for peripheral tumors, but can demonstrate hilar cholangiocarcinoma in most cases and are better than CT to evaluate the intraductal extent of the tumor. Percutaneous cholangiography and/or endoscopic retrograde cholangiopancreatography are the procedures of choice to demonstrate the infiltrating/sclerosing type of cholangiocarcinoma. Typically a malignant stricture tapers irregularly and is associated with proximal ductal dilatation, although it is difficult to differentiate from sclerosing cholangitis, one of the preexisting conditions. Some tumors are seen as intraluminal defects, but mucin, blood clots, calculi, an air bubble, or biliary sludge may have a similar appearance. ERCP/PTC is often performed at the same time as a biliary drainage procedure.

Role of FDG PET in the Diagnosis of Malignant Hepatic Lesions

Differentiated hepatocytes normally have a relatively high glucose-6-phosphatase activity which allows dephosphorylation of intracellular FDG and its egress from the liver. Although experimental studies have shown that glycogenesis decreases and glycolysis increases during carcinogenesis, the accumulation of FDG in hepatocellular carcinoma is variable due to varying degrees of activity of the enzyme glucose-6-phosphatase in these tumors.[68,69] Therefore, it has been predicted that evaluation of liver tumors, especially hepatocellular carcinomas, with FDG PET would require dynamic imaging with blood sampling and kinetic analysis. Kinetic analysis is cumbersome to perform clinically and cannot be performed over the entire body, thus preventing staging. Studies using kinetic analysis have shown that the phosphorylation kinetic constant (k3) is elevated in virtually all malignant tumors including hepatocellular carcinoma. The dephosphorylation kinetic constant (k4) is low in metastatic lesions and cholangiocarcinomas, thus resulting in intralesional accumulation of FDG. But k4 is similar to k3 for hepatocellular carcinoma that do not accumulate FDG.[70–72] Therefore, hepatocellular carcinomas are hypermetabolic, but many do not accumulate FDG due to their inability to retain the FDG taken up. There are three patterns of uptake for hepatocellular carcinoma: FDG uptake higher, equal to, or lower than liver background (55%, 30%, and 15%, respectively). FDG PET detects only 50 to 70% of hepatocellular carcinomas but has a sensitivity greater than 90% for all other primaries (cholangiocarcinoma and sarcoma) and all metastatic tumors to the liver.[73,74] All benign tumors, including focal nodular hyperplasia, adenoma, regenerating nodules, cysts, and hemangiomas, demonstrate FDG uptake at the same level as normal liver, except for rare abscesses with granulomatous inflammation. In addition, a correlation was found between the degree of FDG uptake, including both the standard uptake value (SUV) and k3, and the grade of malignancy.[72,73] Therefore, FDG imaging may have a prognostic significance in the evaluation of patients with hepatocellular carcinoma. Hepatocellular carcinomas that accumulate FDG tend to be moderately to poorly differentiated and are associated with markedly elevated alpha-fetoprotein levels.[75,76] However, FDG PET has limited value for the differential diagnosis of focal liver lesions in patients with chronic hepatitis C virus infection because of the low sensitivity for detection of hepatocellular carcinoma and the high prevalence of this tumor in that population of patients.[77]

There is preliminary evidence that FDG PET imaging may be useful in the diagnosis and management of small cholangiocarcinomas in patients with sclerosing cholangitis.[78] It is more helpful in patients with nodular cholangiocarcinomas than in those with the infiltrating variety. False-positive findings can be seen in patients with biliary stents, probably related to inflammatory changes, as well as in patients with acute cholangitis.

Role of FDG PET in Staging Hepatobiliary Tumors

In patients with hepatocellular carcinoma that accumulate FDG, PET imaging is able to detect unsuspected regional and distant metastases, as with other tumors. In some cases, FDG PET is the only imaging modality that can demonstrate the tumor and its metastases. In a series of 23 patients with hepatocellular carcinoma who underwent FDG PET scanning in an attempt to identify extrahepatic metastases, 13 of the 23 (57%) patients had increased uptake in the primary tumor, and four of those 13 had extrahepatic metastases demonstrated by FDG PET images.[79]

Role of FDG PET in Monitoring Therapy of Hepatobiliary Tumors

Because the majority of patients with hepatocellular carcinoma have advanced-stage tumors and/or underlying cirrhosis with impaired hepatic reserve, surgical resection is often not possible. Therefore, other treatment strategies have been developed, including hepatic arterial chemoembolization, systemic chemotherapy, surgical cryoablation, ethanol ablation, radiofrequency ablation, and in selected cases, liver transplantation. In patients treated with hepatic arterial chemoembolization, FDG PET is more accurate than lipiodol retention on CT in predicting the presence of residual viable tumor. The presence of residual uptake in some lesions can help in guiding further regional therapy.[80–82] It is expected but not yet demonstrated that FDG PET may surpass CT in determining the success of other ablative procedures in these patients.

Unsuspected gallbladder carcinoma is discovered incidentally in 1% of routine cholecystectomies. At present, the majority of cholecystectomies are performed laparoscopically, and occult gallbladder carcinoma found after laparoscopic cholecystectomy has been associated with reports of gallbladder carcinoma seeding of laparoscopic trocar sites.[83,84] Increased FDG uptake has been demonstrated in gallbladder carcinoma[85] and has been helpful in identifying recurrence in the area of the incision when CT could not differentiate scar tissue from malignant recurrence.[86]

Summary

Most malignant hepatic tumors, primary or secondary, are FDG-avid, and most benign processes accumulate FDG to the same level as normal hepatic parenchyma. Approximately one-third of hepatocellular carcinomas do not accumulate FDG and are false-negatives. Therefore, FDG imaging is not recommended for evaluation of focal hepatic lesions in patients with chronic hepatitis C or for screening for hepatocellular carcinoma in a population at increased risk. Small ampullary carcinoma and cholangiocarcinoma of the infiltrating type can be false-negative as well. Foci of inflammation along biliary stents and granulomatous abscesses, including foci of acute cholangitis, accumulate FDG and can be misinterpreted as malignant. FDG imaging can detect unsuspected metastases and aid in monitoring therapy in patients with malignant tumors accumulating FDG, including hepatocellular carcinomas and cholangiocarcinomas.

References

1. Flanagan FL, Dehdashti F, Siegel BA, et al.: Staging of esophageal cancer with ^{18}F-fluorodeoxyglucose positron emission tomography. Am J Roentgenol 1997;168:417–424.
2. Block MI, Patterson GA, Sundaresan RS, et al.: Improvement in staging of esophageal cancer

with the addition of positron emission tomography. Ann Thorac Surg 1997;64:770–776.
3. Luketich JD, Schauer PR, Meltzer CC, et al.: Role of positron emission tomography in staging esophageal cancer. Ann Thorac Surg 1997;64: 765–769.
4. Couper GW, McAteer D, Wallis F, et al.: Detection of response to chemotherapy using positron emission tomography in patients with oesophageal and gastric cancer. Br J Surg 1998;85:1403–1406.
5. Yeung HWD, Macapinlac H, Karpeh M, Rinn RD, Larson SM: Accuracy of FDG PET in gastric cancer: Preliminary experience. Clin Positron Imaging 1998;1:213–221.
6. Kole AC, Plukker JT, Nieweg OE, Vaalburg W: Positron emission tomography for staging of oesophageal and gastroesophageal malignancy. Br J Cancer 1998;78(4):521–527.
7. Fukunaga T, Okazumi S, Koide Y, Isono K, Imazeki K: Evaluation of esophageal cancers using fluorine-18-fluorodeoxyglucose PET. J Nucl Med 1998;39(6):1002–1007.
8. Rankin SC, Taylor H, Cook GJ, Mason R: Computed tomography and positron emission tomography in the pre-operative staging of oesophageal carcinoma. Clin Radiol 1998;53(9): 659–665.
9. McAteer D, Wallis F, Couper G, et al.: Evaluation of 18F-FDG positron emission tomography in gastric and oesophageal carcinoma. Br J Radiol 1999;72:525–529.
10. Luketich JD, Friedman DM, Weigel TL, et al.: Evaluation of distant metastases in esophageal cancer: 100 consecutive positron emission tomography scans. Ann Thorac Surg 1999;68(4): 1133–1136.
11. Flamen P, Lerut A, Van Cutsem E, et al.: Utility of positron emission tomography for the staging of patients with potentially operable esophageal carcinoma. J Clin Oncol 2000;18(18):3202–3210.
12. Rice TW: Clinical staging of esophageal carcinoma. CT, EUS, and PET. Chest Surg Clin N Am 2000;10(3):471–485.
13. Skehan SJ, Brown AL, Thompson M, Young JE, Coates G, Nahmias C: Imaging features of primary and recurrent esophageal cancer at FDG PET. Radiographics 2000;20(3):713–723.
14. Hoegerle S, Altehoefer C, Nitzsche EU: Staging an esophageal carcinoma by F-18 fluorodeoxyglucose whole-body positron emission tomography. Clin Nucl Med 2000;25(3):219–220.
15. Lerut T, Flamen P, Ectors N, et al.: Histopathologic validation of lymph node staging with FDG-PET scan in cancer of the esophagus and gastroesophageal junction: A prospective study based on primary surgery with extensive lymphadenectomy. Ann Surg 2000;232(6):743–752.
16. Flamen P, Lerut A, Van Cutsem E, et al.: The utility of positron emission tomography for the diagnosis and staging of recurrent esophageal cancer. J Thorac Cardiovasc Surg 2000;120(6): 1085–1092.
17. Megibow AJ, Zhou XH, Rotterdam H, et al.: Pancreatic adenocarcinoma: CT versus MR imaging in the evaluation of resectability—report of the Radiology Diagnostic Oncology Group. Radiology 1995;195(2):327–332.
18. Diehl SJ, Lehman KJ, Sadick M, Lachman R, Georgi M: Pancreatic cancer: value of dual-phase helical CT in assessing resectability. Radiology 1998;206:373–378.
19. Lu DSK, Reber HA, Krasny RM, Sayre J: Local staging of pancreatic cancer: Criteria for unresectability of major vessels as revealed by pancreatic-phase, thin section helical CT. Am J Radiol 1997;168:1439–1444.
20. Johnson PT, Outwater EK: Pancreatic carcinoma versus chronic pancreatitis: dynamic MR imaging. Radiology 1999;212(1):213–218.
21. Lammer J, Herlinger H, Zalaudek G, Hofler H: Pseudotumorous pancreatitis. Gastrointest Radiol 1995;10:59–67.
22. Bluemke DA, Cameron IL, Hurban RH, et al.: Potentially resectable pancreatic adenocarcinoma: Spiral CT assessment with surgical and pathologic correlation. Radiology 1995;197:381–385.
23. Bluemke DA, Fishman EK: CT and MR evaluation of pancreatic cancer. Surg Oncol Clinics of North America 1998;7:103–124.
24. Catalano C, Pavone P, Laghi A, et al.: Pancreatic adenocarcinoma: Combination of MR angiography and MR cholangiopancreatography for the diagnosis and assessment of resectability. Eur Radiol 1998;8:428–434.
25. Irie H, Honda H, Kaneko K, et al.: Comparison of helical CT and MR imaging in detecting and staging small pancreatic adenocarcinoma. Abdom Imag 1997;22:429–433.
26. Trede M, Rumstadt B, Wendl, et al.: Ultrafast magnetic resonance imaging improves the staging of pancreatic tumors. Ann Surg 1997;226: 393–405.
27. Hawes RH, Zaidi S: Endoscopic ultrasonography of the pancreas. Gastrointestinal Endoscopy Clinics of North America 1995;5:61–80.
28. Legmann P, Vignaux O, Dousset B, et al.: Pancreatic tumors: Comparison of dual-phase

helical CT and endoscopic sonography. Am J Roentgenol 1998;170:1315–1322.
29. Mertz HR, Sechopoulos P, Delbeke D, Leach SD: EUS, PET, and CT scanning for evaluation of pancreatic adenocarcinoma. Gastrointest Endosc 2000;52(3):367–371.
30. Brandt KR, Charboneau JW, Stephens DH, Welch TJ, Goellner JR: CT- and US-guided biopsy of the pancreas. Radiology 1993;187:99–104.
31. Chang KJ, Nguyen P, Erickson RA, et al.: The clinical utility of endoscopic ultrasound-guided fine-needle aspiration in the diagnosis and staging of pancreatic carcinoma. Gastrointest Endosc 1997;45:387–393.
32. McGuire GE, Pitt HA, Lillemoe KD, et al.: Reoperative surgery for periampullary adenocarcinoma. Arch Surg 1991;126:1205–1212.
33. Tyler DS, Evans DB: Reoperative pancreaticoduodenectomy. Ann Surg 1994;219:211–221.
34. Robinson EK, Lee JE, Lowy AM, et al.: Reoperative pancreaticoduodenectomy for periampullary carcinoma. Am J Surg 1996;172:432–438.
35. Thompson JS, Murayama KM, Edney JA, Rikkers LF: Pancreaticoduodenectomy for suspected but unproven malignancy. Am J Surg 1994;169:571–575.
36. Flier JS, Mueckler MM, Usher P, Lodish HF: Elevated levels of glucose transport and transporter messenger RNA are induced by ras or src oncogenes. Science 1987;235:1492–1495.
37. Monakhov NK, Neistadt EL, Shavlovskil MM, et al.: Physiochemical properties and isoenzyme composition of hexokinase from normal and malignant human tissues. J Natl Cancer Inst 1978;61:27–34.
38. Higashi T, Tamaki N, Honda T, et al.: Expression of glucose transporters in human pancreatic tumors compared with increased F-18 FDG accumulation in PET study. J Nucl Med 1997; 38:1337–1344.
39. Reske S, Grillenberger KG, Glatting G, et al.: Overexpression of glucose transporter 1 and increased F-18 FDG uptake in pancreatic carcinoma. J Nucl Med 1997;38:1344–1348.
40. Bares R, Klever P, Hellwig D, et al.: Pancreatic cancer detected by positron emission tomography with 18F-labelled deoxyglucose: Method and first results. Nucl Med Commun 1993;14:596–601.
41. Bares R, Klever P, Hauptmann S, et al.: F-18-fluorodeoxyglucose PET in vivo evaluation of pancreatic glucose metabolism for detection of pancreatic cancer. Radiology 1994;192:79–86.
42. Stollfuss JC, Glatting G, Friess H, Kocher F, Berger HG, Reske SN: 2-(fluorine-18)-fluoro-2-deoxy-D-glucose PET in detection of pancreatic cancer: Value of quantitative image interpretation. Radiology 1995;195:339–344.
43. Inokuma T, Tamaki N, Torizuka T, et al.: Evaluation of pancreatic tumors with positron emission tomography and F-18 fluorodeoxyglucose: Comparison with CT and US. Radiology 1995;195: 345–352.
44. Kato T, Fukatsu H, Ito K, et al.: Fluorodeoxyglucose positron emission tomography in pancreatic cancer: An unsolved problem. Eur J Nucl Med 1995;22:32–39.
45. Friess H, Langhans J, Ebert M, et al.: Diagnosis of pancreatic cancer by 2[F-18]-fluoro-2-deoxy-D-glucose positron emission tomography. Gut 1995;36:771–777.
46. Ho CL, Dehdashti F, Griffeth LK, et al.: FDG PET evaluation of indeterminate pancreatic masses. Comput Assist Tomogr 1996;20:363–369.
47. Zimny M, Bares R, Fab J, et al.: Fluorine-18 fluorodeoxyglucose positron emission tomography in the differential diagnosis of pancreatic carcinoma: A report of 106 cases. Eur J Nucl Med 1997;24:678–682.
48. Keogan MT, Tyler D, Clark L, et al.: Diagnosis of pancreatic carcinoma: Role of FDG PET. Am J Roentgenol 1998;171:1565–1570.
49. Imdahl SA, Nitzsche E, Krautmann F, et al.: Evaluation of positron emission tomography with 2-[18F]fluoro-2-deoxy-D-glucose for the differentiation of chronic pancreatitis and pancreatic cancer. Br J Surg 1999;86(2):194–199.
50. Delbeke D, Chapman WC, Pinson CW, Martin WH, Beauchamp DR, Leach S: F-18 fluorodeoxyglucose imaging with positron emission tomography (FDG PET) has a significant impact on diagnosis and management of pancreatic ductal adenocarcinoma. J Nucl Med 1999;40: 1784–1792.
51. Rose DM, Delbeke D, Beauchamp RD, et al.: 18Fluorodeoxyglucose-positron emission tomography (18FDG-PET) in the management of patients with suspected pancreatic cancer. Annals of Surg 1998;229:729–738.
52. Wahl RL, Henry CA, Ethrer SP: Serum glucose: Effects on tumor and normal tissue accumulation of 2-[F-18]-fluoro-2-deoxy-D-glucose in rodents with mammary carcinoma. Radiology 1992;183:643–647.
53. Lindholm P, Minn H, Leskinen-Kallio S, et al.: Influence of the blood glucose concentration on FDG uptake in cancer—a PET study. J Nucl Med 1993;34:1–6.

54. Diederichs CG, Staib L, Glatting G, Beger HG, Reske SN: FDG PET: Elevated plasma glucose reduces both uptake and detection rate of pancreatic malignancies. J Nucl Med 1998;39: 1030–1033.
55. Diederichs CG, Staib L, Vogel J, et al.: Values and limitations of FDG PET with preoperative evaluations of patients with pancreatic masses. Pancreas 2000;20:109–116.
56. Zimny M, Buell U, Diederichs CG, Reske SN: False positive FDG PET in patients with pancreatic masses: An issue of proper patient selection? Eur J Nucl Med 1998;25:1352.
57. Shreve PD: Focal fluorine-18-fluorodeoxyglucose accumulation in inflammatory pancreatic disease. Eur J Nucl Med 1998;25:259–264.
58. Diederichs CG, Staib L, Glasbrenner B, et al.: F-18 fluorodeoxyglucose (FDG) and c-reactive protein (CRP). Clin Pos Imaging 1999;2(3): 131–136.
59. Nakata B, Chung YS, Nishimura S, et al.: 18F-fluorodeoxyglucose positron emission tomography and the prognosis of patients with pancreatic carcinoma. Cancer 1997;79:695–699.
60. Zimny M, Fass J, Bares R, et al.: Fluorodeoxyglucose positron emission tomography and the prognosis of pancreatic carcinoma. Scand J Gastroenterol 2000;35:883–888.
61. Frolich A, Diederichs CG, Staib L, et al.: Detection of liver metastases from pancreatic cancer using FDG PET. J Nucl Med 1999;40:250–255.
62. Yeung RS, Weese JL, Hoffman JP, et al.: Neoadjuvant chemoradiation in pancreatic and duodenal carcinoma. A Phase II Study. Cancer 1993;72(7):2124–2133.
63. Jessup JM, Steele G Jr, Mayer RJ, et al.: Neoadjuvant therapy for unresectable pancreatic adenocarcinoma. Arch Surg 1993;128(5):559–564.
64. Maisey NR, Webb A, Flux GD, et al.: FDG PET in the prediction of survival of patients with cancer of the pancreas: A pilot study. Br J Cancer 2000;83:287–293.
65. Franke C, Klapdor R, Meyerhoff K, Schauman M: 18-F positron emission tomography of the pancreas: Diagnostic benefit in the follow-up of pancreatic carcinoma. Anticancer Res 1999;19: 2437–2442.
66. Del Pilar Fernandez M, Redvanly RD: Primary hepatic malignant neoplasms. Radiologic Clinics of North America 1998;36(2):333–348.
67. Oppenheim BE: Liver imaging, in Sandler MP, Coleman RE, Wackers FTJ, et al. (eds): Diagnostic Nuclear Medicine. Baltimore: Williams and Wilkins, 1996, pp 749–758.
68. Weber G, Cantero A: Glucose-6-phosphatase activity in normal, precancerous, and neoplastic tissues. Cancer Res 1955;15:105–108.
69. Weber G, Morris HP: Comparative biochemistry of hepatomas. III. Carbohydrate enzymes in liver tumors of different growth rates. Cancer Res 1963;23:987–994.
70. Messa C, Choi Y, Hoh CK, et al.: Quantification of glucose utilization in liver metastases: Parametric imaging of FDG uptake with PET. J Comput Assist Tomogr 1992;16:684–689.
71. Okazumi S, Isono K, Enomoto D, et al.: Evaluation of liver tumors using fluorine-18-fluorodeoxyglucose PET: Characterization of tumor and assessment of effect of treatment. J Nucl Med 1992;33:333–339.
72. Torizuka T, Tamaki N, Inokuma T, et al.: In vivo assessment of glucose metabolism in hepatocellular carcinoma with FDG PET. J Nucl Med 1995;36:1811–1817.
73. Khan MA, Combs CS, Brunt EM, et al.: Positron emission tomography scanning in the evaluation of hepatocellular carcinoma. J Hepatol 2000; 32:792–797.
74. Delbeke D, Martin WH, Sandler MP, Chapman WC, Wright JK Jr, Pinson CW: Evaluation of benign vs. malignant hepatic lesions with positron emission tomography. Arch Surg 1998;133: 510–515.
75. Iwata Y, Shiomi S, Sasaki N, et al.: Clinical usefulness of positron emission tomography with fluorine-18-fluorodeoxiglucose in the diagnosis of liver tumors. Ann Nucl Med 2000;14:121–126.
76. Trojan J, Schroeder O, Raedle J, et al.: Fluorine-18 FDG positron emission tomography for imaging of hepatocellular carcinoma. Am J Gastroenterol 1999;94:3314–3319.
77. Schroder O, Trojan J, Zeuzem S, Baum RP: Limited value of fluorine-18-fluorodeoxyglucose PET for the differential diagnosis of focal liver lesions in patients with chronic hepatitis C virus infection. Nuklearmedizin 1998;37:279–285.
78. Keiding S, Hansen SB, Rasmussen HH, et al.: Detection of cholangiocarcinoma in primary sclerosing cholangitis by positron emission tomography. Hepatology 1998;28:700–706.
79. Rose AT, Rose DM, Pinson CW, et al.: Hepatocellular carcinoma outcome based on indicated treatment strategy. The American Surgeon 1998;64:1122–1135.
80. Torizuka T, Tamaki N, Inokuma T, et al.: Value of fluorine-18-FDG PET to monitor hepatocellular carcinoma after interventional therapy. J Nucl Med 1994;35:1965–1969.

81. Akuta K, Nishimura T, Jo S, et al.: Monitoring liver tumor therapy with [18F] FDG positron emission tomography. J Comput Assist Tomogr 1990;14:370–374.
82. Vitola JV, Delbeke D, Meranze SG, Mazer MJ, Pinson CW: Positron emission tomography with F-18-fluorodeoxyglucose to evaluate the results of hepatic chemoembolization. Cancer 1996;78: 2216–2222.
83. Drouart F, Delamarre J, Capron JP: Cutaneous seeding of gallbladder cancer after laparoscopic cholecystectomy. N Engl J Med 1991;325: 1316.
84. Weiss SM, Wengert PA, Harkavy SE: Incisional recurrence of gallbladder cancer after laparoscopic cholecystectomy. Gastrointest Endosc 1994;40:244–246.
85. Hoh CK, Hawkins RA, Glaspy JA, et al.: Cancer detection with whole-body PET using 2-[18F]fluoro-2-deoxy-D-glucose. J Comput Assist Tomogr 1993;17:582–589.
86. Lomis KD, Vitola JV, Delbeke D, et al.: Recurrent gallbladder carcinoma at laparoscopy port sites diagnosed by PET scan: Implications for primary and radical second operations. The American Surgeon 1997;63:341–345.

Cases Presentations

Case 6.6.1

History

A 61-year-old male with a 19-year history of prior hepatitis B infection presented with an elevated serum alpha-fetoprotein level of 49.4 ng/ml. A CT scan (Figure 6.6.1A) and FDG PET imaging were performed (Figure 6.6.1B). A selected CT slice from the portal venous phase of enhancement and coronal FDG images acquired with a dedicated PET tomograph (GE Advance) and reconstructed with iterative reconstruction and measured segmented attenuation correction are shown.

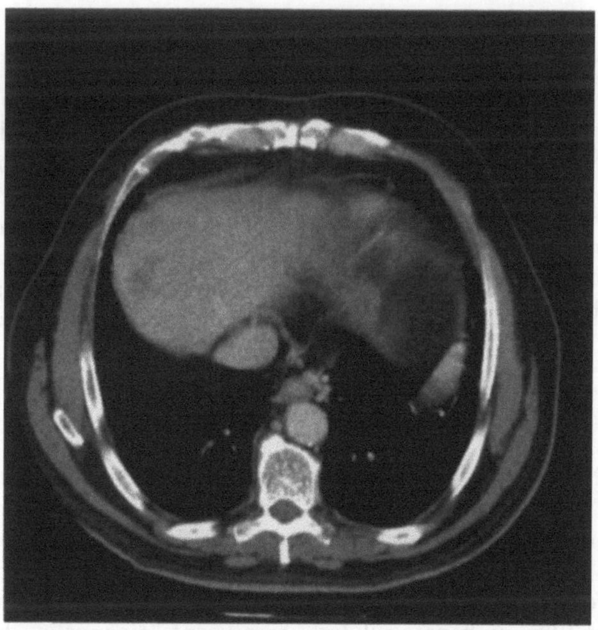

FIGURE 6.6.1A.

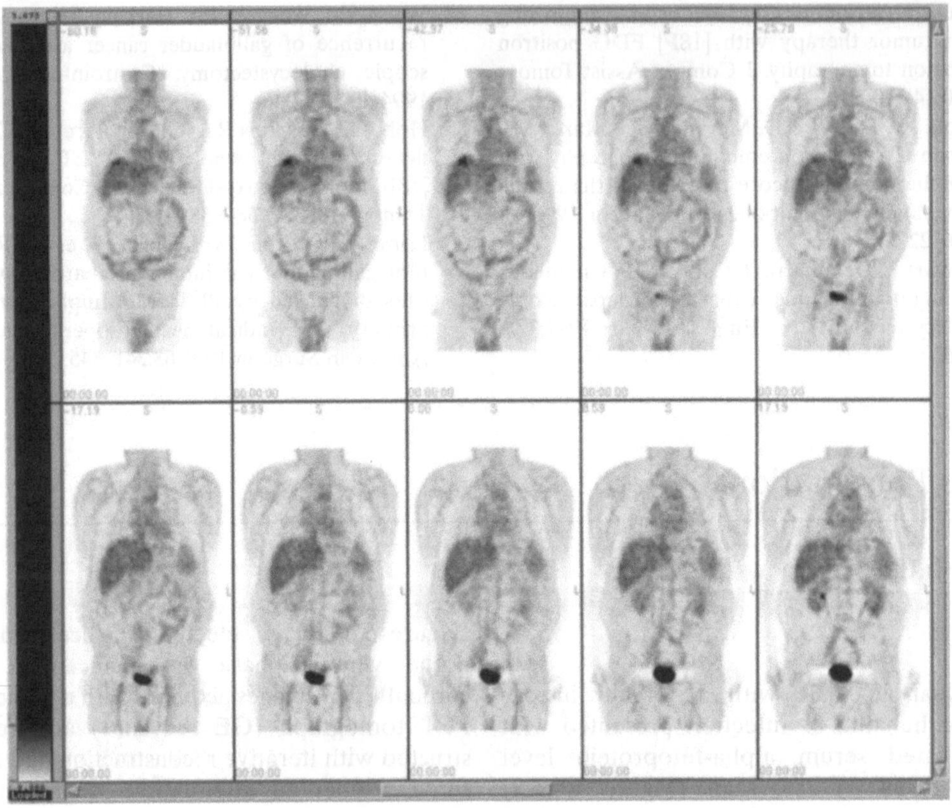

FIGURE 6.6.1B. *(Continued)*

Findings

The CT image demonstrates an area of decreased attenuation in the dome of the liver with a surgical clip present from prior resection. The FDG PET images reveal a focus of markedly increased activity within the dome of the liver congruent with the mass on CT. Normal physiologic uptake is present within the liver, gastrointestinal, and genitourinary systems.

Discussion

The area of increased activity at the dome of the liver on the PET scan is consistent with hepatocellular carcinoma that was confirmed at surgery, during which radiofrequency ablation of this lesion was performed.

The accumulation of FDG in hepatocellular carcinoma is variable due to the differing amounts of glucose-6-phosphatase present. It has been demonstrated that these tumors have increased levels of hexokinase activity and increased glucose metabolism. However, FDG-6-phosphate does not accumulate intracellularly when significant levels of glucose-6-phosphatase activity are present. Studies have shown that FDG accumulation in hepatocellular carcinomas will be greater than in normal liver parenchyma in approximately 50 to 70% of patients, with the remaining patients having uptake equal to (30% of patients) or less than (15% of patients) background liver activity. It has also been proposed that the degree of uptake may be correlated with the degree of malignancy. Benign lesions such as regenerating nodules (which can represent significant diagnostic dilemmas on conventional imaging), focal nodular hyperplasia, adenomas, cysts, and cavernous hemangiomas do not result in increased uptake of FDG (except in rare cases of abscesses with granulomatous inflammation). Therefore, in this case, the increased uptake of FDG is consistent with the diagnosis of hepatocellular carcinoma in a patient with elevated serum alpha-fetoprotein.

Diagnosis

Hepatocellular carcinoma accumulating FDG.

Case 6.6.2

History

A 69-year-old male who had a remote history of colorectal carcinoma and had undergone a partial right hepatic lobectomy for hepatocellular carcinoma one year earlier presented for reassessment. FDG PET imaging performed three years earlier for evaluation of suspected recurrent colorectal carcinoma was normal. A CT scan (Figure 6.6.2A) and FDG imaging (Figures 6.6.2B and C) were performed to assess recurrence. Selected transaxial CT

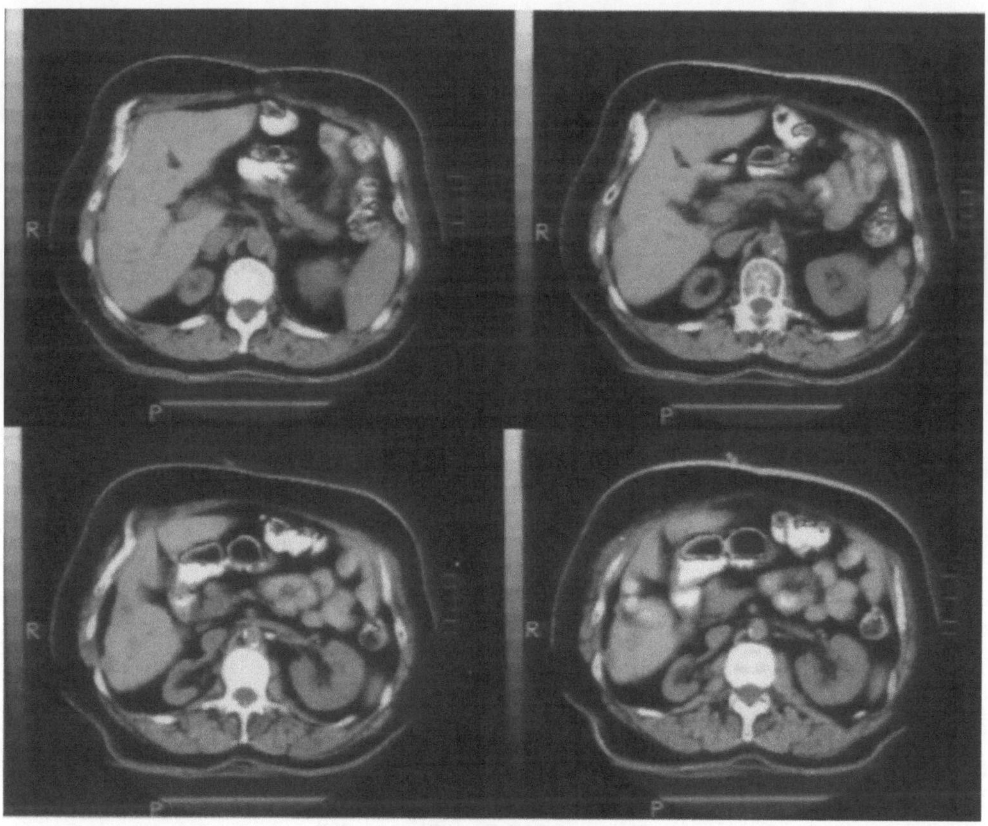

FIGURE 6.6.2A.

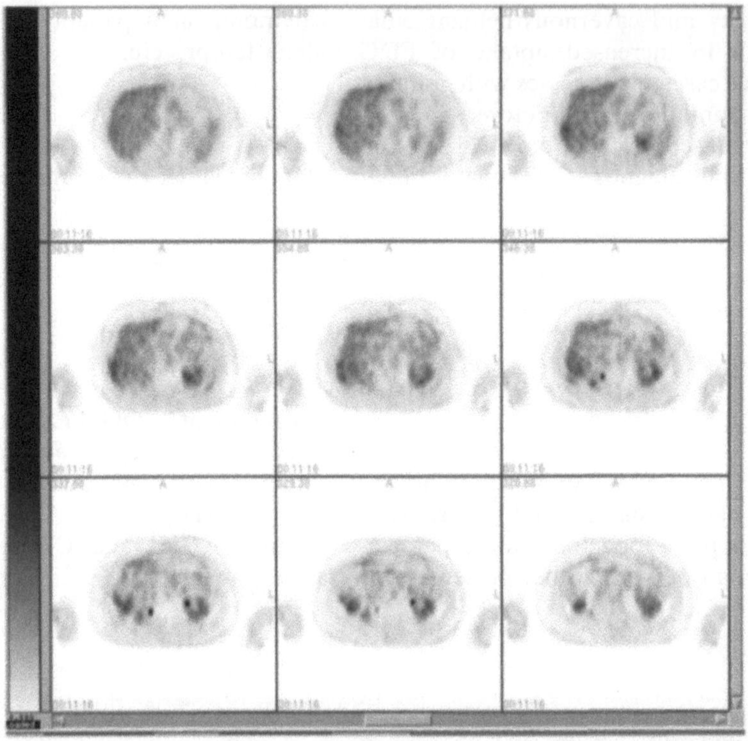

B

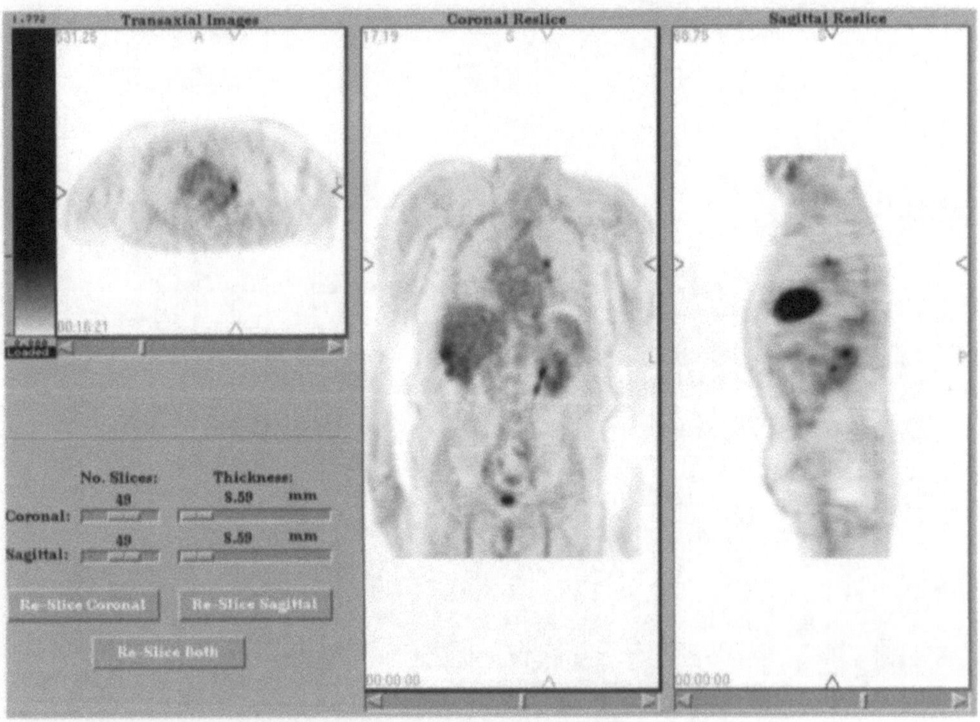

C

FIGURE 6.6.2B,C. (*Continued*)

(Figure 6.6.2A) and FDG PET (Figure 6.6.2B) images through the liver are shown, as well as transaxial, coronal, and sagittal FDG images through the mediastinum (Figure 6.6.2C). The FDG images were obtained with a dedicated PET tomograph (GE Advance) and reconstructed with iterative reconstruction and measured segmented attenuation correction.

Findings

The CT scan shows three low-density lesions at the periphery of the liver. The corresponding transaxial FDG PET images (Figure 6.6.2B) reveal increased uptake in the three hepatic lesions seen on CT. In addition, there is a focus of increased activity in the region of the left pulmonary hilum seen on the coronal images (Figure 6.6.2C). The foci of uptake in the liver and the left pulmonary hilum are new compared to the FDG PET scan performed three years before.

Discussion

The foci of hepatic uptake as well as the focus within the left pulmonary hilum are consistent with recurrent hepatocellular carcinoma at the periphery of the liver and a metastatic focus within the left pulmonary hilum. A subcentimeter lymph node was identified on a chest CT performed subsequently (Figure 6.6.2D), corresponding to the FDG-avid focus in the left pulmonary hilum.

The low attenuation lesions within the resection bed on the CT scan, although suspicious for recurrence, are by no means diagnostic. In general, benign lesions in the liver do not accumulate FDG at levels greater than normal liver background, therefore making the three lesions within the resection bed highly suspicious for recurrence of hepatocellular carcinoma. As discussed in Case 6.6.1, the accumulation of FDG in hepatocellular carcinoma is variable due to the differing amounts of glucose-6-phosphatase present. For the 50 to 70% of hepatocellular carcinomas that do accumulate FDG, FDG PET imaging is also valuable with regard to staging and monitoring therapy. Given that FDG PET images can be obtained over a large portion of the body without additional radiation exposure to the patient, unsuspected metastasis can be identified that would preclude surgical management with curative intent in patients who have a solitary liver tumor. In this particular case, a metastasis was found in the left pulmonary hilum, which precludes regional therapy to the liver. The correspond-

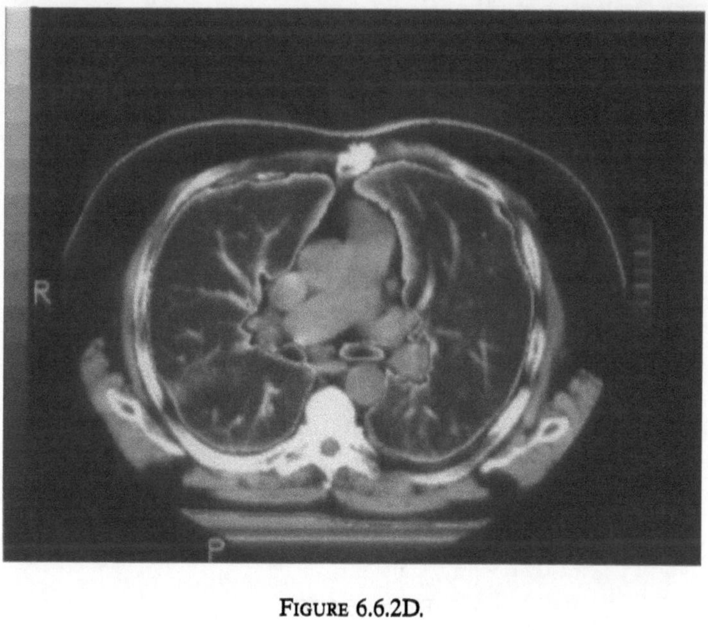

FIGURE 6.6.2D.

ing lymph node seen on the chest CT scan does not meet the size criteria for lymphadenopathy and therefore would not have been diagnosed as potentially malignant on CT alone. Although the impact of FDG PET imaging on management of patients with hepatocellular carcinoma has not been studied in a large series of patients, it has been demonstrated that FDG PET imaging can alter the management in up to 28% of patients evaluated for recurrent or metastatic colorectal carcinoma. The discovery of the previously unsuspected metastasis to the left pulmonary hilum has significant prognostic implications given that this represents a distant metastasis instead of a local recurrence.

Figures 6.6.2E and F illustrate the value of FDG PET imaging in another patient with hepatocellular carcinoma. This 71-year-old patient was treated with left hepatectomy four years ago and left hip surgery for a pathological fracture of the femur due to a metastasis one year ago. She presented with recurrence at the margin of resection of the liver diagnosed on CT. Figures 6.6.2E and F show coronal and orthogonal FDG images through the spine acquired with a dedicated PET tomograph (GE Advance) and reconstructed with iterative reconstruction and attenuation correction. The coronal images demonstrate the large area of uptake in the region of the caudate lobe of the liver, corresponding to the known recurrence, and also a small focus of uptake in the upper thoracic spine (better localized on the orthogonal images), indicating another bone metastasis. This finding spared the patient another surgical intervention to the liver. FDG uptake is also seen surrounding the left proxi-

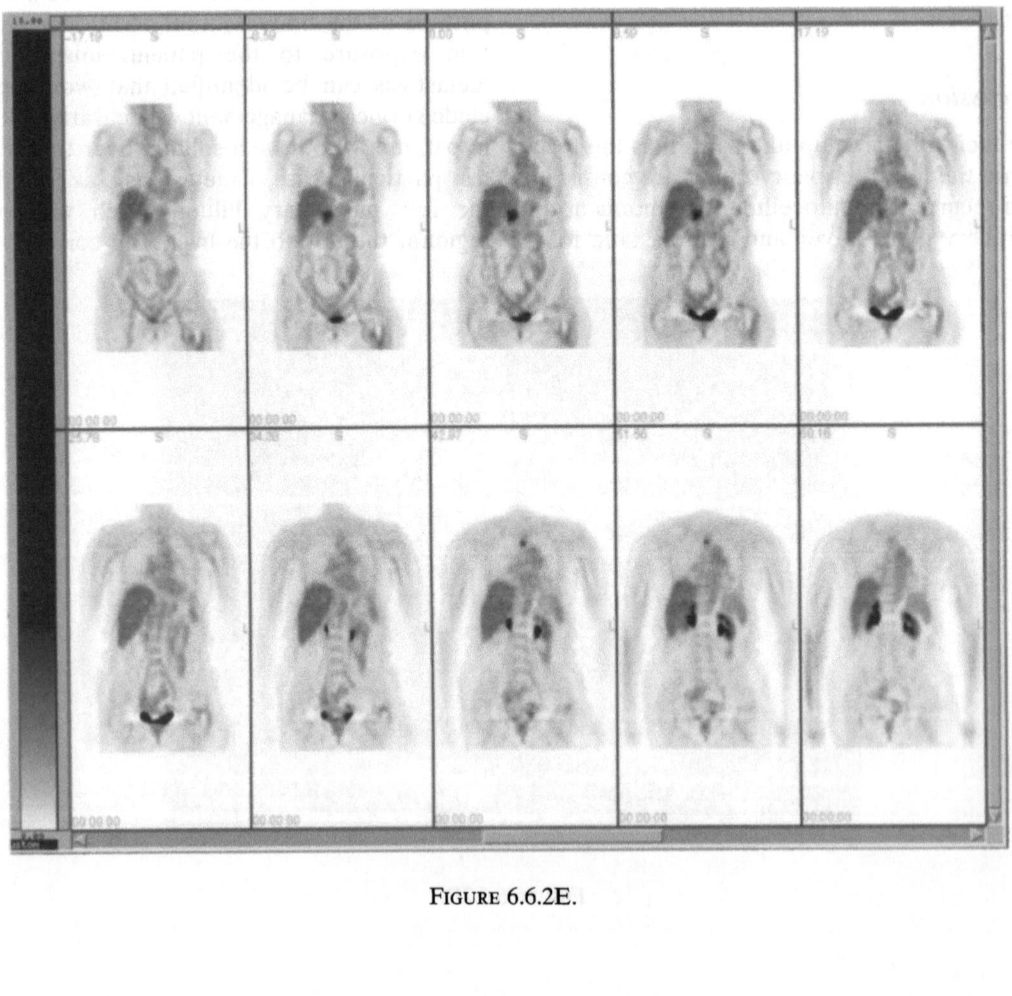

FIGURE 6.6.2E.

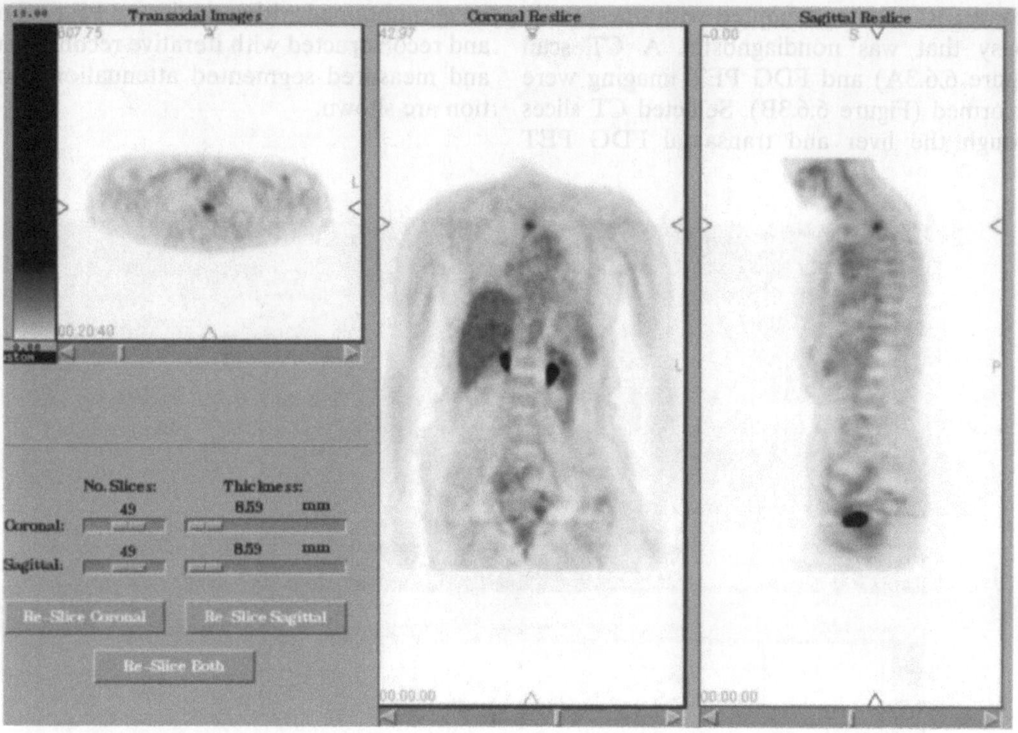

FIGURE 6.6.2F.

mal femur, probably due to inflammatory changes secondary to rod placement (see Case 6.1.3).

Patients with hepatocellular carcinoma can often not tolerate surgical treatment with hepatectomy because of underlying hepatic disease and limited hepatic reserve. Therefore, many of these patients are treated with regional transarterial chemoembolization. The assessment of the presence of residual tumor is problematic with CT, and FDG PET imaging is a promising alternative to monitor treatment of these patients, allowing for identification and guiding further therapy of recurrent or persistent foci of tumors.

Diagnoses

1. Recurrent hepatocellular carcinoma to the liver.
2. Unsuspected metastasis to the left pulmonary hilum.

Case 6.6.3

History

A 57-year-old male presented with jaundice and epigastric pain. An ERCP demonstrated choledocholithiasis that was treated with sphincterotomy. A biliary stent was placed, which did not relieve hyperbilirubinemia. A Whipple procedure was attempted at another institution and was aborted secondary to inflammatory change within the pancreas. A second ERCP was attempted with fine-needle biopsy that was nondiagnostic. A CT scan (Figure 6.6.3A) and FDG PET imaging were performed (Figure 6.6.3B). Selected CT slices through the liver and transaxial FDG PET images obtained with a dedicated PET scanner and reconstructed with iterative reconstruction and measured segmented attenuation correction are shown.

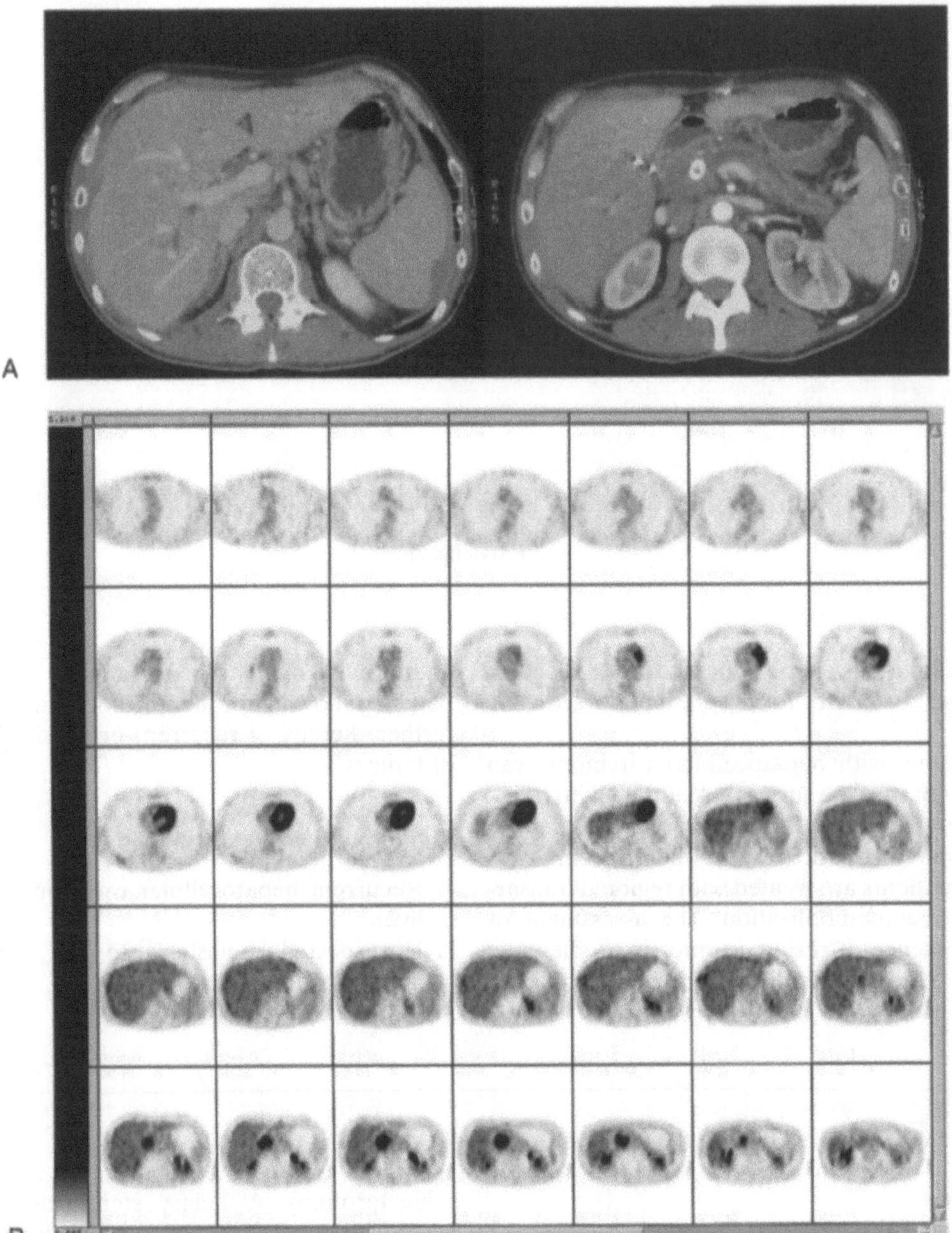

FIGURE 6.6.3A,B.

Findings

The CT images reveal a partially necrotic region in the head of the pancreas that is suggestive of malignancy, although the possibility of chronic pancreatitis is also a consideration (Figure 6.6.3A right).

The FDG PET images reveal markedly increased uptake anterior and medial to the right kidney corresponding to the pancreatic head on CT (Figure 6.6.3B, last row of images). A second focus of uptake is noted adjacent to the surface of the right lobe of the liver, which could retrospectively be identified on the CT scan as a serosal low density on the lateral surface of the liver (Figure 6.6.3A left).

Discussion

These findings are consistent with a carcinoma of the head of the pancreas accompanied by a serosal metastasis on the liver. The patient underwent a Whipple procedure, and tissue obtained at surgery confirmed well-differentiated adenocarcinoma in both locations.

This case demonstrates the difficulty of arriving at a preoperative diagnosis that can be encountered in the setting of possible pancreatic neoplasm. This patient had undergone the typical work-up for evaluation of pancreatic neoplasm, including multiple ERCPs and CTs and even laparotomy without arriving at a final diagnosis. CT has been shown to have an accuracy of 70% in the diagnosis of pancreatic cancer and a positive predictive value of nonresectability of 90%. The diagnosis can be difficult in mass-forming pancreatitis and in cases of enlargement of the pancreatic head without definite signs of malignancy.

ERCP is the other means of evaluating the pancreas and has an accuracy of 80 to 90% in differentiating benign from malignant masses. There is approximately a 10% technical failure rate and up to 8% morbidity (iatrogenic pancreatitis, primarily). Fine-needle biopsy can be performed, although it can result in significant sampling error.

FDG PET imaging has a sensitivity of 85 to 100%, specificity of 67 to 99%, and accuracy of 85 to 93% in several reported series for the preoperative diagnosis of pancreatic carcinoma. FDG imaging is particularly useful in determining the presence of metastatic disease, which can significantly alter surgical management. In one study, surgical management was altered in up to 41% of patients that underwent FDG PET imaging in addition to CT scanning, two-thirds of this group by identifying pancreatic carcinoma preoperatively and one-third of this group by identifying unsuspected metastasis or confirming the benign nature of lesions that were equivocal on CT. Patients with high SUV values within tumors have also been shown to have a significantly shorter survival time. It may be possible to exclude neoplasm in patients with chronic pancreatitis in up to 84 to 100% of those that present with a pancreatic mass.

Figures 6.6.3C and D illustrate the value of FDG PET imaging in another patient who presented with obstructive jaundice and a normal CT scan of the abdomen, other than a stent seen in the pancreatic duct (Figure 6.6.3C). An ERCP allowed placement of the biliary stent but was otherwise nondiagnostic. Figure 6.6.3D shows transaxial FDG PET images acquired with a dedicated PET tomograph (GE Advance) and reconstructed with iterative reconstruction and attenuation correction. A focus of uptake is identified anterior and medial to the upper pole of the right kidney and corresponds to the head of the pancreas on CT. This finding was indicative of a malignant lesion in the pancreas, and there was no evidence of distant metastases. An endoscopic ultrasound demonstrated a 2.6 cm hypoechoic mass in the head of the pancreas, and a biopsy revealed adenocarcinoma.

Limitations of FDG PET imaging are seen with respect to false-negative findings in patients with glucose intolerance and tumors smaller in size than twice the resolution of the PET system used for acquiring the images (less than 1 cm). False-positive findings can be seen in patients with acute inflammatory disease in the abdomen. These patients frequently have

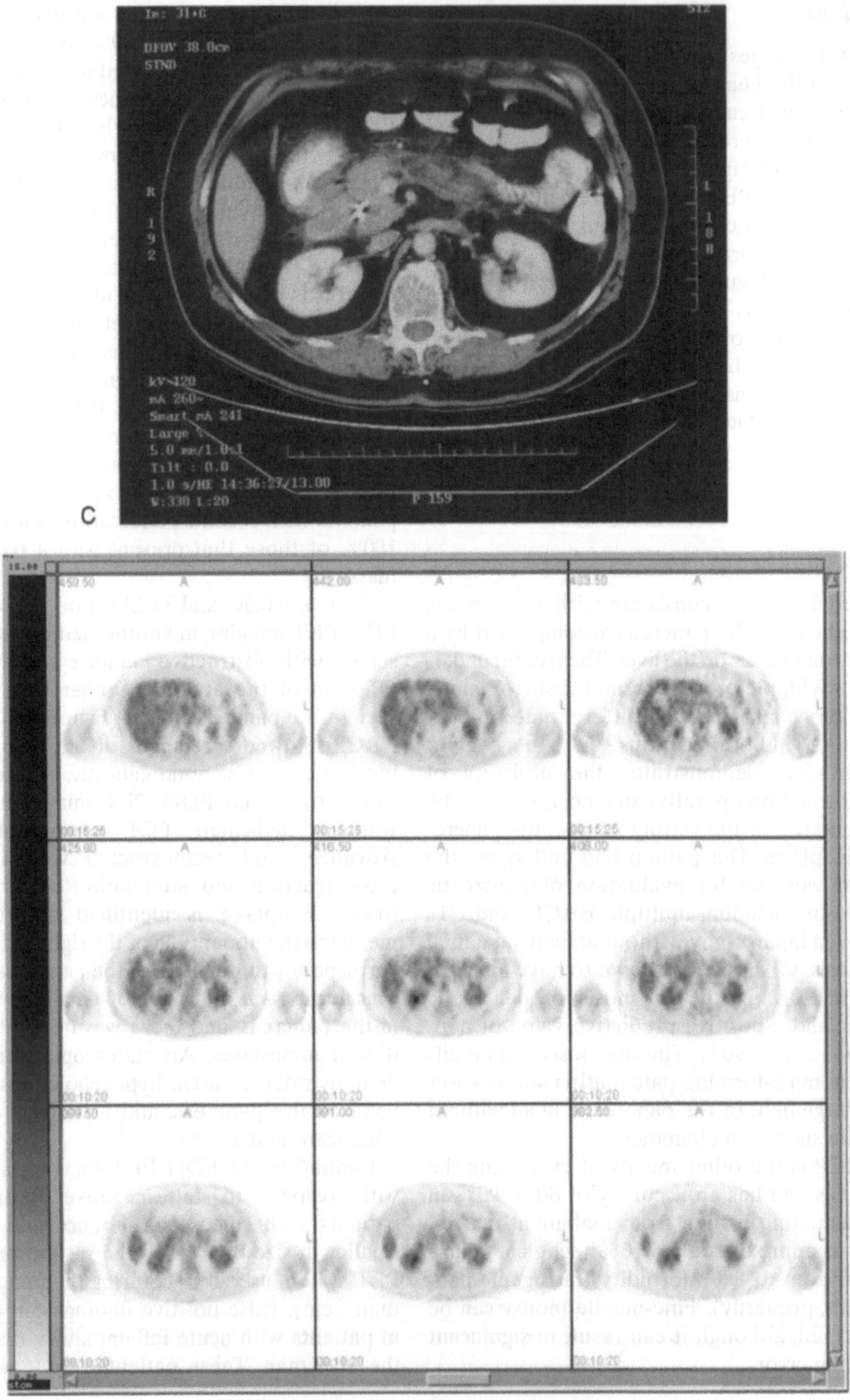

FIGURE 6.6.3C,D.

elevated C-reactive protein. Therefore, FDG PET scans in patients with elevated serum levels of C-reactive protein should be interpreted with care.

Diagnoses

1. Pancreatic carcinoma.
2. Unsuspected serosal metastasis to the liver.

Case 6.6.4

History

A 57-year-old male presented for FDG PET imaging with a history of poorly differentiated adenocarcinoma of the distal esophagus (stage T2). Prior to presentation, the patient had undergone neoadjuvant chemoradiation therapy and was being considered for surgical resection. CT (Figure 6.6.4A) and FDG PET imaging were performed for preoperative staging. Coronal and orthogonal FDG PET images acquired with a dedicated PET tomograph (GE Advance) and reconstructed with iterative reconstruction and measured segmented attenuation correction are shown in Figures 6.6.4B and C, respectively.

Findings

The CT images reveal thickening of the distal esophagus corresponding to the known primary tumor. There is also an indeterminate 8 mm nodule in the right upper lobe of the lung that would preclude surgical therapy if it represented a metastasis.

The FDG PET images reveal increased uptake along the distal esophagus, correlating with the region of the patient's known primary esophageal carcinoma. No abnormal uptake is seen in the right upper lobe of the lung.

Discussion

The absence of FDG uptake in the pulmonary nodule is indicative of a benign lesion. The negative predictive value of FDG PET imaging for pulmonary nodules larger than 1 cm is 95%. However, the size of the nodule in this patient is at the limit of the resolution of the PET technique. A PET tomograph with an intrinsic resolution of 5 mm full-width half maximum has a reconstructed image resolution of approximately 8 mm. Lesions that have less than twice the resolution of the imaging technique suffer from partial volume averaging artifact, meaning that the lesion will be blurred and the degree of uptake will appear decreased

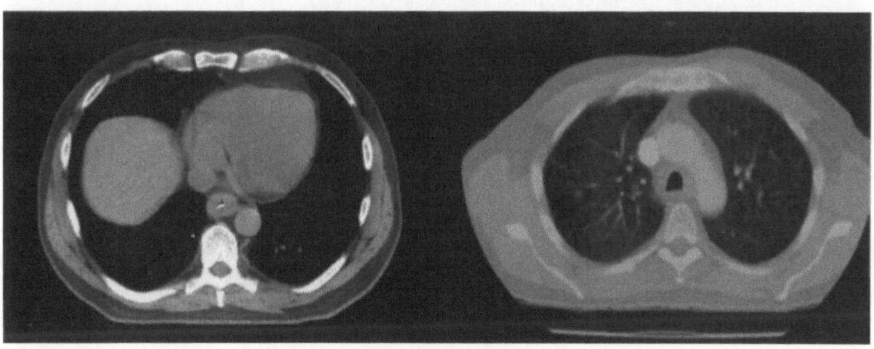

FIGURE 6.6.4A.

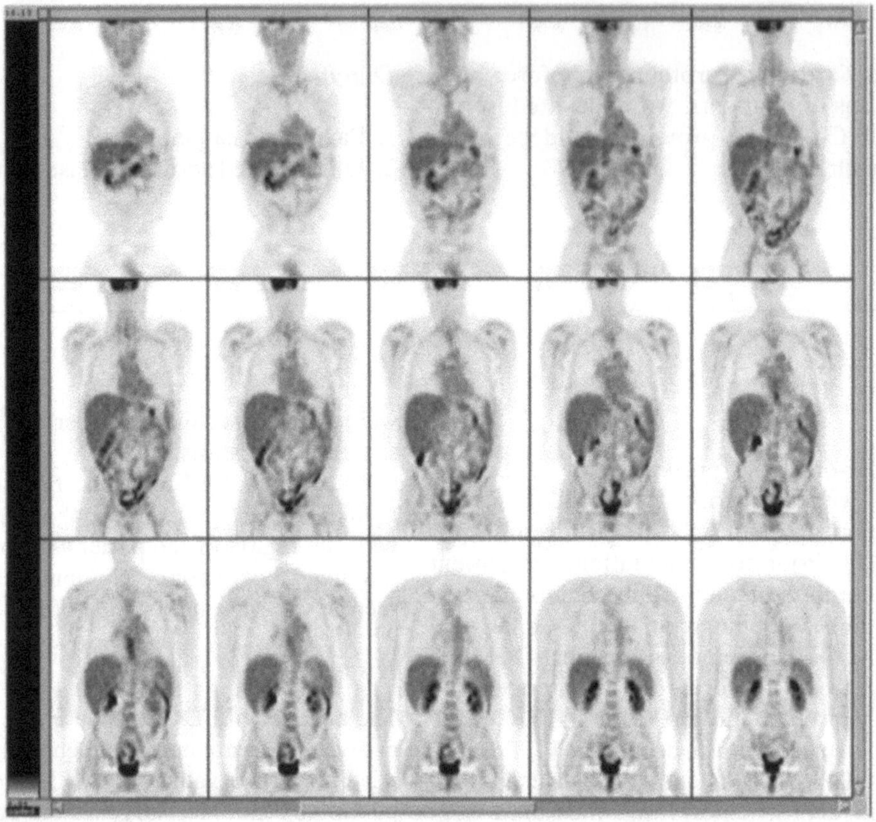

B

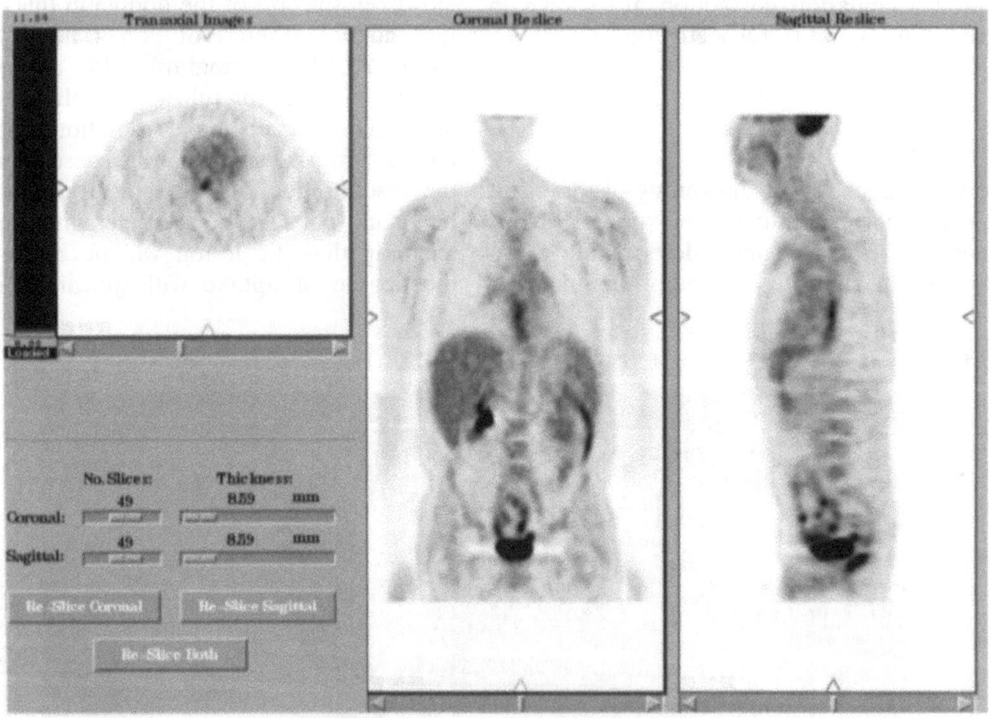

C

FIGURE 6.6.4B,C. (*Continued*)

compared to the actual degree of uptake. Therefore, in this patient, the pulmonary nodule is likely benign, but the negative predictive value is probably less than 95%.

This case demonstrates the value of preoperative FDG PET imaging in the evaluation of esophageal carcinoma. FDG PET is more sensitive than CT at detecting distant metastasis and at least as sensitive as CT in detecting regional metastasis. This is of critical importance since approximately 20% of patients with esophageal cancer being considered for surgical therapy have distant metastases. FDG PET also demonstrates the primary tumor in the vast majority of patients. Both CT and PET are limited by their inability to determine the depth of wall invasion. However, endoscopic ultrasound is a promising new modality in this regard. When FDG PET is performed in addition to CT, ill-advised surgery may be decreased by 90%. PET may play a role in differentiating responders from nonresponders after chemotherapy as well.

Diagnoses

1. Distal esophageal carcinoma without evidence of distant metastases.
2. Probably benign pulmonary nodule; a repeat CT is recommended in six months.

Case 6.6.5

History

A 51-year-old male presented with a complex medical history including adenocarcinoma of the distal esophagus six years prior, which was treated with esophagectomy and gastric pull-through followed by chemotherapy. Two years later the patient underwent a left lower lobe lung resection for adenocarcinoma. A CT scan of the chest and abdomen were performed for follow-up (Figures 6.6.5A and B), and the findings on CT scan triggered the performance of FDG PET imaging. Coronal FDG PET images acquired with a dedicated PET tomograph and reconstructed with iterative reconstruction and measured segmented attenuation correction are shown in Figure 6.6.5C.

Findings

The CT images demonstrate a 1 cm nodule in the apex of the left lung, and on the abdominal CT, there is a 2 cm lesion in the inferior aspect of the right lobe of the liver.

The FDG PET images reveal increased FDG uptake in the left lung nodule seen on CT. Increased FDG uptake is also noted in the anterior chest wall on the right. The hepatic lesion seen on CT did not demonstrate FDG uptake.

Discussion

These findings suggest a pulmonary metastasis at the left apex and a benign hepatic lesion. Both the lung and hepatic lesions were biopsied. The hepatic lesion was benign, and the lung nodule was positive for metastatic adenocarcinoma. The patient reported a traumatic injury two weeks prior, and retrospective review of a chest radiograph reveals a healing right anterolateral rib fracture (Figure 6.6.5D). Therefore, the chest wall lesion seen on PET can be explained by a healing rib fracture.

This case demonstrates the value of preoperative FDG PET in the evaluation of suspected metastatic esophageal carcinoma. As discussed in Case 6.6.4, FDG PET is more sensitive than CT at detecting distant metastasis. In this patient with a history of previous lung resection for adenocarcinoma, FDG uptake in the lung nodule favors a metastasis. The patient was a candidate for resection of the left apical lung nodule in the absence of other metastases, and

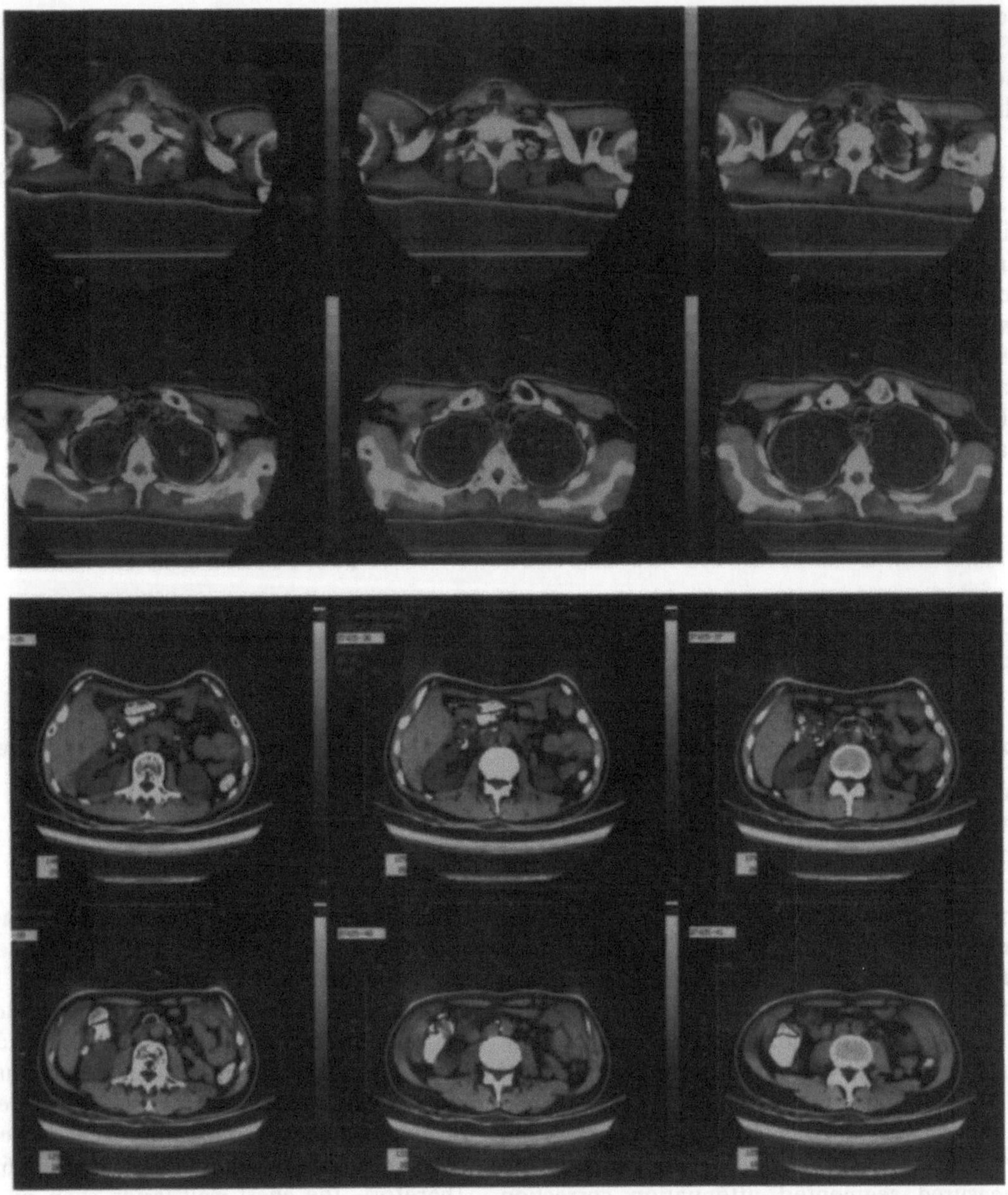

A

B

FIGURE 6.6.5A,B.

therefore, characterization of the 2 cm hepatic lesion became critical.

FDG PET is useful in the characterization of equivocal hepatic lesions, especially in patients with known primary tumors that accumulate FDG. For this population of patients, the most likely differential diagnosis includes benign hepatic lesions and metastases. Benign hepatic lesions, such as cysts, hemangiomas, adenomas, and focal nodular hyperplasia, do not accumulate FDG, and metastases do accumulate FDG. Therefore, the absence of uptake in the hepatic

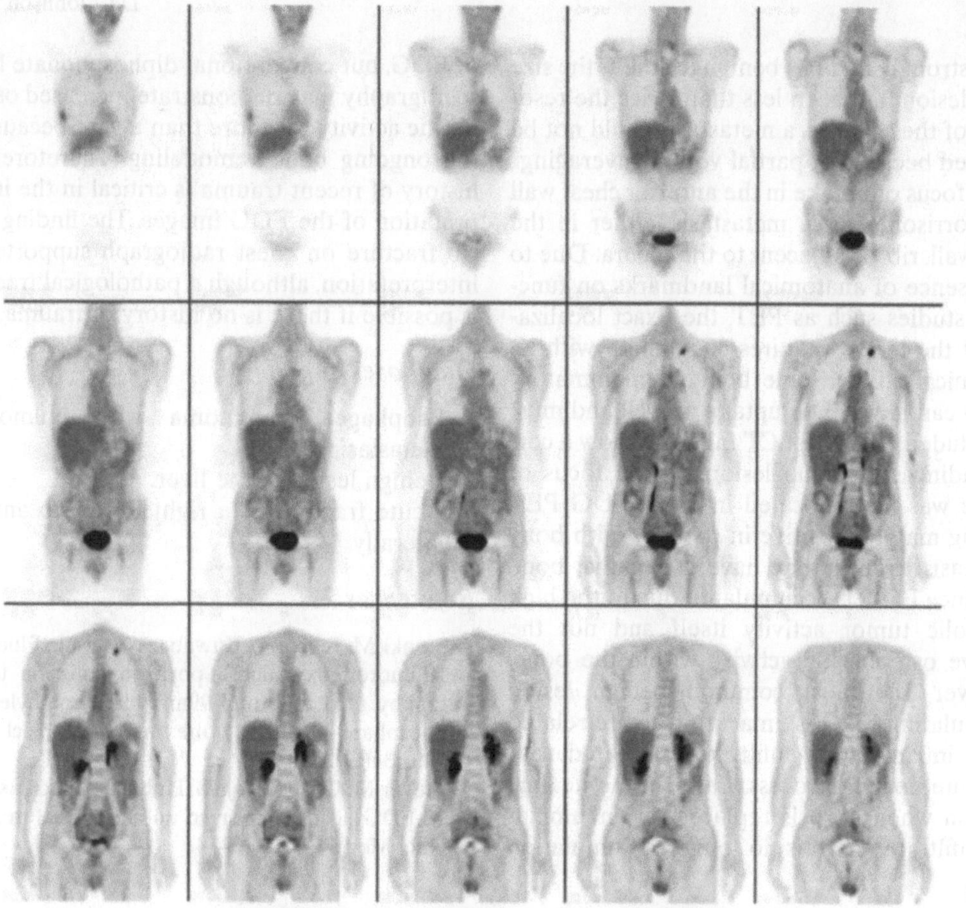

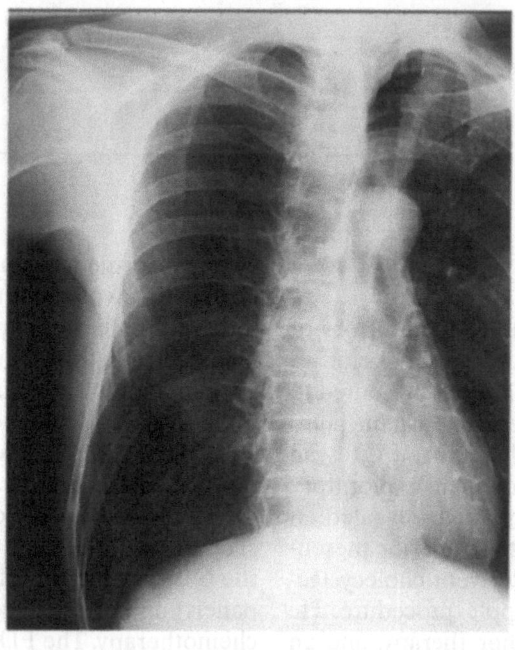

FIGURE 6.6.5C,D.

lesion strongly favors a benign lesion. If the size of the lesion had been less than twice the resolution of the scanner, a metastasis could not be excluded because of partial volume averaging.

The focus of uptake in the anterior chest wall was worrisome for a metastasis, either in the chest wall, rib, or adjacent to the pleura. Due to the absence of anatomical landmarks on functional studies such as PET, the exact localization of the lesion requires correlation with an anatomical study. Some benign inflammatory lesions can have FDG uptake as well and must be excluded. The chest CT failed to show a corresponding soft tissue lesion, so the focus of uptake was likely located in a rib. FDG PET imaging may be positive in patients with bony metastasis even if they have a negative bone scan since FDG is accumulated due to the high metabolic tumor activity itself and not the reactive osteoblastic activity within the bone. However, the most common benign lesion accumulating FDG is an acute fracture related to the inflammatory infiltrate associated with the acute healing process. Later in the healing reaction when fibrosis replaces the inflammatory infiltrate, there is no longer accumulation of FDG, but conventional diphosphonate bone scintigraphy may demonstrate increased osteoblastic activity for more than a year because of the ongoing bone remodeling. Therefore, the history of recent trauma is critical in the interpretation of the FDG images. The finding of a rib fracture on chest radiograph supports the interpretation, although a pathological fracture is possible if there is no history of trauma.[1,2]

Diagnoses

1. Esophageal carcinoma with pulmonary metastasis.
2. Benign lesion in the liver.
3. Acute fracture of a right lower rib anterolaterally.

References

1. Sasaki M, Ichiya Y, Kuwabara Y, et al.: Fluorine-18-fluorodeoxyglucose positron emission tomography in technetium-99m-hydroxymethylenediphosphate negative bone tumors. J Nucl Med 1993;34(2):288–290.
2. Meyer M, Gast T, Raja S, Hubner K: Increased F-18-FDG accumulation in an acute fracture. Clin Nucl Med 1994;19:13–14.

Case 6.6.6

History

A 62-year-old male presented with a history of pancreatic carcinoma. Four months prior to presenting for imaging, the patient presented to an outside institution with epigastric pain, jaundice, and weight loss. At that time, a CT scan revealed a pancreatic mass. An exploratory laparotomy was performed which revealed an adenocarcinoma encasing the superior mesenteric vein. The patient underwent cholecystectomy and a modified Whipple procedure. He was then referred for further therapy, and an abdominal CT scan and FDG PET imaging were performed (Figure 6.6.6, upper panels). Given the involvement of the superior mesenteric vein, palliative chemotherapy began which included radiation therapy and chemotherapy. Three months later, after completion of the radiation and chemotherapy, a follow-up abdominal CT scan and FDG imaging were performed (Figure 6.6.6, lower panels). Figure 6.6.6 shows a selected corresponding transaxial slice through the head of the pancreas on both the CT scan and the FDG image before (upper panels) and after (lower panels) radiation and chemotherapy. The FDG images were acquired with a dedicated PET tomograph (ECAT 933)

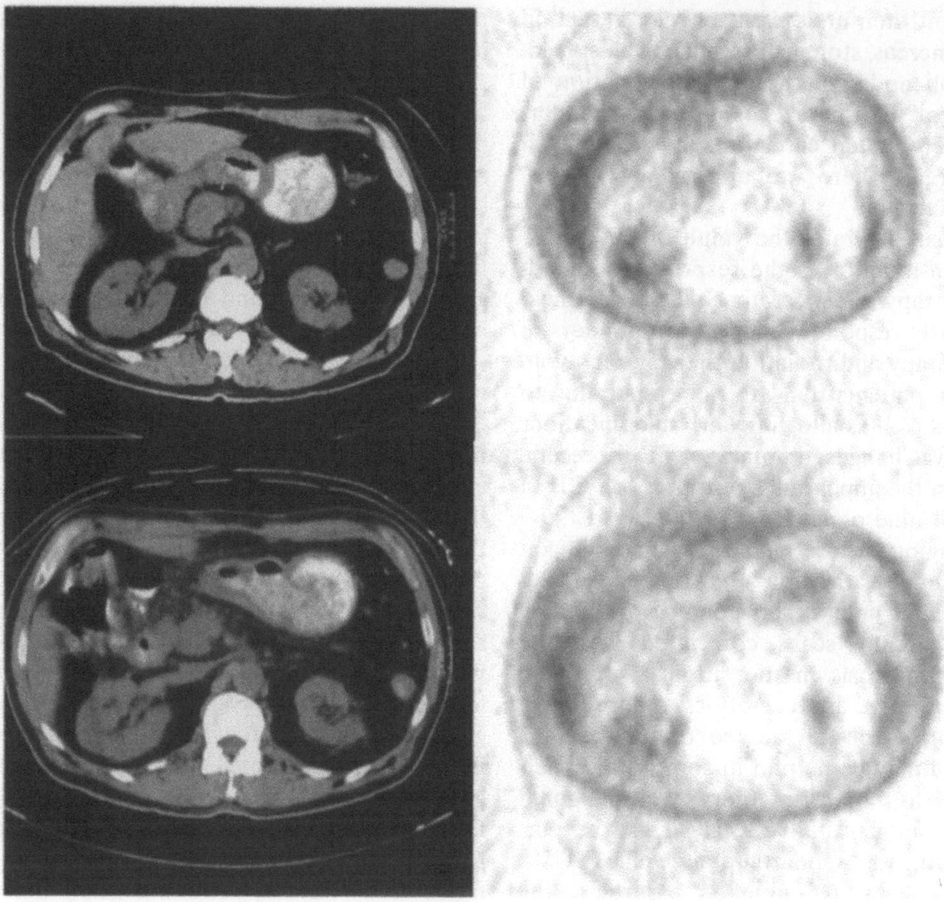

FIGURE 6.6.6.

and reconstructed with filtered back projection without attenuation correction.

Findings

The pretherapy FDG PET image (upper right) reveals increased uptake within the pancreatic mass identified on pretherapy CT scan (upper left). The activity within the pancreatic head had an SUV value measured on the FDG images reconstructed with attenuation correction of 3.3. The CT scan also revealed a hyperdense lesion at the anterior periphery of the right lobe of the liver that was suggestive of a cavernous hemangioma (not shown). The PET scan did not reveal any abnormality in this region.

The follow-up posttherapy CT scan (lower left) reveals a persistent mass in the head of the pancreas, which has not changed significantly in size or appearance. The posttherapy FDG PET image (lower right) reveals no abnormal uptake in the head of the pancreas or elsewhere.

Discussion

The FDG uptake in the head of the pancreas on the pretherapy images confirms the presence of residual tumor after the palliative surgical procedure performed at the time of diagnosis. The absence of FDG uptake after completion of the neoadjuvant chemoradiation therapy indicates a good response to therapy.

The patient then underwent en bloc resection of the pancreas, stomach, small bowel, spleen, and lymph nodes. Pathologic examination of the surgical specimen revealed a 5 cm moderately differentiated carcinoma in the head of the pancreas. There was approximately 80% tumor necrosis.

This case illustrates the value of FDG PET imaging in monitoring the response to neoadjuvant therapy in pancreatic cancer. Identification of early responders and nonresponders to chemotherapy and radiation therapy can avoid toxicity in patients that are not responding to therapy as well as allowing early modifications to therapy. Changes in uptake of FDG precede changes in the appearance of tumors on CT. In a study of nine patients who underwent FDG PET imaging before and after neoadjuvant chemoradiation therapy, the degree of decreased FDG uptake between the pretherapy and posttherapy scans correlated with the degree of necrosis in the surgical specimen. Semiquantitative analysis offers a more objective reporting of the degree of uptake in a lesion and may be helpful in some clinical settings, such as monitoring therapy of malignant lesions. Semiquantitative analysis can be performed using the standard uptake value (SUV).

The degree of FDG uptake measured by the SUV may also have value in predicting survival of patients with pancreatic cancer. Patients with an SUV value of less than 3.0 may have a slight survival advantage. In one study consisting of 14 patients, those with an SUV of greater than 3.0 had a mean survival of 5 months, whereas those with an SUV of less than 3.0 had a survival of 14 months. Another study of 26 patients reports similar findings using a cutoff level of 6.0 for the SUV.

The absence of FDG uptake in the hepatic lesion, in a population of patients with a low incidence of hepatocellular carcinoma, is indicative of a benign lesion. The most common benign lesions in the liver are cysts that can be characterized by ultrasonography if they are larger than 1 cm in size. Cavernous hemangiomas are the second most common benign hepatic lesions. They can be characterized with ^{99m}Tc-labeled red blood cell imaging, T_2-weighted MRI imaging, or delayed contrast-enhanced CT or MRI imaging. ^{99m}Tc-labeled red blood cell imaging is the least expensive alternative and is accurate for lesions larger than 2 cm. If FDG PET imaging is performed, the absence of increased FDG uptake above physiologic hepatic background is compatible with a cavernous hemangioma. In a published series of over 100 patients with hepatic lesions who underwent FDG PET imaging, all benign lesions (including cysts, cavernous hemangiomas, adenomas, focal nodular hyperplasia, hematoma, hamartoma, and remote postsurgical sites) had FDG uptake below or at the level of physiologic uptake in the normal hepatic parenchyma, with the exception of granulomatous lesions, including granulomatous abscesses and occasional postoperative active granulomas.

Diagnoses

1. Pancreatic carcinoma with a good response to neoadjuvant chemoradiation therapy.
2. Benign hepatic lesion.

Case 6.6.7

History

The same patient as in Case 6.6.6 with known pancreatic adenocarcinoma presented four years later for follow-up FDG PET imaging. The patient had been in remission for three years without evidence of disease until the development of a solitary liver metastasis one year ago treated with ongoing chemotherapy. He was referred for CT (Figure 6.6.7A) and FDG PET imaging. Figure 6.6.7B shows coronal FDG PET images acquired with a dedicated PET tomograph (GE Advance) and reconstructed with iterative reconstruction and measured segmented attenuation correction.

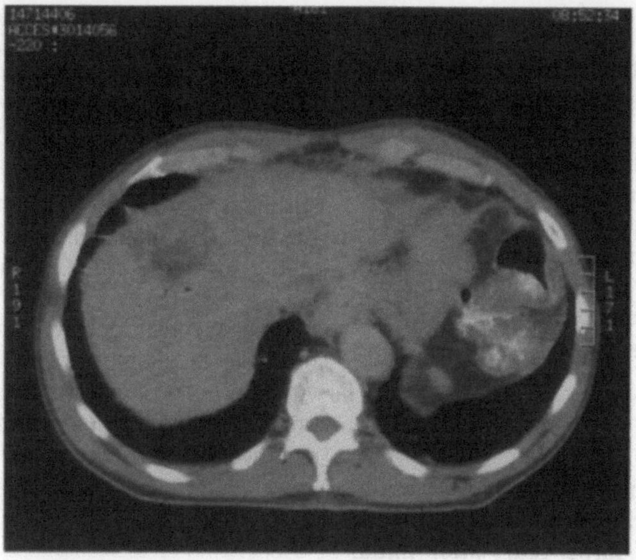

A

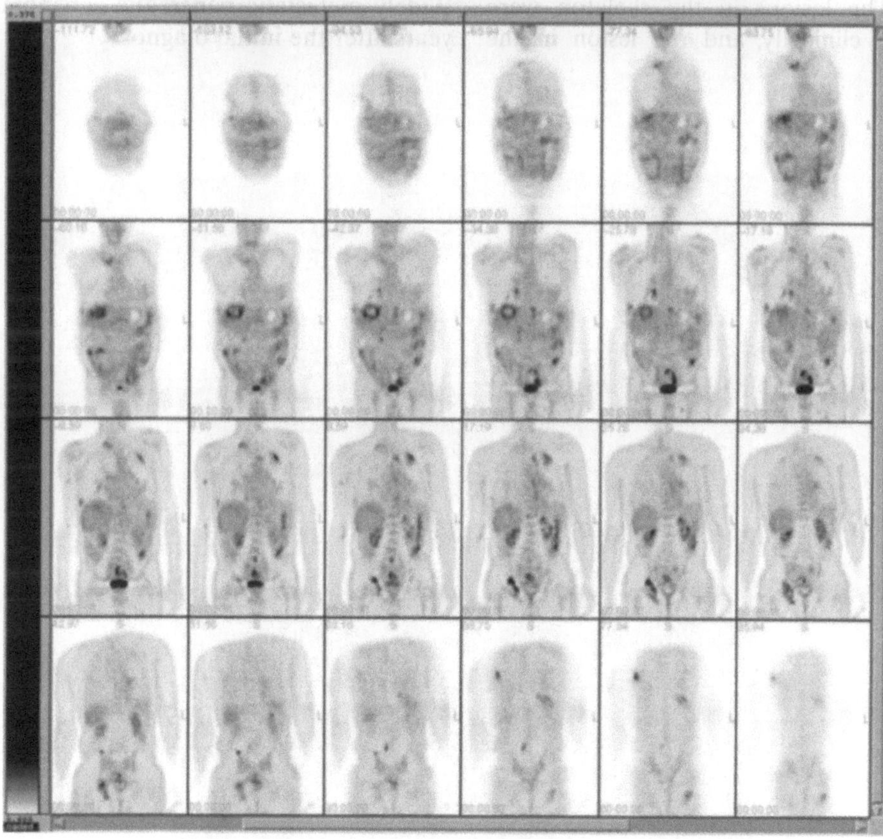

B

FIGURE 6.6.7A,B.

Findings

The CT image shows the known hepatic lesion. The FDG PET images reveal multiple metastatic foci involving the liver, right ischium, right clavicle, ribs, right humerus, and multiple foci throughout the spine. Multiple areas of increased uptake within the abdomen were felt to represent abdominal nodal spread. The lesion in the liver has a photopenic center surrounded by a rim of markedly increased FDG uptake. This indicates central necrosis with a rim of viable tumor.

Discussion

This patient demonstrated a good initial response to therapy; unfortunately, the disease recurred in the liver three years after initial diagnosis. The lesions in the skeleton were unsuspected clinically, and the lesion in the right ischium was confirmed by plain radiograph (Figure 6.6.7C). The patient received focused radiation therapy to the areas of painful bony metastasis.

Pancreatic carcinoma is associated with a poor prognosis, with nearly all patients dying within two years after the initial diagnosis. At the time of diagnosis, the degree of uptake in the primary tumor of this patient was not very severe (SUV = 3.3), and this patient had a long survival despite vascular invasion at the time of diagnosis. This illustrates the previous reports suggesting that the degree of uptake in the primary tumor has prognostic significance.

Diagnosis

Widely metastatic pancreatic carcinoma, four years after the initial diagnosis.

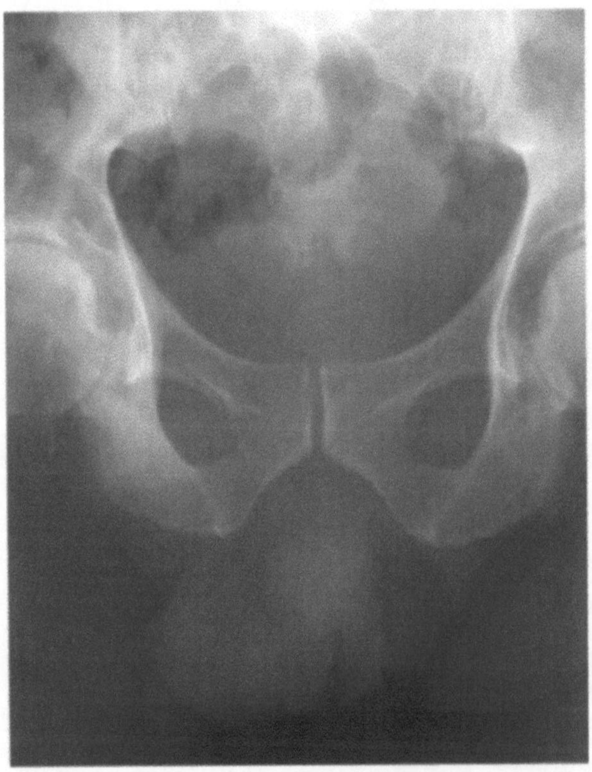

FIGURE 6.6.7C.

Case 6.6.8

History

A 64-year-old male with a history of poorly differentiated gastric adenocarcinoma presented for FDG PET imaging for evaluation of pulmonary nodules seen on CT. The patient's malignancy was discovered during preoperative evaluation for knee arthroplasty when profound microcytic anemia was noted. Subsequent esophagogastroduodenoscopy was performed which revealed multiple gastric polyps, one of which was malignant.

The FDG images were first acquired with a dedicated PET tomograph (ECAT 933) and reconstructed using filtered back projection without attenuation correction (Figure 6.6.8A). FDG images were then obtained with a hybrid dual-head gamma camera operating in the coincidence mode (VG Millenium). The hybrid FDG PET images were reconstructed using an iterative reconstruction algorithm and corrected for attenuation using attenuation maps obtained with an X-ray tube and array of detectors mounted on the gantry of the camera and functioning basically as a third-generation CT scanner. These attenuation maps also provide hybrid CT images for image fusion and anatomical mapping. Figure 6.6.8B, see color plate, shows a corresponding transaxial slice of the hybrid CT (left), hybrid PET (middle), and fusion image (right).

Findings

The FDG PET image reveals multiple foci of increased uptake within the posterior chest wall. This was felt to represent either pleural-based, chest wall, or rib metastasis.

The corresponding hybrid PET image (Figure 6.6.8B, middle) demonstrates the same foci of uptake, although the images are noisier. The fusion image (Figure 6.6.8B, right) clearly shows that the increased uptake seen on the FDG images corresponds to soft tissue nodules seen within the lung on the hybrid CT images.

Discussion

FDG uptake in the pulmonary nodules is indicative of pulmonary metastases. One of these was biopsied and proved to be adenocarcinoma. At the time of interpretation of the FDG PET images, the CT images were not

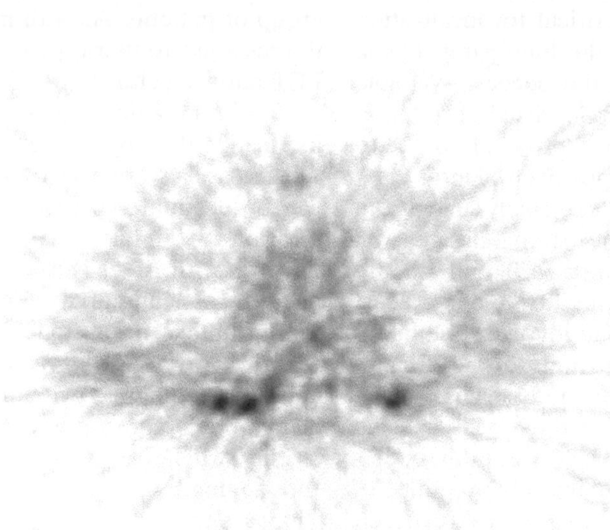

FIGURE 6.6.8A.

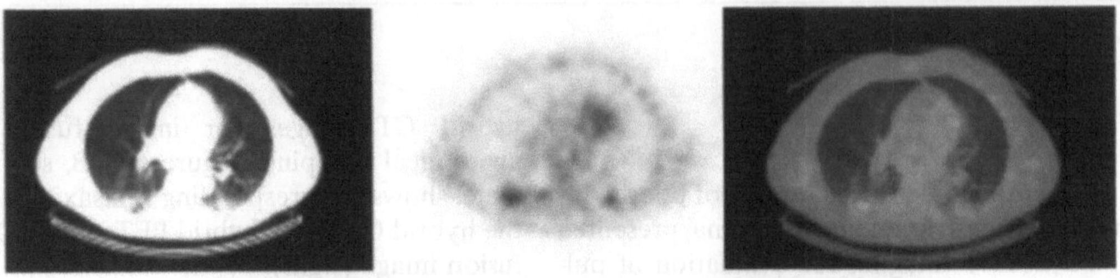

B

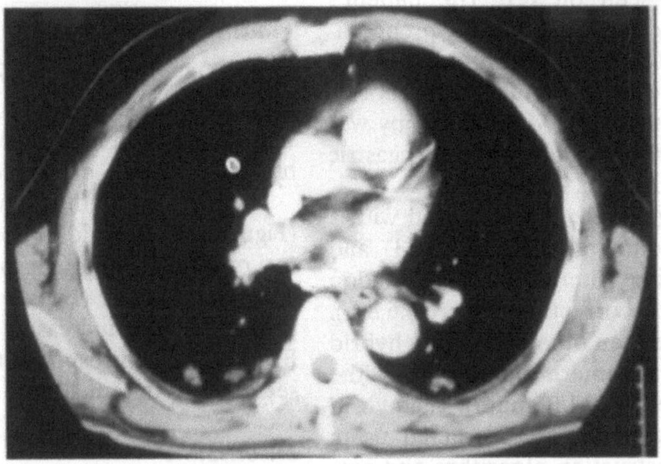

C

FIGURE 6.6.8B,C. (*Continued*) (See color plate)

available for review, and correlation with the hybrid CT images was critical for localization of the foci of uptake in the lung parenchyma. When the dedicated CT did become available for review (Figure 6.6.8C), visual correlation helped for localization of the foci of uptake to nodules adjacent to the posterior pleura.

FDG PET scanning is extremely sensitive in detecting primary gastric carcinomas as well as metastatic disease. Both PET and CT are somewhat limited in the ability to detect local extension and lymph node involvement, possibly secondary to the proximity of the primary tumor, but as for other body malignancies, whole-body FDG PET can detect unsuspected distant metastases. PET is crucial in preoperative evaluation, as approximately one-third of patients undergoing surgery will have occult metastasis. PET may be of even more value in patients who present with recurrence, as distant metastases are even more prevalent in this subgroup of patients. As with many other tumors, the response to therapy can be monitored with PET, allowing either early change to alternative chemotherapeutic regimens or cessation of ineffective therapy.

This case also demonstrates the difficulty that can be encountered in determining the exact location of uptake identified on metabolic imaging with FDG because of the absence of anatomical landmarks. The exact location of foci of uptake in or adjacent to the chest wall requires correlation with a CT scan. The hybrid system is equipped with an X-ray tube and array of detectors mounted on the same gantry as the two heads of the gamma camera and functioning as a third-generation CT scanner. This system allows acquisition of hybrid CT and hybrid PET images sequentially in time and provides fusion anatomical and metabolic images. However, it should be noted that the hybrid PET images are noisier than dedicated PET images, resulting in less sensitivity for the detection of small lesions (less than 15 mm), and the hybrid CT images do not approach the resolution of a modern dedicated CT scanner. Although fusion images certainly improve localization of abnormal hypermetabolic foci, visual correlation with concurrent CT images provides a comparable degree of accuracy in most instances.

Diagnosis

Gastric adenocarcinoma with pulmonary metastases.

Case 6.6.9

History

A 64-year-old male presented with epigastric pain and jaundice. A CT scan of the abdomen revealed biliary ductal dilatation, and an ERCP was subsequently performed with successful stenting of both the right and left hepatic ducts for symptomatic relief of the biliary obstruction. The CT scan of the abdomen is shown in Figure 6.6.9A. Figure 6.6.9B shows transaxial

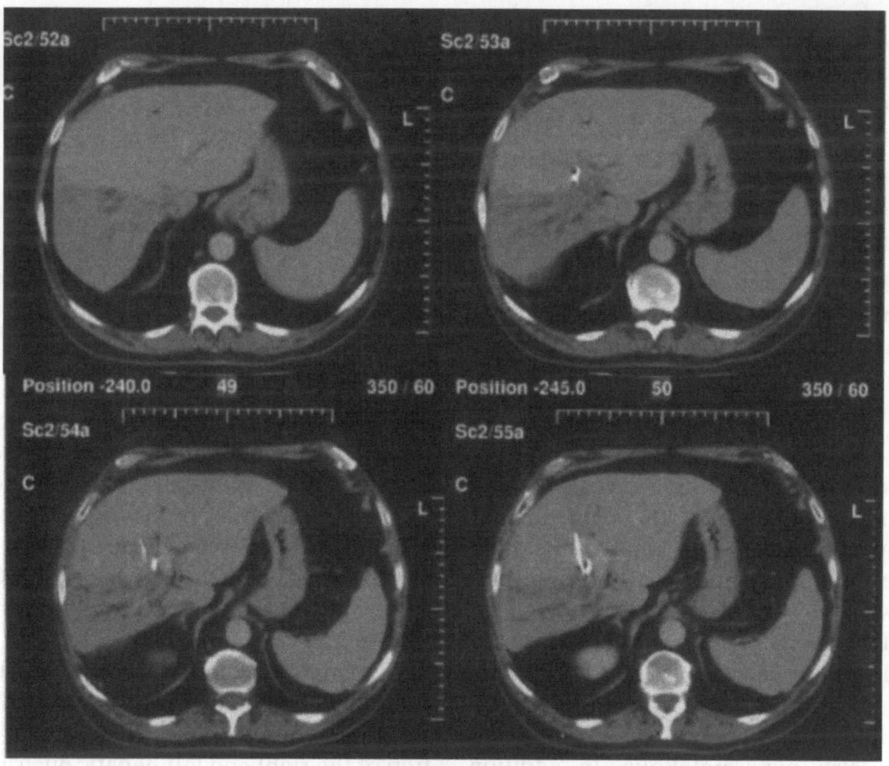

FIGURE 6.6.9A.

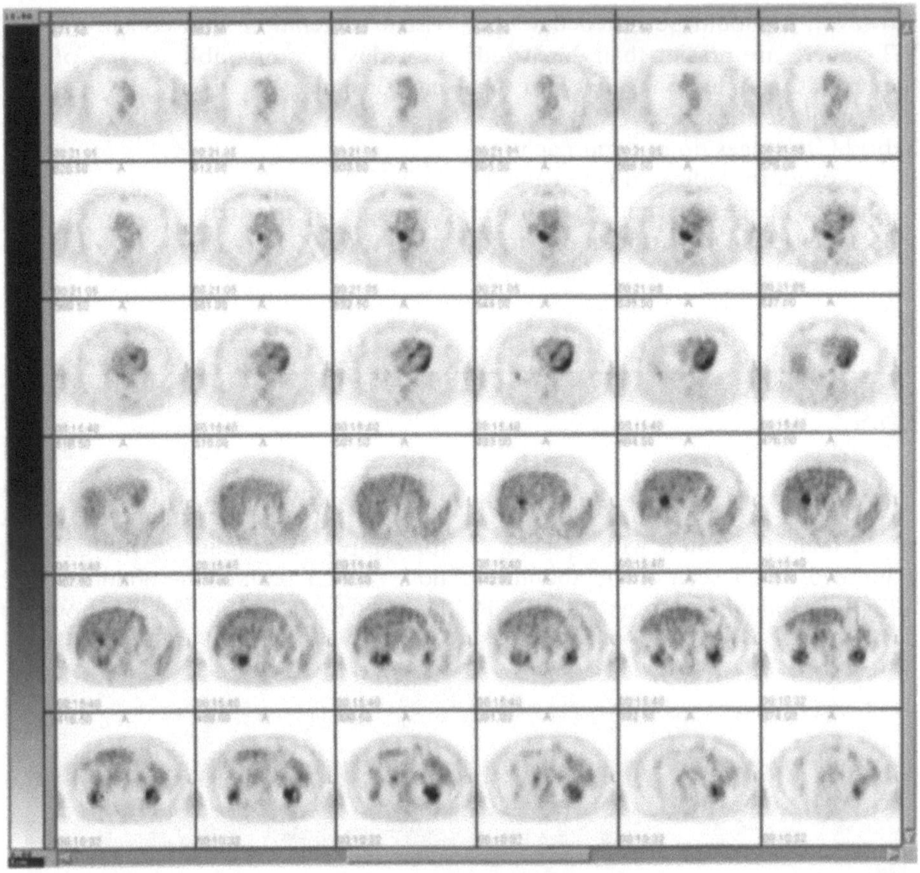

FIGURE 6.6.9B. (*Continued*)

FDG images acquired with a dedicated PET tomograph (GE Advance) and reconstructed with iterative reconstruction and measured segmented attenuation correction.

Findings

The CT scan of the abdomen reveals a subtle mass at the confluence of the right and left hepatic ducts (Figure 6.6.9A) and a small indeterminate pulmonary nodule at the right base (not shown).

The FDG images demonstrate a focus of increased uptake centrally in the liver at the expected location of the bifurcation of the common bile duct. The right basilar pulmonary nodule is also hypermetabolic. In addition, there is a large focus of uptake in the posterior mediastinum, not in the field of view of the abdominal CT.

Discussion

These findings are consistent with a malignant lesion in the liver at the confluence of the hepatic ducts (Klatskin's tumor) and a pulmonary metastasis at the right base. A subsequent chest CT scan (Figure 6.6.9C) revealed a subcarinal nodal mass as well as scar at the right base that demonstrated nodular thickening.

Cholangiocarcinomas are relatively rare tumors with 17,000 cases reported annually in the United States. Tumors that arise at the junction of the right and left hepatic ducts represent approximately 3,000 cases. Primary cholangio-

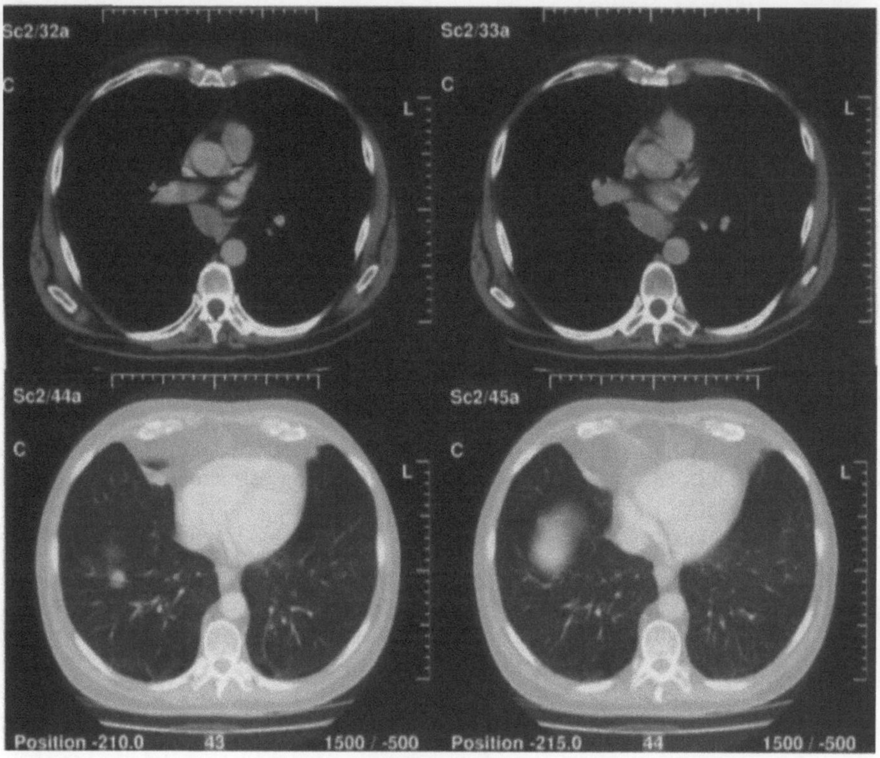

FIGURE 6.6.9C.

carcinomas arising at this location are known as hilar bile duct tumors or more commonly as Klatskin's tumors (Klatskin reported a large series of these patients in 1965). Risk factors for cholangiocarcinomas include sclerosing cholangitis, alpha-1 antitrypsin deficiency, ulcerative colitis, Caroli's disease, choledocal cyst, infestation by the fluke Clonorchis sinensis, cholelithiasis, exposure to Thorotrast, and others. One of five patients with cholangiocarcinomas has a predisposing factor. The majority of these tumors are unresectable at the time of presentation, although patients may survive for some time as these tumors tend to be slow growing.[1–3] Distant metastasis is reportedly relatively rare, although 50% of patients will have local lymph node metastases.

Diagnosis of hilar cholangiocarcinomas using CT or ultrasound can be difficult as the majority of these lesions are isodense. The point at which intrahepatic ductal dilatation begins or where hepatic atrophy can be identified can infer the extent of the tumor.[4–8] MRI can be helpful in some cases with a hypointense central scar identified on T2-weighted images in approximately 25 to 30% of cases.[9] Preliminary evidence exists that FDG PET imaging may be useful in the diagnosis and management of patients with small cholangiocarcinomas and in patients with sclerosing cholangitis.[10]

The FDG images in this patient demonstrate findings compatible with distant metastasis to the right lung base and the posterior mediastinum. The patient was being evaluated for a possible liver transplant prior to FDG imaging; the diagnosis by PET of distant metastases will dramatically alter these plans.

Diagnoses

1. Klatskin's cholangiocarcinoma.
2. Pulmonary and mediastinal metastases.

References

1. Childs T, Hart M: Aggressive surgical therapy for Klatskin tumors. Am J Surg 1993;165(5):554–557.
2. Lillemoe KD: Current status of surgery for Klatskin tumors. Curr Opin Gen Surg 1994;161–167.
3. Gerhards MF, van Gulik TM, Bosma A, et al.: Long-term survival after resection of proximal bile duct carcinoma (Klatskin tumors). World J Surg 1999;23(1):91–96.
4. Meyer DG, Weinstein BJ: Klatskin tumors of the bile ducts: Sonographic appearance. Radiology 1983;148(3):803–804.
5. Tio TL, Reeders JW, Sie LH, et al.: Endosonography in the clinical staging of Klatskin tumor. Endoscopy 1993;25(1):81–85.
6. Hann LE, Greatrex KV, Bach AM, Fong Y, Blumgart LH: Cholangiocarcinoma at the hepatic hilus: sonographic findings. Am J Roentgenol 1997;168(4):985–989.
7. Bloom CM, Langer B, Wilson SR: Role of US in the detection, characterization, and staging of cholangiocarcinoma. Radiographics 1999;19(5):1199–1218.
8. Cha JH, Han JK, Kim TK, et al.: Preoperative evaluation of Klatskin tumor: Accuracy of spiral CT in determining vascular invasion as a sign of unresectability. Abdom Imaging 2000;25(5):500–507.
9. Guthrie JA, Ward J, Robinson PJ: Hilar cholangiocarcinomas: T2-weighted spin-echo and gadolinium-enhanced FLASH MR imaging. Radiology 1996;201(2):347–351.
10. Keiding S, Hansen SB, Rasmussen HH, et al.: Detection of cholangiocarcinoma in primary sclerosing cholangitis by positron emission tomography. Hepatology 1998;28:700–706.

Case 6.6.10

History

A 34-year-old female with a history of sclerosing cholangitis presented with complaints of fevers and weight loss. The patient was diagnosed with primary sclerosing cholangitis six years prior to presentation and was considered for liver transplantation. She was referred for a CT scan (Figure 6.6.10A) and FDG imaging. Figure 6.6.10B shows transaxial FDG images acquired with a dedicated PET tomograph (GE Advance) and reconstructed with iterative reconstruction and measured segmented attenuation correction.

Findings

The CT images reveal increased attenuation in the region of the porta hepatis that was unchanged compared to prior CT scans and was felt to represent fatty sparing (not shown). Dilated, fluid-filled ducts with pneumobilia were noted as well, which represent a new finding when compared with previous studies. The FDG images demonstrate numerous small foci of increased uptake, some of them corresponding to dilated bile ducts.

Discussion

The PET scan was felt to be consistent with malignancy such as cholangiocarcinoma with adjacent spread, although the possibility of an inflammatory process could not be excluded. An open biopsy was subsequently performed that revealed foci of granulomatous inflammation but no evidence of malignancy.

This case illustrates the difficulty that can be encountered when trying to differentiate neoplastic processes from inflammatory processes on FDG PET images. Any acute inflammatory process can demonstrate marked increased FDG uptake secondary to the increased metabolic activity in the region of inflammation. Increased FDG uptake is seen in granulation tissue, healing uninfected wounds, fractures,

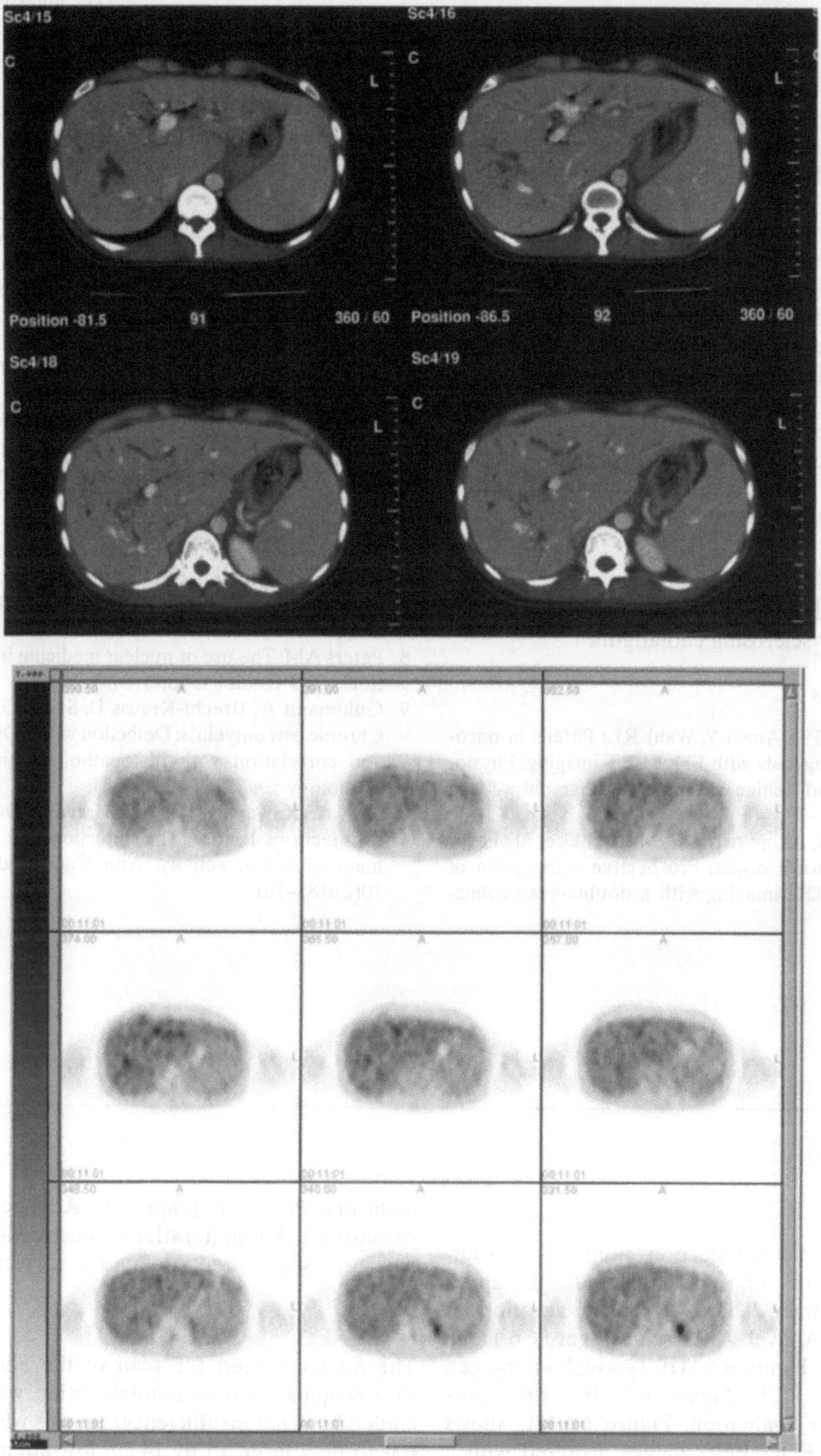

A

B

FIGURE 6.6.10A,B.

recently placed biliary stents, and colostomy sites. It is important to remember that inflammatory processes, with or without associated infection, are always a diagnostic consideration in areas of abnormal accumulation of FDG. Because of this, FDG has been investigated as a marker for some infectious processes, such as osteomyelitis.[1–10] In most cases, correlation with the clinical history and other imaging modalities is helpful for accurate interpretation. In this case, however, the history was not helpful because sclerosing cholangitis is a predisposing factor for cholangiocarcinomas, and these patients experience episodes of cholangitis. Another source of false-positive interpretation is due to inflammatory reaction along the course of biliary stents.

Diagnoses

1. Acute cholangitis.
2. Primary sclerosing cholangitis.

References

1. Shreve PD, Anzai Y, Wahl RL: Pitfalls in oncologic diagnosis with FDG PET imaging: Physiologic and benign variants. Radiographics 1999; 19(1):61–77.
2. Meller J, Altenvoerde G, Munzel U, et al.: Fever of unknown origin: Prospective comparison of [18F] FDG imaging with a double-head coincidence camera and gallium-67 citrate SPET. Eur J Nucl Med 2000;27(11):1617–1625.
3. Stumpe KD, Dazzi H, Schaffner A, von Schulthess GK: Infection imaging using whole-body FDG-PET. Eur J Nucl Med 2000;27(7): 822–832.
4. Kalicke T, Schmitz A, Risse JH, et al.: Fluorine-18 fluorodeoxyglucose PET in infectious bone diseases: Results of histologically confirmed cases. Eur J Nucl Med 2000;27(5):524–528.
5. Robiller FC, Stumpe KD, Kossmann T, Weisshaupt D, Bruder E, von Schulthess GK: Chronic osteomyelitis of the femur: Value of PET imaging. Eur Radiol 2000;10(5):855–858.
6. Bakheet SM, Saleem M, Powe J, Al-Amro A, Larsson SG, Mahassin Z: F-18 fluorodeoxyglucose chest uptake in lung inflammation and infection. Clin Nucl Med 2000;25(4):273–278.
7. Guhlmann A, Brecht-Krauss D, Suger G, et al.: Fluorine-18-FDG PET and technetium-99m antigranulocyte antibody scintigraphy in chronic osteomyelitis. J Nucl Med 1998;39(12):2145–2152.
8. Peters AM: The use of nuclear medicine in infections. Br J Radiol 1998;71(843):252–261.
9. Guhlmann A, Brecht-Krauss D, Suger G, et al.: Chronic osteomyelitis: Detection with FDG PET and correlation with histopathologic findings. Radiology 1998;206(3):749–754.
10. Ichiya Y, Kuwabara Y, Sasaki M, et al.: FDG-PET in infectious lesions: The detection and assessment of lesion activity. Ann Nucl Med 1996; 10(2):185–191.

Case 6.6.11

History

A 70-year-old female presented with a four-month history of right flank and right upper quadrant pain. There was also elevation of serum CEA level. A CT scan (Figure 6.6.11A), MRI scan (Figure 6.6.11B, T_2-weighted image), and FDG PET (Figure 6.6.11C) were performed for evaluation. Figure 6.6.11C shows transaxial FDG PET images acquired with a dedicated PET tomograph (GE Advance) and reconstructed with iterative reconstruction and measured segmented attenuation correction.

Findings

The noncontrasted CT scan of the abdomen (intravenous contrast administration was precluded by renal insufficiency) reveals what was felt to be a large 15 by 14 cm low-attenuation

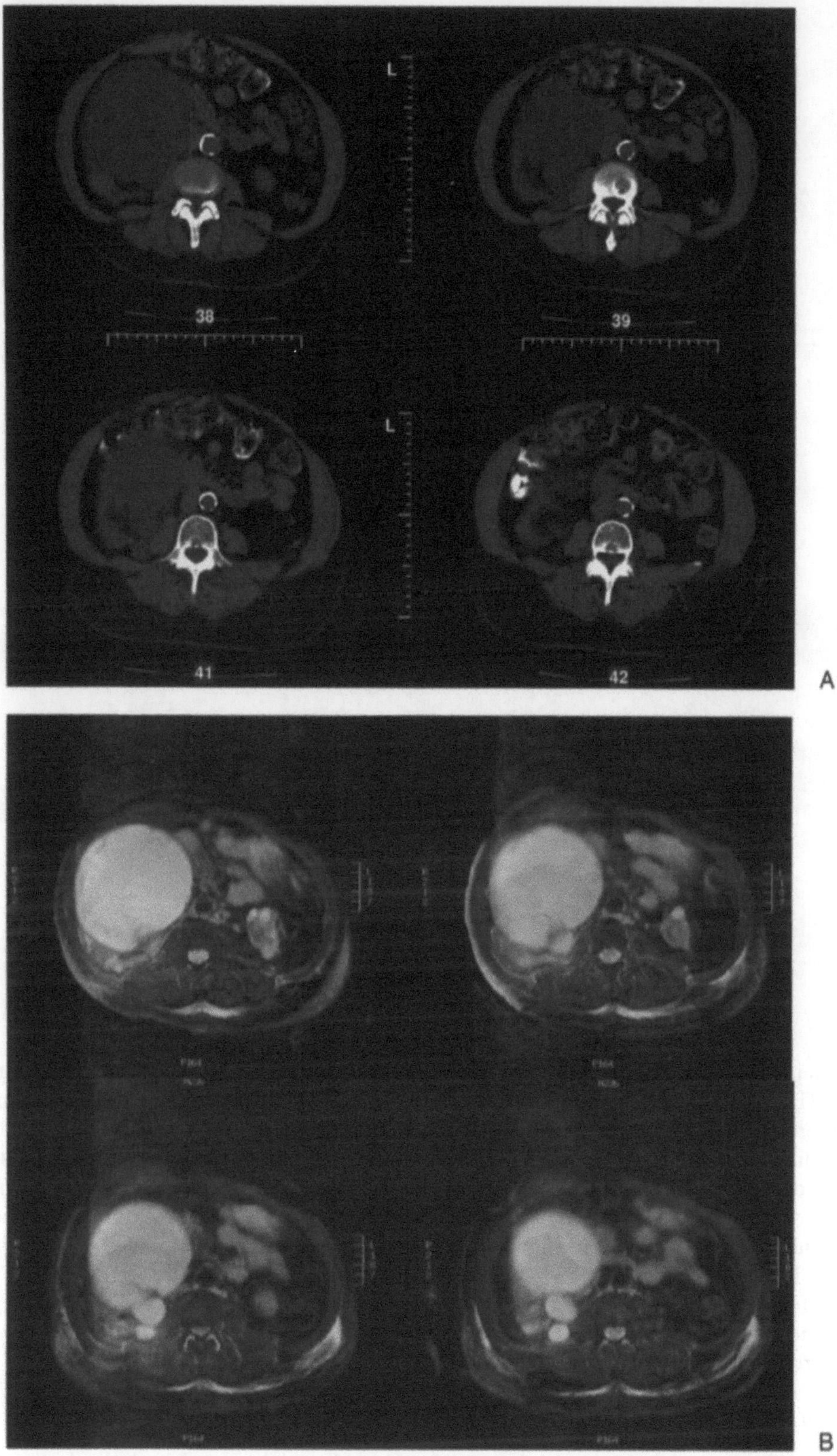

Figure 6.6.11A,B.

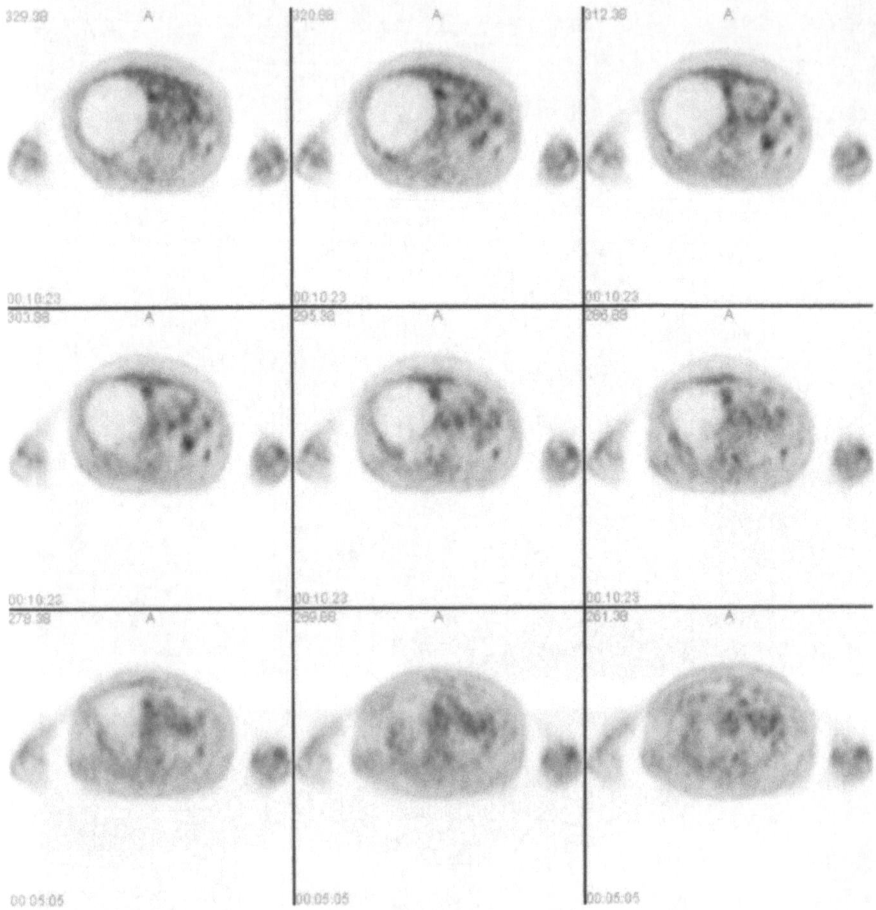

FIGURE 6.6.11C. (*Continued*)

mass replacing the entirety of the right lobe of the liver. The right kidney was felt to be displaced inferiorly by this mass. The MRI scan reveals findings that are consistent with a large cystic mass occupying almost the entirety of the right lobe of the liver. The MRI scan more clearly defined multiple septations (not shown). The FDG PET images reveal a large, photopenic defect consistent with a cystic mass. There are no internal foci of hypermetabolism and no surrounding rim of increased activity.

Discussion

The FDG PET scan was obtained because of the concern for underlying liver malignancy such as mucinous cystadenocarcinoma causing elevated CEA levels. The FDG PET images did not reveal any evidence of increased activity within the mass, favoring a benign cystic mass. Since the patient was becoming increasingly symptomatic, she was explored surgically. At surgery, a large septated renal cystic mass was found that displaced the right lobe of the liver superiorly.

Diagnosis

Complex right renal cyst displacing the liver superiorly.

Case 6.6.12

History

A 61-year-old female presented with right upper quadrant pain. A CT scan (Figure 6.6.12A) and FDG PET imaging (Figures 6.6.12B and C) were performed. Coronal (Figure 6.6.12B) and transaxial (Figure 6.6.12C) FDG images were acquired with a dedicated PET tomograph (Siemens ECAT 933) and reconstructed with filtered back projection without attenuation correction.

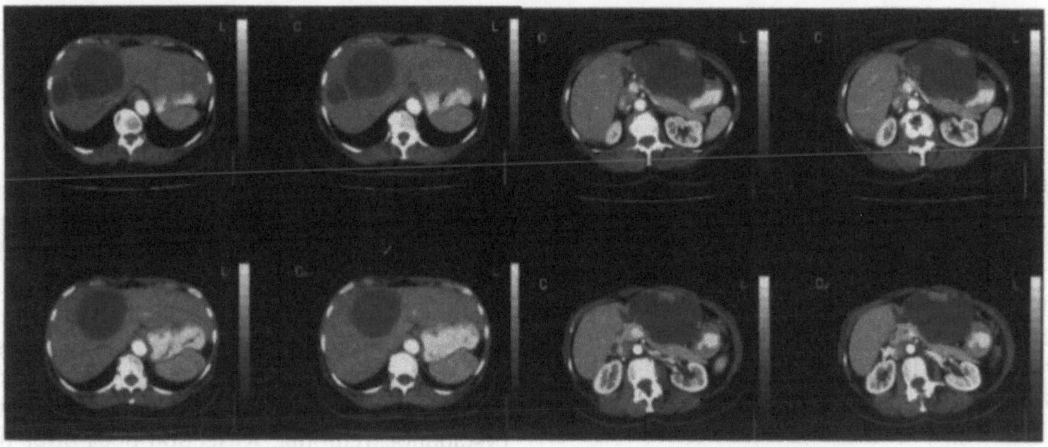
A

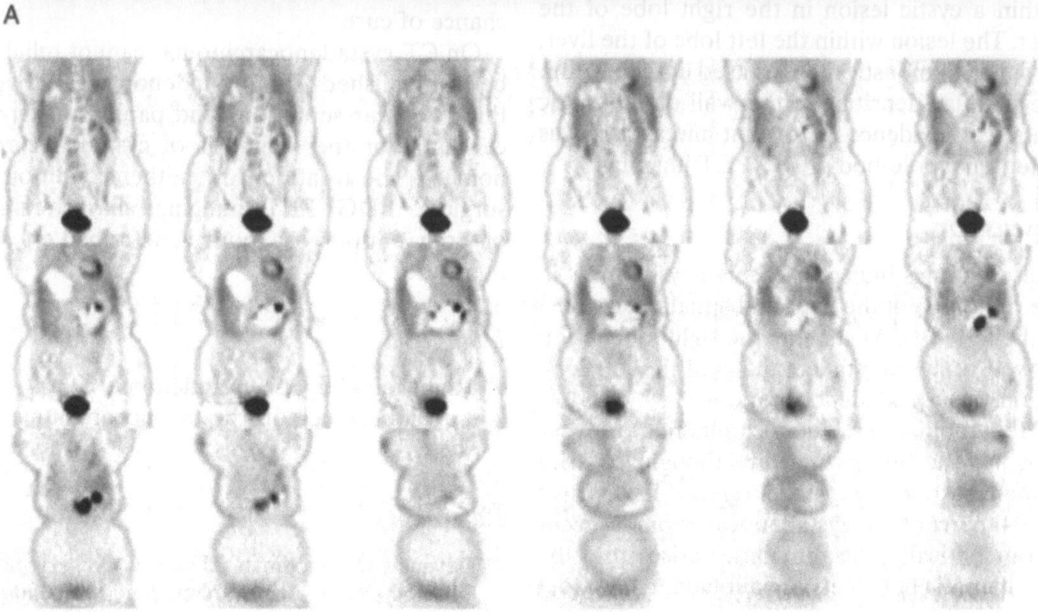
B

FIGURE 6.6.12A,B.

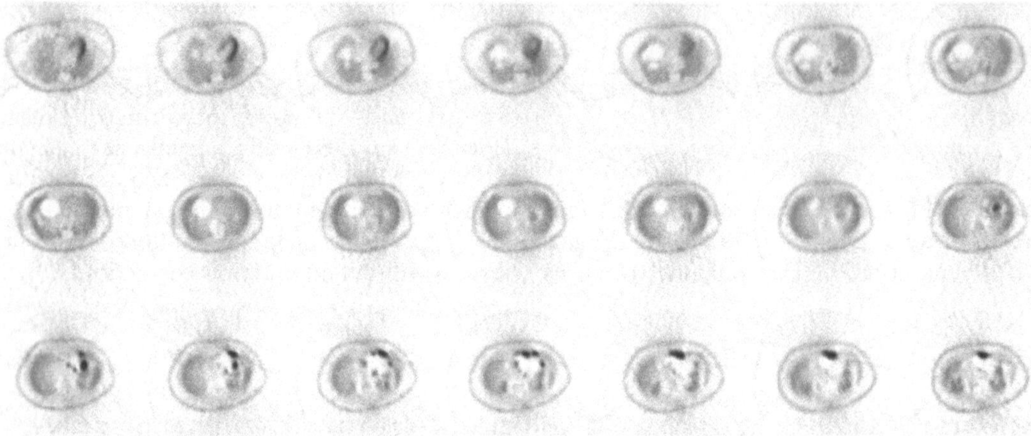

Figure 6.6.12C. (*Continued*)

Findings

The CT scan of the abdomen reveals large, predominately cystic masses within both the left and right lobes of the liver. Septations and peripheral nodular densities are noted in the cystic mass located in the left lobe of the liver.

The FDG PET images reveal no uptake within a cystic lesion in the right lobe of the liver. The lesion within the left lobe of the liver, however, demonstrates increased uptake within the nodular densities in the wall of the cystic mass. No evidence of distant metastasis was noted on whole-body FDG PET imaging.

Discussion

These findings indicate a benign cystic mass in the right lobe of the liver and a malignant mass in the left lobe. At surgery, the right lobe lesion proved to be a cystadenoma, and the left lobe lesion was a cystadenocarcinoma.

Hepatobiliary cystadenocarcinomas are very rare hepatic tumors that are thought to arise from hepatobiliary cystadenomas.[1,2] Eighty-five to 94 percent of cystadenocarcinomas occur intrahepatically; the remainder arise from the extrahepatic bile ducts or gallbladder. Cystadenocarcinomas with ovarian stroma are seen only in women and may develop from preexisting biliary cystadenomas. Cystadenocarcinomas without ovarian stroma may be seen in both men and women and generally have a poorer prognosis (50% mortality). A predisposing condition (that is, preexistent cyst) has been traced to approximately half of those tumors in one series. In general, the prognosis of patients with these tumors is poorer when compared with patients who have pancreatic cystadenocarcinoma. Resection does offer the chance of cure.

On CT, cystadenocarcinomas cannot reliably be distinguished from cystadenomas, although thick nodular septations and papillary excrescences favor the diagnosis of cystadenocarcinoma.[3–5] The treatment for either condition is surgical. FDG PET imaging characteristics of both entities are poorly described in the literature.

Diagnoses

1. Right lobe hepatic cystadenoma.
2. Left lobe mucinous cystadenocarcinoma of the liver.

References

1. Devaney K, Goodman ZD, Ishak KG: Hepatobiliary cystadenoma and cystadenocarcinoma. A light microscopic and immunohistochemical study of 70 patients. Am J Surg Pathol 1994;18(11): 1078–1091.

2. Ishak KG, Willis GW, Cummins SD, Bullock AA: Biliary cystadenoma and cystadenocarcinoma: Report of 14 cases and review of the literature. Cancer 1977;39(1):322–338.
3. Korobkin M, Stephens DH, Lee JK, et al.: Biliary cystadenoma and cystadenocarcinoma: CT and sonographic findings. Am J Roentgenol 1989; 153(3):507–511.
4. Choi BI, Lim JH, Han MC, et al.: Biliary cystadenoma and cystadenocarcinoma: CT and sonographic findings. Radiology 1989;171(1):57–61.
5. Nakajima T, Sugano I, Matsuzaki O, et al.: Biliary cystadenocarcinoma of the liver. A clinicopathologic and histochemical evaluation of nine cases. Cancer 1992;69(10):2426–2432.

6.7
Genitourinary Tract

William H. Martin and Dominique Delbeke

Because FDG is excreted by the kidneys, the high concentration of FDG in the urine may obscure visualization of structures adjacent to the renal collecting system and bladder. With good hydration, the administration of diuretics, and placement of an irrigating urinary catheter, visualization of renal, perirenal, and paravesicular lesions can be improved. The reported experience of FDG PET imaging in patients with genitourinary neoplasms is limited to studies of small populations of patients.[1–3]

Renal and Bladder Tumors

A review of the applications of FDG PET in urological oncology has been published by Hoh et al.[3] FDG seems to accumulate in most renal cell[1,3,4] and bladder carcinomas.[2,5] There is recent evidence that there is a large variability in the degree of accumulation of FDG in renal carcinoma, related to variability in expression of the enzyme glucose-6-phosphatase, as in hepatocellular carcinomas.[6] In a study of 29 patients,[7] the sensitivity of FDG PET imaging was only 77% for detection of the primary tumor; there were six false-negative malignant tumors and three false-positive benign tumors (angiomyolipoma, pericytoma, and pheochromocytoma). High-grade tumors appear to have higher FDG uptake, correlating with higher Glut-1 intensity by peroxidase staining than low-grade tumors.[8] For bladder carcinoma, FDG imaging is limited by urinary excretion of the radiopharmaceutical that prevents distinction of the primary tumor from the surrounding urine activity. In a pilot study of 23 patients,[5] it was possible to detect 18 of 23 primary tumors with ^{11}C-methionine, which may be a more appropriate radiopharmaceutical for evaluation of primary bladder carcinoma.

Prostate Carcinoma

Prostate carcinoma represents 32% of newly diagnosed cancers and 13% of all cancer deaths in men. Despite its reputation as a more indolent malignancy than many others, there is a 55% risk of cancer death within 15 years, even in men with low-grade tumors. Initial staging is performed using clinical assessment, serum PSA determination, transrectal ultrasound, bone scintigraphy, and CT/MR to determine if the patient is a candidate for radiotherapy or radical prostatectomy versus androgen ablation therapy. Twenty percent of newly diagnosed patients have skeletal metastases at presentation, but the remainder require accurate preoperative staging. Transrectal ultrasound has a sensitivity of only 53 to 89%. CT and MR imaging are notoriously inaccurate for detecting low-volume pelvic adenopathy (< 50% and 69%, respectively), and monoclonal antibody scintigraphy is only marginally better. Fifty percent of patients undergoing radical prostatectomy for presumed organ-confined disease are found to have disease beyond the prostate at surgery. To date, no imaging modality has been able to compete with pelvic lymph node dissection for initial staging. Ten-year, disease-free survival drops to

40 to 60% in patients found to have extracapsular disease at surgery.

Following definitive therapy, patients are restaged if serum PSA concentration rises. Differentiating the patients in whom there is local recurrence within the prostate fossa from those with regional nodes or distant metastases affects therapy because the former population is considered for adjuvant external beam radiotherapy (for surgical failures) or salvage prostatectomy/ablation (for radiotherapy failures). It is in restaging that both FDG PET and monoclonal antibody scintigraphy are emerging as useful modalities.

For prostate carcinoma, the primary tumors and pelvic lymph nodes are difficult to image due to the proximity of the bladder. In addition, the uptake appears relatively low in most prostate carcinoma (SUV = 2.5–3.5) and may reflect relatively low metabolism in a slow-growing tumor.[9–12] Patients who have a higher SUV (> 5.0) experience rapid progression of their disease and do not respond well to androgen deprivation or radiation therapy. Relatively high uptake in benign prostatic hyperplasia makes the differentiation of benign from malignant prostatic lesions difficult. The sensitivity of FDG PET imaging is below 50% for detection of local recurrence after radical prostatectomy,[13,14] not much better than monoclonal antibodies in the same study. However, the sensitivity of CT for detection of pelvic prostate metastases is less than 50%.

For skeletal metastases from prostate carcinoma, FDG PET imaging is not as sensitive as bone scintigraphy. A study of 22 patients with over 200 skeletal metastases showed that the sensitivity of PET was only 65%, but the positive predictive value was 98%, an advantage over bone scintigraphy which is very sensitive but poorly specific.[10] The study of Yeh et al.[15] reports a sensitivity of only 18% for detection of skeletal metastases. FDG PET imaging may have a role in the evaluation of indeterminate bone lesions on bone scan. ^{18}F seems to be the most promising radiopharmaceutical in that regard.[16]

FDG PET may also have a role for detection of recurrence in patients with elevated prostatic specific antigen (PSA) and normal CT scan.[3]

Testicular Tumors

Testicular tumors arise most often from totipotential germ cells. Seminomas are the most common testicular tumors (40%), and testicular tumors of other histologies are referred to as nonseminomatous germ cell tumors (NSGCT) because of similarities of prognosis and therapy. They include embryonal carcinomas, choriocarcinomas, mature and immature teratomas, teratocarcinomas, and tumors of mixed histologies. Lymph node metastases are found at the time of diagnosis in approximately two-thirds of patients with NSGCT and one-third of patients with seminomas. Distant metastases most often occur in the lungs, followed by the liver and brain. Various tumor markers may be elevated in testicular carcinoma, for example, alpha-fetoprotein (AFP), human chorionic gonadotropin (HCG), lactic acid dehydrogenase (LDH), and placental alkaline phosphatase (PALP).

For staging regional lymph nodes, CT has limitations related to size criteria. The role of FDG PET in patients with testicular cancer is still under investigation. Preliminary studies suggest that FDG PET may be useful for initial staging after orchiectomy by detecting metastases not seen by conventional imaging.[3] Although FDG PET imaging does not offer an advantage over CT in stage I seminoma (no metastases), it may be helpful to characterize retroperitoneal lesions[17–19] in stage II disease (infradiaphragmatic lymph node metastases). In patients with NSGCT, FDG PET seems to be more sensitive than CT for detection of metastases, but further studies on a larger series of patients are necessary to confirm these data.

FDG PET seems to be promising for predicting response to therapy.[20,21] After chemotherapy, PET may be able to differentiate viable tumor from scar tissue, but not scar tissue from mature teratoma.[22–25] As for other tumors, PET may also be useful for localization of recurrence in patients with rising levels of serum tumor markers.

In summary, FDG PET seems to be helpful in the staging of both seminomas and NSGCT, monitoring the response to therapy, evaluation of residual masses after therapy, and localization of recurrence in patients with rising levels of serum tumor markers.

Ovarian Carcinoma

If nonmelanomatous skin cancers are excluded, ovarian carcinoma is the sixth most common malignancy and the fifth most common cause of cancer deaths in women. Ovarian carcinoma initially spreads to regional organs, then to the peritoneum with drop metastases in the Douglas pouch, to the omentum and subphrenic space. The lymphatic spread occurs via the inguinal, pelvic, and paraaortic lymph nodes. Because of this, patients are generally asymptomatic, 70% presenting with advanced disease. Despite the use of extensive cytoreductive surgery and platinum-based chemotherapy with a response rate of 60 to 80%, five-year survival is only 5 to 20%. In two studies totaling 60 patients evaluated for recurrent ovarian carcinoma, the sensitivity of FDG PET imaging was superior to that of CT for detection of recurrent disease, ranging from 83 to 93% for PET and 67 to 87% for CT. The specificity of PET was 80%, and the specificity of CT was 50%.[26–29] In a recent study of 23 patients undergoing FDG imaging for suspected recurrence of ovarian carcinoma, 18 of whom had only an increased serum CA-125 level, the overall sensitivity and accuracy on a per patient basis was 18 out of 18 (100%) for FDG, while sensitivity and accuracy of conventional imaging was only 6 out of 18 (33%).[30] In these studies and in our own experience, PET identified occult foci that were not seen on CT. False-negative studies have been reported in carcinomatosis. Although experience to date is limited, there is accumulating evidence that FDG imaging is superior to CT and at least equivalent to MRI for the detection of metastatic disease in patients suspected clinically on the basis of elevated serum tumor marker levels to have recurrent ovarian carcinoma.

Carcinoma of the Cervix and Uterus

Cervical carcinoma is the third most common gynecological cancer in the United States. MRI is the most accurate imaging modality for evaluation of local invasion with a staging accuracy of 80 to 92% as compared to 58 to 88% for CT. The sensitivity for detection of nodal metastasis is similar for MRI and CT, approximately 50%.[31,32] Few clinical reports have been reported in the literature evaluating the role of FDG PET imaging in patients with cervical carcinoma.[33–35] In a pilot study of 21 patients, the primary tumor was detected in 76% of the patients without post-void images and in all patients when post-void images were obtained. FDG PET imaging detected lymph node involvement in 86% (6 out of 7) of patients with proven metastases, whereas CT detected nodal involvement in 57% (4 out of 7). In three reports totaling 76 women, FDG PET performed better than CT in the identification of metastasis not only in patients undergoing initial staging (n = 60), but also in patients undergoing restaging for suspected recurrence (n = 16). If these preliminary findings can be confirmed in larger populations, FDG PET may provide incremental diagnostic and prognostic information in the initial staging of patients with advanced disease, thus altering therapy, and may become instrumental in the follow-up of these patients, especially as the combination of chemotherapy to aggressive radiotherapy regimens emerges.

Intrauterine accumulation of FDG uptake has been reported in leiomyoma,[36] gestational sac,[37] and during menstruation[38] that may potentially lead to misinterpretation.

References

1. Wahl RL, Harney J, Hutchins G, Grossman HB: Imaging of renal cancer using positron emission tomography with 2-deoxy-2-(18F)-fluoro-D-glucose: Pilot animal and human studies. J Urol 1991;146:1470–1474.
2. Harney JV, Wahl RL, Liebert M, et al.: Uptake of 2-deoxy, 2-(18F) fluoro-D-glucose in bladder cancer: Animal localization and initial patient positron emission tomography. J Urol 1991;145: 279–283.
3. Hoh CK, Seltzer MA, Franklin J, et al.: Positron emission tomography in urological oncology. J Urol 1998;159:347–356.
4. Montravers F, Grahek D, Kerrou K, et al.: Evaluation of FDG uptake by renal malignancies

(primary tumor or metastases) using a coincidence detection gamma camera. J Nucl Med 2000;41(1):78–84.
5. Ahlstrom H, Malmstrom PU, Letocha H, Andersson J, Langstrom B, Nilsson S: Positron emission tomography in the diagnosis and staging of urinary bladder cancer. Acta Radiol 1996;37(2): 180–185.
6. Hoffman M, Börner AR, Kühnel G, et al.: Interindividual variance of glucose-6-phosphatase (G-6-Pse) expression in renal cell cancer. Eur J Nucl Med 2000;27:104.
7. Bachor R, Kotzerke J, Gottfried HW, Brandle E, Reske SN, Hautmann R: Positron emission tomography in the diagnosis of renal cell carcinoma (German). Urologe A 1996;35:146–150.
8. Miyauchi T, Brown TS, Grossman HB, et al.: Correlation between visualization of primary renal cancer and histopathological findings, abstracted. J Nucl Med 1996;37(suppl):64P.
9. Bender H, Schomburg A, Albers P, Ruhlmann J, Biersack HJ: Possible role of FDG-PET in the evaluation of urologic malignancies. Anticancer Res 1997;17:1655–1660.
10. Effert PJ, Bares R, Handt S, et al.: Metabolic imaging of untreated prostate cancer by positron emission tomography with 18flourine-labeled deoxy-glucose. J Urol 1996;155:994–998.
11. Schreve PD, Grossman PD, Gross MD, Wahl RL: Metastatic prostate cancer: Initial findings of PET with 2-deoxy-2[F-18]fluoro-D-glucose. Radiology 1996;155:994–998.
12. Laudenbacker C, Hofer C, Avril N, et al.: FDG PET for differentiation of local recurrent prostate cancer and scar, abstracted. J Nucl Med 1995;36(suppl):198P.
13. Hofer C, Laubenbacher C, Block T, et al.: Fluorine-18fluorodeoxyglucose positron emission tomography is useless for the detection of local recurrence after radical prostatectomy. Eur Urol 1999;36:31–35.
14. Seltzer MA, Barbaric Z, Belldegrun A, et al.: Comparison of helical computerized tomography, positron emission tomography and monoclonal antibody scans for the evaluation of lymph node metastases in patients with prostate specific antigen relapse after treatment for localized prostate cancer. J Urol 1999;162:1322–1328.
15. Yeh SDJ, Imbriaco M, Garza D, et al.: Twenty percent of bony metastases of hormone resistant prostate cancer are detected by PET-FDG whole body scanning. J Nucl Med 1995;36:198.
16. Silberstein EB, Saenger EL, Tofe AJ, et al.: Imaging of bone metastases with 99m Tc-Sn-EHDP (diphosphonate), 18 F and skeletal radiography. A comparison of sensitivity. Radiology 1973;107:551–555.
17. Cremerius U, Effert PJ, Adam G, et al.: FDG PET for detection and therapy control of metastatic germ cell cancer. J Nucl Med 1998;39: 815–822.
18. Albers P, Bender H, Yilmaz H, et al.: Positron emission tomography in the clinical staging of patients with stage I and II testicular germ cell tumors. Urology 1999;53:808–811.
19. Muller-Mattheis V, Reinhardt M, Gerharz CD et al.: Positron emission tomography with [18 F]-2-fluoro-2-deoxy-D-glucose (18FDG-PET) in diagnosis of retroperitoneal lymph node metastases of testicular tumors. Urologe A 1998;37(6): 609–620.
20. Price P, Jones T: Can positron emission tomography (PET) be used to detect subclinical response to cancer therapy? Europ J Cancer 1995;31A:1924–1927.
21. Reinhardt MJ, Müller-Mattheis VG, Gerharz CD, et al.: FDG-PET evaluation of retroperitoneal metastases of testicular cancer before and after chemotherapy. J Nucl Med 1997;38:99–101.
22. Stomper PC, Kalish LA, Garnick MB, et al.: CT and pathologic predictive features of residual mass histologic findings after chemotherapy for nonseminomatous germ cell tumors: Can residual malignancy or teratoma be excluded? Radiology 1991;181:711–714.
23. Stephens AW, Gonin R, Hutchins GD, Einhorn LH: Positron emission tomography evaluation of residual radiographic abnormalities in post-chemotherapy germ cell tumor patients. J Clin Oncol 1996;14:1637–1641.
24. Wilson CB, Young HE, Ott RJ, et al.: Imaging metastatic testicular germ cell tumours with ^{18}FDG positron emission tomography: Prospects for detection and management. Eur J Nucl Med 1995;22:508–513.
25. Sugawara Y, Zasadny KR, Grossman HJ, et al.: Germ cell tumor: Differentiation of viable tumor, mature teratoma, and necrotic tissue with FDG PET and kinetic modeling. Radiology 1999;211:249–256.
26. Wahl RL, Hutchins D, Robert J, et al.: FDG-PET imaging of ovarian cancer: Initial evaluation in patients, abstracted. J Nucl Med 1991;32:982.
27. Casey MJ, Gupta NC, Muths CK: Experience with positron emission tomography (PET) scans in patients with ovarian cancer. Gynecol Oncol 1994;53:331–338.
28. Hubner KF, McDonald TW, Niethammer JG, et al.: Assessment of primary and metas-

tatic ovarian cancer by positron emission tomography (PET) using 2-[18FDG]deoxy-glucose (2-[18F]FDG). Gynecol Oncol 1993;51:197–204.
29. Bohdewiecz PJ, Scott GC, Juni JE, et al.: Indium-11 OncoScint CR/OV and F-18 FDG in colorectal and ovarian carcinoma recurrences. Early observations. Clin Nucl Med 1995;20:230–236.
30. Kerrou K, Montravers F, Grahek D, Younsi N, de Beco V, Talbot JN: Detection of recurrence of ovarian cancer using [F-18]-FDG scan performed on a dual-head coincidence gamma camera (CDET). Clin Positron Imaging 2000; 3(4):186.
31. Hricak H, Yu KK: Radiology in invasive cervical cancer. Am J Roentgenol 1996;167(5):1101–1108.
32. Yu KK, Forstner R, Hricak H: Cervical carcinoma: Role of imaging. Abdom Imaging 1997; 22(2):208–215.
33. Sugawara Y, Eisbruch A, Kosuda S, Recker BE, Kison PV, Wahl RL: Evaluation of FDG PET in patients with cervical cancer. J Nucl Med 1999; 40(7):1125–1131.
34. Grigsby PW, Dehdashti F, Siegel BA: FDG-PET evaluation of carcinoma of the cervix. Clin Positron Imag 1999;2:105–109.
35. Rose PG, Adler LP, Rodriguez M, Faulhaber PF, Abdul-Karim FW, Miraldi F: Positron emission tomography for evaluating para-aortic nodal metastasis in locally advanced cervical cancer before surgical staging: A surgicopathologic study. J Clin Oncol 1999;17(1):41–45.
36. Holder WD Jr, White RL Jr, Zuger JH, Easton EJ Jr, Greene FL: Effectiveness of positron emission tomography for the detection of melanoma metastases. Ann Surg 1998 May; 227(5):764–769; discussion 769–771.
37. Alibazoglu H, Kim R, Ali A, Green A, LaMonica G: FDG uptake in gestational sac. Clin Nucl Med 1997;22(8):557.
38. Yasuda S, Ide M, Takagi S, Shohtsu A: Intrauterine accumulation of F-18 FDG during menstruation. Clin Nucl Med 1997;22(11):793.

Case Presentations

Case 6.7.1

History

Eight months ago, a right orchiectomy revealed a large mixed nonseminomatous high-grade germ cell tumor in this 20-year-old male who now presents with a rising serum alphafetoprotein level at the completion of induction chemotherapy. A recent CT scan of the chest, abdomen, and pelvis was interpreted as negative for metastatic disease. FDG images were first acquired with a dedicated PET tomograph (ECAT 933) and reconstructed using filtered back projection without attenuation correction. Figure 6.7.1A, see color plate, shows orthogonal images through the spine (top left = transaxial, bottom = coronal, top right = sagittal). FDG images were then obtained with a hybrid dual-head gamma camera operating in the coincidence mode (VG Millenium). The hybrid FDG PET images were reconstructed using an iterative reconstruction algorithm and corrected for attenuation using attenuation maps obtained with an X-ray tube and array of detectors mounted on the gantry of the camera and functioning as a third-generation CT scanner. These attenuation maps also provide hybrid CT images for image fusion and anatomical mapping. Figure 6.7.1B shows transaxial images of the hybrid CT (left), hybrid PET (middle), and fusion image (right).

Findings

Both the FDG PET and FDG hybrid PET images show a moderate-sized focus of markedly increased activity between the lower poles of the kidneys. Physiologic FDG uptake in the bone marrow is unusually low in this patient, and therefore, it is difficult to definitively localize the abnormality to the prevertebral soft tissues versus the spine, even on the sagittal image that is optimal for that purpose. The PET images shown have not been corrected for attenuation, but the hybrid PET images have been corrected, demonstrating that attenuation correction was not helpful.

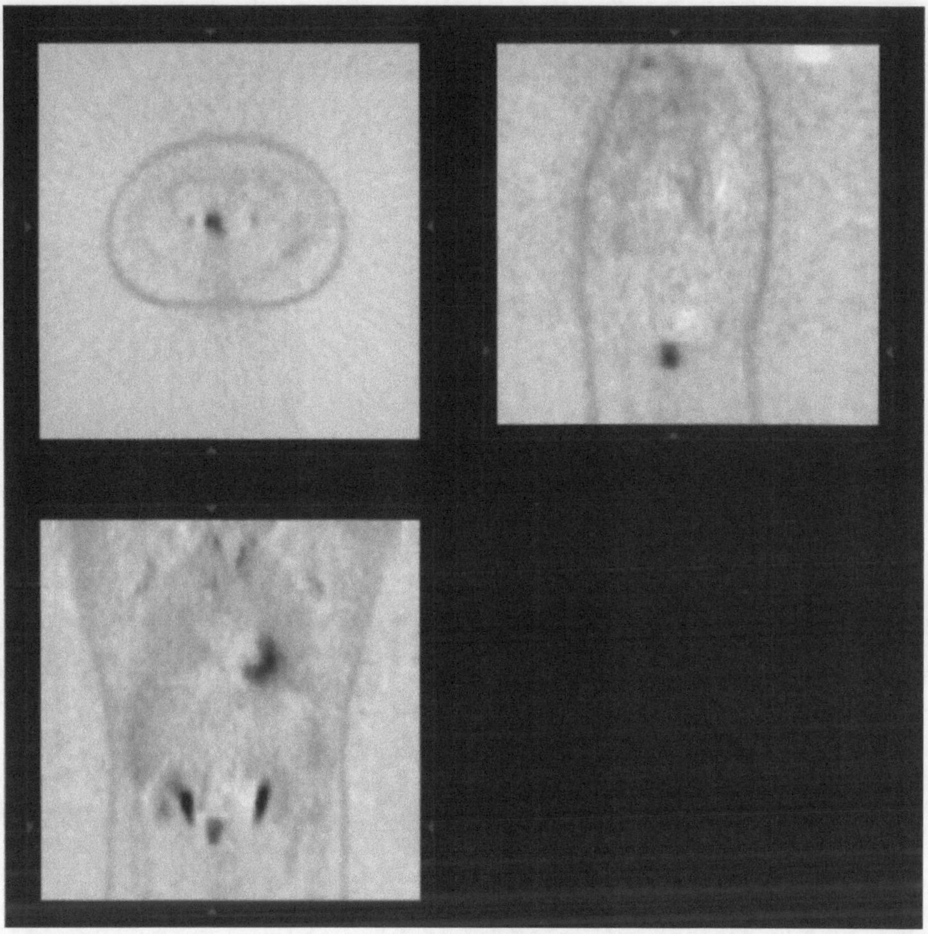

FIGURE 6.7.1A.

However, the fused anatomic/functional images acquired with the hybrid imaging system place the focus of abnormal FDG activity within the right anterior aspect of a mid-lumbar vertebral body.

Discussion

The FDG images acquired with the dedicated PET camera are diagnostic of a solitary metastasis, but localization was difficult due to the unusually low uptake in the bone marrow, resulting in poor delineation of the spine. In this example, fusion of CT and FDG metabolic data acquired with the integrated hybrid imaging system allows accurate localization of the metastasis to a lumbar vertebral body, which was confirmed on a subsequent MRI. Such systems will become more prevalent as their utility is further demonstrated by cases such as this.

Germ cell cancers of the testis are rare malignancies that occur most commonly in young men. With appropriate staging and therapy, cure rate approaches 95%. There is only limited experience with the use of FDG PET imaging in the staging and follow-up of patients with testicular tumors. Preliminary studies suggest that FDG PET may be useful for initial staging after orchiectomy by detecting metastases not

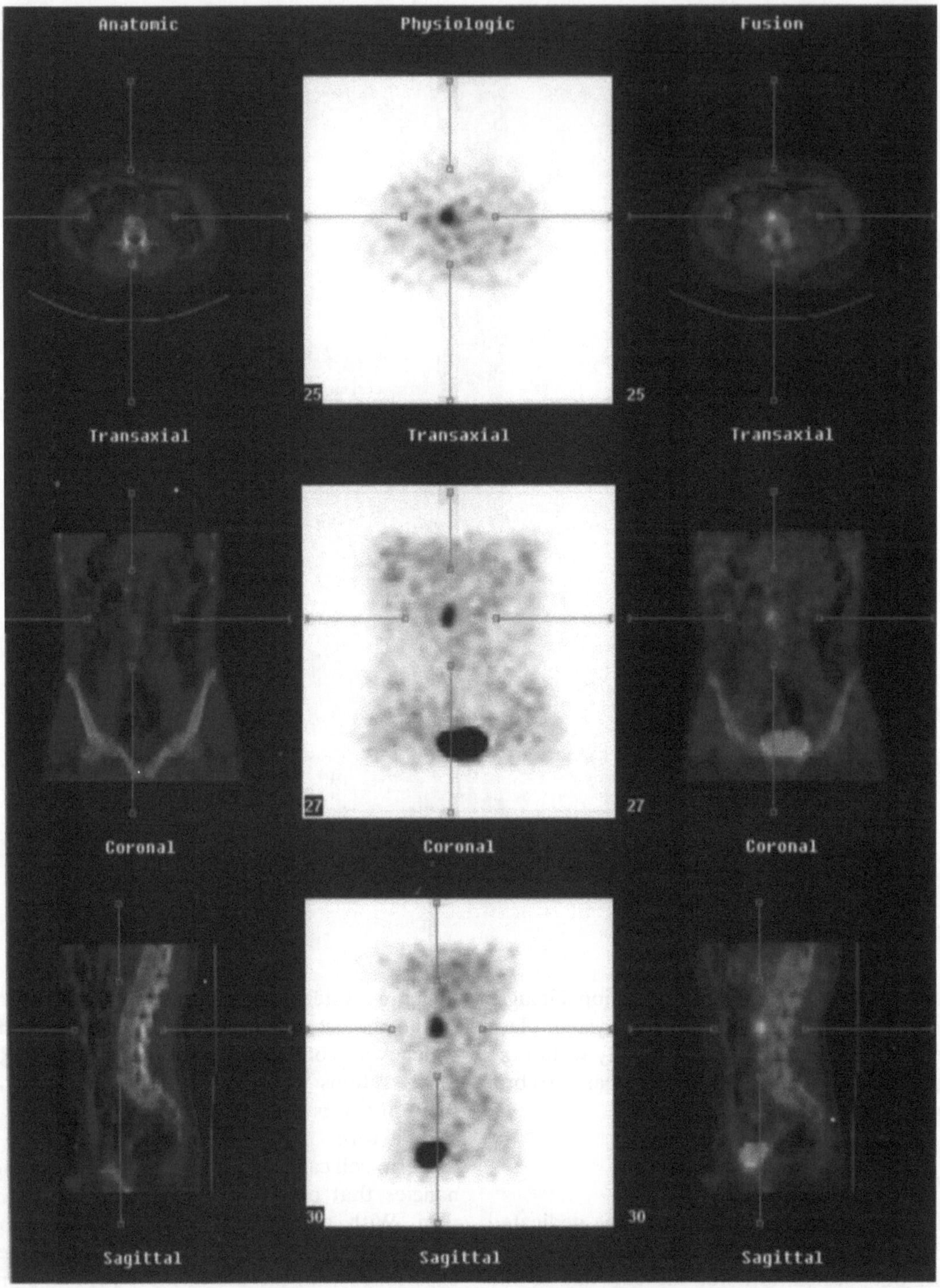

FIGURE 6.7.1B. (*Continued*) (See color plate)

seen by conventional imaging, but it cannot replace retroperitoneal lymph node dissection for staging purposes. In patients with stage II seminomas (infradiaphragmatic lymph node metastases), FDG PET imaging may aid in the characterization of retroperitoneal lesions detected by CT. In patients with nonseminomatous germ cell tumors, several reports indicate that FDG PET is more sensitive than CT for detection of metastases, particularly with high-grade lesions.

FDG PET imaging seems to be promising for predicting response to therapy. After chemotherapy, PET is able to differentiate viable tumor from scar tissue, especially if the scan is delayed for two to three weeks after completion of therapy. FDG PET imaging is not sensitive for the detection of mature teratoma and cannot reliably differentiate scar tissue from mature teratoma. As with other neoplasms, PET has been found useful for localization of recurrence in patients with rising levels of serum tumor markers, as in this example. In this patient, the promotion from stage II to stage IV by PET changes the prognosis dramatically.

Diagnosis

Testicular germ cell tumor metastatic to the spine.

Case 6.7.2

History

A 66-year-old male, who 16 years earlier had undergone a right nephrectomy for a 13 cm clear cell adenocarcinoma, was found on chest radiograph to have a new nodular mass in the right pulmonary hilum. A CT scan at an outside institution showed a 4 cm right hilar mass, a 3.5 cm left adrenal mass, and a 6 cm mass in the tail of the pancreas. Transbronchial biopsy revealed only inflammatory cells, but a percutaneous biopsy of the pancreatic mass was compatible with metastatic renal cell carcinoma (RCC). Figures 6.7.2A and B show coronal and transaxial FDG PET images acquired with a dedicated PET tomograph (GE Advance) and reconstructed with iterative reconstruction and measured segmented attenuation correction.

Findings

Findings are the following: (1) The right hilar mass is markedly hypermetabolic; (2) the left adrenal mass demonstrates marked increased FDG uptake seen on the coronal images (bottom row, second image from the left) and transaxial images (top row on the right); (3) a large focus of moderately increased activity is present in the left abdomen anterior to the kidney and medial to the spleen, congruent with the pancreatic mass best seen on the transaxial images (middle row on the right); (4) right renal activity is absent due to prior nephrectomy; (5) asymmetrical uptake in the neck; and (6) mild uptake in the spleen.

Discussion

The pancreatic biopsy material was reviewed by a university pathologist and confirmed to be a renal cell carcinoma metastasis. The pancreatic mass is hypermetabolic, consistent with malignancy, and the hypermetabolic left adrenal mass is also a metastatic lesion.

RCC often displays atypical behavior with 10% recurring more than ten years after nephrectomy. It commonly metastasizes to the lung (55%), and often metastasizes to the liver, bone, and adrenal (20 to 25%). Metastasis to the contralateral kidney occurs in 10%, and metastasis to other organs occurs in 5%. RCC is one of the few neoplasms reported to metastasize to pancreatic parenchyma. In this patient, surgical resection of the pancreatic and

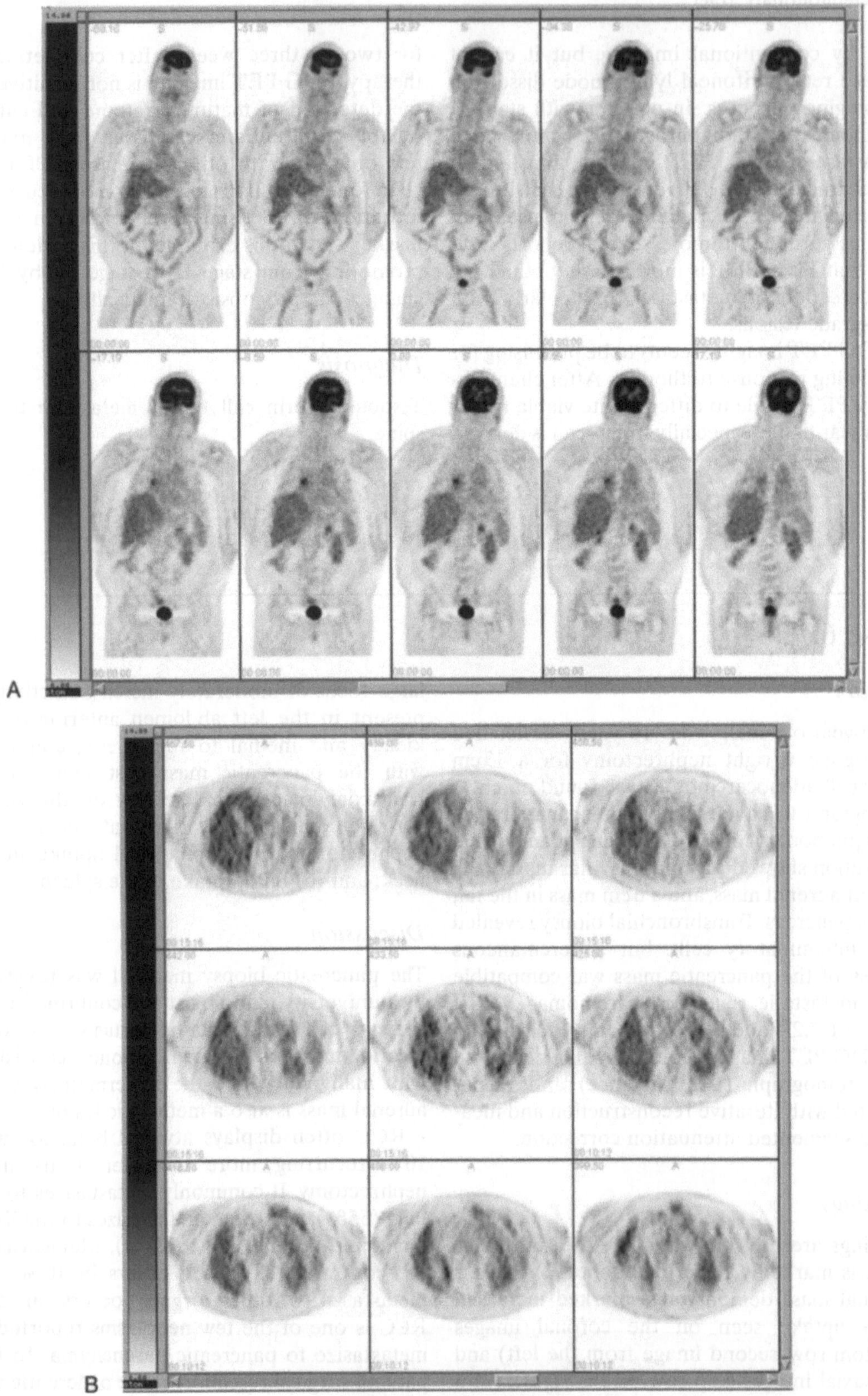

FIGURE 6.7.2A,B.

adrenal lesion was considered, but only if the lung lesion was not a metastasis. Its hypermetabolism was consistent with malignancy, but a stage I lung cancer cannot be differentiated from metastatic disease by FDG PET imaging. Adrenal metastasis is not uncommon in either bronchogenic or renal carcinoma. Resection of the hilar mass revealed only inflammatory granulomatous tissue and anthracosis. Active granulomatous lesions represent the majority of the few false-positive PET findings.

Although several patients with sizeable RCC have been reported to have false-negative FDG PET imaging, PET is positive in 77 to 90%[1,2] and is highly accurate in the assessment of indeterminate renal cysts. In patients with indeterminate renal cysts, a positive PET scan obviates the need for cyst aspiration, and a negative PET allows noninvasive radiographic follow-up.[3] However, due to the physiologic presence of FDG in urine, identification of small RCC may be difficult, and renal abnormalities such as hydronephrosis may cause false-positives.[4] In equivocal circumstances, the administration of furosemide with repeat imaging 30 minutes later may be advantageous. As with other neoplasms, FDG PET imaging is more specific than CT in defining metastatic lymphadenopathy and is more sensitive in the detection of distant metastases. Preliminary evidence indicates that FDG PET may have a role in monitoring the response to therapy, especially in cases of persistent posttherapeutic mass.[5]

Relatively mild-to-moderate diffuse splenic activity is not uncommon and is nonspecific, just as in ^{67}gallium scintigraphy. Focal abnormalities and more intense uptake in an enlarged spleen may be indicative of neoplastic involvement, especially in patients with lymphoma. Despite the asymmetry, the cervical activity is most likely related to benign skeletal muscle uptake.

Diagnoses

1. Metastatic renal cell adenocarcinoma.
2. False-positive inflammatory lung lesion.

References

1. Montravers F, Grahek D, Kerrou K, et al.: Evaluation of FDG uptake by renal malignancies (primary tumor or metastases) using a coincidence detection gamma camera. J Nucl Med 2000;41(1):78–84.
2. Bachor R, Kotzerke J, Gottfried HW, Brandle E, Reske SN, Hautmann R: Positron emission tomography in the diagnosis of renal cell carcinoma (German). Urologe A 1996;35:146–150.
3. Goldberg MA, Mayo-Smith WW, Papanicolaou N, Fischman AJ, Lee MJ: FDG PET characterization of renal masses: Preliminary experience. Clin Radiol 1997;52(7):510–515.
4. Zhuang H, Duarte PS, Pourdehnad M, Li P, Alavi A: Standardized uptake value as an unreliable index of renal disease on fluorodeoxyglucose PET imaging. Clin Nucl Med 2000;25(5):358–360.
5. Mankoff DA, Thompson JA, Gold P, Eary JF, Guinee DG Jr, Samlowski WE: Identification of interleukin-2-induced complete response in metastatic renal cell carcinoma by FDG PET despite radiographic evidence suggesting persistent tumor. Am J Roentgenol 1997;169(4):1049–1050.

Case 6.7.3

History

A 62-year-old diabetic man presented with a one-year history of progressive left ankle pain without precedent trauma. Two years earlier he had undergone nephrectomy for a 6 cm clear cell carcinoma. An ankle MRI demonstrated a 3.7 cm osseous mass with intermediate T1 and T2 signal, exhibiting cortical destruction involving the distal anterolateral left tibia with an

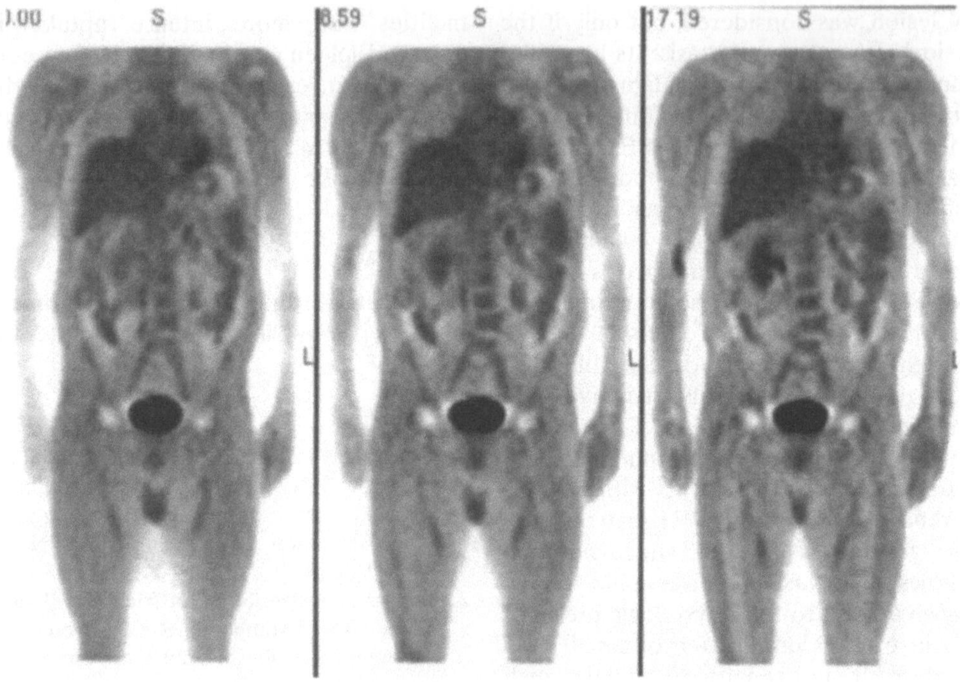

FIGURE 6.7.3A.

adjacent 1 cm similar lesion. Bone scintigraphy revealed no additional abnormalities, and CT of the brain, chest, abdomen, and pelvis were interpreted as normal except for surgical absence of the left kidney. A needle biopsy of the left tibia was consistent with clear cell renal cell carcinoma (RCC). Coronal FDG PET images of the body (Figure 6.7.3A) and lower legs (Figure 6.7.3B) are displayed. The FDG images were acquired with a dedicated PET tomograph (GE Advance) and reconstructed with iterative reconstruction and measured segmented attenuation correction.

Findings

Fasting plasma glucose was 150 mg/dl at the time of FDG administration. Foci of increased activity are identified at the distal left tibia congruent with the lesions seen on MRI. There are also two foci of relatively mild uptake in the mediastinum, one of which is congruent with a normal-sized left paratracheal lymph node and the other is congruent with a calcified node in the aortopulmonary window. No left renal activity is present. Note that the inactive marrow of the mid-to-distal femurs and the tibiae are normally photopenic as compared to active vertebral marrow. Mildly increased appendicular skeletal muscle uptake is noted.

Discussion

This diabetic's fasting glucose was only mildly elevated at the time of FDG administration; it is important to measure each patient's serum glucose prior to FDG administration because of the diminished sensitivity for detection of tumor in the face of hyperglycemia. Some investigators administer small doses of intravenous regular insulin if fasting plasma glucose is above 180 mg/dl, aiming to decrease it to less than 140 mg/dl prior to FDG administration. Although this maneuver may improve detection of some neoplastic deposits, the resultant

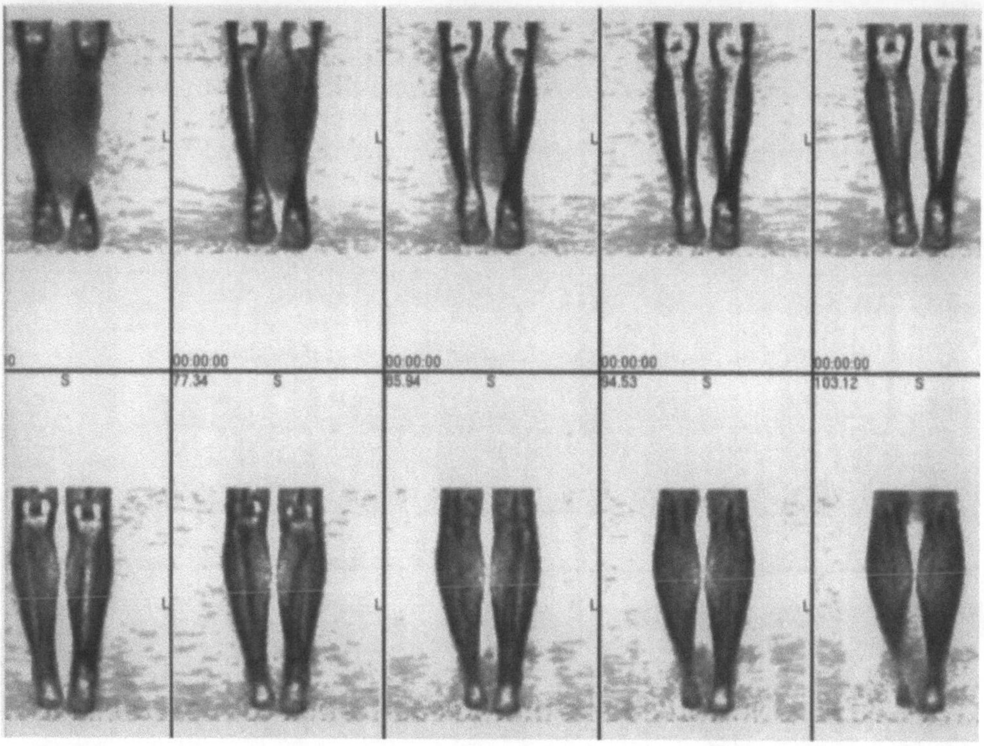

FIGURE 6.7.3B.

increased skeletal muscle uptake may interfere with tumor identification at some sites.

The known metastatic sites were easily demonstrated to be markedly hypermetabolic by FDG PET imaging, but only after the examination was tailored according to the patient's history; most PET centers do not routinely image the mid-to-distal legs. Similar procedural alterations are sometimes necessary in the occasional patient with melanoma or lymphoma. Any additional metastases can be expected to be similarly hypermetabolic. The only findings of interest are the two mediastinal foci, but uptake is only mild and barely above that of physiologic mediastinal activity. In view of the mild degree of uptake and the calcification of one of the nodes (on CT), it is likely that these nodes are inflammatory rather than neoplastic. The patient underwent limb salvage surgery, and repeat FDG PET imaging four months later (Figures 6.7.3C and D) was essentially unchanged. The mediastinal nodes exhibited a similar degree of uptake but were no larger, and there were no additional lesions noted. Only mildly increased benign uptake is present in the postoperative distal tibia. In this case, the high sensitivity and specificity of FDG PET imaging for the identification of RCC metastatic disease allowed the surgical oncologist to confidently proceed with an aggressive surgical procedure.

Incidentally noted is obvious diffusely increased activity within the musculature of the left arm (related to use of a crutch) and the right calf (related to differential weight bearing). Patients with lower limb injuries or during the postoperative period may preferentially use the unaffected extremity. As FDG accumulates in activated muscular groups, the unaffected limb will demonstrate more FDG uptake than the neglected limb. If the patient uses crutches, muscular groups of both upper extremities and both pectoralis may also demonstrate markedly increased FDG uptake that can be confused with malignancy. The pertinent history and symmetric appearance of

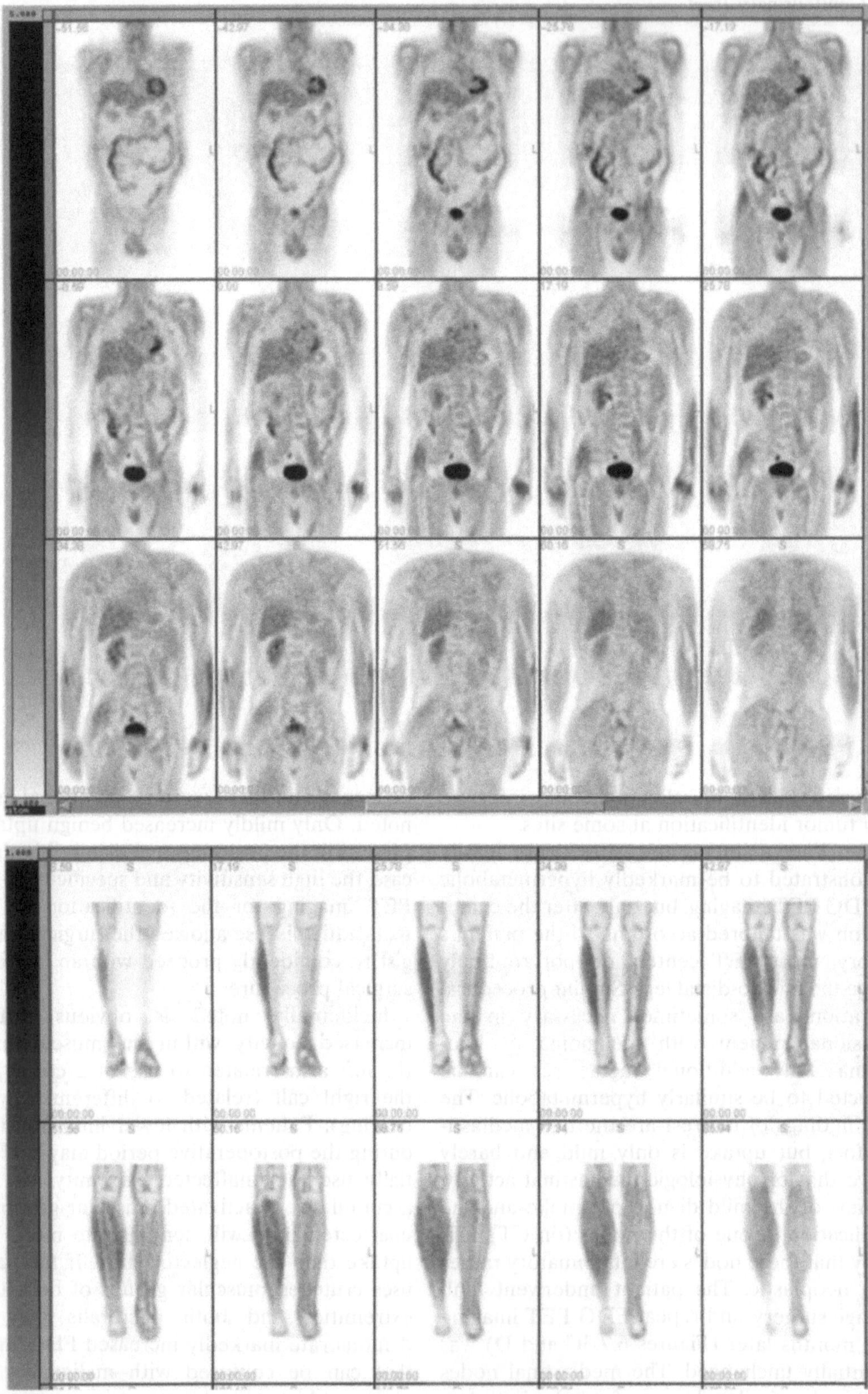

C

D

FIGURE 6.7.3C,D.

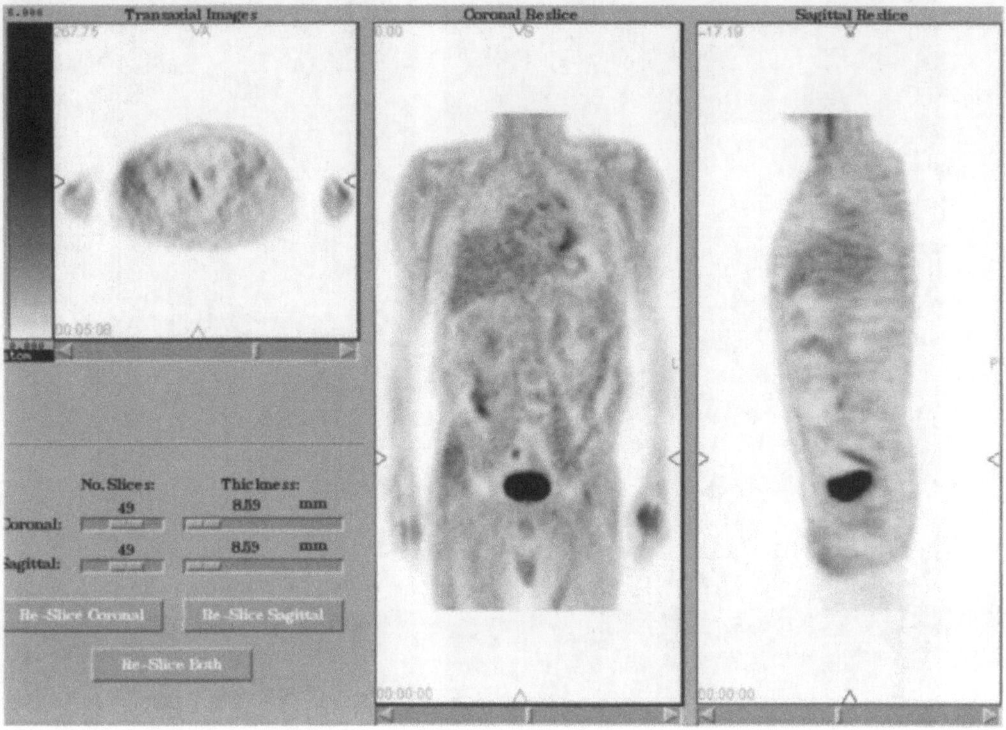

FIGURE 6.7.3E.

muscular compartments are helpful for correct interpretation.

Another incidental finding on the coronal images is the focus of uptake seen above the bladder and to the right. The focality on the coronal images is worrisome for a metastasis. Two alternative diagnostic possibilities should be considered in that location: focal retention of urine in the ureter or physiologic uptake in the sigmoid colon. In this case, the sagittal image (Figure 6.7.3E) clearly demonstrates a tubular pattern of uptake diagnostic of physiologic colonic activity.

Diagnoses

1. Isolated tibial metastases from renal cell carcinoma.
2. Postoperative crutch artifact.
3. Benign mediastinal lymphadenopathy.

Cases 6.7.4

History

A 61-year-old female with a three-year history of recurrent ovarian carcinoma was referred for assessment of a rising serum Ca-125 level. She had been off chemotherapy for one year. A CT of the abdomen and pelvis was interpreted as showing no evidence of disease (Figure 6.7.4A). Figure 6.7.4B shows transaxial FDG images acquired with a full ring dedicated PET

A

B

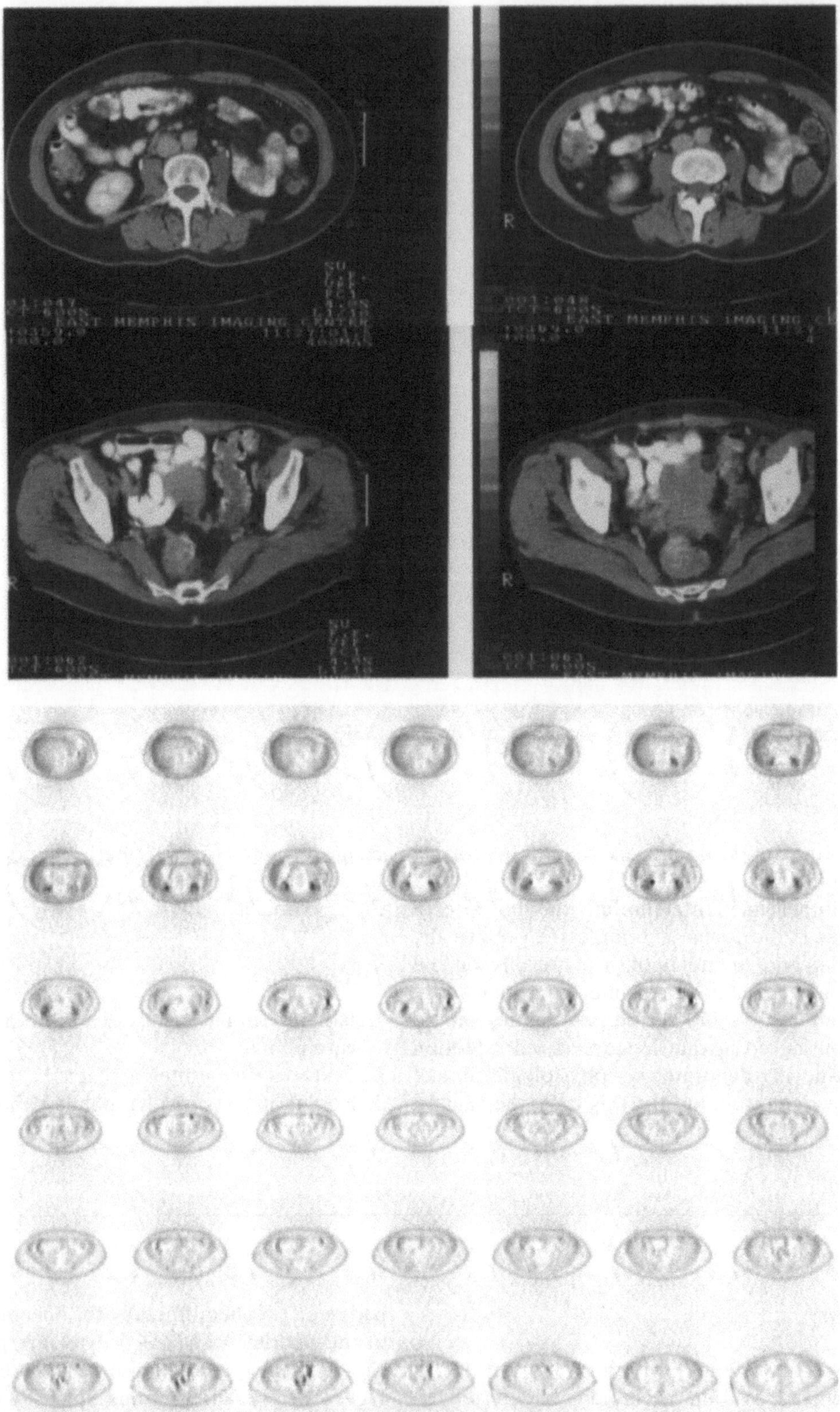

FIGURE 6.7.4A,B.

tomograph (Siemens ECAT 933) and reconstructed with filtered back projection without attenuation correction.

Findings

The FDG images were acquired with an irrigating urinary catheter in place, thus explaining the absence of urinary bladder activity. Physiologic activity is present within the renal pelves and calyces. Immediately inferior to the lower pole of the left kidney is an abnormal focus of markedly increased FDG activity (Figure 6.7.4B, third row of images). In retrospect, this corresponds to a small soft tissue mass on CT (Figure 6.7.4A, upper left image). There are also several other small foci of increased activity in the pelvis. The two more posterior of these likely represent a small amount of activity in the bladder surrounding the urinary catheter balloon, but the more anterior focus on the left corresponds to a cystic-appearing lesion recognized in retrospect on the CT in the left adnexal area (Figure 6.7.4A, lower right image).

Discussion

CT is notoriously inaccurate in detecting recurrent and/or metastatic ovarian carcinoma. Recognizing small, slightly enlarged nodes and differentiating them from nonopacified loops of bowel are challenging. In this patient, two metastatic deposits could be identified by CT retrospectively, when careful correlation is made with the PET images.

If nonmelanomatous skin cancers are excluded, ovarian carcinoma is the sixth most common malignancy and the fifth most common cause of cancer deaths in women, with over 23,000 cases diagnosed in the United States annually. Although only 25% of ovarian carcinomas are diagnosed before there has been spread to the pelvis, the five-year survival for these stage I patients is 95%. In a study of 85 patients with suspicious adnexal masses, PET identified only four of eight malignant tumors and failed to detect the two borderline low-grade tumors.[1] Several false-positive interpretations occurred with cystadenomas, a teratoma, a benign thecoma, and three inflammatory lesions. MR imaging did not improve sensitivity and increased specificity only from 78 to 86%. For this reason, FDG PET has not been promoted for initial staging, and no modality has been shown to be effective for screening asymptomatic women. At present, all patients suspected to harbor a primary ovarian carcinoma will undergo laparotomy regardless of the results of PET or other imaging.

Whereas PET may not play a role in initial preoperative staging, recent studies report a high sensitivity of 80 to 100% for the detection of metastatic disease in patients suspected of harboring recurrent ovarian cancer, including patients with elevated serum CA-125 levels but negative CT scans. However, disseminated peritoneal carcinomatosis and micrometastatic disease have been missed by FDG PET in several reports.[2] In this patient, the absence of organ and extraabdominal involvement allowed confident reexploration for debulking prior to institution of second-line chemotherapy. There is preliminary evidence that effective surgical cytoreduction at recurrence may offer a survival advantage (24 months versus 10 months).[3]

For patients with ovarian carcinoma, evaluation of the pelvis is critical. Marked FDG uptake in the bladder may obscure evaluation of the pelvis. To minimize activity in the bladder in general, the patient should be well hydrated before FDG administration and void just before acquisition of the emission scan. It is also preferable to start the emission scan on the pelvis. Attenuation correction of the images is important to reduce the high activity artifact in structures such as the bladder and ureters. On images without attenuation correction, soft tissue attenuation is more severe in the lateral projection than in the anteroposterior projection, producing positive and negative image artifact. Correction for attenuation optimally used in conjunction with iterative reconstruction overcomes this problem. Even when attenuation correction is performed on images reconstructed with filtered back projection, the quality of the images is often sufficient for clinical purposes. Bladder catheterization with irrigation has been recommended for optimal evaluation of the pelvis but can often be avoided if attenuation correction is performed. The images of this patient were acquired with an older model of PET tomograph when iterative reconstruction algorithm was not available and the transmission images had to be acquired prior to FDG administration. As discussed in Case 6.1.3, this can provide suboptimal images with attenuation correction. Therefore, an irrigating urinary catheter was placed in this patient that was critical for detecting pelvic metastatic deposits.

Diagnosis

Metastatic ovarian carcinoma, occult by CT.

References

1. Fenchel S, Kotzerke J, Stohr I, et al.: Preoperative assessment of asymptomatic adnexal tumors by positron emission tomography and F-18 fluorodeoxyglucose. Nuklearmedizin 1999;38:101–107.
2. Karlan BY, Hawkins R, Hoh C, et al.: Whole-body positron emission tomography with 2-[18F]-fluoro-2-deoxy-D-glucose can detect recurrent ovarian carcinoma. Gynecol Oncol 1993;51(2): 175–181.
3. Gadducci A, Iacconi P, Fanucchi A, Cosio S, Teti G, Genazzani AR: Surgical cytoreduction during second-look laparotomy in patients with advanced ovarian cancer. Anticancer Res 2000;20: 1959–1964.

Case 6.7.5

History

In June 2000, a 75-year-old female with a history of recurrent breast and ovarian cancer presented with a rising serum CA-125 level and left leg swelling. In 1992, she had undergone right mastectomy for carcinoma, and in 1994, she was found at laparotomy to have bilateral poorly differentiated serous adenocarcinoma of the ovaries. Immediately after completing combination chemotherapy, she developed a left iliac nodal recurrence that was resected and irradiated. The patient developed recurrent ovarian carcinoma in 1996 and again in 1997, at a left iliac node and the cecum, respectively. In March 1999, a chest wall recurrence of her breast carcinoma occurred; this was resected and treated with radiation and tamoxifen. In May 2000, a bone scintigraphy, brain MRI, and chest radiograph were interpreted as normal. A CT of the abdomen and pelvis revealed a stable large left parapelvic cyst but new mild dilatation of the left ureter. Coronal FDG PET images (Figure 6.7.5) acquired with a dedicated full ring tomograph (GE Advance) and reconstructed using an iterative algorithm and segmental attenuation correction are displayed.

Findings

The FDG images demonstrate a small focus of markedly increased activity at the distal left ureter. The central photopenia of the left kidney suggests left hydronephrosis, but in this case was due to the long-standing parapelvic cyst.

Discussion

In view of the dilated collecting system seen on CT and the elevated serum tumor marker levels, the abnormal FDG focus in the pelvis is most consistent with a recurrent deposit of ovarian carcinoma. Repeat images acquired after voiding (not shown) were unchanged, making ureteral retention of radioactive urine a less likely explanation. This maneuver, in addition to using an indwelling irrigating urinary catheter during acquisition, may be helpful in detecting metastatic deposits in the lower abdomen and pelvis adjacent to the renal collecting system. This is especially important in patients with genitourinary tumors but may also be useful in patients with colorectal carcinoma or lymphoma. Laparotomy revealed recurrent tumor along the left pelvic sidewall

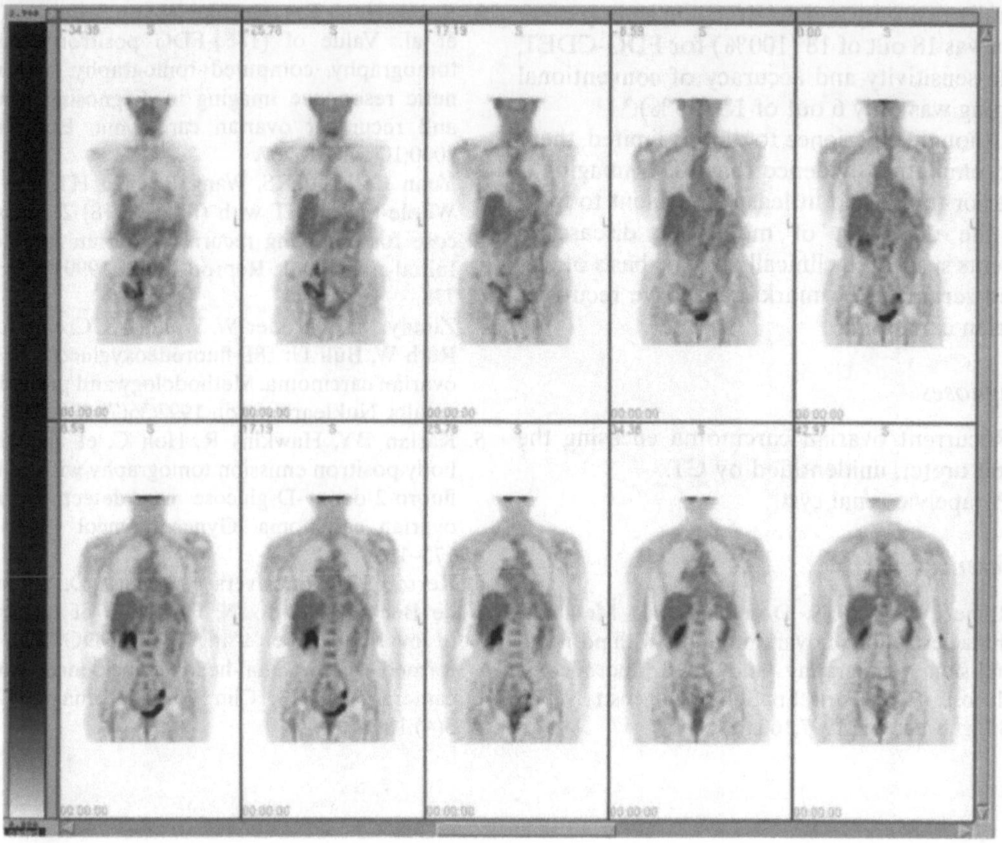

FIGURE 6.7.5.

encasing the iliac vessels and the ureter with histology most compatible with recurrent ovarian carcinoma.

Romer et al.[1] localized recurrent ovarian carcinoma in four of five cases, but disseminated peritoneal carcinomatosis in two patients was not detected using FDG PET. In the follow-up of 11 patients for recurrent ovarian carcinoma, Kubik-Huch et al.[2] detected recurrent disease in ten of ten patients for a sensitivity of 100%, specificity of 50%, and accuracy of 90%; CT and MRI had accuracies of 43% and 89%, respectively. They felt that PET and MRI were similar in their abilities to detect recurrent disease, but FDG has a potential advantage in its larger field of view. Yuan et al.[3] found that FDG PET demonstrated findings that correlated with the surgical-pathologic findings in all five of their patients suspected of having recurrent ovarian carcinoma, including two with elevated serum CA-125 levels but negative CT findings; CT had a sensitivity of only 60% in these five patients. In another series of nine patients with suspected recurrence, FDG PET was found to be highly accurate.[4] In an early study of 13 patients,[5] all the patients thought to have recurrence clinically had positive findings on FDG PET, but five of six with negative PET scans had microscopic foci of residual tumor at surgery. Other instances of failure to identify microscopic disease or low-grade ovarian malignancies have been reported.[4] In a recent study of 23 patients imaged with a hybrid dual-head gamma camera (FDG-CDET) for suspected recurrence of ovarian carcinoma, 18 of whom had only an increased serum CA-125 level, the overall sensitivity and accuracy on a per patient basis was 18 out of 18 (100%) for FDG-CDET, while sensitivity and accuracy of conventional imaging was only 6 out of 18 (33%).[6]

Although experience to date is limited, there is accumulating evidence that FDG imaging is superior to CT and at least equivalent to MRI for the detection of metastatic disease in patients suspected clinically on the basis of elevated serum tumor markers to have recurrent ovarian carcinoma.

Diagnoses

1. Recurrent ovarian carcinoma encasing the left ureter, unidentified by CT.
2. Parapelvic renal cyst.

References

1. Romer W, Avril N, Dose J, et al.: Metabolic characterization of ovarian tumors with positron-emission tomography and F-18 fluorodeoxyglucose. Rofo Fortschr Geb Rontgenstr Neuen Bildgeb Verfahr 1997;166:62–68.
2. Kubik-Huch RA, Dorffler W, von Schulthess GK, et al.: Value of (18F)-FDG positron emission tomography, computed tomography, and magnetic resonance imaging in diagnosing primary and recurrent ovarian carcinoma. Eur Radiol 2000;10(5):761–767.
3. Yuan CC, Liu RS, Wang PH, Ng HT, Yeh SH: Whole-body PET with (fluorine-18)-2 deoxyglucose for detecting recurrent ovarian carcinoma. Initial report. J Reprod Med 1999;44(9):775–778.
4. Zimny M, Schroder W, Wolters S, Cremerius U, Rath W, Bull U: 18F-fluorodeoxyglucose PET in ovarian carcinoma: Methodology and preliminary results. Nuklearmedizin 1997;36(7):228–233.
5. Karlan BY, Hawkins R, Hoh C, et al.: Whole-body positron emission tomography with 2-[18F]-fluoro-2-deoxy-D-glucose can detect recurrent ovarian carcinoma. Gynecol Oncol 1993;51(2):175–181.
6. Kerrou K, Montravers F, Grahek D, Younsi N, de Beco V, Talbot JN: Detection of recurrence of ovarian cancer using [F-18]-FDG scan performed on a dual-head coincidence gamma camera (CDET). Clin Positron Imaging 2000; 3(4):186.

Case 6.7.6

History

A 76-year-old woman presented with a rising serum Ca-125 level and a contrasted CT of the abdomen and pelvis showing no evidence of metastatic disease. Two years prior she had undergone resection of an ovarian adenocarcinoma followed by combination chemotherapy. Coronal and transaxial FDG PET images (Figures 6.7.6A and B) acquired with a dedicated full ring PET tomograph (GE Advance) and reconstructed using an iterative algorithm and measured segmented attenuation correction are displayed.

Findings

Physiologic areolar activity is seen symmetrically. A small focus of increased activity is present on the anterior surface of the right hepatic lobe, suggestive of a serosal metastasis. An additional focus of increased activity is identified within the spleen. A focal area of increased activity in the pelvis to the right of the bladder is also present.

Discussion

Periareolar activity is a frequent physiologic finding and should not be mistaken for a breast lesion. FDG imaging demonstrates splenic and hepatic metastases unsuspected by CT, and metastatic disease may be present within the pelvis as well. Without close correlation with a contemporary contrasted CT of the pelvis, it is difficult to judge whether the pelvic abnormality is related to metastatic ovarian carcinoma

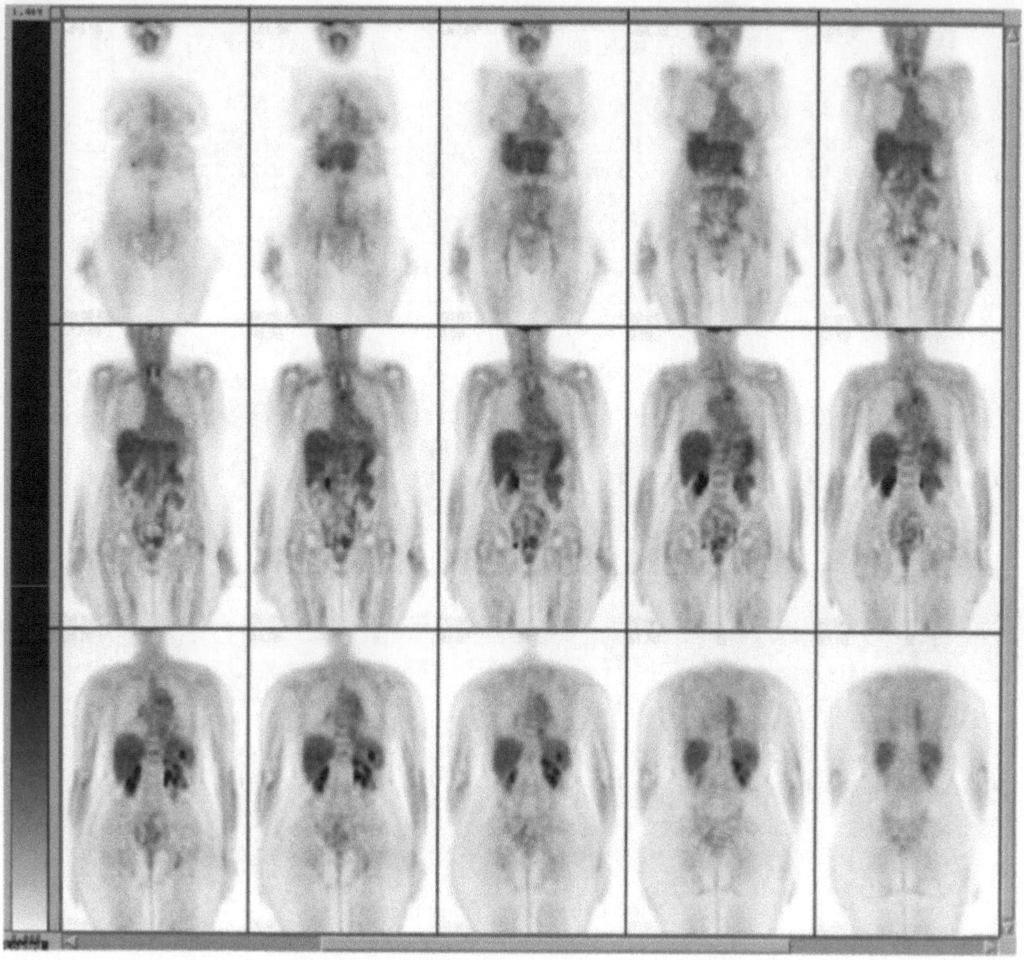

FIGURE 6.7.6A.

or physiologic sigmoid activity. Although CT is not sensitive for the detection of pelvic nodal metastases in women with recurrent ovarian carcinoma, lesions mistaken for unopacified bowel or nodes smaller than 1 cm in diameter can often be recognized in retrospect after close correlation with the PET scan.

Although there is preliminary evidence that FDG PET is more sensitive for the detection of recurrent ovarian carcinoma in patients presenting with elevated serum tumor markers (see Discussion, Case 6.7.5), there is little evidence to suggest that FDG PET is sensitive for the detection of low-volume disease in patients in clinical complete remission after primary chemotherapy. Approximately half of these patients with a complete response are found to have persistent/recurrent disease at the time of second-look laparotomy (or laparoscopy). However, because there is no well-demonstrated survival advantage for patients undergoing second-look surgery and because half of patients found to be negative at second-look surgery recur, the use of routine second-look surgery is controversial. It is doubtful that FDG PET will be able to replace second-look

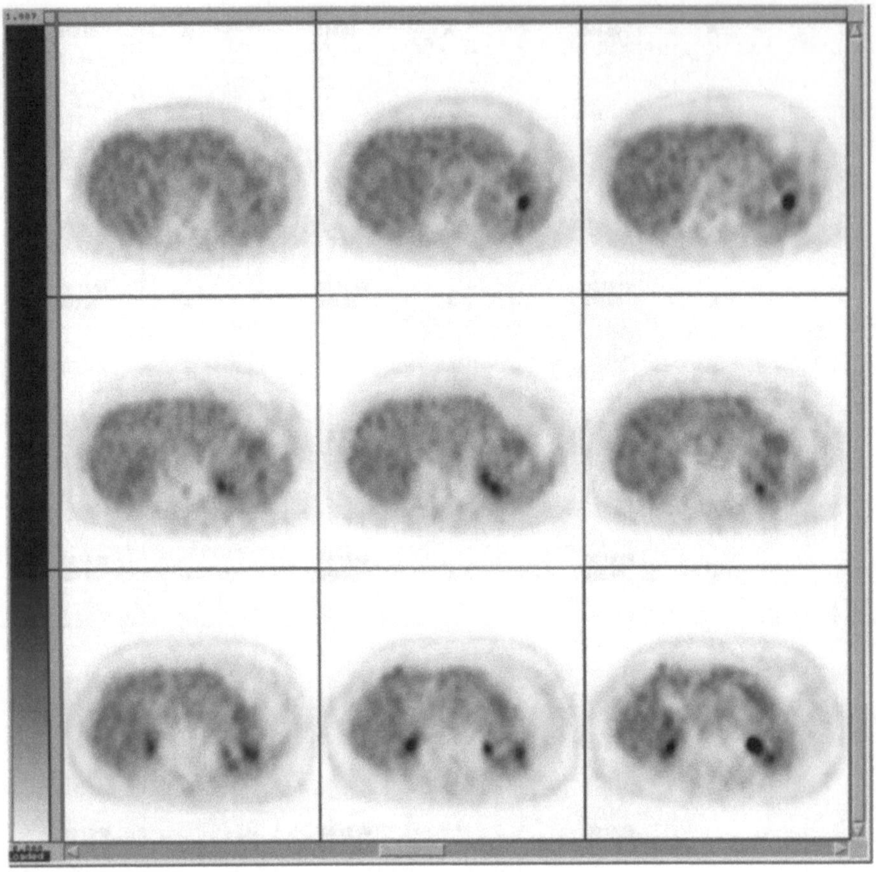

FIGURE 6.7.6B. (*Continued*)

surgery in the patients that such a procedure is deemed advisable.[1]

Diagnosis

Metastatic ovarian carcinoma, occult by CT.

Reference

1. Chu CS, Rubin SC: Second-look laparotomy for epithelial ovarian cancer: A reappraisal. Curr Oncol Rep 2001;3:11–18.

Case 6.7.7

History

In January 2001, a 66-year-old man with a history of poorly differentiated prostate carcinoma was referred for FDG PET imaging due to a progressively rising serum prostate specific antigen (PSA). At the time of his initial diagnosis in January 1996, he was treated with pelvic radiotherapy followed by antiandrogen therapy. He has not experienced skeletal metastases but was first noted to have liver metastases in 1998, which at that time were unresponsive to cytotoxic therapy. In May 1999, a metastasis at the tip of the right hepatic lobe and another in the left lobe were treated with percutaneous CT-guided radiofrequency ablation. Due to the finding of FDG hypermetabolism at the right lobe lesion accompanied by a rising serum PSA, the radiofrequency ablation of the right lobe lesion was repeated in September 1999. In January 2000, both lesions had decreased in size and appeared by CT to be cystic, consistent with necrosis. The serum PSA had dropped from 65 ng/ml to undetectable. During October and November 2000, the serum PSA again rose to 4–12 ng/ml at which time the right lobe and left lobe radiofrequency ablations were repeated. Since the last radiofrequency ablation, serum PSA continued to rise to 17 and then to 41 ng/ml. He is currently being treated with investigational systemic cytotoxic therapy and androgen ablative therapy. CT of the head, thorax, and pelvis are reported to be negative for metastatic disease. Selected current axial CT images of the liver (Figure 6.7.7A) and transaxial (Figure 6.7.7B) FDG PET images acquired with a dedicated full ring PET tomograph (GE Advance) and reconstructed using an iterative algorithm and segmented attenuation correction are displayed.

Findings

No extrahepatic abnormal hypermetabolic foci are noted. Physiologic activity is noted in the stomach and spleen, and a discrete photopenic focus is identified in the left lobe congruent with the radiofrequency ablation-treated partially necrotic lesion seen on CT. However, posterior to the photopenia, there is a similar-sized focus of increased activity. Similarly, at the tip of the right lobe, there is a photopenic focus congruent with the lesion seen on CT, and a hypermetabolic focus is identified immediately

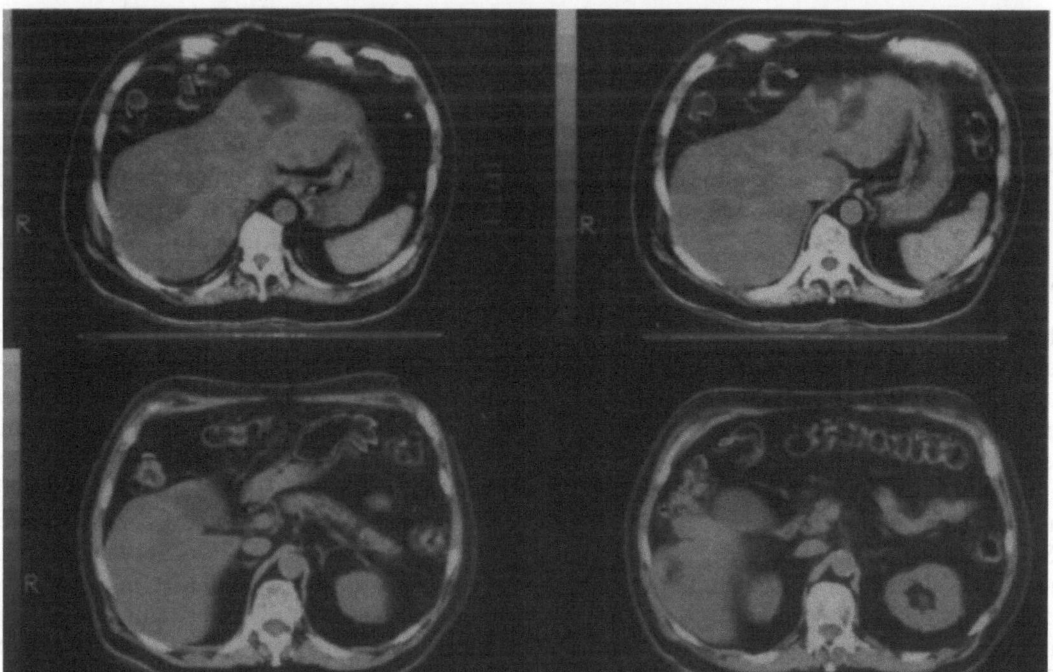

FIGURE 6.7.7A.

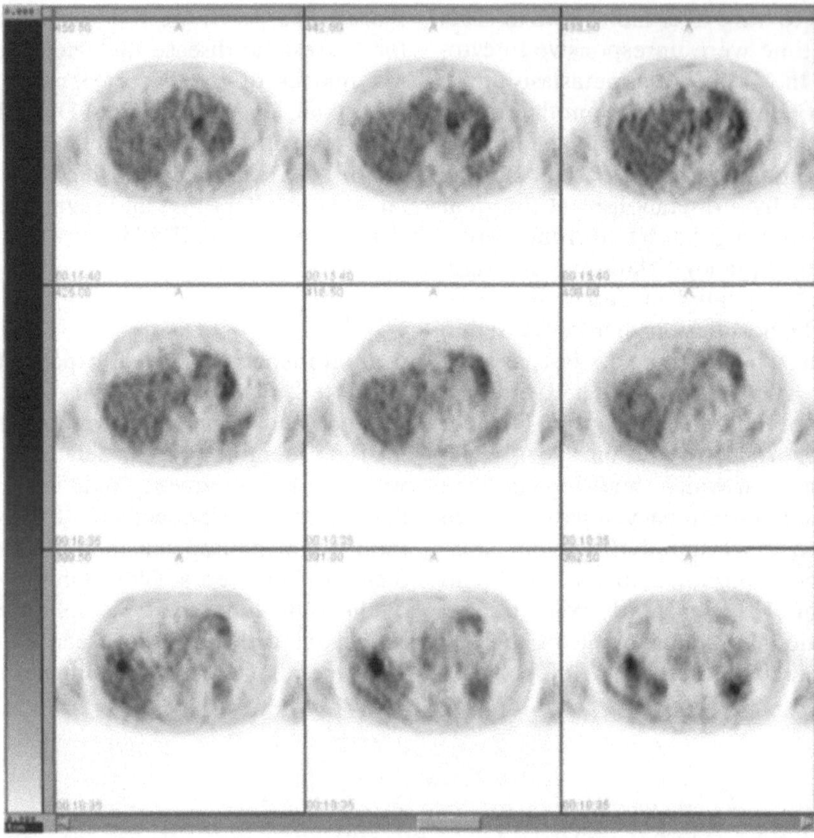

FIGURE 6.7.7B. *(Continued)*

medial to the photopenia. There is no definite CT lesion identified corresponding to either of the hypermetabolic foci seen with PET.

Discussion

These findings are most consistent with adequate treatment of the right and left lobe metastases demonstrated by the photopenic necrosis seen with FDG imaging, but there is also evidence of adjacent recurrent or persistent viable neoplasm, thus accounting for the persistent and progressive rise in serum PSA concentration. Prior success was documented by absence of persistent activity at the left lobe lesion in September 1999, and the fall in PSA to an undetectable level in January 2000, after repeat radiofrequency ablation of the right lobe lesion identified as hypermetabolic by PET.

Radiofrequency ablation is emerging as a new therapeutic method for management of primary and secondary unresectable liver cancers with minimal local and systemic complications. The technique is performed intraoperatively, laparoscopically, or percutaneously using CT or ultrasound guidance. Insertion of a needle electrode emitting radiofrequency waves into the tumor achieves total necrosis in 80% of masses by thermal ablation. Hepatic metastases and primary hepatic tumors are being treated aggressively more often and with good immediate results (tumor control in over 90%) and improved disease-free and overall survival. To date, CT and MR imaging have generally been used in combination with clinical parameters for judging the success of radiofrequency ablation therapy and detection of recurrence, but the optimal technique for monitoring the response of these hepatic neoplasms to radiofrequency ablation therapy is yet to be determined.

In colon cancer, FDG PET imaging has been shown to be superior to CT in distinguishing viable tumor from posttreatment scar and monitoring the response of hepatic metastases to surgical resection; it is also better than CT for monitoring the response of hepatocellular carcinoma to transarterial chemoembolization. Therefore, it is expected that PET will emerge as the pre-eminent modality for detecting recurrent/persistent tumor following radiofrequency ablation of hepatic metastases and guiding further radiofrequency ablation therapy, as demonstrated by this patient.

At present, conventional bone scintigraphy, CT, and ^{111}In-capromab pendetide scintigraphy represent the standard of care for detection of metastatic prostate cancer in patients with a rising serum PSA following radical prostatectomy or radiation therapy. None of these modalities is sensitive for detection of pelvic metastatic deposits, and there is little information regarding the sensitivity of ^{111}In-capromab or FDG scintigraphy for the detection of distant metastases, although neither are especially sensitive for detection of bone metastases. In this particular patient, the hepatic metastases are FDG-avid, so the utility of PET is obvious. In light of evidence that tumors with higher histological Gleason grades have higher degrees of FDG accumulation, it is possible that the tumors that tend to metastasize distantly, that is, the less-differentiated tumors, may be reliably detectable with FDG imaging.

Diagnosis

Recurrent hepatic metastases from prostate carcinoma, postradiofrequency ablation.

Case 6.7.8

History

A 77-year-old woman with invasive carcinoma of the cervix presented for restaging six months following completion of radiation therapy. In addition to CT of the chest, abdomen, and pelvis, FDG PET images were acquired with a dedicated full ring tomograph (GE Advance) and reconstructed using an iterative algorithm and segmental attenuation correction. Axial CT images of the thorax (Figure 6.7.8A) and axial (Figure 6.7.8B) and coronal FDG images (Figure 6.7.8C) are displayed.

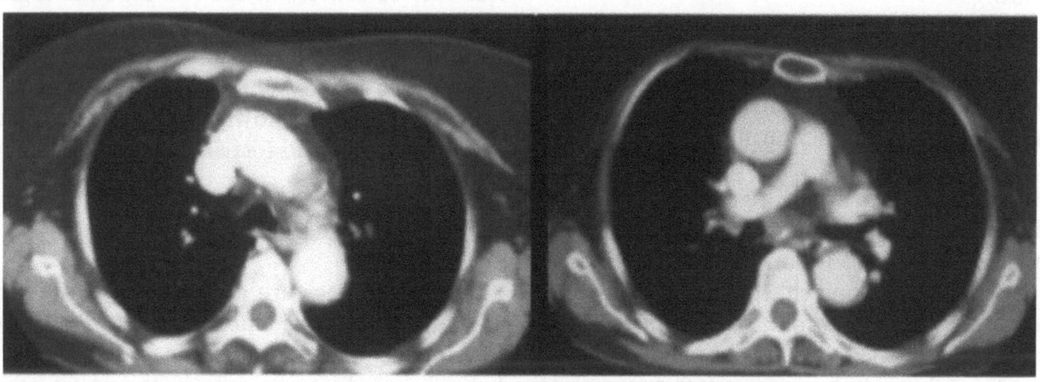

FIGURE 6.7.8A.

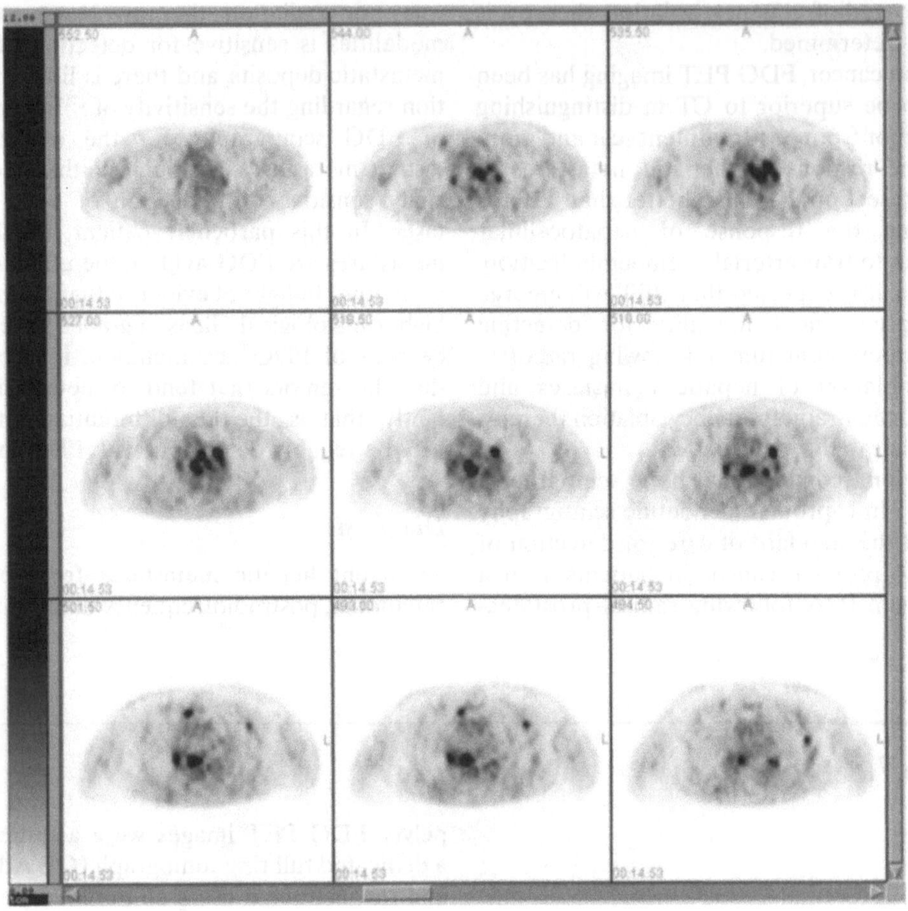

FIGURE 6.7.8B.

Findings

Multiple foci of markedly increased FDG uptake are present in the mediastinum and pulmonary hila, congruent with lymph nodes seen on CT, one of them measuring 2 cm in size. The axial PET images demonstrate that several other foci are located at the chest wall bilaterally; corresponding abnormalities are not seen on the CT images. Relatively mild activity is seen within the stomach, spleen, and bowel at an intensity similar to that of physiologic liver activity. There is a large focus of intense pelvic activity with a photopenic center superior to the bladder, and there are two superficial anterior foci of activity in the left inguinal region. Bilateral ureteral activity should not be mistaken for nodal metastases. A 2 cm low-attenuation mass was noted by CT within the caudate lobe (not shown), but no corresponding hypermetabolic focus is seen on the FDG images.

Discussion

The PET findings are consistent with multiple metastases to the mediastinum and ribs, as well as two left inguinal metastatic nodes. The large hypermetabolic focus seen in the pelvis corresponds to a large partially necrotic retrouterine

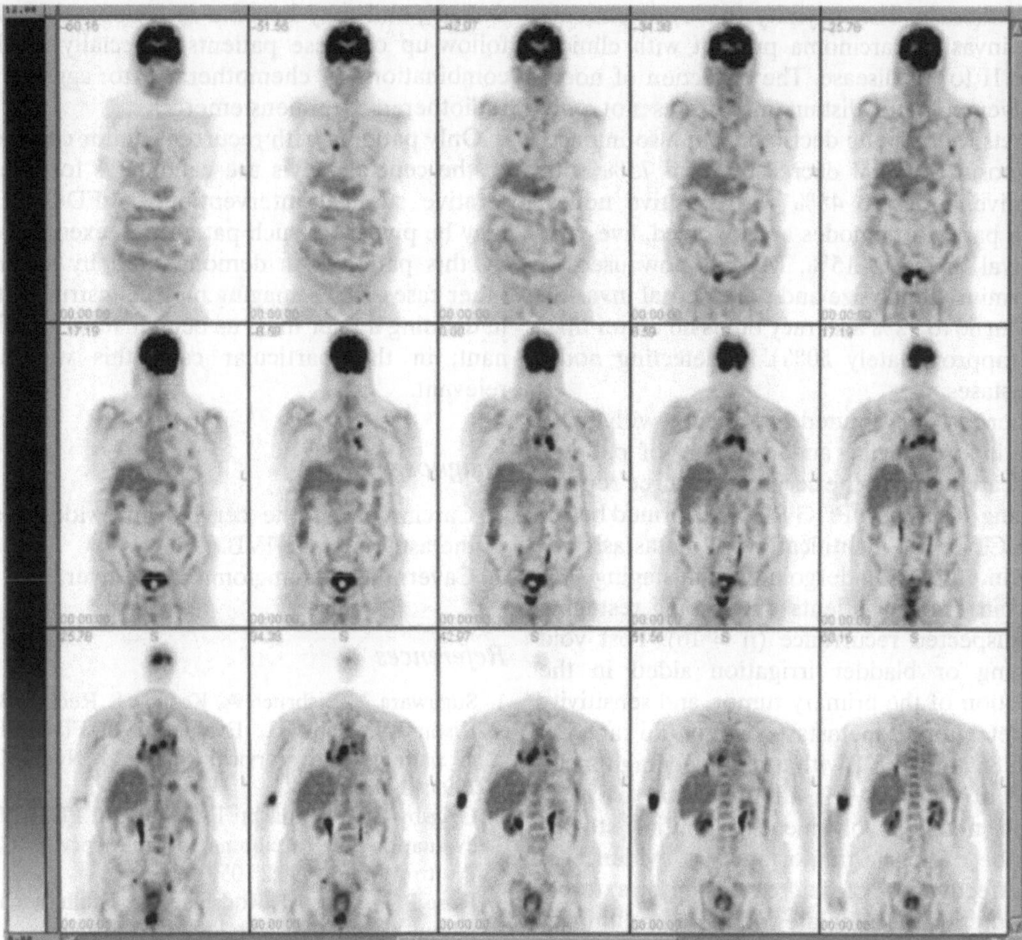

FIGURE 6.7.8C.

mass seen on CT and described as 50% smaller than on the previous CT, representing a partial response to radiotherapy. The absence of hypermetabolism at the caudate lobe of the liver where a low-attenuation mass was identified is consistent with a benign mass, most likely a cavernous hemangioma.

Cervical cancer is the sixth most common solid malignancy in women and the third most common gynecological cancer with almost 13,000 new cases of invasive disease annually. With early detection, the prognosis of preinvasive disease has improved, but the overall five-year survival of 70% for invasive cervical cancer has not changed in over 20 years. Thirteen percent of patients present with advanced disease, experiencing a 50 to 62% five-year survival for stage III and 20% five-year survival for stage IV disease. Internationally recognized guidelines for the diagnosis and pretreatment staging of carcinoma of the cervix include clinical exam, conization, colposcopy, sigmoidoscopy, cystoscopy, and limited conventional imaging with chest X-ray, IVP, and skeletal survey. Identification of nodal metastases is not addressed by conventional staging of this disease, but the clinical staging is inaccurate in 50 to 67% of patients thought to have stage II to IV disease. The majority (62%) of patients with invasive carcinoma present with clinical stage II to IV disease. The detection of nodal involvement and distant metastases not only impacts therapeutic decisions, but also impacts prognosis. Survival decreases from 75% with negative nodes to 45% with positive nodes; when para-aortic nodes are involved, five-year survival drops to 15%. MRI is now used to determine tumor size and parametrial invasion with an 80 to 92% accuracy but is no better than CT (approximately 50%) in detecting nodal metastases.

There is only limited experience with FDG PET in the staging and restaging of patients with carcinoma of the cervix.[1-3] In three reports totaling 76 women, FDG PET performed better than CT in the identification of metastasis not only in patients undergoing initial staging (n = 60), but also in patients undergoing restaging for suspected recurrence (n = 16). Post void imaging or bladder irrigation aided in the detection of the primary tumor, and sensitivity for detection of metastases was in the range of 75 to 86% for PET with a relatively high mean SUV of 10.3 +/- 3.2. Identification of para-aortic nodal involvement at initial staging may be of special importance as evidence of the effectiveness of field extension of external radiotherapy accumulates. If these preliminary findings can be confirmed in larger populations, FDG PET may provide incremental diagnostic and prognostic information in the initial staging of patients with advanced disease, thus altering therapy, and may become instrumental in the follow-up of these patients, especially as the combination of chemotherapy to aggressive radiotherapy regimens emerges.

Only patients with recurrent tumor confined to the central pelvis are candidates for exenterative surgical intervention, so FDG PET may be pivotal in such patients, as exemplified by this patient. As demonstrated by several other cases, FDG imaging may be instrumental in defining a liver mass as benign versus malignant; in this particular case, this was not relevant.

Diagnoses

1. Carcinoma of the cervix with widespread metastases, stage IVB.
2. Cavernous hemangioma of the liver.

References

1. Sugawara Y, Eisbruch A, Kosuda S, Recker BE, Kison PV, Wahl RL: Evaluation of FDG PET in patients with cervical cancer. J Nucl Med 1999;40:1125–1131.
2. Grigsby PW, Dehdashti F, Siegel BA: FDG-PET evaluation of carcinoma of the cervix. Clin Positron Imag 1999;2:105–109.
3. Rose PG, Adler LP, Rodriguez M, Faulhaber PF, Abdul-Karim FW, Miraldi F: Positron emission tomography for evaluating para-aortic nodal metastasis in locally advanced cervical cancer before surgical staging: A surgicopathologic study. J Clin Oncol 1999;17(1):41–45.

6.8 Lymphoma

William H. Martin, Amy B. Gibson, and Dominique Delbeke

Although the incidence of Hodgkin's disease (HD) and non-Hodgkin's lymphoma (NHL) is only 8% of all malignancies, they are potentially curable malignancies. The extent of the disease is the most important factor influencing relapse-free and total survival of patients.[1,2] Conventional methods for staging (CT and ^{67}gallium imaging) have limitations.[3–7] Although ^{67}gallium plays a role in the evaluation of the presence of viable tumor in residual posttherapy masses, it is not superior to CT in initial staging of untreated lymphoma.[7]

Both HD and NHL exhibit marked FDG uptake, and FDG imaging is useful both for staging and monitoring therapy.[8–21] Several of these studies have shown that there is a correlation between the degree of FDG uptake and the grade of the lymphoma.[10–13] However, there is a large overlap between low-grade and high-grade lymphoma. The same is true for ^{67}gallium scintigraphy.

Because lymphoma is not treated surgically and all presumed lesions cannot be biopsied from an ethical and practical point of view, the true sensitivity, specificity, and accuracy of the imaging modalities used for staging cannot be evaluated. Data found in the literature usually compare two imaging modalities: Concordant sites of disease are considered true disease, and discordant sites are discriminated by biopsy, when possible, or by clinical and radiological follow-up.

Staging Lymphoma

One of the most important factors influencing relapse-free and total survival of lymphoma patients, besides histology, is extent of disease, and accurate initial staging is essential for optimizing patient therapy and determining prognosis.[1] Therapeutic implications for patients with HD and NHL emphasize the importance of initial staging accuracy. Patients diagnosed with stage I or II HD and some subgroups of NHL may receive local external radiotherapy alone or in combination with chemotherapy, while those with stage III or IV disease are typically treated with chemotherapy.[2] Prognostic implications are equally important with stage being consistently identified as a major prognostic factor in all lymphomas and HD.

Conventional modalities for staging lymphoma include physical examination, computed tomography (CT) of the chest, abdomen, and pelvis, and bone marrow biopsy. Although CT is the best imaging technique to provide detailed information about the relationship between organs and vascular structures, CT criteria for pathologic adenopathy are based on size alone, which is a major limitation. Benign lymph node enlargement may lead to overstaging, while small malignant lymph nodes may not be recognized, resulting in understaging. In addition, CT has limited sensitivity for detection of spleen, liver, and bone marrow involvement. Equivocal CT lesions are common and frequently require additional imaging or biopsy. This prolongs the staging workup and adds to patient expense and morbidity. Patients who are understaged may receive inadequate therapy for their disease, jeopardizing the opportunity for remission or cure. Conversely, overstaged patients may receive unnecessarily aggressive or investigational therapy and be given an overly grim prognosis.

Although scintigraphy with ^{67}gallium is sometimes included in the initial staging of patients with lymphoma, it has many limitations. These include suboptimal photon energy leading to noisy images, variable uptake of gallium by tumor, particularly low-grade NHL, limited detection of abdominal disease secondary to marked physiologic hepatic and colonic activity, and the potential for false-positive findings related to infectious or inflammatory processes. ^{67}Gallium scintigraphy is inconvenient for the patient since multiple visits to the imaging facility on consecutive days are typically required. In addition, the value of ^{67}gallium scintigraphy is not in the initial staging of patients with lymphoma, but in the evaluation of the response to treatment and assessment of residual mass after therapy. However, a pretherapy scan is necessary to confirm that the tumor is ^{67}gallium-avid before trusting follow-up ^{67}gallium scans as an accurate measure of tumor response.

Evaluation of lymphomatous involvement of the bone marrow requires invasive bone marrow aspiration and biopsy; the sensitivity of bone marrow aspiration and biopsy for detecting bone marrow disease is limited by sampling error. Several studies have shown lymphoma present in only one sample of bilateral iliac crest biopsy in 22 to 30% of NHL patients.[22–25] Bone scintigraphy is unreliable for demonstration of skeletal involvement because of its low sensitivity.[26–29] Although MRI appears to be the most sensitive imaging technique, whole-body MRI is not applicable as a screening technique and should be reserved for areas that are clinically suspect.[30,31]

Many of these limitations of conventional staging modalities for lymphoma can be overcome with the use of FDG PET. Unlike CT, functional imaging with FDG PET imaging directly identifies increased metabolic activity in malignant tissue and does not depend on anatomical distortion or enlargement for determination of abnormalities. Compared with ^{67}gallium, FDG is avidly trapped by virtually all lymphomas, although the degree of FDG uptake does seem to correlate with the histological grade of malignancy and proliferation rate.[10,13] Although physiologic gastrointestinal activity does occur with FDG, the better quality of the images usually allows differentiation of physiologic activity in the bowel from abdominal and pelvic lesions. With FDG PET imaging, most of the skeleton is imaged during scanning, enabling noninvasive detection of focal bone marrow disease that may be missed through sampling error with standard iliac crest biopsy.

The high accuracy of FDG PET imaging for staging lymphoma was first demonstrated in a pilot study of 16 patients by Newman et al.[4] Several subsequent studies on larger numbers of patients, including a review of 45 patients imaged at Vanderbilt University,[32] confirm the value of FDG PET in evaluating the extent of lymphoma in nodal stations,[15] extranodal sites,[16] and bone marrow.[17,18] These studies demonstrate that both CT and FDG PET imaging detect additional nodal sites involved, compared to each modality alone. However, FDG PET imaging is superior to CT for detection of extranodal lymphoma. FDG PET is also suitable for identifying osseous involvement with a high positive predictive value[33] and is more sensitive and specific than bone scintigraphy. Compared to bone marrow biopsy, FDG PET imaging can detect bone marrow involvement when the posterior iliac crest biopsy is normal.[17,18] In these studies, FDG PET led to a change in staging in 7 to 16% of patients. Two studies report a change in therapy in 13% and 14% of the patients, respectively.[32,34] In addition, the degree of FDG uptake appears to be a prognostic factor.[9] Hoh et al.[14] have demonstrated the cost-effectiveness of PET as compared to conventional staging modalities by comparing the actual cost in a group of 18 patients ($36,250 for PET and $66,292 for conventional staging modalities).

Monitoring Therapy and Detection of Persistent or Recurrent Lymphoma

Although the sensitivity of CT and FDG imaging may be comparable in staging untreated lymphoma, CT is unable to distinguish between active or recurrent disease and residual scar tissue after therapy. In a study of 34 patients with lymphoma, 32 had a residual mass on CT after therapy. Of these 32 patients, FDG PET imaging showed no residual uptake in 17 patients and accurately predicted complete remission.[20] In a study of 32 patients with aggressive NHL and a residual mass after completion of therapy, 89% (8 out of 9) patients with a positive PET have relapsed as compared to less than 10% of patients with a negative PET.[35]

In patients with NHL, standard chemotherapy causes a rapid decrease in tumor FDG uptake as early as seven days after treatment and continues to decline during therapy. The uptake at 42 days was superior to the uptake at 7 days posttherapy in predicting the long-term outcome.[21] A study of 28 patients evaluated early during chemotherapy with FDG has demonstrated that the progression-free survival at one and two years was 20% and 0%, respectively for FDG-positive patients and 87% and 68% for FDG-negative patients.[36]

Delbeke et al.[37] reported a change of management in 15 out of 45 (30%) patients evaluated with FDG PET in their follow-up of therapy for lymphoma by avoiding biopsy in patients with residual but nonviable mass on CT at the end of therapy or by diagnoses of recurrence.

Summary

FDG PET imaging is recommended for staging lymphoma in addition to CT and other conventional staging modalities because it can detect additional nodal and extranodal lymphomatous lesions, as well as bone marrow involvement even if bone marrow biopsy is negative. During chemotherapy, FDG PET imaging can identify the responders early in the course of treatment, allowing alterations in the chemotherapy regimen as indicated. Finally, FDG PET can differentiate scarring from persistent or recurrent tumor in residual masses after the end of treatment and allows improved discrimination of rebound thymic hyperplasia from viable lymphoma. Because of the superior resolution of FDG images compared to ^{67}gallium scintigraphy, FDG imaging (when available) is replacing ^{67}gallium for evaluation of patients with lymphoma.

References

1. Jotti G, Bonandonna G: Prognostic factors in Hodgkin's disease: Implications for modern treatment. Anticancer Res 1998;8:749–760.
2. Armitage JO: Drug therapy: Treatment of non-Hodgkin's lymphoma. N Engl J Med 1993;328: 1023–1030.
3. Castellino RA, Blank N, Hoppe RT, Cho C: Hodgkin's disease: Contribution of chest CT in the initial staging evaluation. Radiology 1986; 160:603–605.
4. Newman JS, Francis IR, Kaminske MS, Wahl RL: Imaging of lymphoma with PET with 2-[f-18]fluoro-2-deoxyglucose: Correlation with CT. Radiology 1994;190:111–116.
5. Neumann CH, Robert NJ, Canellos G, Rosenthal D: Computed tomography of the abdomen and pelvis in non-Hodgkin lymphoma. J Comput Assist Tomgr 1983;7:846–850.
6. Munker R, Stengel A, Stabler A, Hiller E, Brehm G: Diagnostic accuracy of ultrasound and computed tomography in the staging of Hodgkin's disease. Cancer 1995;76:1460–1466.
7. Front D, Bar-Shalom R, Epelbaum R, et al.: Early detection of lymphoma recurrence with gallium-67 scintigraphy. J Nucl Med 1993;34:2101–2104.
8. Paul R: Comparison of fluorine-18-2-fluorodeoxyglucose and gallium-67 citrate imaging for detection of lymphoma. J Nucl Med 1987;28: 288–292.
9. Okada J, Yoshikawa K, Imazeki K, et al.: The use of FDG-PET in the detection and management of malignant lymphoma: Correlation of uptake with prognosis. J Nucl Med 1991;32:686–691.
10. Okada J, Yoshikawa K, Imazeki K, et al.: Positron emission tomography using fluorine-18fluorodeoxyglucose in malignant lymphoma: A comparison with proliferative activity. J Nucl Med 1992;33:325–329.
11. Leskinen-Kallio S, Rudsalainen U, Nagren K, Teras M, Joensuu H: Uptake of carbon-11

methionine and fluorodeoxyglucose in non-Hodgkin's lymphoma: A PET study. J Nucl Med 1991;32:1211–1218.

12. Lapela M, Leskinen S, Minn HR, et al.: Increased glucose metabolism in untreated non-Hodgkin's lymphoma: A study with positron emission tomography and fluorine-18 fluorodeoxyglucose. Blood 1995;86:3522–3527.
13. Rodriguez M, Rehn S, Ahlström H, Sunolstrom C, Glimelius B: Predicting malignancy grade with PET in non-Hodgkin's lymphoma. J Nucl Med 1995;36:1790–1796.
14. Hoh CK, Gaspy J, Rosen P, et al.: Whole body FDG-PET imaging for staging of Hodgkin's disease and lymphoma. J Nucl Med 1997;38: 343–348.
15. Moog F, Bangerter M, Diedrichs CG, et al.: Lymphoma: Role of whole-body 2-deoxy-2-[F 18]fluoro D-glucose (FDG) PET in nodal staging. Radiology 1997;203:795–800.
16. Moog F, Bangerter M, Diedrichs CG, et al.: Extranodal malignant lymphoma: Detection with FDG-PET versus CT. Radiology 1998;206: 475–481.
17. Carr R, Barrington SF, Madan B, et al.: Detection of lymphoma in bone marrow by whole-body positron emission tomography. Blood 1998;91:3340–3346.
18. Moog F, Bangerter M, Kotzerke J, Guhlmann A, Frickhofen N, Reske SN: 18-F fluorodeoxyglucose-positron emission tomography as a new approach to detect lymphomatous bone marrow. J Clin Oncol 1998;16:603–609.
19. Stumpe KD, Urbinelli M, Steinert HC, Glanzmann C, Buck A, von Schulthess GK: Whole-body positron emission tomography using fluorodeoxyglucose for staging of lymphoma: Effectiveness and comparison with computed tomography. Eur J Nucl Med 1998;25:721–728.
20. De Wit M, Bumann D, Beyer W, Herbst K, Clausen M, Hossfeld DK: Whole-body positron emission tomography (PET) for diagnoses of residual mass in patients with lymphoma. Ann Oncol 1997;8(Suppl):57–60.
21. Romer W, Hanauske AR, Ziegler S, et al.: Positron emission tomography in non-Hodgkin's lymphoma: Assessment of chemotherapy with fluorodeoxyglucose. Blood 1998;91:4464–4471.
22. Brunning RD, Bloomfield CD, McKenna RW, Peterson L: Bilateral trephine bone marrow biopsies in lymphoma and other neoplastic disease. Ann Intern Med 1975;82:375.
23. Ebie N, Loew JM, Gregory SA: Bilateral trephine bone marrow biopsies for staging non-Hodgkin's lymphoma: A second look. Hematol Pathol 1989;3:29.
24. Haddy TB, Parker RI, Magrath IT: Bone marrow involvement in young patients with non-Hodgkin's lymphoma: The importance of multiple bone marrow samples for accurate staging. Med Pediatr Oncol 1989;17:418.
25. Juneja SK, Wolf MM, Cooper IA: Value of bilateral bone marrow biopsy specimens in non-Hodgkin's lymphoma. J Clin Pathol 1990;43:630.
26. Landgren O, Axdorph U, Jacobson H, et al.: Routine bone scintigraphy is of limited value in the clinical assessment of untreated patients with Hodgkin's disease. Med Oncol 2000;17:174–178.
27. Orzel J, Sawaf NW, Richardson ML: Lymphoma of the skeleton: Scintigraphic evaluation: Am J Rehabil 1988;150:1095–1099.
28. Schechter JP, Jones SE, Woolfenden JM, et al.: Bone scanning in lymphoma. Cancer 1976;38: 1142–1146.
29. Ferrant A, Rodhain J, Michaux JL, Piret L, Maldaque B, Sokal G: Detection of skeletal involvement in Hodgkin's disease: A comparison of radiography, bone scanning, and bone marrow biopsy in 38 patients. Cancer 1975;35: 1346–1353.
30. Shields AF, Porter BA, Olson DO, et al.: The detection of bone marrow involvement by lymphoma using magnetic resonance imaging. J Clin Oncol 1987;5:225–230.
31. Altenhoefer C, Blum U, Bathmann J, et al.: Comparative diagnostic accuracy of magnetic resonance imaging and immunoscintigraphy for detection of bone marrow involvement in patients with malignant lymphoma. J Clin Oncol 1997;15:1754–1760.
32. Delbeke D, Kovalsky E, Cerci R, Martin WH, Kinney M, Greer J: 18F-fluorodeoxyglucose imaging with positron emission tomography for initial staging of Hodgkin's disease and lymphoma. J Nucl Med 2000;41:275P.
33. Moog F, Kotzerke J, Reske SN: FDG PET can replace bone scintigraphy in primary staging of malignant lymphoma. J Nucl Med 1999;40: 1407–1413.
34. Bangerter M, Moog F, Buchmann I, et al.: Whole-body 2-[18F]-fluoro-2-deoxy-D-glucose positron emission tomography (FDG PET) for accurate staging of Hodgkin's disease. Ann Oncol 1998; 9(10):1117–1122.
35. Mikhaeel NG, Timothy AR, Hain SF, O'Doherty MJ: 18-FDG-PET for the assessment of residual masses on CT following treatment of lymphomas. Ann Oncol 2000;11(Suppl):147–150.

36. Jerusalem G, Beguin Y, Fassotte MF, et al.: Persistent tumor 18F-FDG uptake after a few cycles of polychemotherapy is predictive of treatment failure in non-Hodgkin's lymphoma. Haematologica 2000;85(6):613–618.

37. Delbeke D, Kovalsky E, Cerci R, Martin WH, Kinney M, Greer J: 18F-fluorodeoxyglucose imaging with positron emission tomography in the follow-up of patients with lymphoma. J Nucl Med 2000;41:70P.

Cases Presentations

Case 6.8.1

History

A 35-year-old female presented with a six-month history of fatigue and low back pain. Two years earlier, she had received radiation therapy for NHL involving the neck and chest. FDG PET imaging was performed using a dual-head gamma camera operating in the coincidence mode (hybrid PET). The gamma camera is equipped with an X-ray tube and an array of detectors functioning basically as a third-generation CT scanner (VG Millenium). This system allows acquisition of CT transmission images that allow attenuation correction and provide low dose X-ray CT images for generation of fusion images and anatomical mapping. Coronal hybrid PET images with attenuation correction are shown in Figure 6.8.1A, and selected transaxial images with corresponding hybrid CT (left), FDG hybrid PET (middle left), fusion images (middle right), and high-resolution CT images (right) are shown in Figure 6.8.1B, see color plate. Figure 6.8.1C shows images from dedicated high-resolution CT performed six months earlier and interpreted as normal at that time. The image on the left corresponds to the upper panel images from the hybrid system, and the image on the right corresponds to the lower panel images.

Findings

No abnormalities are identified in the neck or chest. Within the lower abdomen and pelvis,

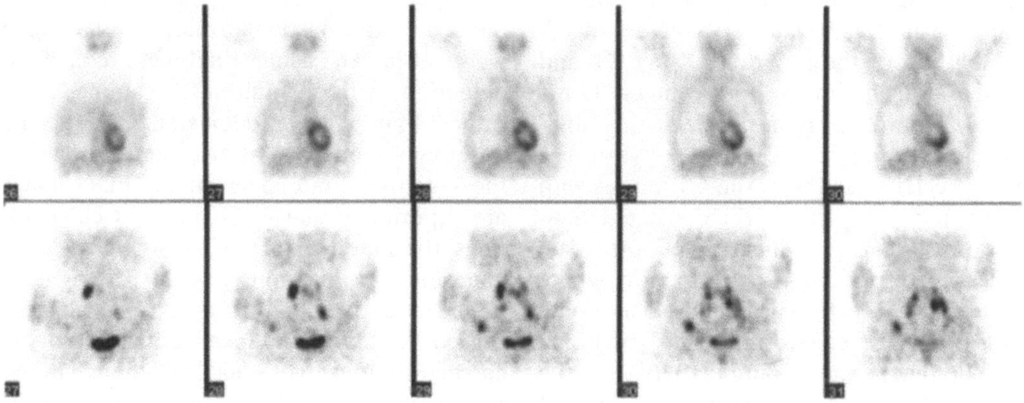

FIGURE 6.8.1A.

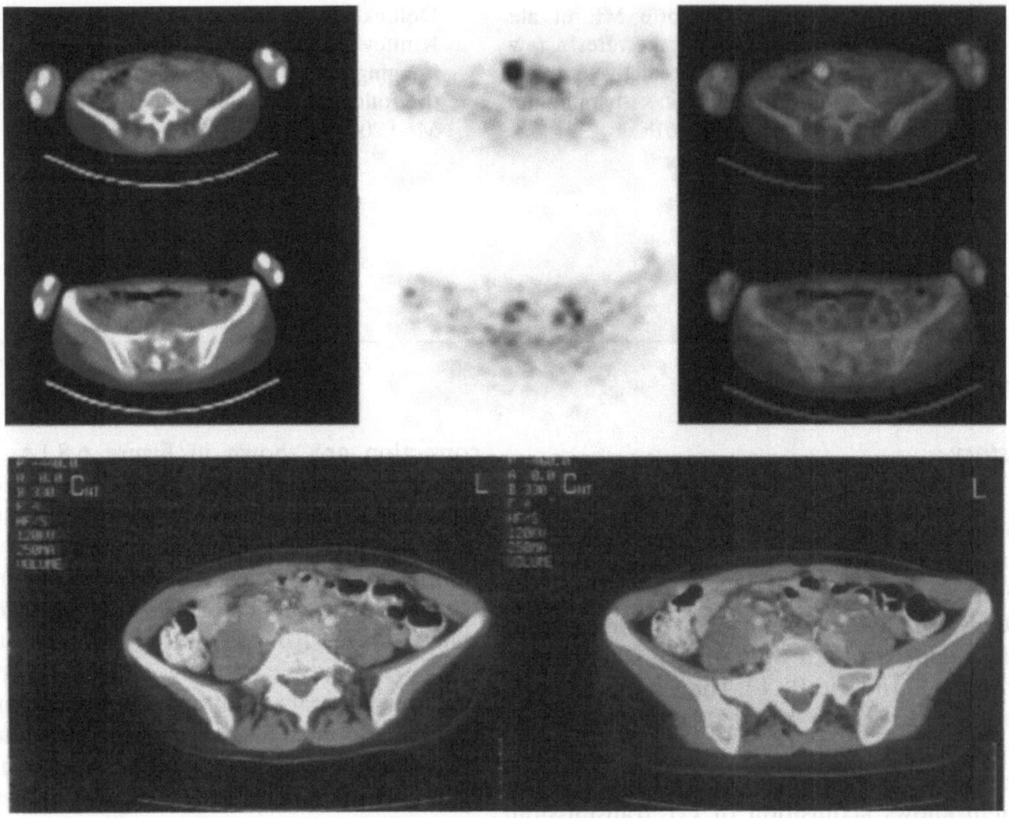

B

C

FIGURE 6.8.1B,C. *(Continued)*

there are multiple foci of abnormal FDG activity congruent with periaortic, pelvic, and iliac lymphadenopathy seen on the CT transmission image. The adenopathy is not well seen on the hybrid CT images because of the relatively low resolution of the low dose X-ray CT and the lack of oral and intravenous contrast. However, they are well seen on the dedicated high-resolution CT (Figure 6.8.1C). The hybrid CT allowed precise selection of the CT images with abnormal foci of uptake on the dedicated high-resolution CT and identification of soft tissue densities, corresponding to the foci of uptake that were retrospectively diagnosed as nodal masses. Biopsy revealed malignant lymphoma with pathologic features similar to those in the primary neck and chest masses at the time of diagnosis.

Discussion

The abnormal foci of activity in the abdomen and pelvis represent lymphomatous nodal disease. In this particular case, the FDG images were obtained using dual-head coincidence detection with a multihead gamma camera rather than with a dedicated PET scanner. Although numerous studies have shown that the sensitivity and specificity of FDG imaging are superior to that of CT in many clinical settings, the inability of FDG imaging to provide anatomic localization remains a significant impairment in maximizing its clinical use. In regard to anatomic localization, attenuation correction improves anatomic delineation of mediastinum from lungs and lungs from liver. Therefore, images with attenuation correction are easier to interpret than images without attenuation correction, especially for the inexperienced reader, and lesions can be located more accurately. The model of gamma camera used for this patient is equipped with an X-ray tube and array of detectors on the gantry, which function essentially like a third-generation CT scanner. This system allows for acquisition of attenuation maps for attenuation correction.

In this particular case, the major diagnostic challenge was the foci of uptake in the abdomen. Precise localization of these foci was critical since they could represent physiologic bowel uptake or uptake in involved nodal groups. The fusion of anatomical and metabolic images and visual correlation with the dedicated high-resolution CT scan were critical in accurately localizing the uptake to nodal groups. Although the nodal groups cannot be clearly identified on the low resolution CT images without contrast provided by the hybrid system, it does allow precise selection of the appropriate slices for review on the dedicated high-resolution CT scan, with oral and IV contrast that matches up with the area of increased metabolism.

Some studies suggest that the detectability of lesions is not improved on images with attenuation correction as compared to images without attenuation correction, and if a lesion is not detected on FDG images, it cannot be localized on the fusion of anatomical and metabolic images. The limit of detectability is in the 5 to 10mm range for dedicated PET tomographs and in the 15 to 20mm range for hybrid gamma cameras.[1]

Diagnosis

Recurrent non-Hodgkin's lymphoma after therapy.

Reference

1. Delbeke D, Martin WH, Patton JA, Sandler MP: Value of iterative reconstruction, attenuation correction, and image fusion in the interpretation of FDG PET images with an integrated dual-head coincidence camera and x-ray-based attenuation maps. Radiology 2000;218:163–171.

Case 6.8.2

History

A 17-year-old female with nodular sclerosing Hodgkin's lymphoma recently diagnosed by biopsy of an enlarged right cervical lymph node presented for staging, including CT (Figure 6.8.2A) and FDG imaging (Figure 6.8.2B). FDG images were acquired with a dedicated PET tomograph (Siemens ECAT 933) and reconstructed with filtered back projection without attenuation correction.

Findings

In addition to lesions in the neck and mediastinum (not shown), the CT demonstrates a 3cm by 2cm enhancing lesion within the right lobe of the liver, adjacent to the inferior vena cava. A ^{99m}Tc-labeled red blood cell SPECT study (not shown) was unable to differentiate the mass from the inferior vena cava secondary to poor spatial resolution and therefore was nondiagnostic for a cavernous hemangioma. On the FDG PET images, there is marked FDG uptake in the lesions of the neck and mediastinum, as well as physiological myocardial uptake, but no abnormal uptake in the hepatic lesion seen on CT.

Discussion

Benign hepatic lesions include cavernous hemangioma, cyst, adenoma, and focal nodular hyperplasia, none of which accumulate FDG.

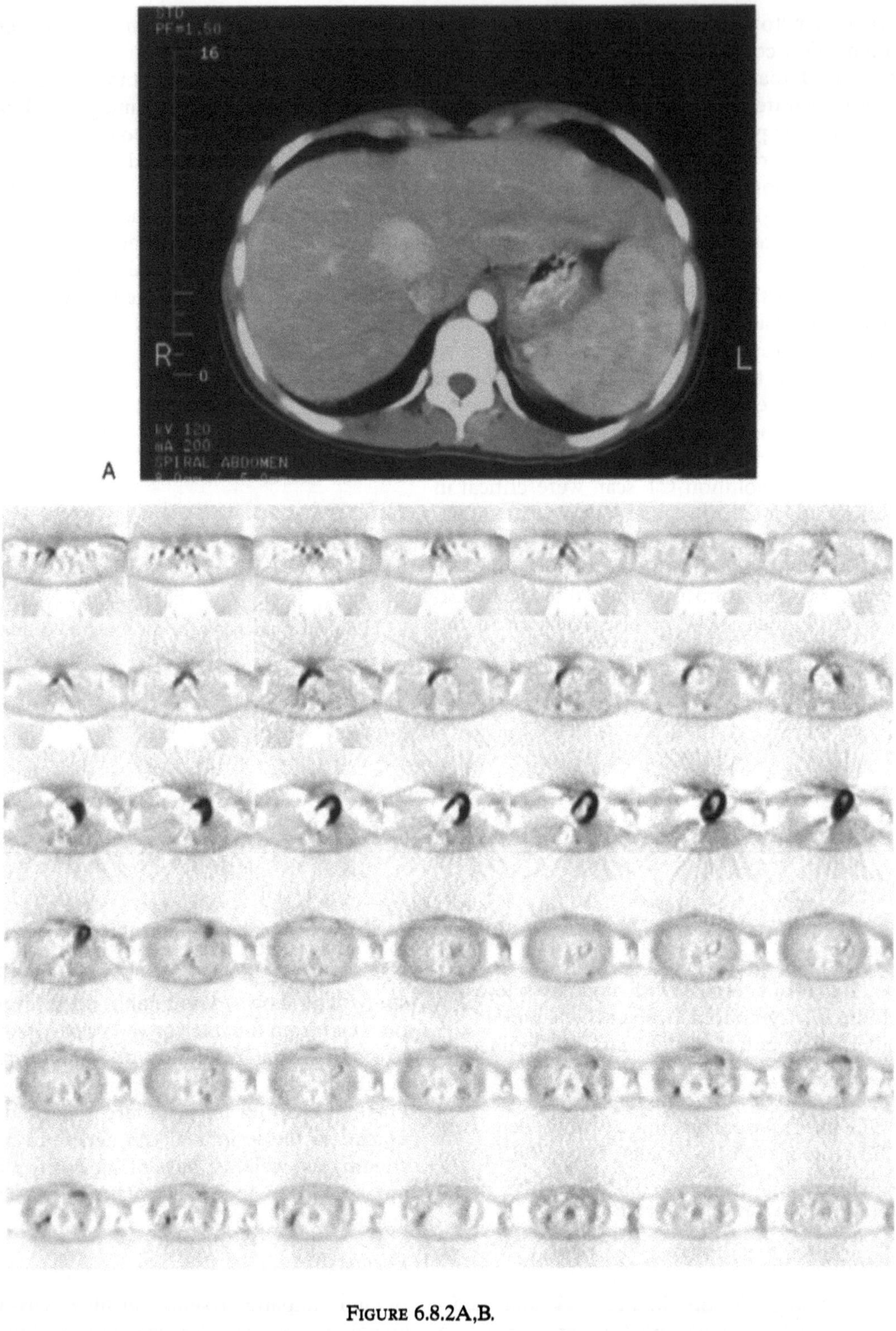

FIGURE 6.8.2A,B.

Since the lymphomatous nodes above the diaphragm are FDG-avid, the absence of FDG accumulation in the hepatic lesion is indicative of a benign process.

Although FDG imaging has been found to be most useful in the restaging of patients with recurrent disease and monitoring the effect of therapy, it may also play an important role in the initial staging of patients with Hodgkin's disease and non-Hodgkin's lymphoma. Patients with involvement of lymphoid tissue on one side of the diaphragm are classified as stage I or II according to the number of nodal stations involved. Involvement of lymphoid tissue on two sides of the diaphragm is classified as stage III, and systemic involvement is classified as stage IV. A and B characterize patients without and with symptoms. Accurate staging is critical for optimizing therapy and determining prognosis. FDG PET imaging allowed accurate classification of this patient as stage IIA (asymptomatic involvement of two or more lymph node stations on the same side of the diaphragm), instead of stage IVA (asymptomatic systemic involvement). She was treated accordingly and is still currently in remission three years later.

Diagnoses

1. Stage IIA nodular sclerosing Hodgkin's lymphoma.
2. Benign hepatic mass.

Case 6.8.3

History

A 50-year-old male was recently diagnosed with diffuse large transformed cell lymphoma by biopsy of a hepatic lesion. A CT scan (Figure 6.8.3A) and FDG imaging (Figures 6.8.3B and C) were performed for staging. Coronal FDG PET images acquired with a dedicated PET tomograph (Siemens ECAT 933) and reconstructed with filtered back projection without attenuation correction are shown in Figure 6.8.3B, and orthogonal images through the right kidney in are shown in Figure 6.8.3C. Two months following the end of therapy, follow-up CT (Figure 6.8.3D) and FDG PET (Figure 6.8.3E) images were obtained.

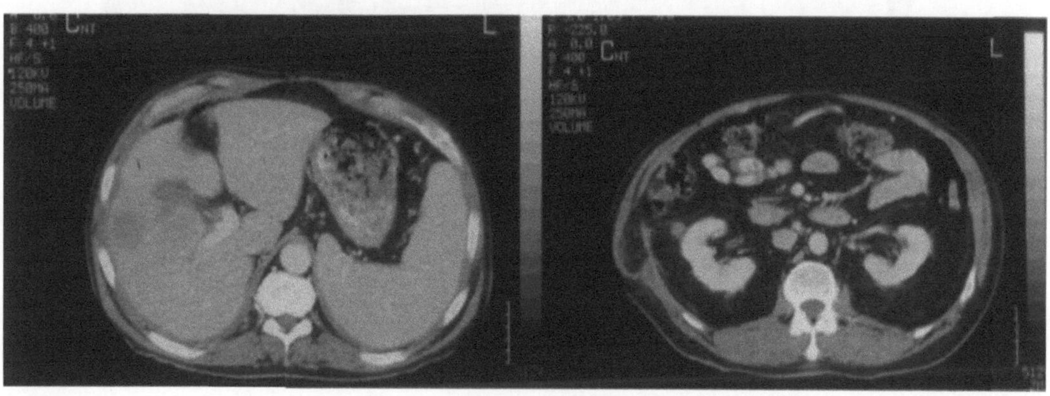

FIGURE 6.8.3A.

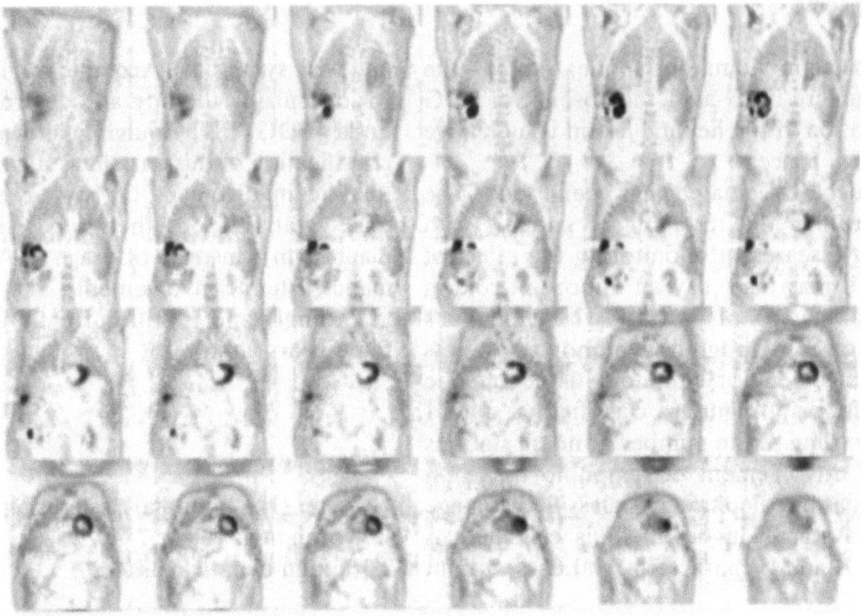
B

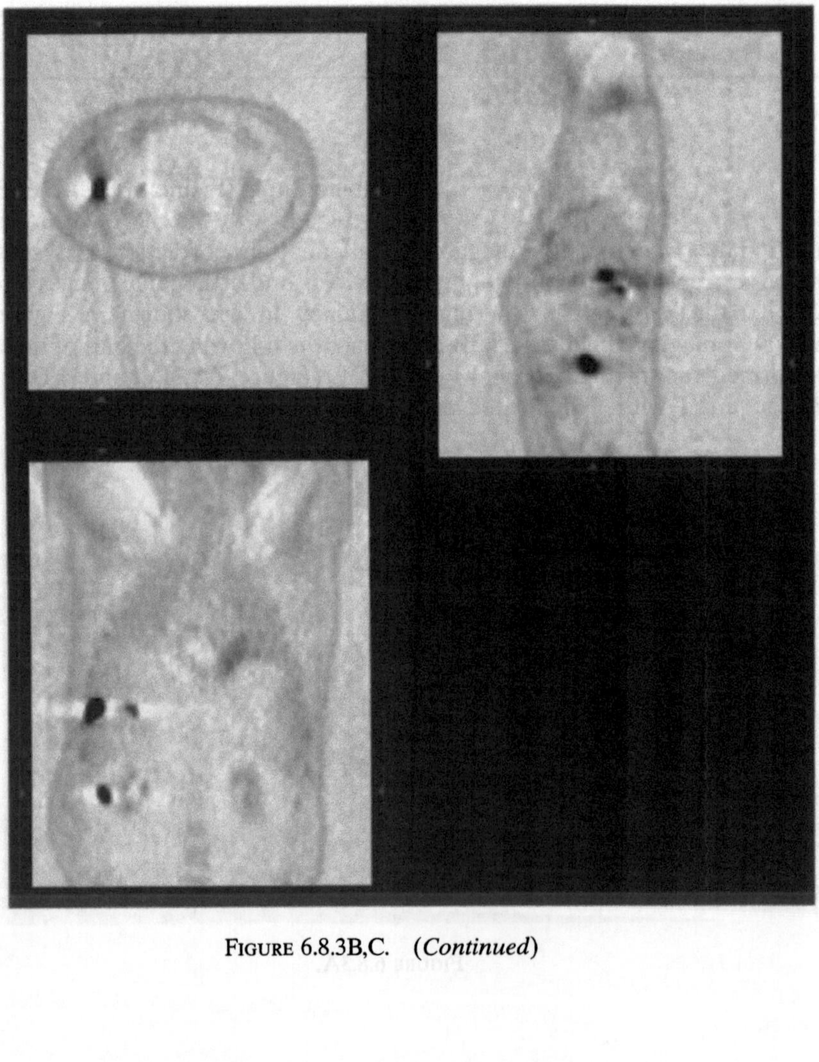
C

FIGURE 6.8.3B,C. (*Continued*)

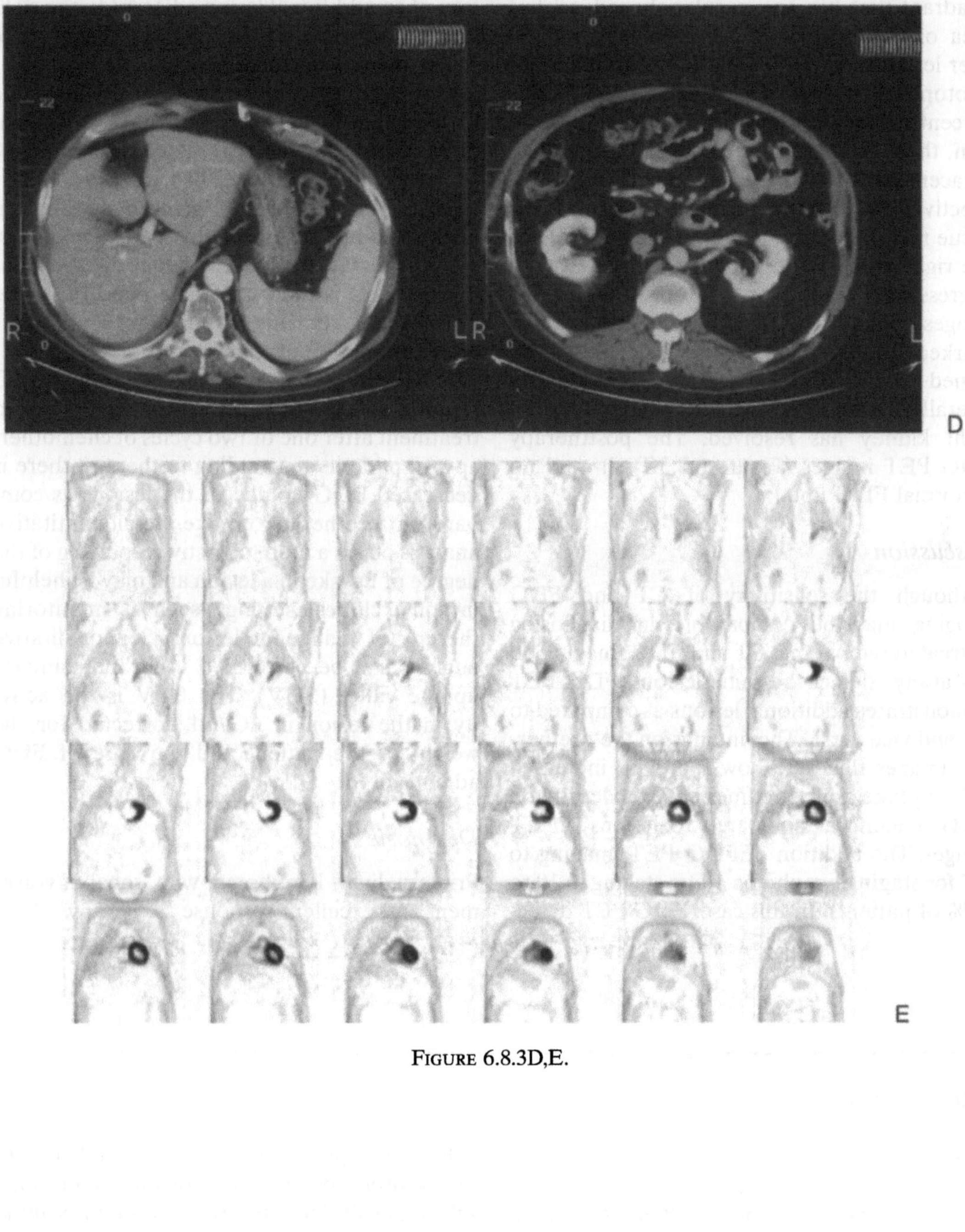

FIGURE 6.8.3D,E.

Findings

The CT image on page 315 (Figure 6.8.3A) shows a hypodense lesion in the right lobe of the liver, diagnosed as lymphoma by biopsy. This lesion extended to the inferior tip of the liver and had areas of necrosis and hemorrhage (not shown on Figure 6.8.3A). On the FDG PET images (Figures 6.8.3C and D), there is a region of marked uptake in the right upper quadrant that has an irregular-shaped, central area of photopenia. It is congruent with the liver lesion seen on CT, and the central area of photopenia on FDG PET images corresponds to central necrosis and hemorrhage. In addition, there is a focal lesion of marked uptake adjacent to the right kidney, which was retrospectively seen on the CT images as a small soft tissue nodule located lateral to the mid-pole of the right kidney. The patient was treated with aggressive chemotherapy. The posttherapy CT images (Figure 6.8.3D) of the liver show marked improvement of the lesion but continued to demonstrate an abnormal density laterally in the liver; the lesion lateral to the right kidney has resolved. The posttherapy FDG PET images (Figure 6.8.3E) showed no abnormal FDG uptake.

Discussion

Although the sensitivity of CT and FDG imaging may be comparable in diagnosing untreated lymphoma, CT and FDG imaging do not always detect the same lesions. FDG PET demonstrates additional lesions as compared to CT and vice versa. The findings on the pretherapy images illustrate how foci with increased FDG uptake are sometimes easy to identify on FDG imaging as compared to lesions on CT images. The addition of FDG PET imaging to CT for staging lymphoma alters staging in 10 to 20% of patients. In this case, FDG PET detection of an additional lesion adjacent to the right kidney did not alter the stage IV diagnosis of this patient as diagnosed by hepatic biopsy.

However, it is well known that CT is unable to distinguish between active or recurrent disease and residual scar tissue after therapy. Metabolic imaging with FDG is helpful in this regard. The absence of glucose metabolism in the residual lesion of this patient indicates scar tissue rather active residual disease after therapy and is indicative of a good response. The patient remains in remission two years after completion of therapy.

FDG PET imaging is also accurate to differentiate responders from nonresponders to treatment after one or two cycles of chemotherapy. In patients responding to therapy, there is decreased FDG uptake in the lesions as compared to pretherapy uptake. Semiquantitative analysis offers a more objective reporting of the degree of uptake in a lesion and may be helpful in some clinical settings, such as monitoring therapy of malignant lesions. Semiqualitative analysis can be performed using the standard uptake value (SUV). The SUV is the activity in the lesion in uCi/ml, corrected for the weight of the patient and the dose of FDG administered.

Diagnosis

Primary liver lymphoma with renal involvement and excellent response to therapy.

Case 6.8.4

History

A 31-year-old HIV-positive male presented with progressive, severe diffuse bone pain. Six months earlier a diagnosis of intermediate-grade non-Hodgkin's lymphoma had been made by biopsy of a soft tissue mass over the mandible. Since that time, he had undergone several courses of chemotherapy. A recent CT of the chest, abdomen (Figure 6.8.4A), and pelvis was reported to be unremarkable except for shotty axillary adenopathy and mild splenomegaly. He was referred for bone scintigraphy (Figure 6.8.4B) and FDG imaging (Figures 6.8.4C and D). Coronal (Figure 6.8.4C) and transaxial (Figure 6.8.4D) FDG PET images acquired with a dedicated PET tomograph (GE Advance) and reconstructed with iterative reconstruction and measured segmented attenuation correction are displayed.

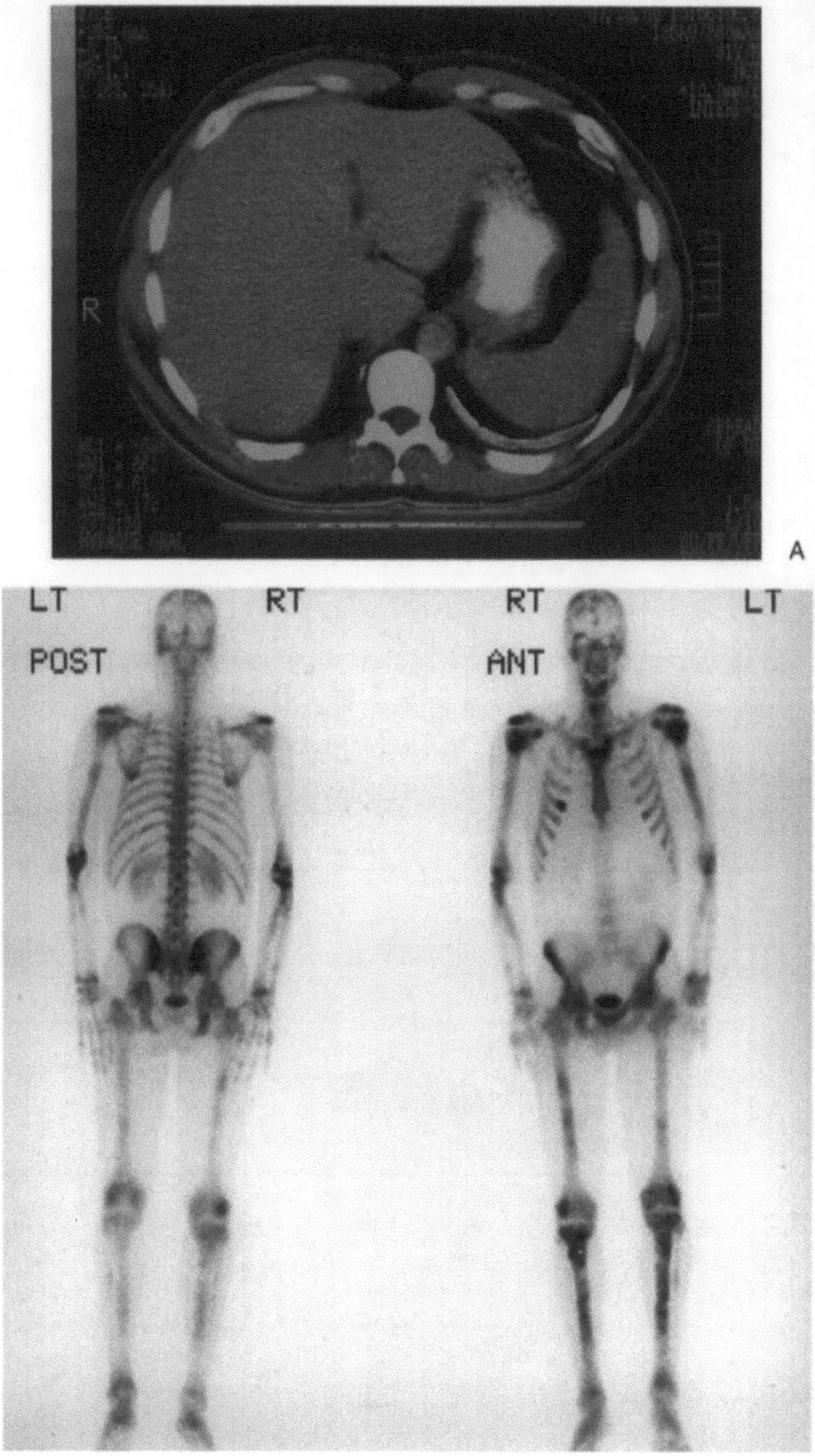

A

B

FIGURE 6.8.4A,B.

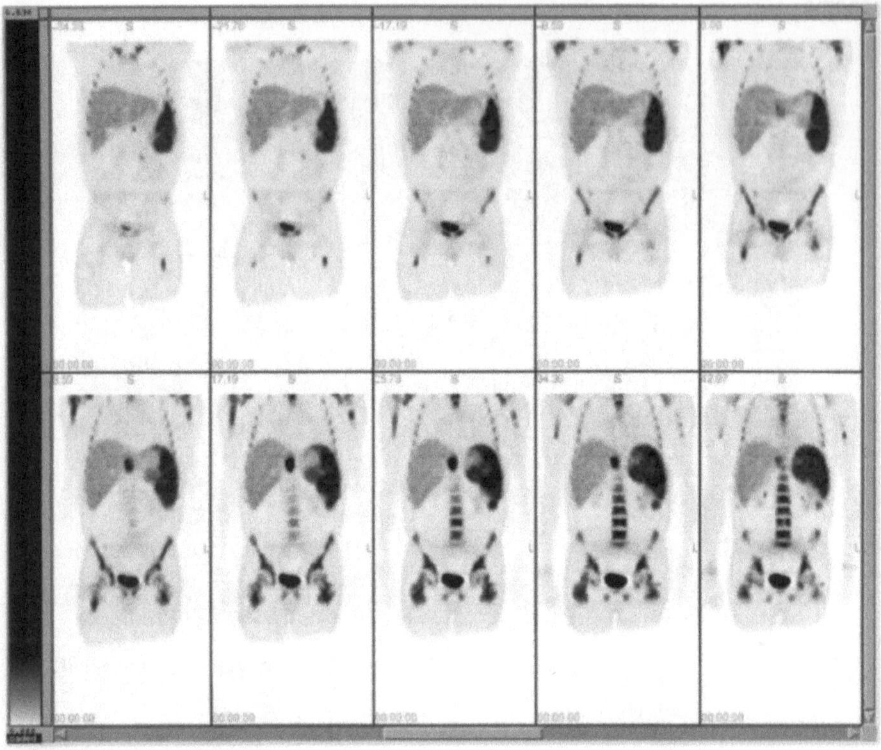

C

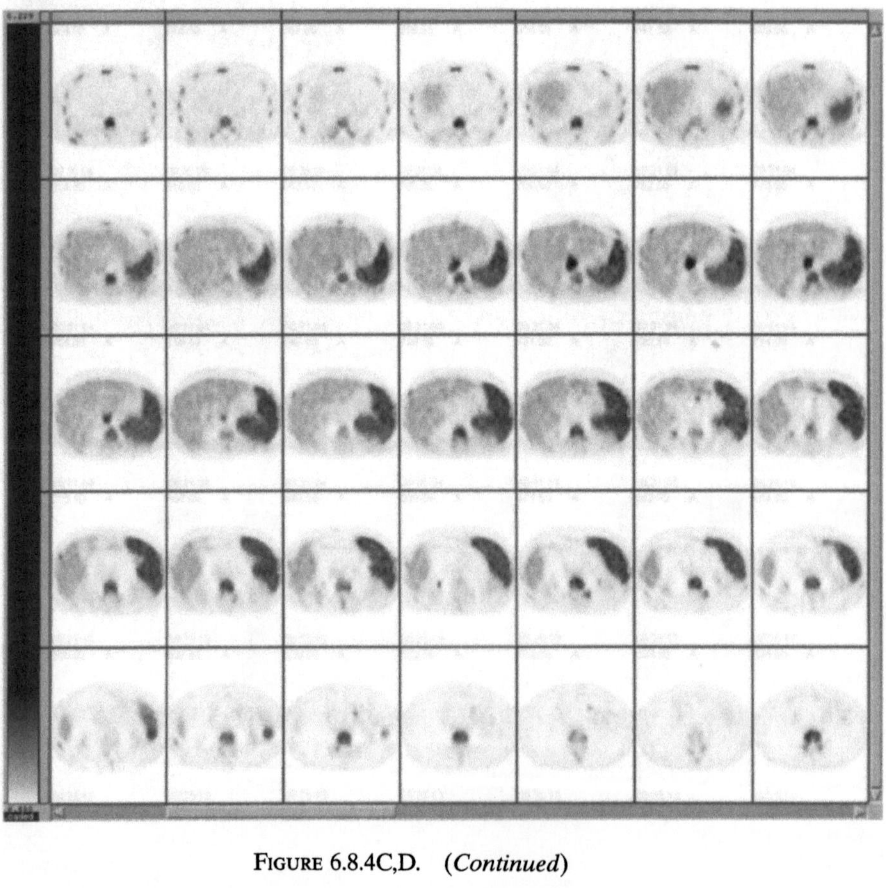

D

FIGURE 6.8.4C,D. (*Continued*)

Findings

The CT image shows normal liver and spleen. The bone scintigraphy is suggestive of metastatic disease involving the skull left humerus, both femurs, and both tibiae. The FDG images reveal markedly increased marrow activity in a homogenous fashion throughout the spine and pelvis. Patchy inhomogeneous activity is also seen within the femurs, humeri, and forearms as well as several ribs. There is diffusely increased activity throughout an enlarged spleen, and a large focus of markedly increased uptake is seen in a paravertebral location, probably corresponding to the caudate lobe of the liver.

Discussion

Although diffusely increased marrow activity can be seen in patients with reactive bone marrow hyperplasia secondary to pancytopenia and for several weeks following chemotherapy, especially if granulocyte-stimulating factor has been administered, the focal activity seen within the marrow of the extremities is abnormal and consistent with widespread neoplastic involvement. This makes the diffuse vertebral activity likely to also be due to lymphomatous infiltration rather than mere hyperplasia. The abdominal foci of increased activity are due to retroperitoneal and mesenteric malignant lymphadenopathy. A blind biopsy of the iliac crest revealed sheets of monomorphic, monoclonal transformed B-cells consistent with Burkitt's lymphoma. The patient declined further assessment as well as any further therapy.

Similar to the situation seen in patients with organ transplants and patients with various immunodeficiency syndromes, patients with AIDS have an increased risk of high-grade non-Hodgkin's lymphoma (NHL), and lymphoma may be the initial AIDS-defining event. NHL is the second most common malignancy affecting patients infected with the HIV, and Burkitt's lymphoma is the most common variety.[1] There is preliminary evidence that the incidence of AIDS-related lymphoma is decreasing with more prevalent use of highly active antiretroviral therapy. Chemotherapy has been used in these patients with modest success, but the prognosis remains worse than for immunocompetent patients. As with other lymphomas, accurate staging is important; FDG PET provides significant incremental value in the staging of patients with NHL, as is evidenced by this patient.

Diagnosis

AIDS-related non-Hodgkin's lymphoma with diffuse marrow and splenic infiltration.

Reference

1. Powles T, Matthews G, Bower M: AIDS related systemic non-Hodgkin's lymphoma. Sex Transm Infect 2000;76:335–341.

Case 6.8.5

History

A 10-year-old male presented for evaluation of a posttransplant lymphoproliferative disorder diagnosed at the time of a recent tonsillectomy, performed because of persistent bilateral cervical lymphadenopathy. Five years earlier he had undergone orthotopic heart transplantation for a dilated cardiomyopathy. Figure 6.8.5 shows coronal FDG PET images acquired with a dedicated PET tomograph (GE Advance) and reconstructed with iterative reconstruction and measured segmented attenuation correction.

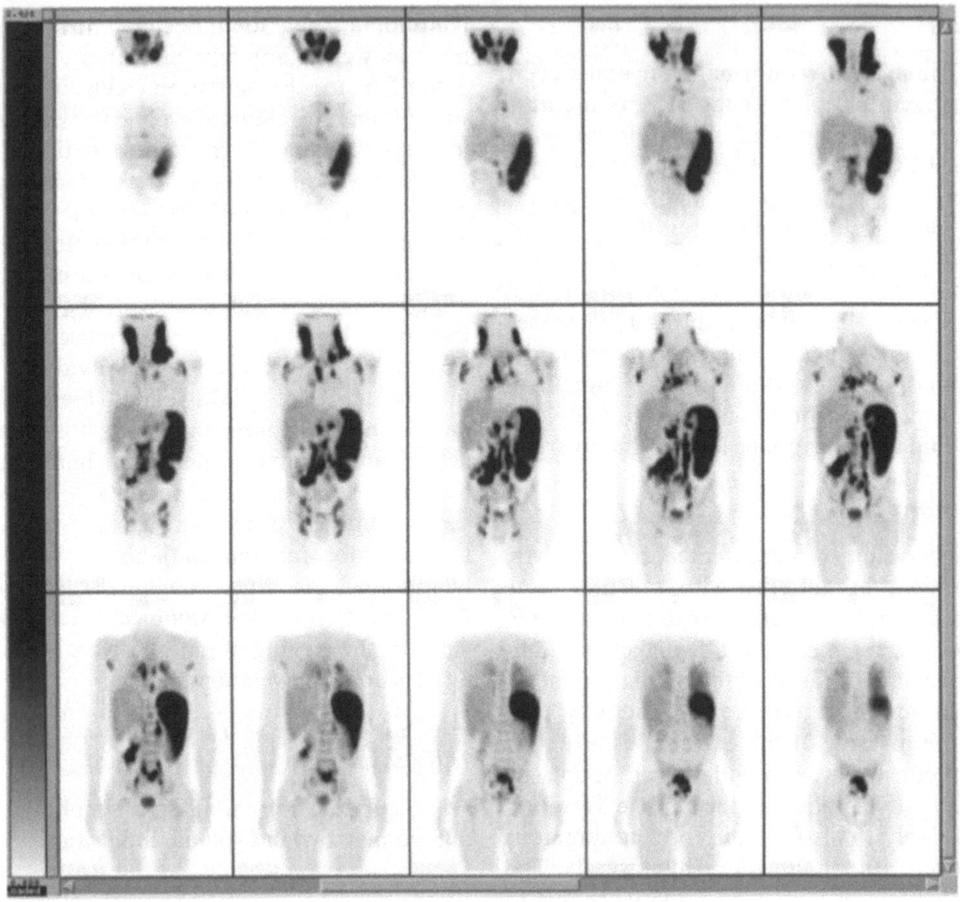

FIGURE 6.8.5.

Findings

Markedly increased abnormal FDG activity is seen throughout essentially all lymphoid tissue, including the neck, axillae, mediastinum, mesenteric and retroperitoneal abdominal regions, and inguinal/iliac/femoral nodal groups. The spleen is dramatically enlarged with intensely increased activity. No abnormal hepatic activity is identified, but abnormalities of the renal cortices cannot be excluded due to marked physiologic activity within the collecting system. There is mild diffusely increased activity at the posterior left lung. No definite abnormalities are identified within the bone marrow.

Discussion

The PET findings are congruent with the findings at CT, demonstrating innumerable enlarged cervical, mediastinal, subcarinal, diaphragmatic, para-aortic and mesenteric abdominal nodes, and inguinal nodes. Although numerous peripheral splenic low-attenuation abnormalities were initially thought to represent infarcts, the PET findings are strongly suggestive of diffuse lymphomatous involvement of the spleen. The left posterior left lung activity noted on PET is congruent with atelectasis seen on CT. Diffuse rather than focal abnormalities seen with PET, as with ^{67}gallium and other modalities, are generally benign but require radiographic correlation. PET is not intended to supplant CT and other radiographic modalities, but rather to compliment them.

Posttransplant lymphoproliferative disorder, varying from a mononucleosis-like syndrome to malignant non-Hodgkin's lymphoma, is a well-recognized severe complication occurring in allograft recipients treated with immunosuppressive therapy.[1] It accounts for 15 to 25% of the neoplasms arising in this population as opposed to less than 5% of the general population. The incidence varies with the organ transplanted (1 to 2% of renal transplants but as high as 6% of lung and heart transplant recipients) and the severity of the immunosuppressive regimen. Some of these patients will respond to reduction in their immunosuppressive regimen, but mortality may be as high as 80% in patients with monoclonal B-cell lymphomas, such as this patient. Burkitt's lymphoma and posttransplant lymphoma have been associated with evidence of Epstein-Barr virus (EBV) infection, and there is preliminary evidence that both heart and lung allograft recipients who experience posttransplant primary EBV infection are at greatest risk for development of lymphoproliferative disease. In this particular patient, FDG PET imaging will be used to monitor response to combination chemotherapy after there is clinical evidence of remission.

Diagnoses

1. Posttransplantation malignant lymphoproliferative disorder with diffuse splenic involvement.
2. Posterobasilar left lung atelectasis.

Reference

1. Zangwill SD, Kichuk MR, Garvin JH, et al.: Incidence and outcome of primary Epstein-Barr virus infection and lymphoproliferative disease in pediatric heart transplant recipients. J Heart Lung Transplant 1998;17:1161–1166.

Case 6.8.6

History

A 62-year-old female with a history of recurrent Hodgkin's lymphoma presented for restaging. Three years earlier she had experienced a complete remission of nodular sclerosing Hodgkin's disease following conventional chemotherapy. Eighteen months later she relapsed with ^{67}gallium-negative cervical lymphadenopathy, again achieving a complete remission. She experienced a second relapse a year later. At that time, she received aggressive chemotherapy followed by stem cell transplantation approximately six months prior to this presentation. A CT of the neck (not shown) was interpreted as showing no evidence of disease. Coronal FDG PET images (Figure 6.8.6) are displayed. The FDG PET images were acquired using a full ring dedicated tomograph (GE Advance) and reconstructed using an iterative algorithm and segmented attenuation correction.

Findings

The CT images demonstrate mild paratracheal and azygoesophageal adenopathy (not shown). Scattered ill-defined pulmonary nodules are worrisome for lymphatic infiltration versus posttransplant infection. The liver and spleen are unremarkable, but there is left para-aortic adenopathy (1.3 cm) and a 1 cm aortocaval node. Subtle sclerotic foci throughout the thoracic spine are worrisome for lymphomatous infiltration.

The FDG PET images reveal multiple foci of increased activity throughout the mediastinum

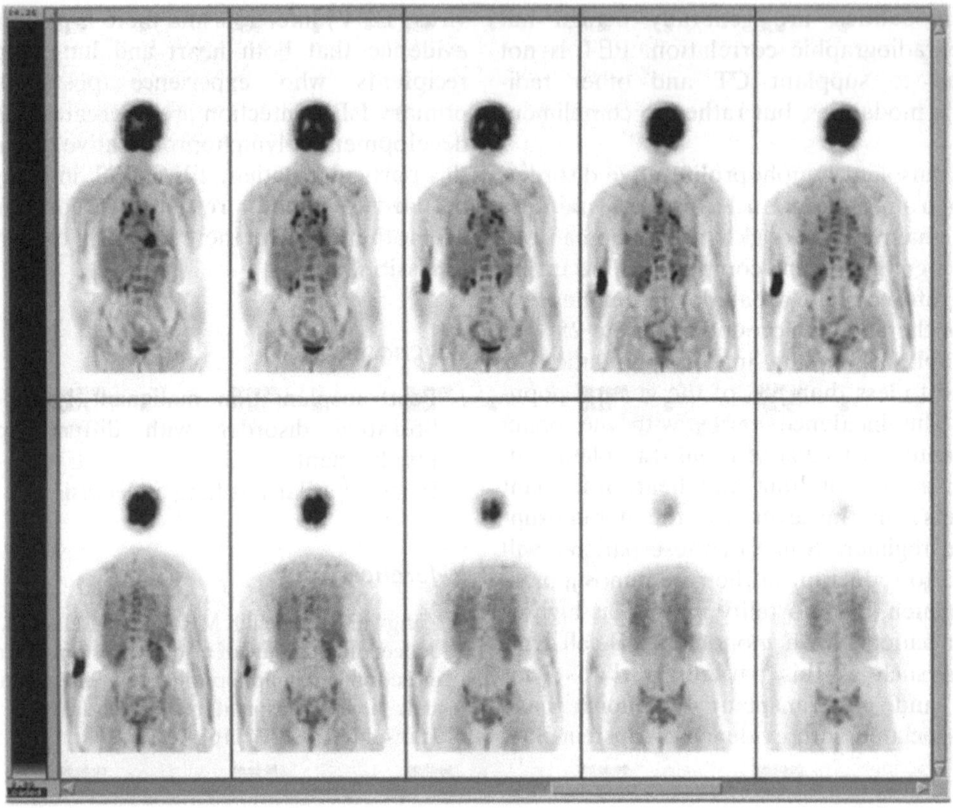

FIGURE 6.8.6.

including the paratracheal, hilar, subcarinal, and azygoesophageal nodes. The lung nodules are not definitely identified on the PET images, but there are abnormal foci within the abdomen in the left para-aortic region and aortocaval region, congruent but somewhat more extensive than what is seen on the CT images. Heterogeneous activity is seen throughout the thoracic and upper lumbar spine. Although it is difficult to differentiate posterior mediastinal tumor from vertebral involvement on the coronal views, the two can be easily separated on the sagittal views (not shown) where the mild physiologic uptake within the marrow functions as a useful landmark.

Discussion

Despite high dose chemotherapy and stem cell marrow transplantation, this patient has experienced rapid progression of his NHL, as evidenced by widespread nodal disease both above and below the diaphragm. Although many of these lymph nodes are visible by CT, they are equivocal for neoplastic involvement on the basis of size. Furthermore, possible marrow disease identified by CT is unequivocal by FDG PET. Several investigators have reported superior detection of recurrent lymphoma by FDG PET as compared to CT with higher sensitivity, specificity, and accuracy. FDG PET has been found to be cost-effective and results in an alteration in management in a significant minority of patients. Although ^{67}gallium scintigraphy is generally sensitive for detection of high-grade lymphoma, this case illustrates why FDG PET is emerging as the modality of choice for the evaluation of lymphoma recurrence as well as at initial staging.

Bone marrow involvement with lymphoma is associated with a less favorable prognosis. Bone marrow biopsy, the standard technique for diagnosing marrow disease, is associated with a high rate of false-negative results. Comparing PET with marrow biopsy in two separate reports totaling 128 patients (77 NHL and 51 Hodgkin's disease), there were 20 concordant positives and 83 concordant negatives (80% concordance). However, FDG PET revealed focal regions of increased activity in 18 (14%) biopsy-negative patients, whereas only 7 (5%) patients had positive biopsies but negative PET scans. Although these preliminary findings need to be confirmed in a larger population, our experience at Vanderbilt University has been similar. Performance of FDG PET as part of the standard staging protocol in patients with lymphoma may reduce the need for routine bone biopsies while, at the same time, improving staging.

Diagnosis

Unexpected widespread non-Hodgkin's lymphoma, post–stem cell transplantation.

Case 6.8.7

History

A 66-year-old man presented with abdominal fullness and a new abdominal bruit. Ten years earlier a localized low-grade follicular non-Hodgkin's lymphoma of the small bowel had been resected and was followed with adjuvant combination chemotherapy; he had experienced no recurrence. An ultrasound performed to exclude a possible abdominal aortic aneurysm revealed an 18 cm spleen containing a 14 by 12 cm hypoechoic mass, which was confirmed by CT. Laparotomy and splenectomy revealed a transformed high-grade NHL with features of Burkitt's lymphoma involving the spleen, a peritoneal nodule, and several mesenteric nodes. A CT was interpreted as no evidence of disease (Figure 6.8.7A). On physi-

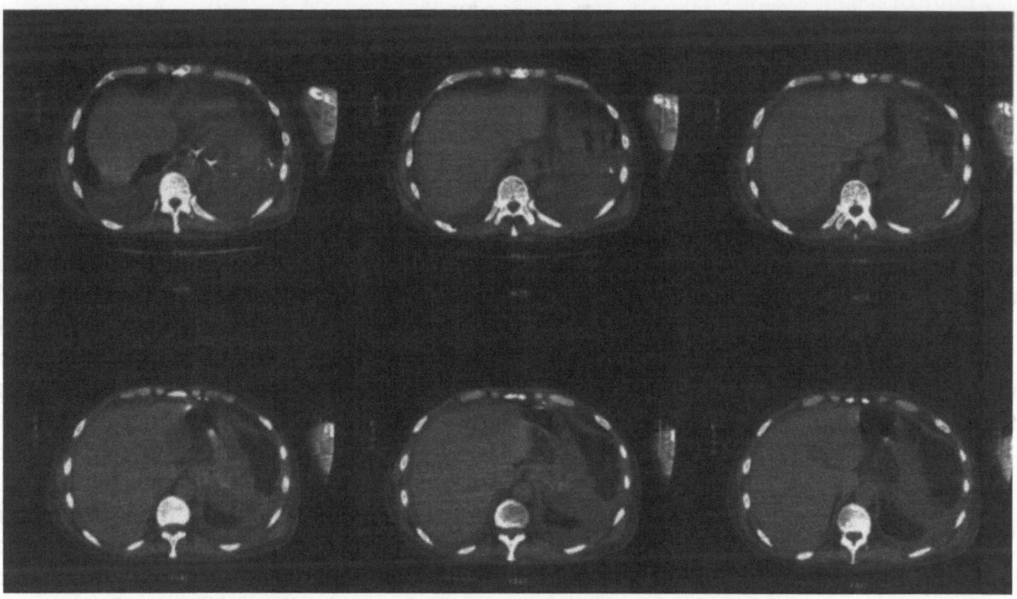

FIGURE 6.8.7A.

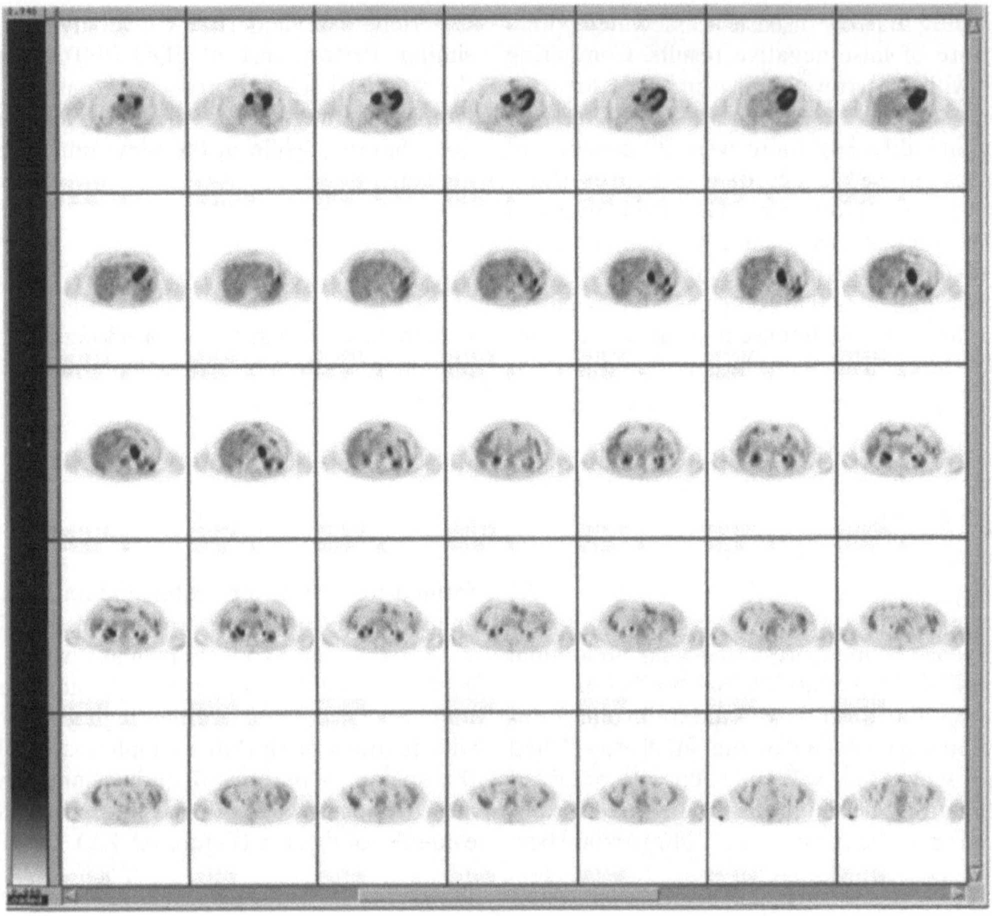

FIGURE 6.8.7B.

cal examination, there was a cutaneous nodule adjacent to the left nares and another nodule above the base of the penis. Staging transaxial and coronal FDG PET images (Figures 6.8.7B and C) acquired on a dedicated full ring tomograph (GE Advance) and reconstructed using an iterative algorithm and segmented attenuation correction are displayed.

Findings

Multiple foci of increased uptake are present. The myocardial, bowel, and genitourinary tract (GU) activity, including bilateral ureteral activity, is physiologic. Although there is mild diffuse activity present within the splenic bed similar to that of physiologic liver activity, there is also a relatively large focus of markedly increased activity present consistent with persistent high-grade neoplasm. Additional foci of abnormal activity consistent with high-grade lymphoma are present at the (1) right mid-lung, (2) inferior right mediastinum at the cardiophrenic angle, (3) left upper para-aortic nodal region, (4) left iliac nodal region, (5) mid-portion of the right lobe of the liver, (6) superficial anterior

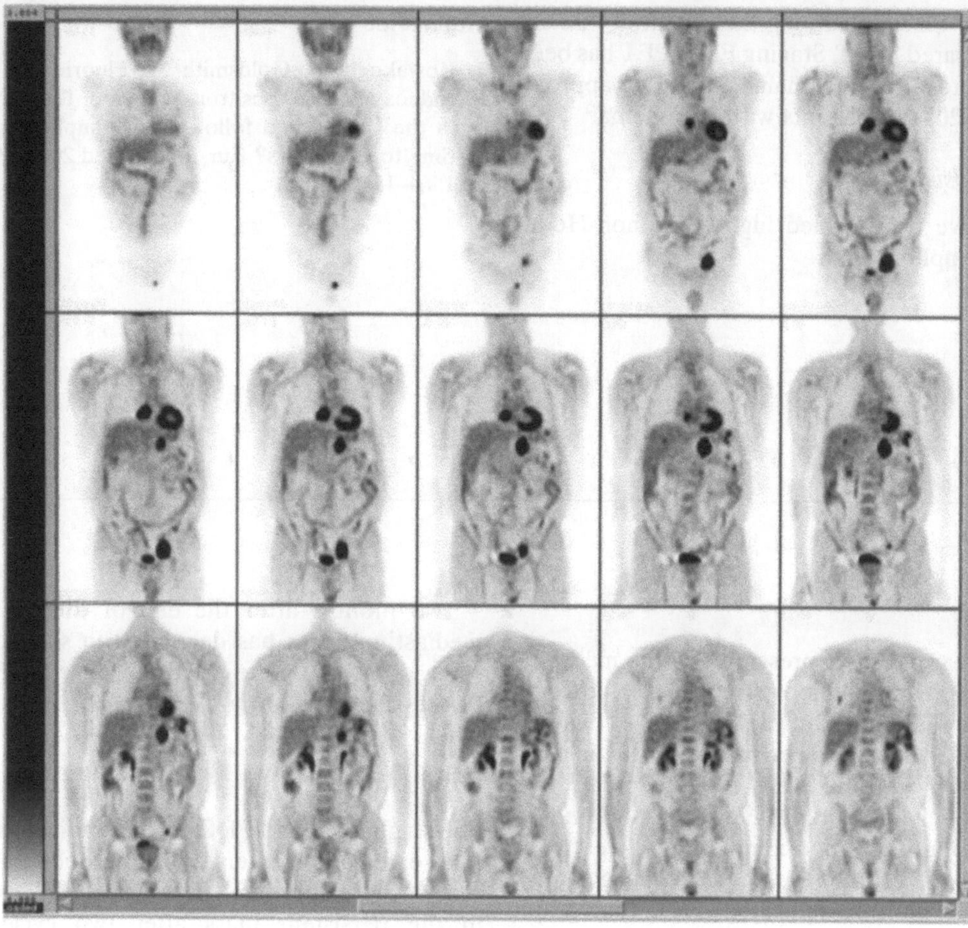

FIGURE 6.8.7C.

left upper thigh, (7) base of the penis, and (8) upper left lip (not in field of view of the images shown).

Discussion

Although FDG PET has a sensitivity of over 90% for the detection of NHL, the degree of activity tends to be lower in low-grade lymphomas than in high-grade lymphomas, and the sensitivity for the detection of low-grade NHL is significantly less than 90%. Due to considerable overlap, however, semiquantitative FDG PET cannot be used to differentiate low-grade from high-grade NHL.

Both biopsy-proven skin lesions are identified by FDG PET involving the left upper lip and at the base of the penis. There appears to be persistent lymphoma at the splenectomy site, but previously unidentified disease is present within the lung, mediastinum, liver (not seen on CT), abdominal nodal regions, and iliac nodal region. Therefore, this patient was found, by FDG PET, to have much more extensive disease than was identified by CT and at laparotomy. He was started on aggressive combination chemotherapy, and FDG PET represents an ideal modality for monitoring his response to therapy. This case is an excellent example of the utility of the high sensitivity and specificity of FDG PET in defining the extent of disease, as compared to CT. Staging FDG PET has been shown to alter the management of approximately 20% of patients with lymphoma.[1]

Diagnosis

Extensive transformed high-grade non-Hodgkin's lymphoma.

Reference

1. Kostakoglu L, Goldsmith SJ: Fluorine-18 fluorodeoxyglucose positron emission tomography in the staging and follow-up of lymphoma: Is it time to shift gears? Eur J Nucl Med 2000;27(10): 1564–1578.

Case 6.8.8

History

A 24-year-old male presented with a mediastinal mass, and a biopsy revealed Hodgkin's disease. CT (not shown) and FDG imaging (Figure 6.8.8A) were performed for staging. CT and FDG imaging were repeated after two cycles of chemotherapy (Figures 6.8.8B and C) and two months after completion of treatment (Figures 6.8.8D and E). The FDG images were acquired with a dedicated PET tomograph (GE Advance) and reconstructed with iterative algorithm and measured segmented attenuation correction.

Findings

The staging CT scan of the chest (not shown) was very similar to the CT obtained after two cycles of chemotherapy (Figure 6.8.8B), revealing a 4cm lobulated soft tissue mass in the upper left mediastinum. The staging FDG PET images (Figure 6.8.8A) demonstrate a lobulated area of increased uptake in the left mediastinum corresponding to the mass on CT.

After two cycles of chemotherapy, the mediastinal mass on CT (Figure 6.8.8B) is unchanged, but the FDG images (Figure 6.8.8C) are normal with no abnormal uptake corresponding to the mass. Physiologic FDG uptake is seen in the brain, myocardium, and urinary tract.

Two months after the end of therapy, the mediastinal mass has decreased in size somewhat on CT (Figure 6.8.8D), and the FDG images are still normal.

Discussion

The staging CT and FDG images indicate stage II disease (involvement of lymph node on one side of the diaphragm). The absence of uptake in the persistent mass after two cycles of chemotherapy predicts a good response to chemotherapy, and the absence of uptake after completion of therapy confirms the good response to treatment, even in the presence of a residual mass on CT.

Anatomical imaging with CT has limitations to predict tumor response to chemotherapy. It usually takes several months before a mass decreases in size, even if it does respond to therapy. Identification of patients with poor response to therapy early into the course of treatment allows appropriate modifications of therapy and avoids unnecessary morbidity associated with an ineffective treatment. Physiological changes occur before anatomical changes, and therefore, functional imaging with radiopharmaceuticals is more appropriate in that regard. Studies using ^{67}gallium have demonstrated that after two cycles of chemotherapy, the absence of ^{67}gallium uptake in tumors that

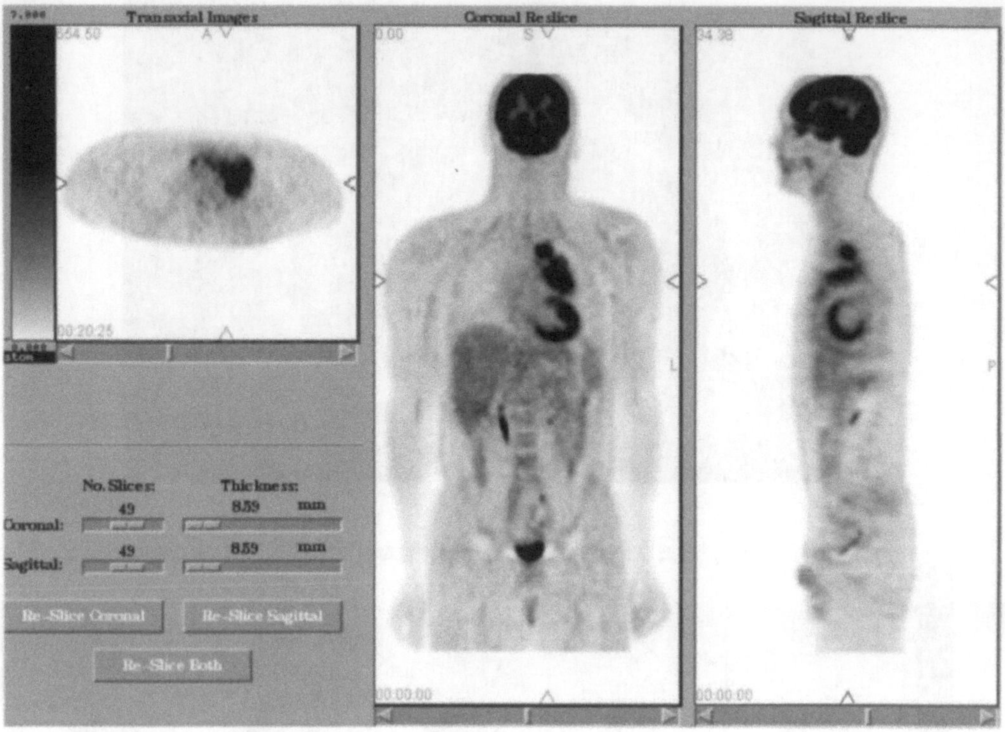

FIGURE 6.8.8A.

were ^{67}gallium-avid prior to therapy was associated with remission after completion of therapy in over 90% of the patients, as compared to less than 20% of patients with ^{67}gallium-avid lymphoma after two cycles of therapy.[1] However, the resolution of ^{67}gallium images is limited, and high uptake in the normal liver and colon often precludes adequate evaluation of the abdomen and pelvis. In addition, ^{67}gallium scintigraphy is a procedure that takes several days, requiring multiple visits from the patient to the clinic. Preliminary studies suggest that FDG imaging can attain the same goal, providing higher resolution images with a lower background activity in normal liver parenchyma and colon, allowing evaluation of the abdomen and pelvis, and being completed in two hours.[2] A study of 28 patients evaluated early during chemotherapy with FDG has demonstrated that the progression-free survival at one and two years was 20% and 0%, respectively, for FDG-positive patients and 87% and 68% for FDG-negative patients.[3]

Bulky disease is common in patients with lymphoma, and the presence of a residual mass on CT after completion of therapy is the rule rather than the exception. If the residual masses are scarring tissue, no further treatment is necessary, but if they contain viable tumor, additional treatment is required. The limitations of CT to differentiate post-therapy fibrous residual masses from residual or recurrent tumor are well recognized. ^{67}Gallium scintigraphy is more accurate than CT in that regard and has been used for that purpose in the past ten years. More recently, studies have demonstrated that FDG imaging can be used for the same purpose with advantages over ^{67}gallium scintigraphy, as outlined previously.[4–6] In a study of 32 patients with aggressive NHL and a residual mass after completion of therapy, 89% (8 out of 9) patients with a positive PET have relapsed as compared to less than 10% of patients with a negative PET.[7]

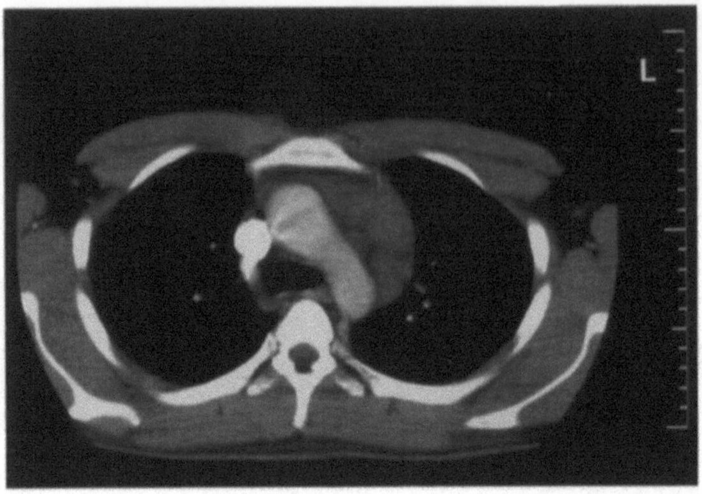

B

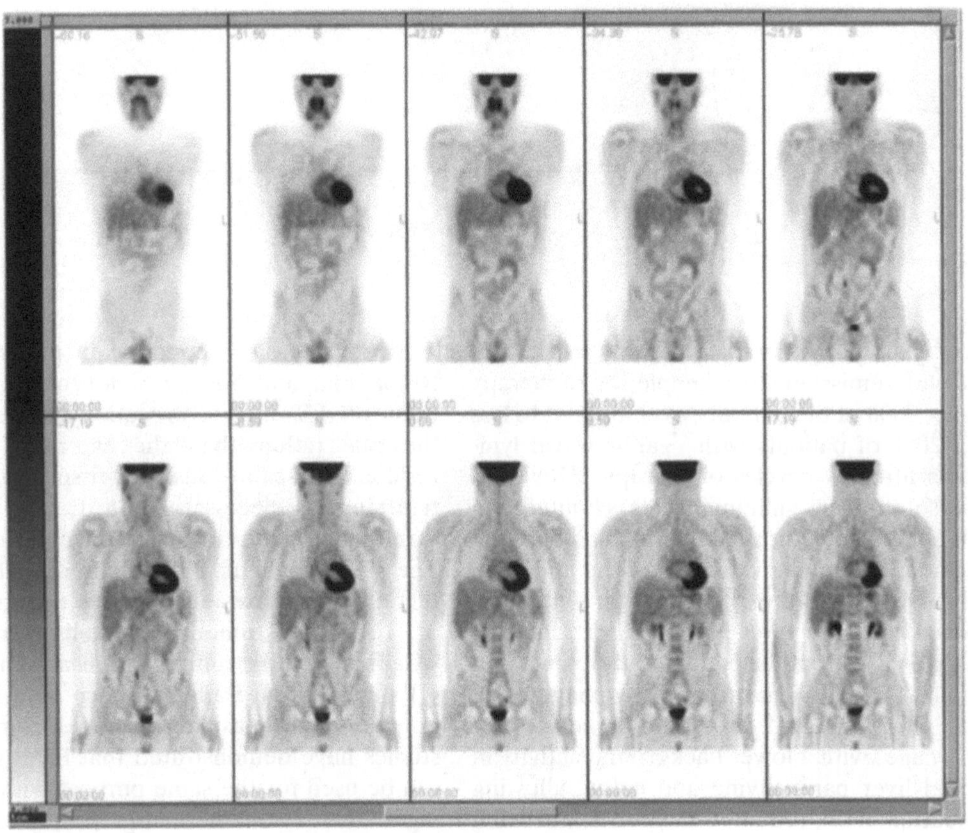

C

FIGURE 6.8.8B,C. (*Continued*)

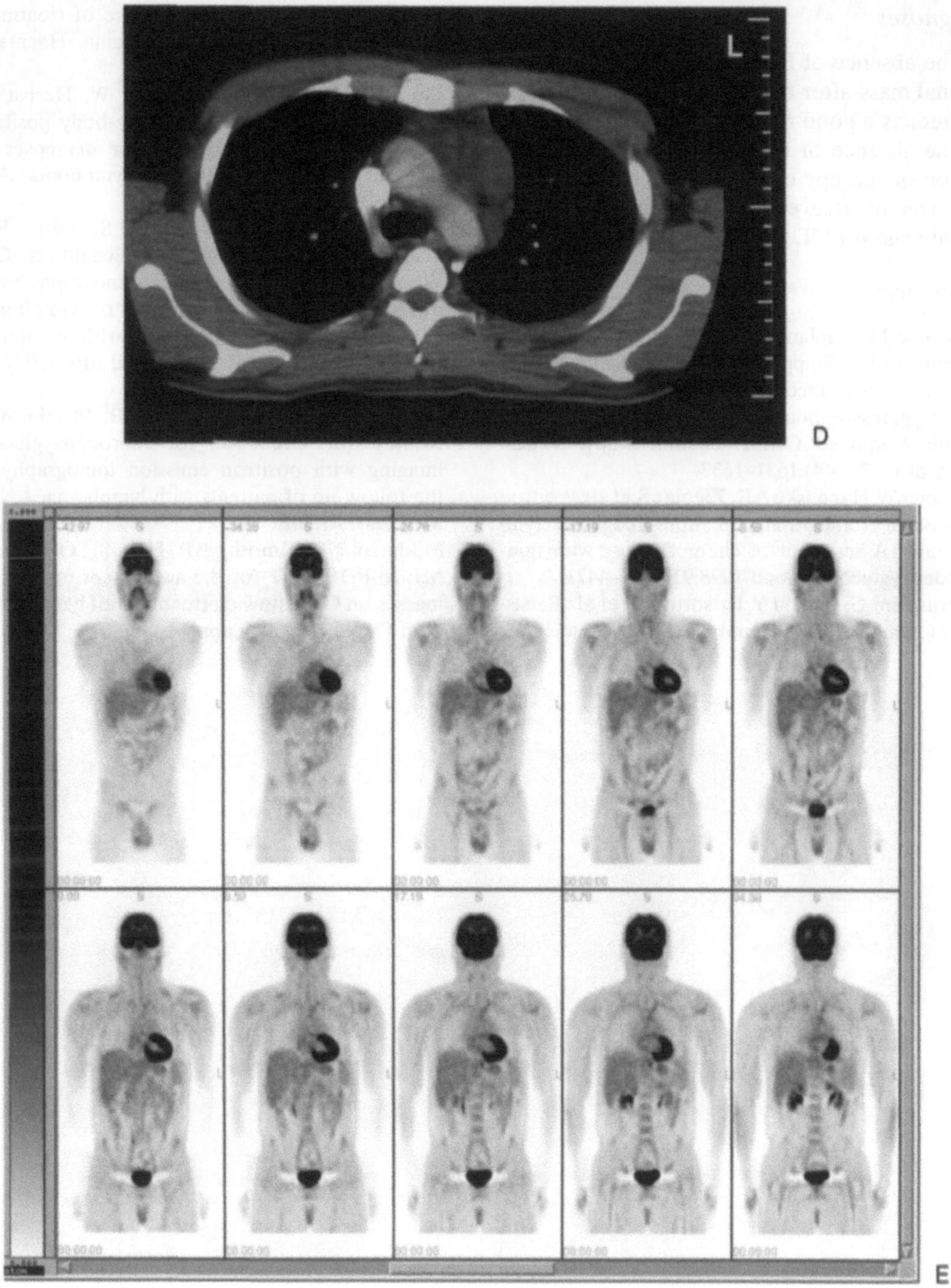

FIGURE 6.8.8D,E.

Diagnoses

1. The absence of FDG uptake in the mediastinal mass after two cycles of chemotherapy predicts a good response to chemotherapy.
2. The absence of FDG uptake after completion of therapy confirms the good response to treatment, even in the presence of a residual mass on CT.

References

1. Janicek M, Kaplan W, Neuberg D, Canellos GP, Shulman LN, Shipp MA: Early restaging gallium scans predict outcome in poor-prognosis patients with aggressive non-Hodgkin's lymphoma treated with high-dose CHOP chemotherapy. J Clin Oncol 1997;15(4):1631–1637.
2. Romer W, Hanauske AR, Ziegler S, et al.: Positron emission tomography in non-Hodgkin's lymphoma: Assessment of chemotherapy with fluorodeoxyglucose. Blood 1998;91:4464–4471.
3. Jerusalem G, Beguin Y, Fassotte MF, et al.: Persistent tumor 18F-FDG uptake after a few cycles of polychemotherapy is predictive of treatment failure in non-Hodgkin's lymphoma. Haematologica 2000;85(6):613–618.
4. De Wit M, Bumann D, Beyer W, Herbst K, Clausen M, Hossfeld DK: Whole-body positron emission tomography (PET) for diagnoses of residual mass in patients with lymphoma. Ann Oncol 1997;8(Suppl):57–60.
5. Stumpe KD, Urbinelli M, Steinert HC, Glanzmann C, Buck A, von Schulthess GK: Whole-body positron emission tomography using fluorodeoxyglucose for staging of lymphoma: Effectiveness and comparison with computed tomography. Eur J Nucl Med 1998;25:721–728.
6. Delbeke D, Kovalsky E, Cerci R, Martin WH, Kinney M, Greer J: 18F-fluorodeoxyglucose imaging with positron emission tomography in the follow-up of patients with lymphoma. J Nucl Med 2000;41:70P.
7. Mikhaeel NG, Timothy AR, Hain SF, O'Doherty MJ: 18-FDG-PET for the assessment of residual masses on CT following treatment of lymphomas. Ann Oncol 2000;11(Suppl):147–150.

6.9 Melanoma

Stanley L. Pope, William H. Martin, and Dominique Delbeke

Melanoma is the most aggressive of skin cancers and is increasing in frequency, particularly in Caucasians in areas of high sun exposure. The classification of melanomas is based on the depth of invasion in the dermis as well as the thickness of the tumor.[1,2] Melanoma frequently spreads to regional lymph nodes once the vertical growth phase develops and then is likely to metastasize to any organ. The peak for metastases is during the first and second year after diagnosis. The presence of lymph node metastases is well established as a crucial prognostic indicator of this disease. Melanoma can metastasize to virtually any organ; the most frequent metastatic sites are the skin and lymph nodes, lungs, liver, brain, and skeleton. The presence of systemic metastases is associated with a very poor prognosis and mean survival of less than six months. Accurate staging of disease extent in malignant melanoma remains problematic.

Early Stage Melanoma

For early stage melanoma, staging of regional lymph nodes is critical for determining the prognosis and therapy. Because FDG PET has well-known limitations for detection of microscopic metastases, sentinel lymph node mapping, resection, and histological examination have become the standard of care. The sentinel node is the first draining node of the lymphatic bed draining a malignant tumor. If the sentinel node is free of tumor, the remainder of the nodes in that basin are likely to be free of tumor, which obviates more radical lymph node dissection.[3] Lymphoscintigraphy for sentinel node identification and intraoperative mapping with a gamma probe have now become the standard of care at many institutions.

High-Risk Melanoma

A pilot study of patients with high-risk melanoma (thickness > 1.5 mm) suggested that FDG PET imaging was useful in detecting subclinical lymph nodes noninvasively, as well as metastases to other organs.[4] In a study of 33 patients with 53 lesions, FDG PET imaging had a sensitivity of 92% and specificity of 77% without clinical information and 100% with clinical information.[5] The findings on PET images affected therapy in 4 out of 29 (14%) patients. Subsequent studies have demonstrated the high accuracy of FDG PET to identify both nodal and visceral metastases from melanoma.[6–14] False-positive findings have included other malignancies, Warthin's tumor, leiomyoma of the uterus, endometriosis, and inflammatory lesions; false-negatives have included skin lesions without mass effects and lesions smaller than 5 mm in size. As for other tumors, detection of cerebral metastases is limited by the high background of FDG uptake in the gray matter.[10] MRI is the best imaging modality to detect cerebral metastases. In a prospective study of 100 patients with high-risk melanoma (thickness > 1.5 mm) comparing FDG PET imaging and conventional diagnostic methods, FDG PET was superior to conventional diagnostic methods in staging melanoma at primary diagnosis and during follow-up, both on a patient basis and a lesion basis.[10] Potentially, patients that have a negative FDG PET scan could be followed by close clinical observation. However, including FDG PET in the primary staging of melanoma is still debated because of the limitations for detection of micrometastases. Although controversy still exists, combining sentinel lymph node localization and biopsy with whole-body FDG PET imaging may optimize initial staging of high-risk melanoma. Cost-benefit and outcome analyses have not yet been reported. However, a 1996–1997 retrospective study of the inclusion of FDG PET in the staging of patients with suspected or metastatic melanoma demonstrated a saving of $1,800 per patient, a net savings-to-cost ratio of more than two.[15]

Summary

FDG PET imaging has proven beneficial in the assessment of patients with high-risk melanoma and patients with suspected recurrent or metastatic disease. At present, it is not typically used in the initial evaluation of patients with low-to-intermediate risk melanoma.

References

1. Breslow A: Thickness, cross sectional areas and depth of invasion in the prognosis of cutaneous melanoma. Annals of Surg 1970;172:902–908.
2. Clark WH, From L, Bernardino EA, Mihm MC: The histogenesis and biologic behavior of primary human malignant melanoma of the skin. Cancer Res 1969;29:705–706.
3. Morton DL, Wen DR, Wong JH, et al.: Technical details of intraoperative lymphatic mapping for early stage melanoma. Arch Surg 1992;127:391–399.
4. Gritters LS, Francis IR, Zasadny KR, Wahl RL: Initial assessment of positron emission tomography using 2-fluoro-18-fluoro-2-deoxy-D-glucose in the imaging of malignant melanoma. J Nucl Med 1993;34:1420–1427.
5. Steinert HC, Huch-Boni RA, Buck A, et al.: Malignant melanoma: Staging with whole-body positron emission tomography and 2-[F-18]-fluoro-2-deoxy-D-glucose. Radiology 1995;195: 705–709.
6. Boni R, Boni RA, Steinert H, et al.: Staging of metastatic melanoma by whole-body positron emission tomography using 2-fluorine-18-fluoro-2-deoxy-D-glucose. Br J Dermatol 1995;132:556–562.
7. Blessing C, Feine U, Geiger L, Carl M, Rassner G, Fierlbeck G: Positron emission tomography and ultrasonography. A comparative retrospective study assessing the diagnostic validity in lymph node metastases of malignant melanoma. Arch Dermatol 1995;131:1394–1398.
8. Damian DL, Fulham MJ, Thompson E, Thompson JF: Positron emission tomography in the detection and management of metastatic melanoma. Melanoma Res 1996;6:325–329.
9. Wagner JD, Schauwecker D, Hutchins G, Coleman JJ III: Initial assessment of positron emission tomography for detection of non-palpable regional lymphatic metastases in melanoma. J Surg Oncol 1997;64:181–189.
10. Rinne D, Baum RP, Hor G, Kaufmann R: Primary staging and follow-up of high risk melanoma patients with whole-body 18F-fluorodeoxyglucose positron emission tomography: Results of a prospective study of 100 patients. Cancer 1998;82:1664–1671.
11. Macfarlane DJ, Sondak V, Johnson T, Wahl RL: Prospective evaluation of 2-[18F]-2-deoxy-D-glucose positron emission tomography in staging of regional lymph nodes in patients with cutaneous malignant melanoma. J Clin Oncol 1998;16:1770–1776.
12. Holder WD Jr, White RL Jr, Zuger JH, Easton EJ Jr, Greene FL: Effectiveness of positron emission tomography for the detection of melanoma metastases. Ann Surg 1998;227:764–769.
13. Steinert HC, Voellmy DR, Trachsel C, et al.: Planar coincidence scintigraphy and PET in staging malignant melanoma. J Nucl Med 1998;39: 1892–1897.
14. Wagner JD, Schauwecker D, Davidson D, et al.: Prospective study of fluorodeoxyglucose-positron emission tomography imaging of lymph node basins in melanoma patients undergoing sentinel node biopsy. J Clin Oncol 1999;17: 1508–1515.
15. Valk PE, Segall GM, Johnson DL, et al.: Cost-effectiveness of whole-body FDG PET imaging in metastatic melanoma, abstracted. J Nucl Med 1997;38(Suppl):89P.

Case Presentations

Case 6.9.1

History

A 75-year-old male who underwent resection of a melanoma from his upper back two years earlier was found to have multiple pulmonary nodules on chest radiograph. At the time of initial diagnosis, he was treated with a wide excision of the primary, and the sentinel node was negative for malignancy. A recent CT scan had not been performed at the time of referral. Coronal FDG PET images acquired with a dedicated PET tomograph (GE Advance) and reconstructed with iterative reconstruction and with measured segmented attenuation correction are shown in Figures 6.9.1A and B.

Findings

There are multiple foci of abnormally increased activity throughout the chest, abdomen, and pelvis. A lesion involving the soft tissues of the upper back, just to the right of the midline, most likely represents a subcutaneous metastasis. Additional foci of abnormal uptake of FDG are

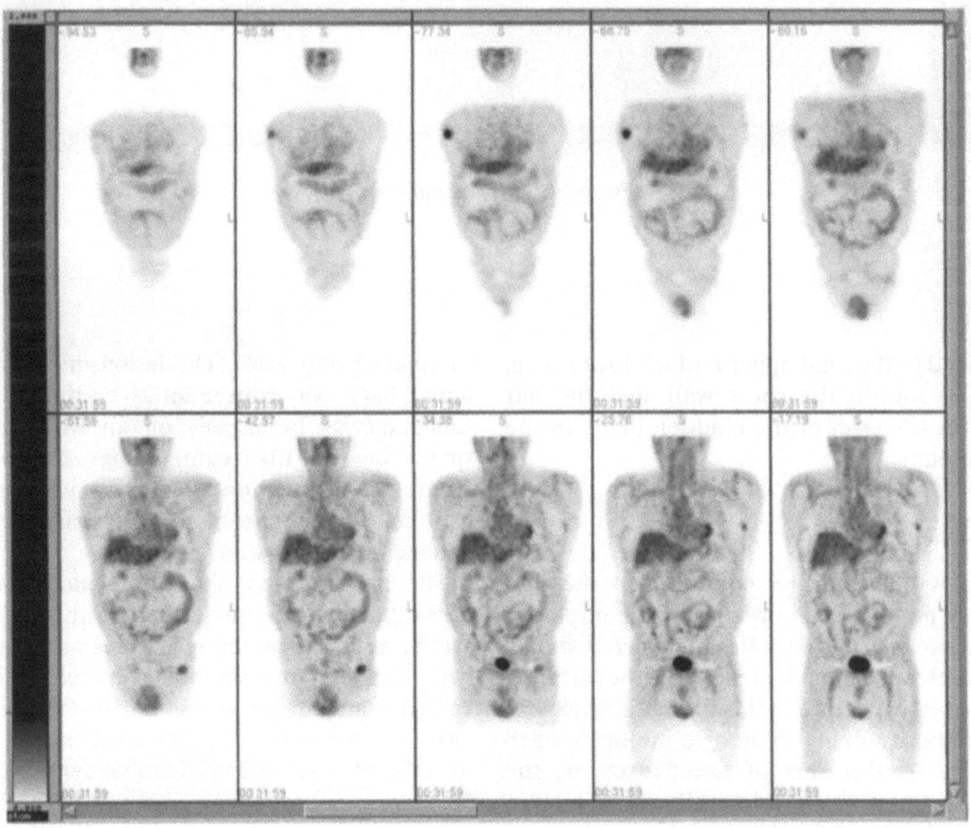

FIGURE 6.9.1A.

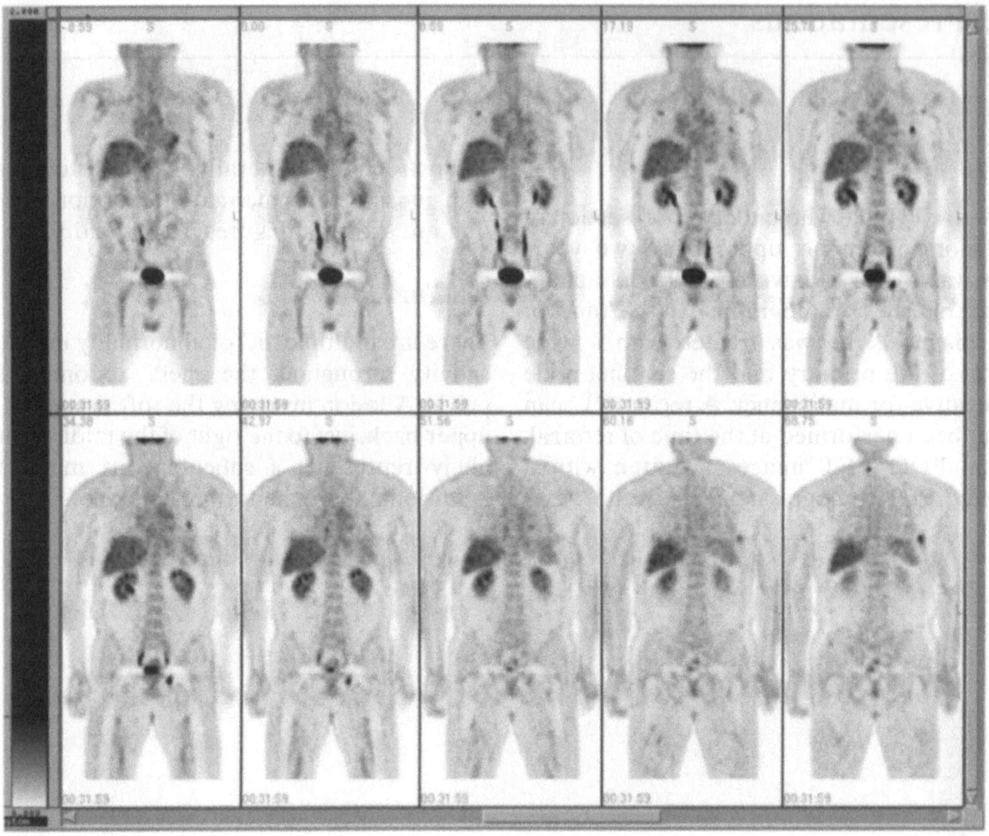

FIGURE 6.9.1B. *(Continued)*

identified in the right upper and left lower lung, multiple foci in the chest wall, and the left pelvis at the level of the bladder, likely in the acetabulum.

Discussion

The FDG PET images confirm that the pulmonary nodules seen on chest radiograph are metastatic, but there is also unexpected widely metastatic melanoma present, demonstrating the aggressive nature of this unpredictable neoplasm and its ability to involve multiple organ systems. At the time of initial excision, the primary lesion was histologically classified as a level IV lesion with a depth of 3 mm. This generally carries a poor prognosis with a five-year survival of only 50%. The lesion involving the upper back was subsequently confirmed as a subcutaneous metastasis on an MRI of the spine. Sagittal T1-weighted images shown in Figure 6.9.1C, without (left) and with (right) gadolinium enhancement, demonstrate the enhancing subcutaneous nodule.

The most frequent sites of melanoma metastasis following treatment of the primary disease are the skin, subcutaneous tissues, and regional lymph nodes, but melanoma can metastasize to virtually any organ or tissue. Autopsy series have demonstrated adrenal involvement in 36 to 54% of cases, bowel involvement in 26 to 58% of cases, lung involvement in 70 to 87% of cases, liver involvement in 54 to 77% of cases, brain involvement in 36 to 54% of cases, and

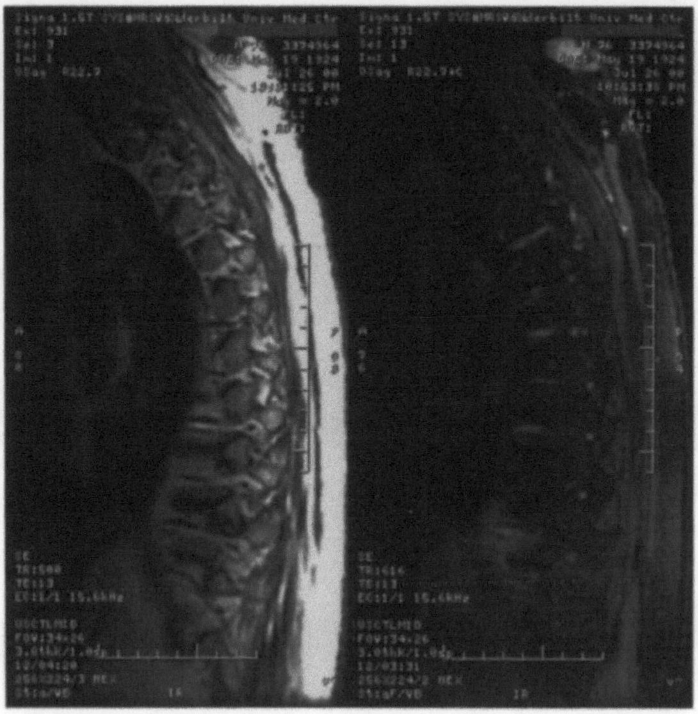

FIGURE 6.9.1C.

bone involvement in 23 to 49% of cases. In this case, the metastatic sites were multiple, including subcutaneous tissues, lungs, and skeleton (ribs and acetabulum).

In the clinical setting of high-grade melanoma with suspected metastases, FDG PET imaging performed early in the evaluation can save time and resources by identifying diffuse metastases that may not all be seen by conventional modalities. Identifying the extent or stage of disease at this point can spare the patient additional CT or MRI scans and further invasive procedures. FDG PET imaging can be used to follow the progression of disease and its response to therapies such as chemotherapy, immunotherapy, or radiation therapy.

Diagnosis

Widely metastatic melanoma.

Case 6.9.2

History

A 37-year-old female, who underwent excision of an intermediate-grade melanoma of the left thigh three years earlier, followed by inguinal lymphadenectomy three months later for recurrence, was found to have three low-density lesions in the liver and a 2 cm left inguinal nodal mass on CT scan (Figure 6.9.2A). Figures 6.9.2B and C show transaxial (Figure 6.9.2B) and coronal (Figure 6.9.2C) images through the pelvis acquired with a dedicated PET tomograph (Siemens ECAT 933) and reconstructed with filtered back projection without attenuation correction.

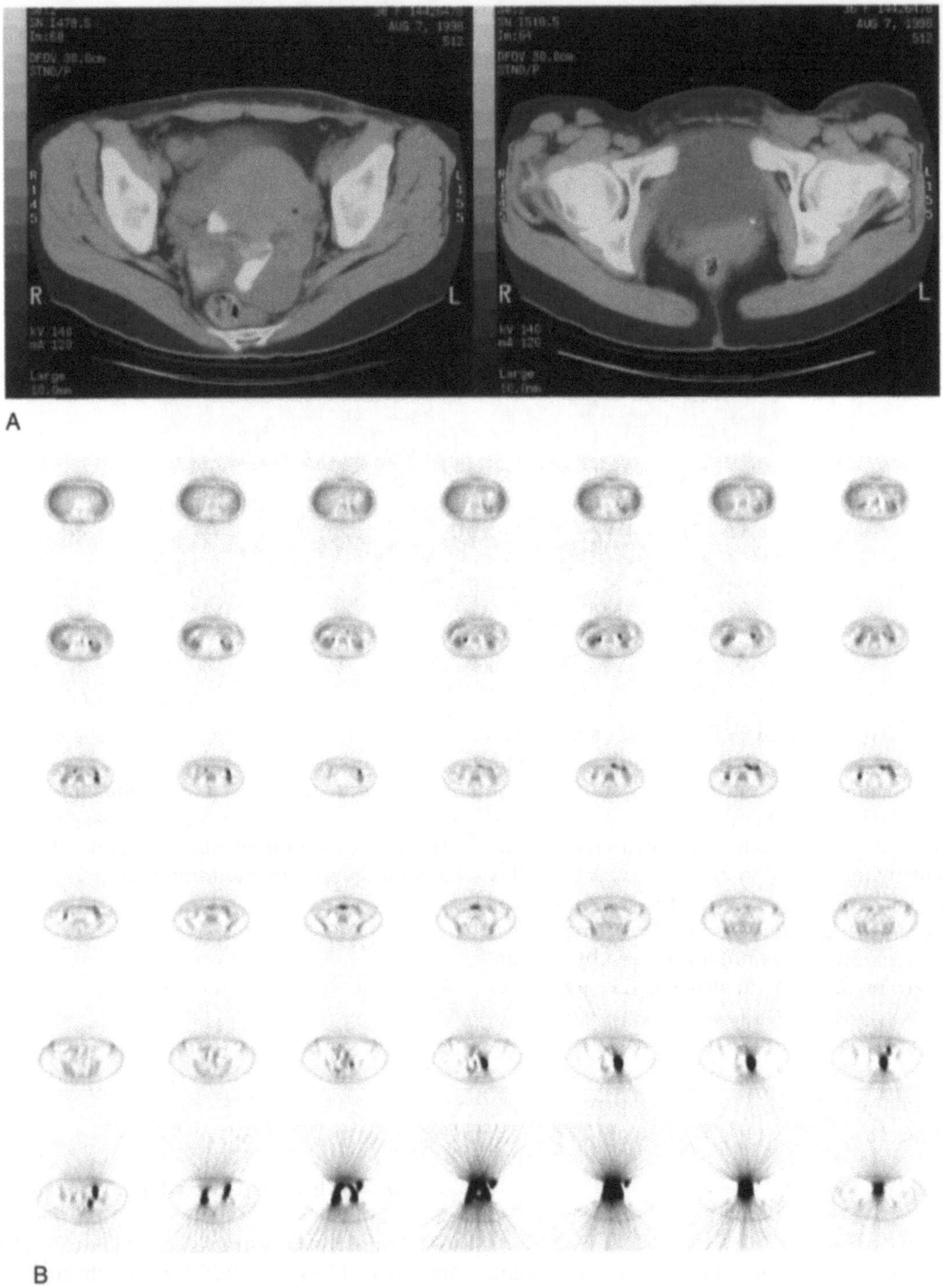

FIGURE 6.9.2A,B.

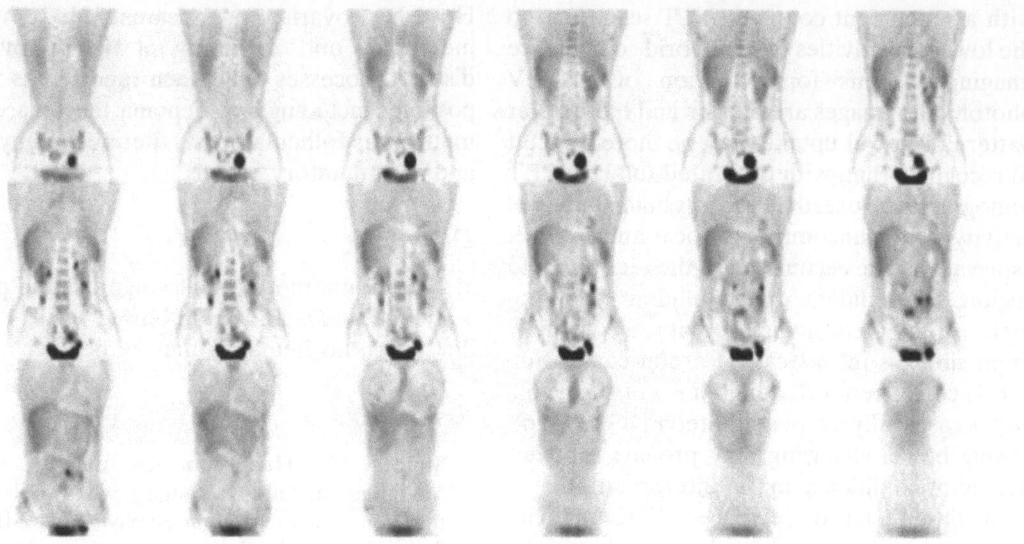

FIGURE 6.9.2C.

Findings

An abnormal focus of increased activity is identified in the left inguinal region corresponding to the nodal mass on CT. There is also increased uptake seen in the left pelvis, posterior and superior to the bladder and corresponding to a mass seen on CT. An additional focus of activity is seen in the mid-abdomen on the right, and other foci of activity are seen in the upper anterior abdomen, best seen on the third row of the transaxial images. No abnormal foci are identified in the liver.

Discussion

These findings indicate metastases in the left inguinal region and left adnexal mass. The foci of activity seen in the mid-abdomen and upper abdomen were initially thought to represent physiologic bowel activity. At laparotomy, the patient was found to have ten small metastases distributed throughout the small bowel, the largest one nearly obstructing the distal ileum. The three suspicious low-density hepatic lesions identified by CT but negative by FDG PET imaging were proven to be cavernous hemangiomas by ^{99m}Tc-labeled red blood cell scintigraphy.

Metastatic melanoma deposits are often resected when feasible with reasonable disease-free intervals followed by repeated limited resections. The ability of FDG PET imaging to accurately identify foci of recurrent disease, while also excluding other lesions as benign, helps greatly in surgical planning and determining the need for additional chemotherapy and/or immunotherapy. In a series of 48 patients who underwent FDG PET imaging for recurrence, FDG PET was superior to CT with sensitivities of 100% by patients and 91% by lesions as compared to 80% by patients and 58% by lesions for CT.[1]

At autopsy, melanoma metastatic to bowel is seen in up to 58% of patients; lymphoma may also metastasize to the bowel. The mechanism of physiologic FDG bowel uptake remains controversial, but it can usually be recognized by its relatively low intensity (as compared to tumor) and tubular pattern. The ability to follow suspicious abdominal FDG activity in sequential sections in three orthogonal planes is often helpful and can be correlated visually with a concurrent contrasted CT scan. Due to the lower sensitivities of the hybrid coincidence imaging systems for detection of 511keV photons, the images are noisier and the tubular pattern of bowel uptake may be more difficult to recognize than with dedicated full ring PET tomographs. Nevertheless, physiologic bowel activity is not uncommonly focal and intense, especially at the cecum and in the rectosigmoid region, so confident discrimination of pathologic from physiologic activity is virtually impossible, as in this case. Careful correlation with a concurrent CT, a high level of suspicion, and occasionally a repeat limited FDG PET following bowel cleansing may provide a higher degree of confidence in the interpretation.

In this scenario, increased FDG activity congruent with an adnexal mass should be considered metastasis until proven otherwise. However, ovarian adenocarcinoma is hypermetabolic, and a variety of benign ovarian disease processes have been reported as false-positives, including cystadenoma, thecoma, endometrioma, follicular cyst, uterine leiomyoma, and inflammatory lesions.

Diagnoses

1. Melanoma metastatic to inguinal and pelvic lymph nodes and small bowel.
2. Cavernous hemangiomas in the liver.

Reference

1. Steinert HC, Huch-Boni RA, Buck A, et al.: Malignant melanoma: Staging with whole-body positron emission tomography and 2-[F-18]-fluoro-2-deoxy-D-glucose. Radiology 1995;195: 705–709.

Case 6.9.3

History

A 53-year-old male with melanoma is referred for staging. Two years earlier a left upper extremity melanoma and metastatic axillary nodes were resected. Six months later he underwent splenectomy and right adrenalectomy for recurrent disease. CT (Figure 6.9.3A) and FDG imaging acquired with a dedicated PET tomograph (Siemens ECAT 933) and

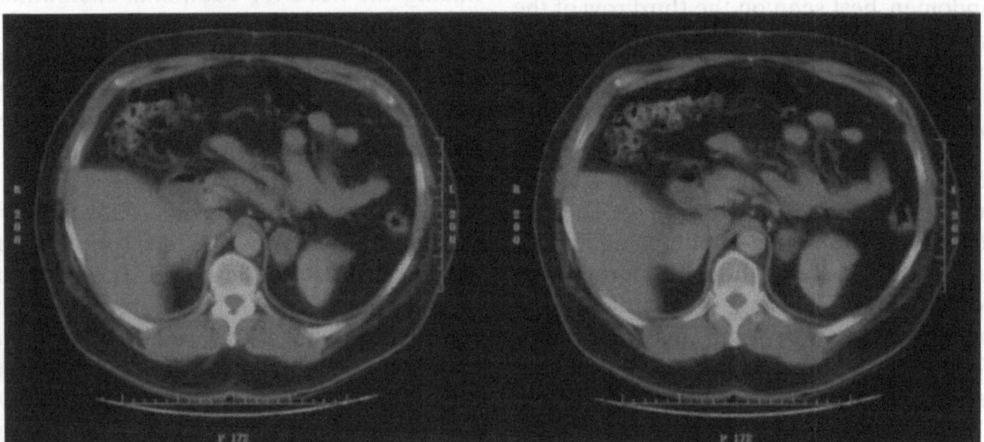

FIGURE 6.9.3A.

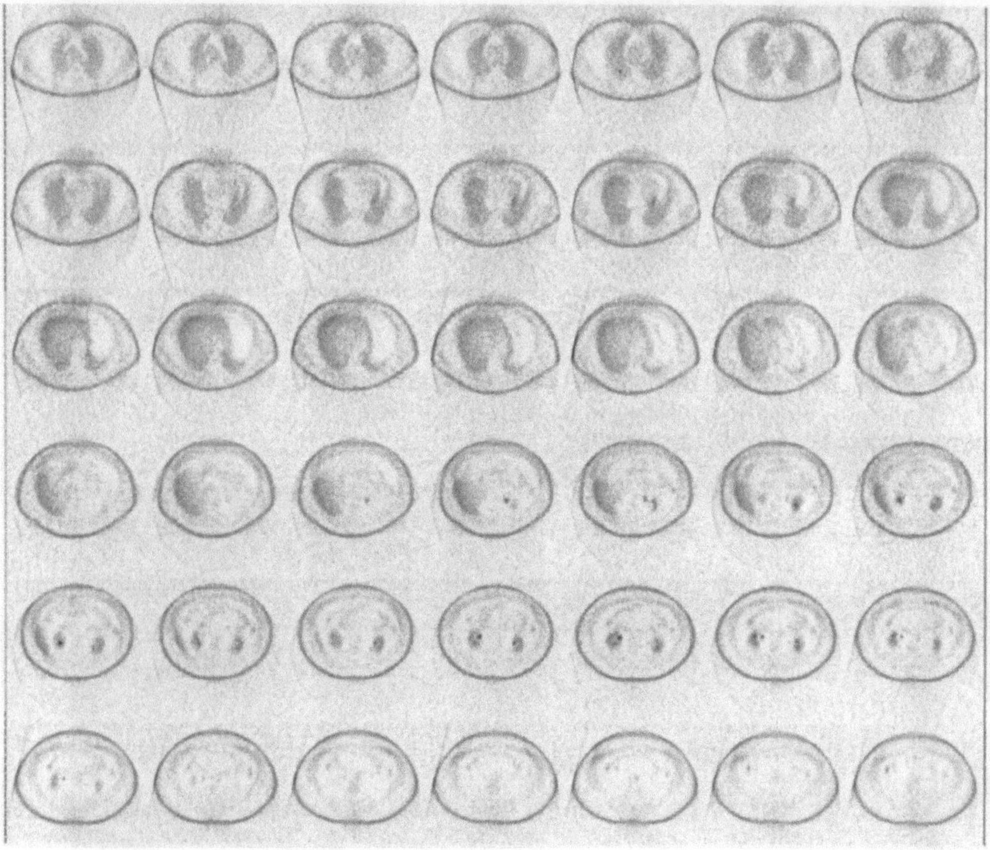

FIGURE 6.9.3B.

reconstructed with filtered back projection without attenuation correction are displayed. Figures 6.9.3B and C show transaxial FDG PET images (Figure 6.9.3B) and orthogonal images through the left adrenal (Figure 6.9.3C).

Findings

The CT scan demonstrates a 1 to 2 cm adrenal mass on the left. The FDG PET images demonstrate increase physiological activity within the renal collecting systems, whose presence can function as a useful landmark. A focus of abnormal uptake is seen in the expected location of the left adrenal gland superior and just medial to the left kidney. No other abnormalities were identified on whole-body FDG images.

Discussion

The left adrenal lesion identified on CT scan correlates with the focus of increased uptake on the FDG images, consistent with metastatic disease to the left adrenal gland.

Adrenal involvement with melanoma metastasis occurs in 36 to 54% of cases and is a common site of metastasis from other malignant neoplasms, especially from lung and breast primaries and lymphoma. Incidental adrenal masses are identified in approximately 2% of patients undergoing CT imaging for other reasons. Conventional CT and MR protocols with and without intravenous contrast administration are unable to accurately differentiate benign from malignant adrenal lesions,[1] although CT imaging protocols with delayed washout images and specific MRI sequences

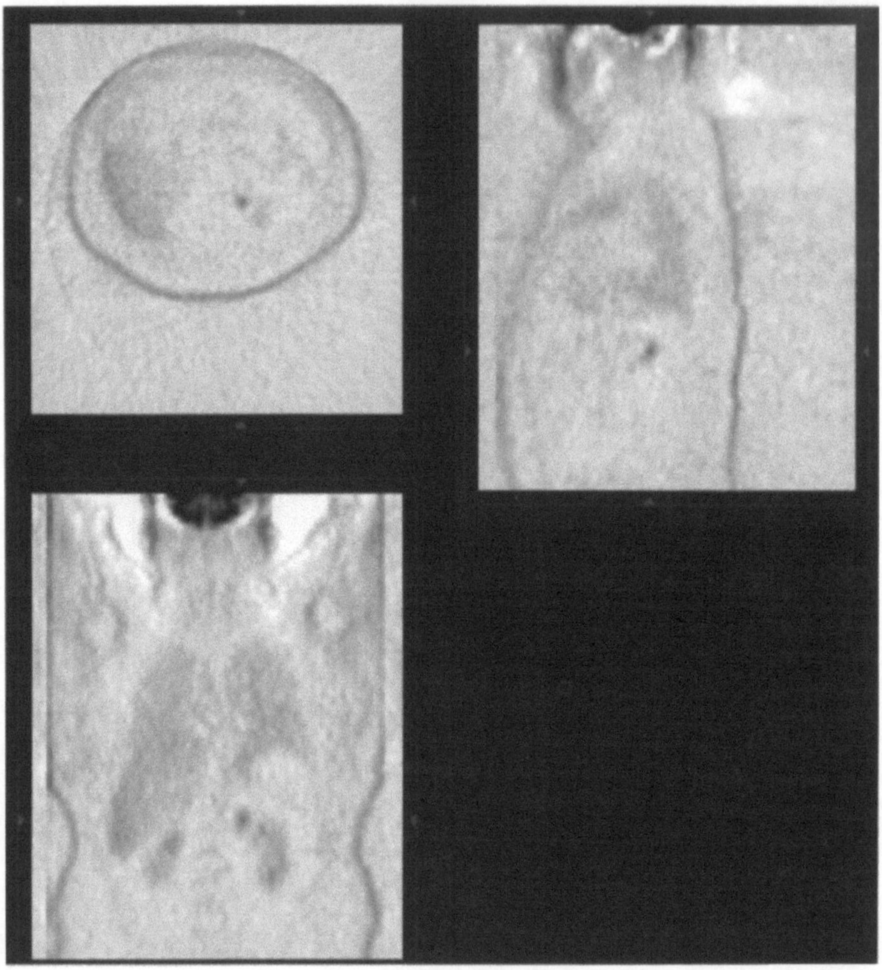

FIGURE 6.9.3C. (*Continued*)

have made great progress in differentiation. Incidental adrenal lesions identified on CT scan are rarely malignant in the patient without a known primary malignancy. However, the chance of malignancy rises significantly in the patient with known malignancy, 27 to 36%. Invasive percutaneous needle biopsy is often used in this clinical situation. In a series of 20 patients with 24 incidental adrenal masses and a known malignancy, FDG PET imaging was able to separate benign (n = 10) from malignant lesions (n = 14) in all cases.[2] In a prospective series of 27 patients with lung cancer and 33 adrenal masses ranging from 1 to 9 cm in size, FDG PET imaging demonstrated 100% sensitivity for detection of metastatic involvement with 80% specificity. The two false-positive PET findings were identified because a percutaneous fine-needle biopsy was negative.[3] However, fine-needle biopsy may be falsely negative in up to 7% of cases due to sampling error.[4]

There are several advantages to FDG PET imaging in this patient. First, PET imaging can distinguish between benign and malignant lesions with a high degree of accuracy. If the new adrenal lesion failed to demonstrate increased FDG uptake, the clinician may choose to monitor the benign lesion and not subject the patient to surgery or biopsy. Second,

PET imaging may identify additional lesions other than the left adrenal lesion. If additional metastases are identified, the treatment strategy may change, that is, local resection versus systemic chemotherapy, immunotherapy, or radiation therapy.

Diagnosis

Melanoma metastatic to the left adrenal gland.

References

1. Porte HL, Ernst OJ, Delebecq T, Metois D, Lemaitre LG, Wurtz AJ: Is computed tomography guided biopsy still necessary for the diagnosis of adrenal masses in patients with resectable non-small-cell lung cancer? Eur J Cardiothorac Surg 1999;15:597–601.
2. Boland GW, Goldberg MA, Lee MJ, et al.: Indeterminate adrenal mass in patients with cancer: Evaluation at PET with 2-[F-18]-fluoro-2-deoxy-D-glucose. Radiology 1995;194:131–134.
3. Erasmus JJ, Patz EF Jr, McAdams HP, et al.: Evaluation of adrenal masses in patients with bronchogenic carcinoma using ^{18}F-fluorodeoxyglucose positron emission tomography. Am J Roentgenol 1997;168:1357–1360.
4. Welch TJ, Sheedy PF, Stephens DH, Johnson CM, Swensen SJ: Percutaneous adrenal biopsy: Review of a 10-year experience. Radiology 1994;193:341–344.

Case 6.9.4

History

A 58-year-old male presented with anemia and melena. Three years ago a melanoma on his back was resected. Seven months prior to presentation, metastatic right axillary nodes were resected followed by high-dose interferon therapy. The CT scan performed at the time of presentation was interpreted as negative for metastases (not shown). Figure 6.9.4 shows transaxial FDG PET images acquired with a dedicated PET tomograph (Siemens ECAT 933) and reconstructed with filtered back projection without attenuation correction.

Findings

The FDG PET images demonstrate multiple foci of uptake scattered throughout the abdomen. The largest cluster is located on the midline in front of the spine at the level of the hila of the kidneys. Correlation with the CT scan demonstrates peripancreatic, mesenteric, and retroperitoneal mildly enlarged lymph nodes seen retrospectively. Some foci are located along the bowel. A focus of uptake is also seen in the posterior mediastinum.

Discussion

These findings indicate widely metastatic melanoma to mediastinal, retroperitoneal, peripancreatic, and mesenteric lymph nodes. With the history of melena, the foci of focal uptake along the bowel are likely bowel metastases, although physiologic bowel uptake can occasionally be focal. Subsequently, endoscopic biopsy of a duodenal lesion was positive for melanoma. This patient's primary melanoma resection proved to be 1.6 mm in depth, a Clark level III. With the axillary nodal metastasis, the patient would be classified as stage III with a five-year survival of 36 to 40%. With distant metastases demonstrated by PET, the patient is stage IV with a median survival of 7.5 months and a five-year survival of only 6%.

Metastasis to the bowel from melanoma occurs in 26 to 58% of patients. FDG PET imaging was able to identify metastatic lesions that the CT scan failed to identify, specifically by identifying tumor tissue in mildly enlarged lymph nodes not deemed pathologic by CT. This information is helpful in treatment planning and strategy, in this case preventing unnecessary resection of the duodenal metastasis.

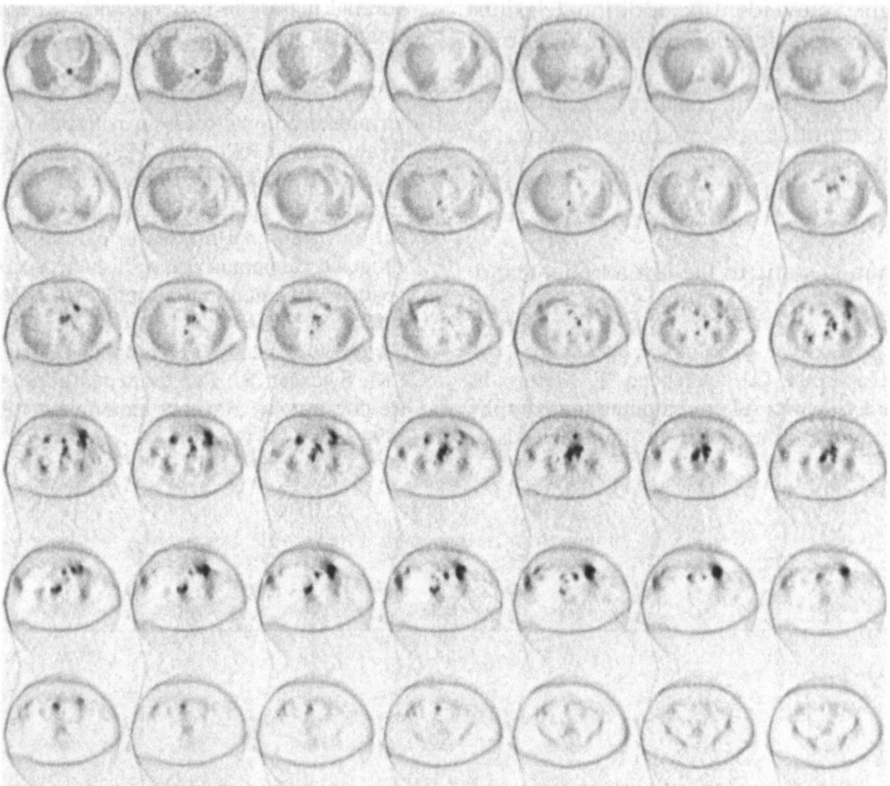

FIGURE 6.9.4.

In the past, ^{67}gallium scintigraphy was utilized for detection of recurrent or metastatic melanoma. The advantage of FDG PET imaging over ^{67}gallium scintigraphy is the better tumor-to-background ratio with PET and better resolution of the images. Although physiologic gastrointestinal activity can be occasionally problematic with FDG PET imaging, with ^{67}gallium scintigraphy the high background activity in the liver and colon often prevents evaluation of the abdomen and pelvis. Therefore, PET is able to detect smaller lesions with greater specificity.

Diagnosis

Melanoma with small bowel metastasis and extensive lymphatic metastases in the abdomen.

Case 6.9.5

History

A 62-year-old male presented with a palpable nodule in the right frontoparietal scalp. Ten months ago, biopsy of a left axillary mass revealed metastatic melanoma. The primary lesion at that time was not apparent, so he underwent axillary dissection followed by radiotherapy and interferon therapy. Staging consisted of bone scintigraphy (Figure 6.9.5A),

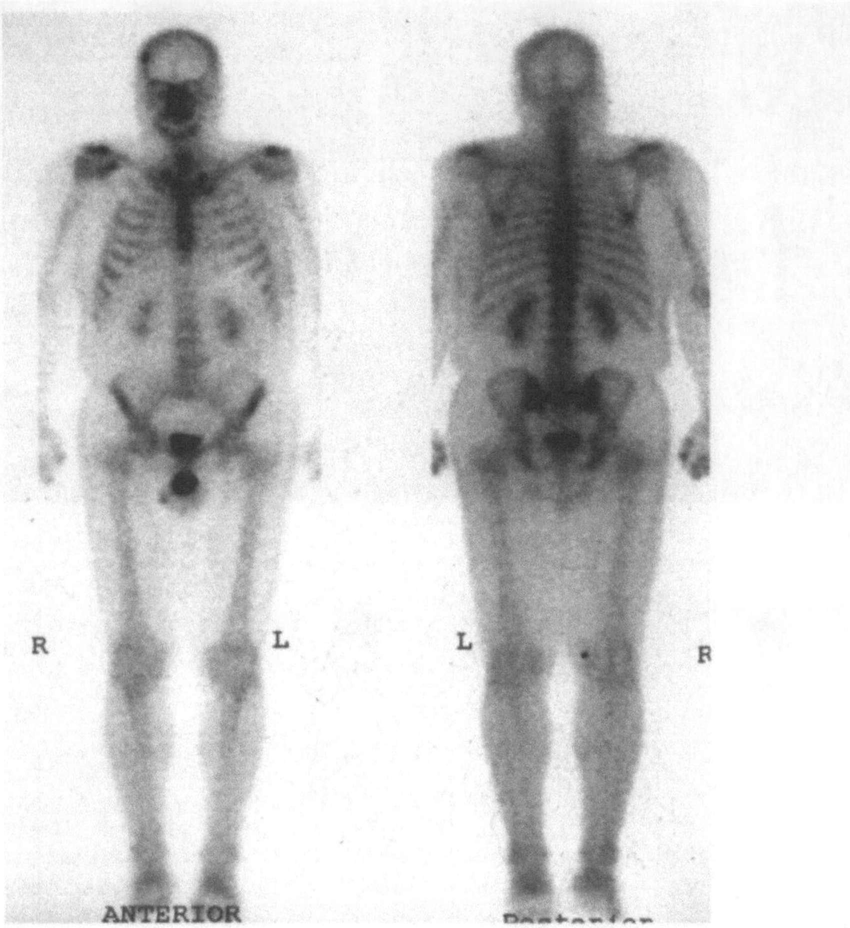

FIGURE 6.9.5A.

CT scan of the head (Figure 6.9.5B, bone window), and FDG PET imaging (Figures 6.9.5C, D, and E). FDG images were acquired with a dedicated PET tomograph (GE Advance) and reconstructed with iterative reconstruction and measured segmented attenuation correction. Coronal FDG PET images are shown in Figures 6.9.5C and D, and transaxial images through the brain are shown in Figure 6.9.5E.

Findings

The bone scan demonstrates increased uptake of the radiopharmaceutical in the right frontoparietal region corresponding to the palpable nodule. The CT scan of the head reveals a 1.5 cm lytic lesion in the same region within the right frontal bone with overlying soft tissue swelling. There is also a 1 cm lytic area in the occipital region that is worrisome for metastatic disease. The FDG images demonstrate increased glucose metabolism in the right frontal lytic lesion. The occipital lesion that was identified on CT but not on the bone scintigraphy was not seen on the FDG images. Markedly increased activity is also identified at the infrahilar region of the right lung. Several foci of faint activity are identified at the left supraclavicular region and the left upper posterior soft tissues of the thorax. There are also large foci of increased activity within the

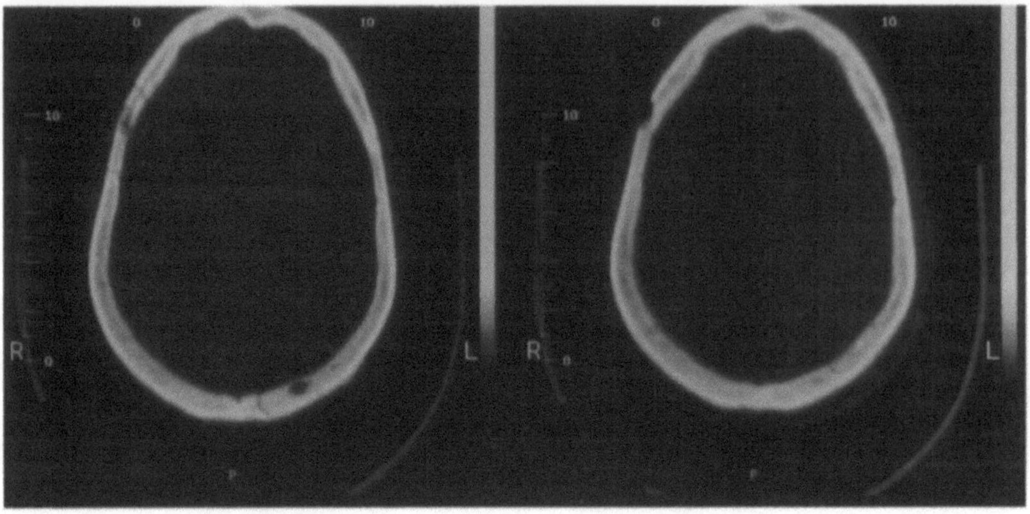

B

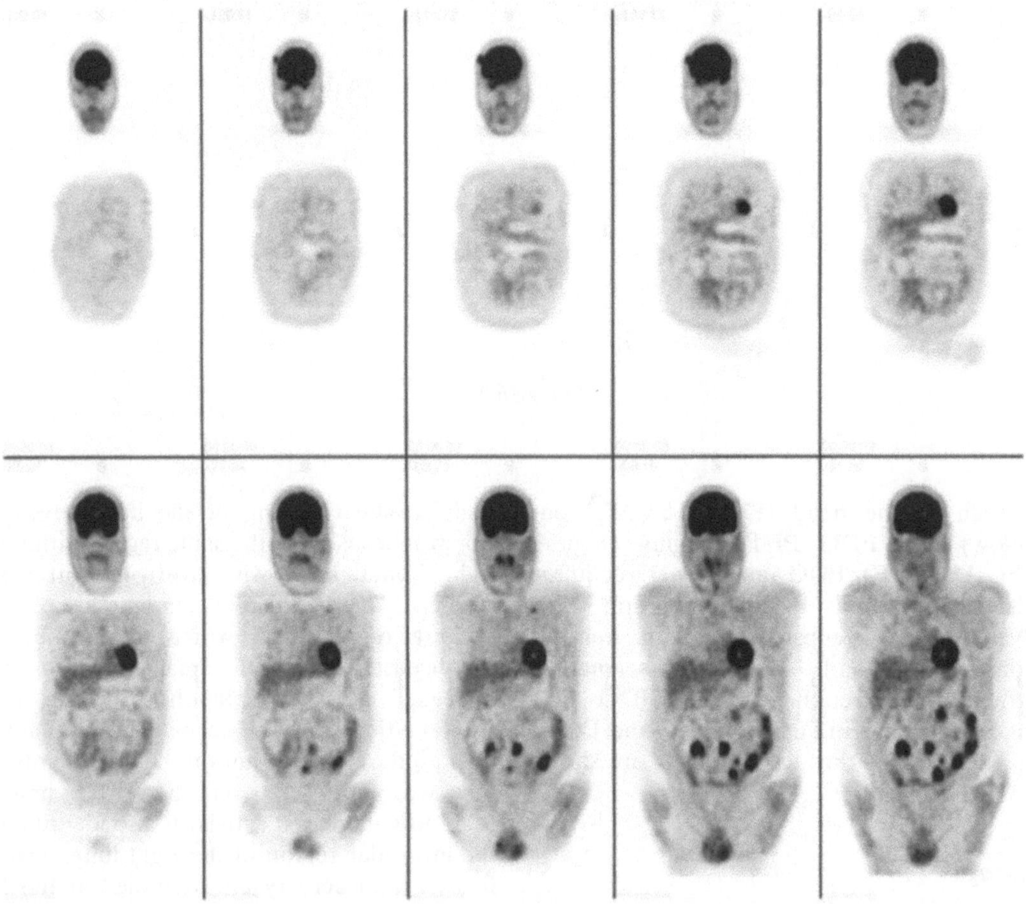

C

FIGURE 6.9.5B,C.

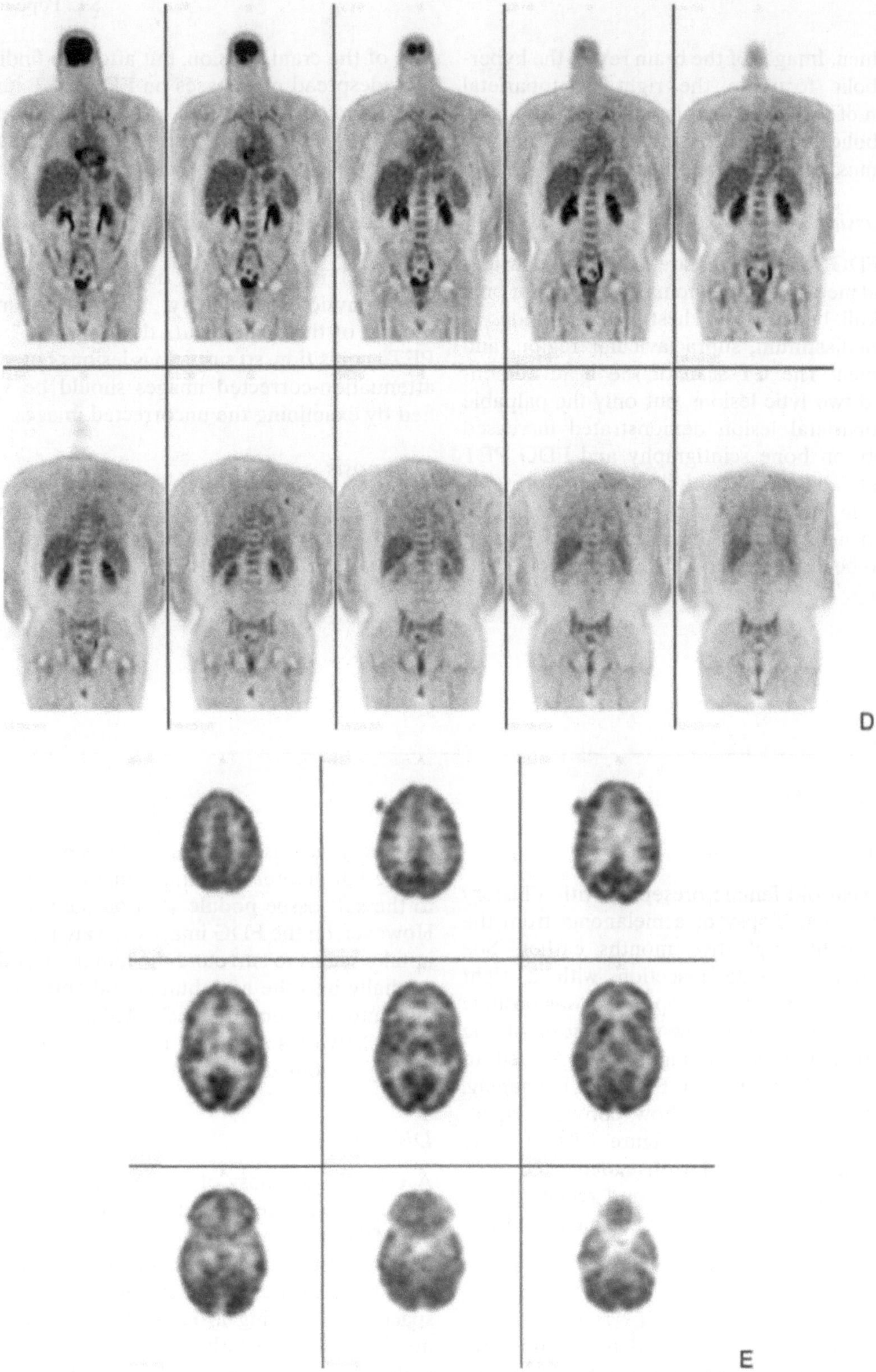

FIGURE 6.9.5D,E.

abdomen. Images of the brain reveal the hypermetabolic focus in the right frontoparietal region of the scalp and also unexpected hypermetabolic foci in the right basal ganglia, left thalamus, and right occipital cortex.

Discussion

The FDG PET images are indicative of widespread metastatic melanoma involving not only the skull, but also the chest wall and nodes of the mediastinum, supraclavicular region, and abdomen. The CT scan of the head demonstrated two lytic lesions, but only the palpable frontoparietal lesion demonstrated increased activity on bone scintigraphy and FDG PET images. The occipital lytic lesion represents a benign lesion such as a venous lake rather than a metastatic lesion. Initially, the patient was to be evaluated by neurosurgery for resection of the cranial lesion, but after the findings of widespread metastases on FDG PET imaging, his management was altered to only provide systemic therapy and avoid unnecessary surgery.

Although MRI is the modality of choice for the detection of intracerebral neoplasm, several unexpected cerebral metastases were identified with PET in this patient, despite the adjacent high physiologic activity. Not infrequently, motion of the head occurs during whole-body PET acquisition, so suspicious lesions noted on attenuation-corrected images should be verified by examining the uncorrected images.

Diagnosis

Unexpected widespread metastatic melanoma including involvement of the subcutaneous tissues, skull, brain, chest, and abdomen.

Case 6.9.6

History

A 32-year-old female presented with a history of excisional biopsy of a melanoma from the lower right thigh five months earlier. She underwent a wide resection with a right inguinal sentinel node biopsy that was positive for melanoma. A follow-up CT scan of the abdomen and pelvis (Figure 6.9.6A) led to further evaluation with FDG PET imaging. Figures 6.9.6B and C show coronal (Figure 6.9.6B) and transaxial (Figure 6.9.6C) FDG PET images acquired with a dedicated PET tomograph (GE Advance) and reconstructed with iterative reconstruction and measured segmented attenuation correction.

Findings

The CT images of the pelvis demonstrate a soft tissue nodular density posterior to the left proximal femur. The FDG images demonstrate markedly increased FDG metabolism posterior to the left greater trochanter that corresponds to the soft tissue nodule seen on the CT scan. However, on the FDG images, the area of FDG uptake seems to surround the femur, extending medially into the acetabulum and anterolaterally into the femoral neck. Mildly increased FDG activity is also seen in the soft tissues of the right groin and medial thigh.

Discussion

A CT-guided biopsy of the lesion posterior to the right femur revealed metastatic melanoma. An MRI of the pelvis (Figure 6.9.6D) confirms the soft tissue lesion posterior to the left femur and demonstrates its extension into the joint space and tracking around the femoral neck medially and anteriorly. There is also abnormal high attenuation signal just above the femoral head extending to the posterior acetabulum,

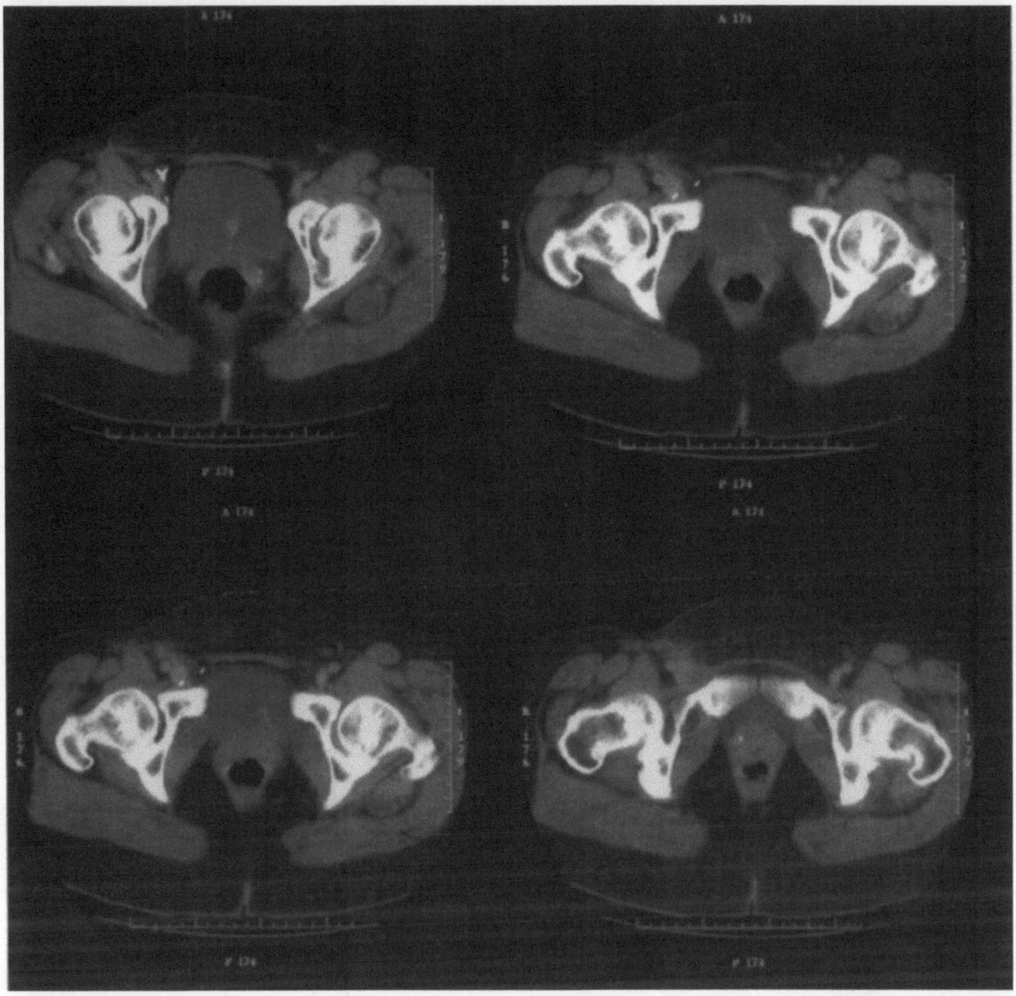

FIGURE 6.9.6A.

and a high intensity lesion in the acetabulum measuring 1.4 by 1.0 cm is consistent with osseous involvement by the melanoma. In addition, within the greater trochanter, there is a 9 mm cystic lesion which demonstrates high intensity on the T2-weighted images and low intensity on the T1-weighted images, similar to the rest of melanoma lesions. Both, T1-weighted and T2-weighted images demonstrate low attenuation abnormalities involving the anterior bone marrow of the intertrochanteric region. The FDG PET findings were suspicious for osseous involvement and led to the confirmatory MRI. FDG PET imaging also excluded metastases outside the pelvis. Although the patient had skeletal extension and was not amendable to surgery, local radiation therapy was an option for her in addition to systemic therapy. If she had widespread metastases, radiation therapy would not have been as useful.

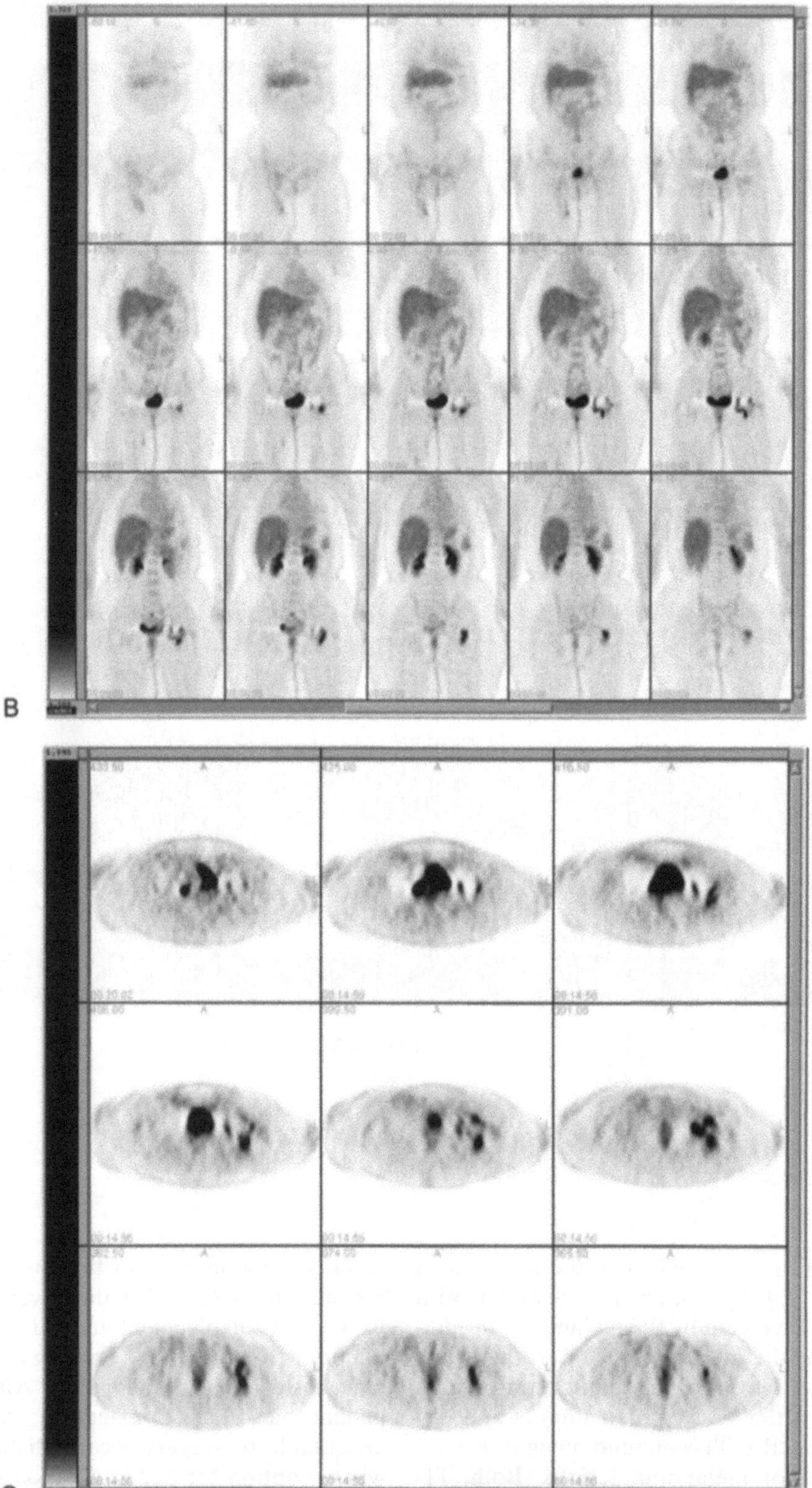

Figure 6.9.6B,C. *(Continued)*

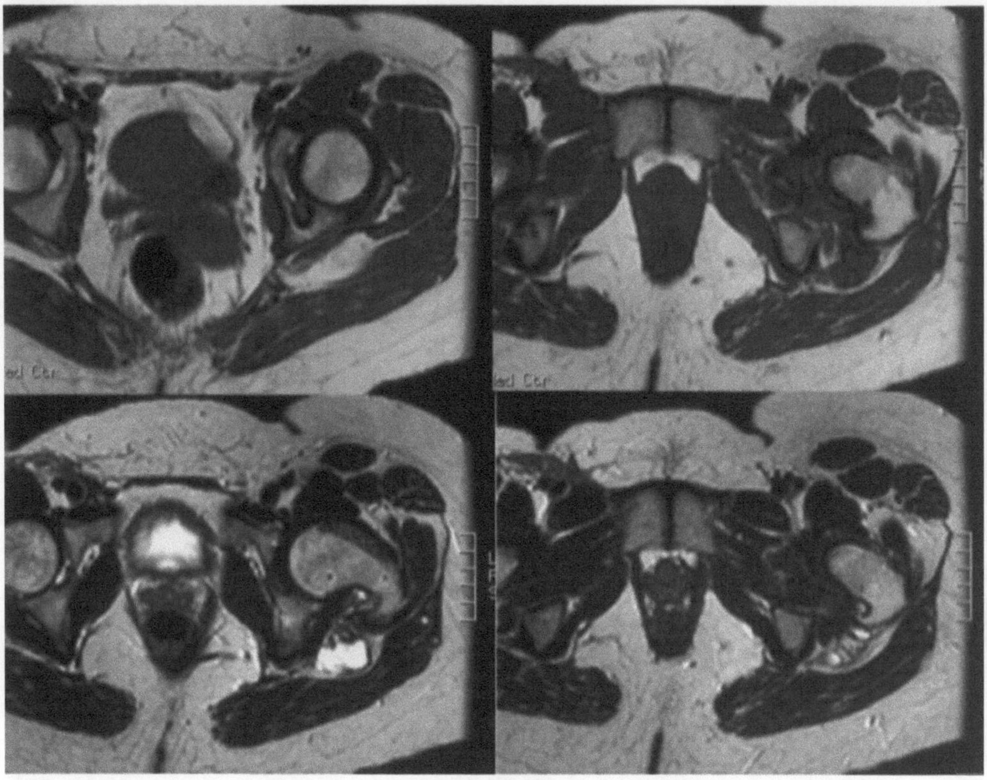

FIGURE 6.9.6D.

The mild activity seen in the right groin and right medial thigh likely represents postsurgical changes from the recent lymphadenectomy. Surgical and nonsurgical wounds can be confounding factors and lead to false-positive interpretations, especially with cutaneous tumors such as melanoma. A brief history and physical examination can often prevent interpretive errors with PET.

Diagnoses

1. Metastasis to the soft tissue posterior to the left femur.
2. Osseous involvement of the acetabulum and left greater trochanter.
3. Postsurgical changes in the right medial thigh due to recent lymphadenectomy.

Case 6.9.7

History

A 39-year-old male presented for restaging six months after a melanoma resected from the right foot. Two months later a recurrence in his right femoral, inguinal, and iliac lymph nodes documented with FDG PET imaging required lymphadenectomy. The FDG images were first acquired with a dedicated PET tomograph (GE Advance) and were reconstructed using itera-

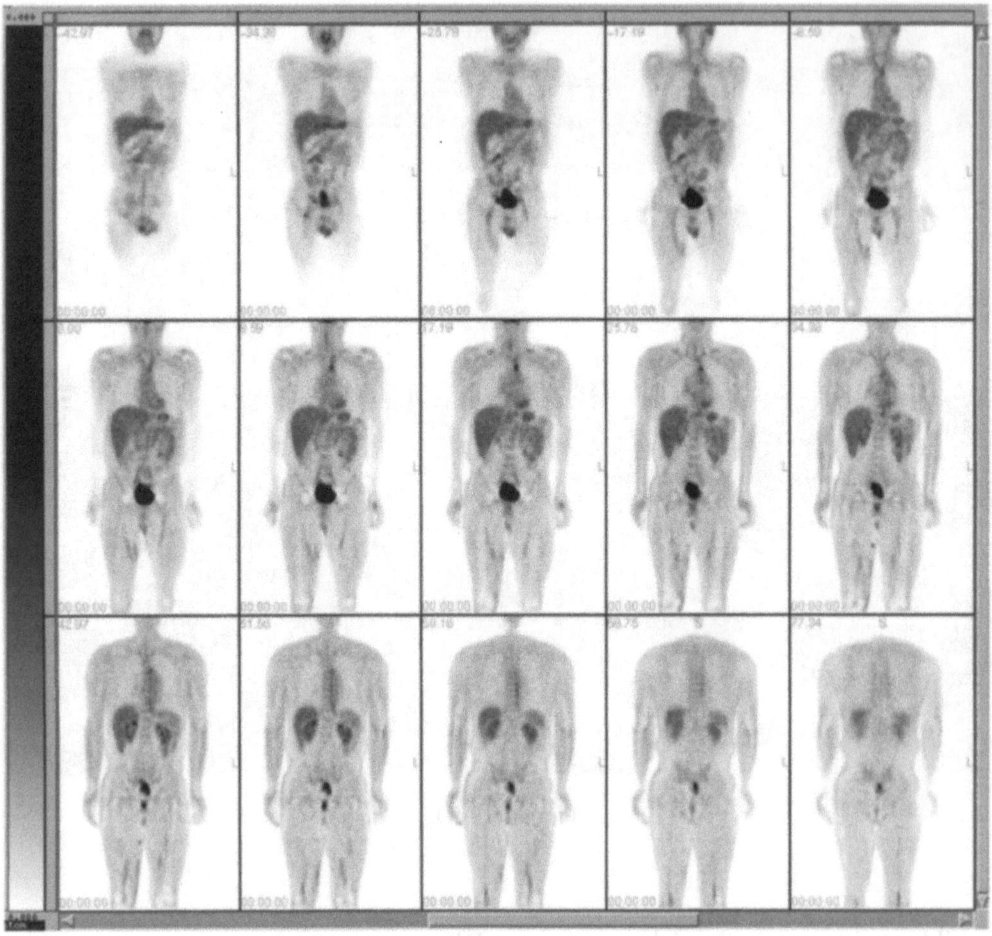

FIGURE 6.9.7A.

tive reconstruction and measured segmented attenuation correction (Figure 6.9.7A coronal images). FDG images were then obtained over the pelvis with a hybrid dual-head gamma camera operating in the coincidence mode (VG Millenium). The hybrid FDG PET images were reconstructed using an iterative reconstruction algorithm and corrected for attenuation using attenuation maps obtained with an X-ray tube and array of detectors mounted on the gantry of the camera and functioning as a third-generation CT scanner. These attenuation maps also provide hybrid CT images for image fusion and anatomical mapping. Figure 6.9.7B shows coronal hybrid PET images, and Figure 6.9.7C, see color plate, shows a transaxial image through the right inguinal region of the hybrid CT (left), hybrid PET (middle), and fusion image (right).

Findings

The FDG PET images demonstrate a focus of uptake located in the upper mediastinum just to the left of the midline and three foci in the right lower pelvis and thigh: one focus to the right of the lower portion of the bladder, a second focus in the anterior right femoral region, and a third focus in the subcutaneous tissue medially at the level of the mid-thigh. The focus in the chest was new as compared

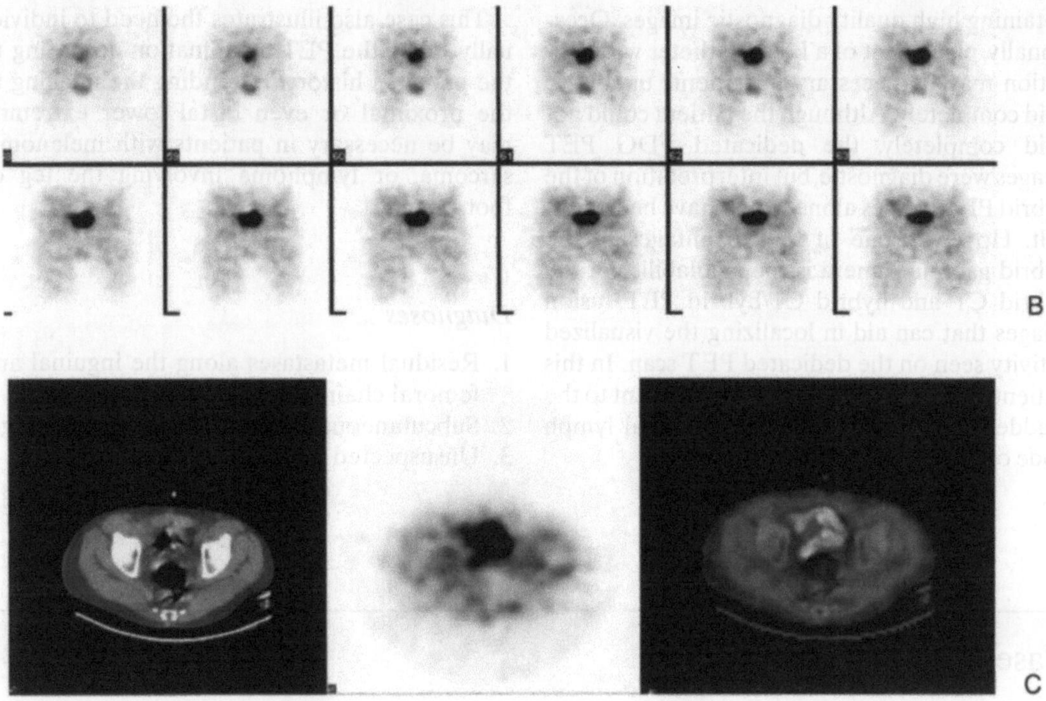

FIGURE 6.9.7B,C. (See color plate)

to the previous PET scan, and the foci in the right lower pelvis and upper thigh were already present but less numerous than on the FDG PET images obtained prior to the wide lymphadenectomy.

On the hybrid FDG images of the pelvis, only the focus to the right of the bladder is identified. The fusion hybrid CT/PET images demonstrate that the focus of increased uptake adjacent to the bladder corresponds to an enlarged lymph node on the CT portion of the study.

Discussion

The abnormal uptake in the chest is worrisome for a metastasis in a mediastinal lymph node. The three foci in the lower pelvis and upper thigh indicate residual lymph node metastases in the right inguinal and femoral regions, as well as a subcutaneous metastasis.

This case illustrates the role of FDG PET imaging for evaluation of residual metastases after lymphadenectomy. In addition, because it is a whole-body technique, FDG PET imaging provides an evaluation of the entire body for detection of distant metastases, for example, in the mediastinum in this patient.

On the hybrid PET images, only the focus of uptake to the right of the bladder is identified because the two other foci are probably below the resolution of the hybrid system, as previously discussed in other cases. In addition, on the hybrid PET images, the focus of uptake seen in the right inguinal region is difficult to separate from bladder uptake. The lower pelvis can be a difficult region to evaluate because of physiologic excretion of FDG by the kidneys, resulting in a variable degree of activity within the ureters and bladder. Keeping the patient well hydrated and obtaining postvoid images are critical to obtaining high quality diagnostic images. Occasionally, placement of a Foley catheter with irrigation may be necessary in patients unable to void completely. Although the patient could not void completely, the dedicated FDG PET images were diagnostic, but interpretation of the hybrid PET images alone would have been difficult. However, one of the advantages of the hybrid gamma camera is the availability of the hybrid CT and hybrid CT/hybrid PET fusion images that can aid in localizing the visualized activity seen on the dedicated PET scan. In this patient, the focus of FDG uptake adjacent to the bladder corresponds to a right inguinal lymph node on the hybrid CT.

This case also illustrates the need to individually tailor the PET examination according to the patient's history. Extending the imaging to the proximal or even distal lower extremity may be necessary in patients with melanoma, sarcoma, or lymphoma involving the leg or foot.

Diagnoses

1. Residual metastases along the inguinal and femoral chain after lymphadenectomy.
2. Subcutaneous metastasis in the medial thigh.
3. Unsuspected mediastinal metastasis.

Case 6.9.8

History

A 78-year-old female with a history of melanoma presented with a right inguinal adenopathy and subcutaneous lesions on the right lower extremity. Approximately four years earlier, a malignant melanoma was resected from her medial right heel, and the pathology revealed a Clark's level IV with a depth of 0.4 cm. She subsequently had a negative CT scan of the chest and a normal bone scintigraphy and liver scan. Figures 6.9.8A and B show transaxial FDG images of the chest and abdomen (Figure 6.9.8A) and coronal images of the thighs (Figure 6.9.8B) acquired with a dedicated PET tomograph (Siemens ECAT 933) and reconstructed using filtered back projection without attenuation correction.

Findings

The FDG PET images reveal multiple foci of increased metabolic activity. On the coronal images of the thighs, foci of FDG uptake are identified in the right groin and subcutaneous tissue medial thigh, corresponding to the lesions known by physical examination. Additional foci of uptake are seen in the left lower extremity but are not in the field of view of the images. On the transaxial chest images, a focus of uptake is noted in the left lower neck (Figure 6.9.8A, second row), left mid-lung field centrally (Figure 6.9.8A, third row), subcutaneous tissue of the right upper back (Figure 6.9.8A, first row), and right chest just below the axilla (Figure 6.9.8A, third row). No abnormal activity is seen in the abdomen or upper pelvis.

Discussion

The FDG images demonstrated increased glucose metabolism in the palpable lesions in the right groin and new subcutaneous lesions on the right thigh. An inguinal lymph node was resected, and pathologic examination revealed metastatic melanoma. The PET images reveal the extent of metastatic disease with involvement of the subcutaneous tissues of the right upper back and right chest below the axilla, as well as pulmonary involvement and nodal involvement in the neck.

A CT scan of the abdomen identified a 6 by 4 cm cystic adnexal mass that did not show increased metabolic activity on the PET scan, suggesting a benign process rather than metastatic involvement with melanoma.

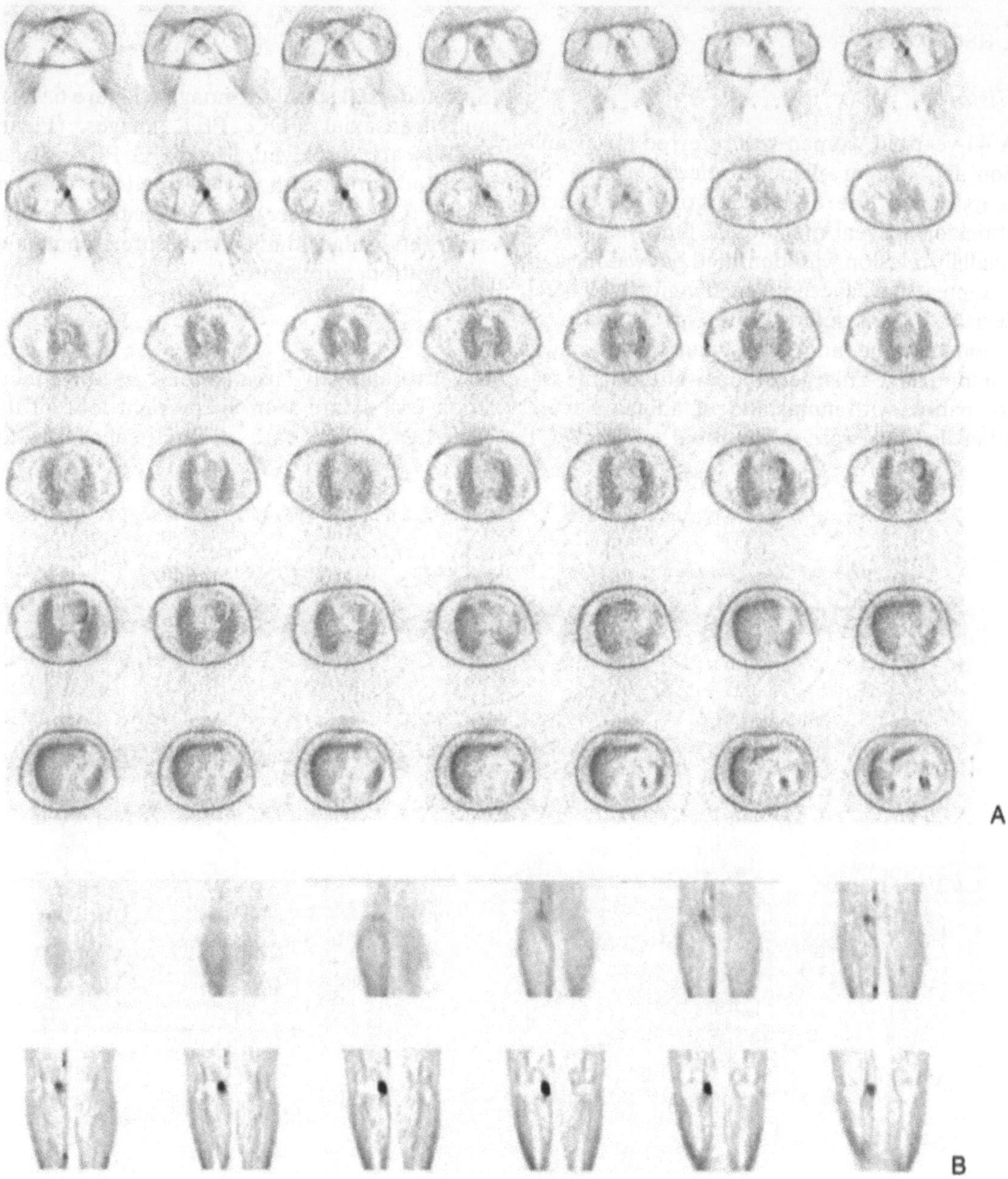

FIGURE 6.9.8A,B.

Regardless, because of the detection of distant metastases, PET changed the stage of this patient's melanoma from III to IV, thus changing the prognosis and therapy.

Diagnosis

Melanoma with distant nodal and subcutaneous metastases.

Case 6.9.9

History

A 44-year-old woman was referred for evaluation and staging of metastatic melanoma. Six years earlier she had undergone left enucleation for a uveal melanoma. One year ago, a small liver lesion was identified but was thought to represent a cavernous hemangioma by MRI. Serial CT scans demonstrated no change in the lesion until one month ago when the lesion was noted to have enlarged; biopsy at that time was compatible with metastatic melanoma. Several other lesions were also noted on that CT. Selected axial spiral CT images (Figure 6.9.9A) and transaxial FDG PET images (Figure 6.9.9B) are displayed. The FDG PET images were acquired with a dedicated PET tomograph (GE Advance) and reconstructed using an iterative algorithm and measured segmented attenuation correction.

Findings

Several relatively large (2 to 3cm) low attenuation lesions are seen in the right lobe of the liver, and there are several subcentimeter

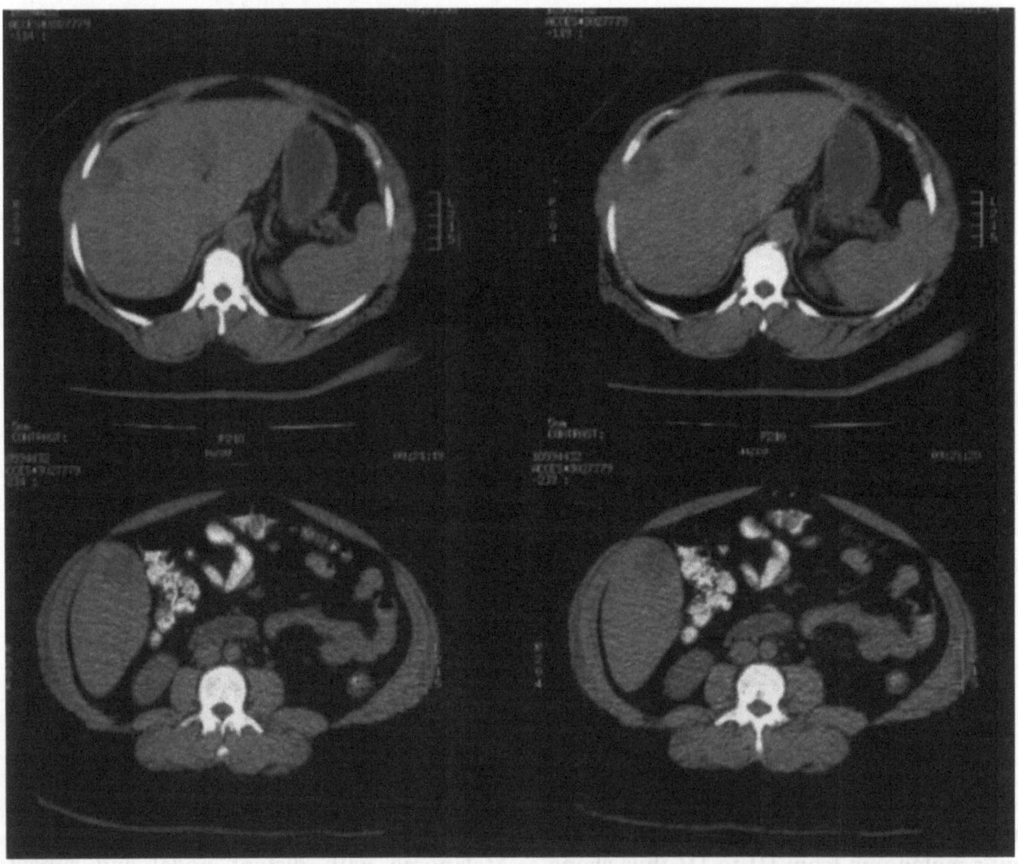

FIGURE 6.9.9A.

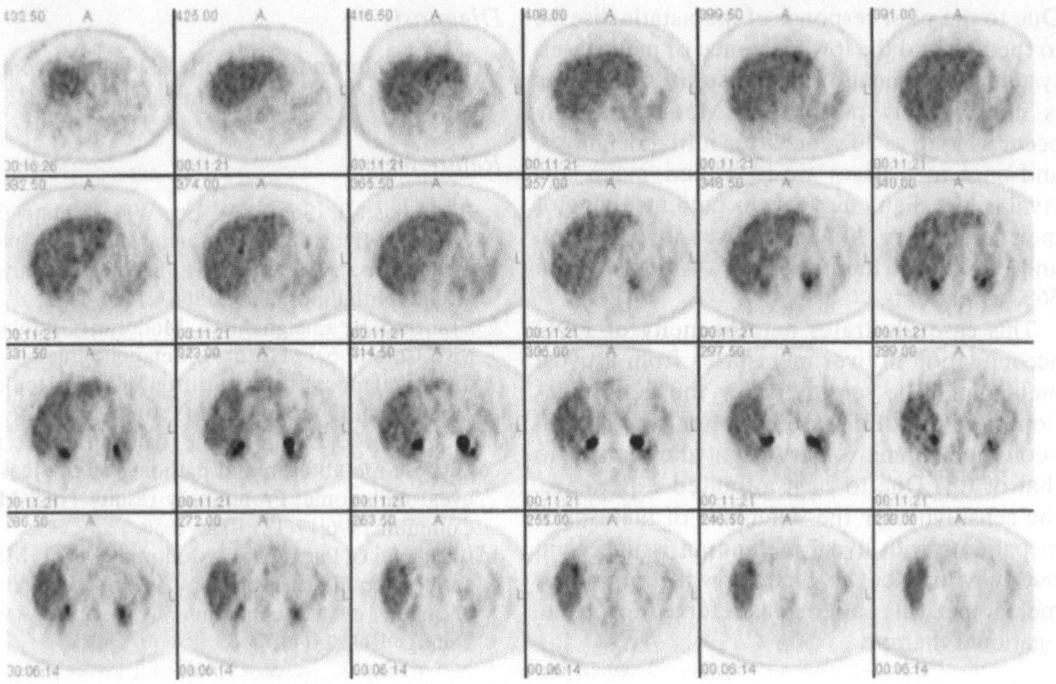

FIGURE 6.9.9B.

lesions as well involving both the right and left lobes. No adenopathy is identified. The PET images demonstrate a single hypermetabolic focus near the inferior tip of a Riedel's right lobe. There may also be a small additional focus at the posterior tip, but the other lesions seen more superiorly on CT are not FDG-avid. No extrahepatic abnormal foci are identified.

Discussion

The liver lesion biopsied was not the lesion found to be hypermetabolic by PET, so the melanoma hepatic metastases in this patient are heterogeneous in respect to FDG accumulation. There are numerous other examples of tumor heterogeneity. For instance, some metastatic carcinoid lesions will express somatostatin receptors and some will not, even in the same patient, likely related to dedifferentiation. Similar heterogeneity is seen with Iodine-131 in differentiated thyroid carcinoma and with monoclonal antibody expression in various neoplasms. There is evidence that uveal melanoma cells may spontaneously transform their cytologic phenotype, resulting in a more aggressive variant.[1] Primary uveal melanoma was first imaged with FDG PET in 1990, but there are no reports of FDG-imaged metastases. In two separate reports totaling 17 patients, one group of investigators has reported that only slightly more than 50% of primary uveal melanomas larger than 7.5 mm in diameter are visualized with FDG PET for reasons yet to be ascertained.[3,4]

Uveal melanoma represents only 12% of all melanomas but is the most common primary intraocular malignancy of adults. The diagnosis is based on ophthalmologic and ultrasonographic findings with a 95% accuracy. CT and/or MR may be necessary for staging and excluding extraocular extension. Only 1 to 2% present with metastases, and metastases develop in only 1 to 2% of patients per year.

Due to the poor response of metastatic disease to therapy and the low incidence of metastases, systematic evaluation for distant metastases is not typically performed. Metastases may occur as long as 30 years after initial diagnosis, and once metastases are identified, mean survival is less than one year. In patients dying of melanoma, over 90% have liver involvement, and the liver is the initial site of metastasis in 56% of patients.

This case illustrates heterogeneity of FDG accumulation in liver metastases from a uveal melanoma. The sensitivity for the determination of extent of disease in patients with cutaneous melanoma is very high and similar to that of CT. Due to such a limited experience, the sensitivity for the detection of metastases in patients with uveal melanoma is uncertain but may not be as high as with cutaneous melanoma. This patient was referred for investigational therapy.

Diagnosis

Ocular melanoma with both FDG-positive and FDG-negative hepatic metastases.

References

1. Bechrakis NE, Sehu KW, Lee WR, Damato BE, Foerster MH: Transformation of cell type in uveal melanomas: A quantitative histologic analysis. Arch Ophthalmol 2000;118(10):1406–1412.
2. Brancato R, Lucignani G, Modorati G, Gilardi MC, Colombo F, Fazio F: Metabolic imaging of uveal melanoma using positron emission tomography. Arch Ophthalmol 1990;108(3):326–327.
3. Modorati G, Lucignani G, Landoni C, et al.: Glucose metabolism and pathological findings in uveal melanoma: Preliminary results. Nucl Med Commun 1996;17(12):1052–1056.
4. Lucignani G, Paganelli G, Modorati G, et al.: MRI, antibody-guided scintigraphy, and glucose metabolism in uveal melanoma. J Comput Assist Tomogr 1992;16(1):77–83.

6.10 Miscellaneous Tumors

William H. Martin and Dominique Delbeke

Thyroid Carcinoma

The most frequent forms of thyroid carcinoma are differentiated tumors, papillary or follicular, having a good prognosis even in the presence of lung metastases. The diagnosis of primary thyroid carcinoma is based on history, physical examination, laboratory testing, ultrasound, thyroid scintigraphy with ^{99}Tc-pertechnetate, and biopsy. Most studies evaluating FDG PET imaging in the preoperative diagnosis of patients with suspected thyroid carcinoma have demonstrated increased uptake in most malignant lesions (papillary, follicular, Hurthle cell, anaplastic, and medullary carcinoma) with little overlap with the degree of uptake in benign lesions.[1–4] However, one study has reported overlap of FDG uptake between benign (nodular goiters and follicular adenomas) and malignant lesions.[5] Therefore, evaluation of thyroid nodules with FDG imaging is not recommended because the specificity is too low to differentiate reliably malignant from benign nodules. However, if there is a focus of increased uptake in the thyroid gland on FDG images performed for other reasons, further evaluation is recommended.

More data are available for the diagnosis of recurrent and metastatic disease. Conventionally, patients with thyroid carcinoma are followed for recurrence using serial serum thyroglobulin levels and radioiodine whole-body scintigraphy. Further functional imaging studies are recommended in patients with rising thyroglobulin levels and normal radioiodine scintigraphy. Although metastases of differentiated thyroid carcinoma trap radioiodine, Hurthle cell, medullary, and anaplastic carcinomas are usually not radioiodine-avid. The first systematic investigation comparing radioiodine scintigraphy and FDG PET imaging was published by Feine et al.[6] These authors described different combinations of patterns of uptake in both papillary and follicular carcinomas, and all four Hurthle cell carcinomas were FDG positive and radioiodine negative. Their study was confirmed by others,[7–12] concluding that FDG imaging is particularly helpful in patients with elevated serum thyroglobulin levels and negative radioiodine scans. The sensitivity of FDG PET imaging in a selected population of patients with elevated serum thyroglobulin levels and negative radioiodine scans varies between 50 and 82%. This, too, has been confirmed by other studies, one of which concluded that FDG PET imaging in this selected population changed the management in 50% of the patients.[13–16] Dietlein et al.[17] compared the value of radioiodine, ^{99m}Tc-sestamibi, and FDG imaging in the follow-up of patients with differentiated thyroid carcinoma. The sensitivity was 50% for FDG or ^{99m}Tc-sestamibi alone, 61% for radioiodine alone, and up to 86% for FDG and radioiodine combined. The similarity of sensitivity between ^{99m}Tc-sestamibi and FDG may be explained on the basis of the mechanism of uptake of these radiopharmaceuticals compared to radioiodine.[18,19] Sources of misinterpretation for evaluation of metastases in the neck are foci of physiologic muscular FDG uptake and laryngeal uptake.

Metastases from thyroid carcinoma most commonly affect the lymph nodes, lungs, and skeleton. These patients have a good chance of curative treatment if these metastases are small and are radioiodine-avid. FDG imaging can localize metastases that are not radioiodine-avid prior to surgery or radiotherapy or prior to redifferentiation therapy with retinoic acid if they are multiple.[20]

Most FDG PET imaging studies of patients with thyroid carcinoma have been performed in the absence of thyroid stimulating hormone (TSH) stimulation, this being considered an advantage over radioiodine scintigraphy which does require either thyroid hormone withdrawal or the administration of human recombinant TSH for optimal sensitivity. There are preliminary reports suggesting that TSH stimulation may enhance FDG uptake by malignant thyroid tumors and thus improve the sensitivity for detection of recurrent and/or metastatic disease.[21,22]

Medullary carcinoma may occur sporadically or in a familial pattern, either in association with the syndrome of multiple endocrine neoplasia (MEN), type 2, or without MEN characteristics. Lymph node involvement is an important prognostic factor, and presurgical staging is more relevant than with differentiated thyroid carcinoma. The most important tumor markers for medullary thyroid carcinoma are calcitonin and CEA plasma levels. Several radiopharmaceuticals, such as ^{131} or ^{123}I-metaiodobenzylguanidine (MIBG), ^{111}In-octreotide, ^{99}Tc DMSA, and radiolabeled anti-CEA monoclonal antibodies, are available for functional imaging, but detection of small lesions remains problematic. Although FDG uptake in medullary thyroid carcinomas seems to be variable,[23,24] for FDG-avid tumors, PET is more sensitive for detection of small lesions because of the higher resolution of this technique compared to SPECT. In view of the respectable but relatively low sensitivity of conventional techniques in detecting medullary carcinoma of the thyroid, FDG PET imaging is being used with good success.[25]

In summary, radioiodine scintigraphy is the preferred modality for the detection of recurrent/metastatic differentiated thyroid carcinoma due to its identification of tumor treatable with high dose radioiodine administration. In patients suspected of metastatic disease but in whom radioiodine imaging is unrevealing, FDG PET imaging offers high sensitivity and specificity for detection of metastases which may then be treated by surgical resection or external radiotherapy. TSH stimulation by thyroid hormone withdrawal or administration of rhTSH may enhance sensitivity. FDG imaging is also helpful in patients with Hurthle cell carcinoma, medullary carcinoma, and anaplastic carcinoma.

Pheochromocytoma, Neuroblastoma, and Carcinoid Tumors

FDG imaging is also an option for neuroendocrine tumors that fail imaging by other more conventional radiopharmaceuticals: For example, pheochromocytomas that are negative with MIBG and ^{111}In-octreotide can be successfully imaged with FDG.[26] Although 90% of pheochromocytomas are reported to be benign, the proportion of patients with metastatic malignant disease has increased to almost 50% with longer periods of follow-up. The most frequent sites of spread are bone (44%), liver and lymph nodes (37%), and lungs (27%). Extra-adrenal paragangliomas are metastatic in almost half of patients. The sensitivity of ^{131}I-MIBG scintigraphy is reported to be 80 to 90% for the detection of pheochromocytoma and paraganglioma and their metastases with a specificity of 95%. Similarly, the sensitivity of ^{111}In-octreotide imaging for pheochromocytoma and paraganglioma detection is approximately 90%. However, in a relatively large series of pheochromocytoma patients, investigators have noted an 88% sensitivity for detection of malignant pheochromocytoma and its metastases, with a 58% sensitivity for benign tumors using FDG PET imaging. All MIBG-negative tumors in this series demonstrated intense FDG uptake.[27]

Neuroblastoma is the most common solid extracranial malignancy of childhood. As with pheochromocytoma, the conventional radiopharmaceuticals to image these neuroendocrine tumors are ^{131}I-MIBG and ^{111}In-octreotide. Shulkin et al.[28] have compared FDG and MIBG imaging in 17 patients; FDG tumor uptake was present in 16 of these patients, both in the primary tumor and the metastases. The uptake was more variable after therapy. The tumor of one patient was FDG-avid but failed to accumulate MIBG. However, the quality of the ^{131}I-MIBG images was rated superior to FDG images in 13 patients (81%).

There is controversy in the literature about the sensitivity of FDG imaging for detection of carcinoid tumors,[29,30] but at least in some reports, ^{111}In-octreotide scintigraphy is more sensitive than FDG PET imaging. FDG positive/octreotide negative tumors tend to be less differentiated and may have a less favorable prognosis.

Indeterminate Adrenal Masses

Incidentally discovered adrenal masses in patients without a history of malignancy are rarely metastatic. However, an adrenal mass detected in a patient with cancer has a 27 to 36% probability of being malignant.[31] Therefore, it is important to be able to accurately differentiate benign from malignant adrenal lesions in patients with a history of malignancy. Conventional CT with and without intravenous contrast cannot differentiate adrenal metastases from benign nonhyperfunctioning adenomas, but more specific CT protocols, including delayed washout images[32] and MRI imaging with T2-weighted imaging, are promising.[33] In a study with a limited number of patients, FDG PET imaging had 100% accuracy in identifying 14 malignant and 10 benign adrenal lesions.[34] In a group of 80% patients with bronchogenic carcinoma and adrenal masses on CT, the sensitivity and specificity of FDG PET imaging was 100% and 33%, respectively, to predict malignancy.[35] These data predict that FDG PET imaging could be used to avoid biopsy in this population.

Musculoskeletal Tumors

Musculoskeletal neoplasms include soft tissue sarcomas, primary osseous sarcomas, and skeletal metastases. Soft tissue sarcomas arise from mesenchymal structures anywhere in the body and represent 1% of all malignant tumors. Soft tissue sarcomas are usually heterogeneous histologically and have a heterogenous behavior. The grade of malignancy is of great prognostic significance. Rhabdomyosarcoma, neuroblastoma, and extraosseous Ewing's sarcomas are usually high-grade tumors, and myxoid liposarcomas are usually low-grade tumors. Soft tissue sarcomas are known to invade surrounding structures and metastasize distantly, usually to the lungs. The therapeutic regimen is dictated by the grade of the tumor and the presence of metastases. Skeletal metastases are frequent in patients with carcinoma, especially from the prostate, breast, lung, thyroid, and kidneys.

Differentiation of Benign from Malignant Tumors

Because activated muscles have increased FDG uptake, it is important to maintain patients being evaluated for musculoskeletal tumors in a relaxed resting state before and after FDG administration. FDG should be injected in the unaffected limb. A study by Griffeth et al.[36] of 19 patients demonstrated that FDG PET could be useful in differentiating benign from malignant soft tissue masses. There is some debate in the literature related to some overlap between benign and malignant lesions by visual examination and tumor/background ratios (TBR).[37,38] Some studies recommend using SUV for semiquantitative evaluation; others have found that TBRs were more reliable and demonstrated improved correlation with response to neoadjuvant chemotherapy as compared to SUV.[39,40] A TBR > 3.0 appears to be highly predictive of malignancy. However, correlation with anatomical images is critical for optimal interpretation. Most recently, 202 patients with suspected primary bone tumors were evaluated using FDG PET imaging and TBRs, and all patients underwent biopsy.[41,42] There were 70 high-grade sarcomas, 21 low-grade sarcomas, 12 metastases, and 99 benign disease processes. Although sarcomas had higher TBRs than did benign lesions, aggressive benign lesions such as giant cell tumor could not be differentiated from sarcomas. High-grade sarcomas had a higher TBR (mean 11.9) than did low-grade sarcomas (mean 6.8). No false-negative findings occurred with osteosarcoma, Ewing's sarcoma, malignant fibrous histiocytoma, or angiosarcoma, but FDG images were falsely negative in six low-grade chondrosarcomas and two of six plasmacytomas. Using a TBR of 3.0 for malignancy, FDG PET imaging was 93% sensitive but with only 67% specificity, indicating that differentiation of benign from malignant tumors is imperfect.

Several studies have shown that the degree of FDG uptake appears to correlate with the grade of the sarcoma.[43–45] Because soft tissue sarcomas are often inhomogeneous with large areas of necrosis and hemorrhage, FDG PET imaging can guide the biopsy to a region with the highest grade tumor.

For accurate interpretation, keep in mind the increased physiologic FDG uptake in the epiphyseal growth plates of children and the increased uptake seen in stimulated or hyperplastic bone marrow. False-positive findings can be seen with recent fracture, insertion tendonitis, uptake at venous valves, bacterial or fungal osteomyelitis, sarcoid involvement, and peritumoral inflammatory processes.

Monitoring Therapy and Detection of Recurrence

The response to preoperative neoadjuvant chemotherapy is an important prognostic factor in osteogenic and Ewing's sarcoma.[46] The failure rate increases in patients treated with limb salvage instead of amputation when there is a poor response to chemotherapy.[47] Many investigators now believe that monitoring preoperative tumor response to neoadjuvant chemotherapy is mandatory before surgical resection, especially if a limb salvage procedure is planned. Jones et al.[48] have demonstrated changes in FDG uptake during and after neoadjuvant therapy in soft tissue and musculoskeletal sarcomas. The changes depend on the neoadjuvant therapy administered (chemotherapy or radiotherapy and hyperthermia); persistent uptake with benign therapy-related fibrous tissue may occur. Similar findings have been reported by another group of investigators who performed FDG PET imaging to evaluate the response to hyperthermic isolated limb perfusion for locally advanced soft tissue sarcomas.[49] Some authors have found that the accuracy of FDG PET imaging to differentiate responders from nonresponders is approximately 90%.[39] They conclude that limb salvage is not recommended in poor responders to neoadjuvant chemotherapy. Other investigators have reached the same conclusions after demonstrating that FDG PET imaging can identify all responders and 80% of nonresponders.[50] FDG PET imaging is also accurate to differentiate relapse from posttherapeutic changes, especially when anatomical imaging is limited due to changes related to therapy and surgical reconstruction.[51]

FDG PET Imaging to Detect Skeletal Metastases

Conventional diphosphonate bone scintigraphy is highly sensitive for detection of osteoblastic metastases but is considered less sensitive than MRI for osteolytic metastases.[52–54] Bone scintigraphy remains the best imaging modality to detect bone metastases from prostate and breast carcinoma because of its high sensitivity. However, it does not differentiate benign from malignant lesions because both cause bone remodeling. FDG PET imaging appears promising in that regard,[55] and although less sensitive than bone scintigraphy for detection of skeletal metastases of prostate[56,57] and breast carcinoma,[53] FDG PET imaging is more specific. However, for lung carcinoma and lymphoma, FDG PET imaging seems to be more sensitive than bone scintigraphy.[58–60] A recent study of 70 patients reports the comparison of FDG PET imaging and bone scintigraphy for the detection metastases of primary osseous tumors.[61] The sensitivity, specificity, and accuracy of FDG PET imaging in the detection of metastases from Ewing's sarcoma were superior to those of bone scintigraphy (100%, 96%, and 97% and 68%, 87%, and 82%, respectively). However, FDG PET imaging was less sensitive than bone scintigraphy for the detection of metastases from osteosarcoma (none of the five osseous metastases were detected by

FDG PET imaging). In our experience, FDG PET imaging demonstrates bone metastases from various primaries, including hepatocellular carcinoma, that were unsuspected clinically and sometimes negative on bone scan.

Fibrous dysplasia and Paget's disease, among other benign entities, can have marked FDG uptake and be false-positive.[62] Bone lesions with an active inflammatory process, such as osteomyelitis, healing fractures, and healing bone infarcts, demonstrate FDG uptake as well. The performance of FDG PET imaging has even been suggested for the detection of chronic osteomyelitis.[63]

^{18}F-soduim fluoride seems to be a promising agent to detect skeletal metastases. Benign lesions demonstrate uptake as with ^{99m}Tc-diphosphonates because uptake of both radiopharmaceuticals depend on bone mineralization. However, the better anatomical resolution with ^{18}F allows better differentiation of benign from malignant lesions and improved sensitivity to detect metastases.[64–66]

Summary

In summary, FDG PET imaging may provide important diagnostic and prognostic information in patients with soft tissue sarcomas and may be useful (1) in differentiating malignant from benign skeletal lesions, (2) diagnosing skip lesions and occult distant metastases at initial staging and detecting recurrences of sarcoma during follow-up, and (3) accurately guiding biopsy of large and/or heterogeneous sarcomas. Aggressive benign tumors such as giant cell tumors and some aneurysmal bone cysts, which also require wide excision, are highly FDG-avid.

For skeletal metastases, bone scintigraphy is more sensitive than FDG PET imaging to detect osteoblastic metastases (for example, prostate and breast carcinoma), but FDG PET imaging has a better sensitivity to detect osteolytic metastases (for example, lymphoma). ^{18}F seems to be the most promising radiopharmaceutical to accurately detect bone metastases, although only improved anatomical location allows differentiation of benign from malignant lesions.

References

1. Bloom AD, Adler LP, Shuck JM: Determination of malignancy of thyroid nodules with positron emission tomography. Surgery 1993;114:728–735.
2. Sasaki M, Ichiya Y, Kuwabara Y, et al.: An evaluation of FDG-PET in the detection and differentiation of thyroid tumors. Nucl Med Comm 1997;18:957–963.
3. Uematsu H, Sadato N, Ohtsubo T, et al.: Fluorine-18-fluorodeoxyglucose PET versus thallium-201 scintigraphy evaluation of throid tumors. J Nucl Med 1998;39:453–459.
4. Gasparoni P, Rubello D, Ferlin G: Potential role of fluorine-18-deoxyglucose (FDG) positron emission tomography (PET) in the staging of primitive and recurrent medullary thyroid carcinoma. J Endocrinol Invest 1997;20:527–530.
5. Uchida Y, Matsuno N, Minoshima S, et al.: Diagnostic value of ^{18}F-FDG PET in primary and metastatic thyroid cancer. J Nucl Med 1995; 36:196P.
6. Feine U, Lietzenmayer R, Hanke J-P, et al.: Fluorine-18-FDG and iodine-131-iodide uptake in thyroid cancer. J Nucl Med 1996;37:1468–1472.
7. Joensuu H, Ahonen A: Imaging of metastases of thyroid carcinoma with fluorine-18 fluorodeoxyglucose. J Nucl Med 1987;28:910–914.
8. Joensuu H, Ahonen A, Klemi PJ: 18F-fluorodeoxyglucose imaging in preoperative diagnosis of thyroid malignancy. Eur J Nucl Med 1988;13:502–506.
9. Sisson JC, Ackermann R, Meyer MA, Wahl RL: Uptake of FDG by thyroid cancer: Implications for diagnosis and therapy. J Clin Endocrinol Metab 1993;77:1090–1094.
10. Scott GC, Meier DA, Dickinson CZ: Cervical lymph node metastasis of thyroid papillary carcinoma imaged with fluorine-18-FDG, technetium-99m-pertechnetate and iodine-131-sodium iodide. J Nucl Med 1995;36:1843–1845.
11. Grunwald F, Menzel C, Bender H, et al.: Comparison of 18-FDG-PET with 131-iodine and 99mTc-sestamibi scintigraphy in diffentiated thyroid cancer. Thyroid 1997;7:327–335.
12. Grunwald F, Schomburg A, Bender H, et al.: Fluorine-18 fluorodeoxyglucose positron emission tomography in the follow-up of differentiated thyroid cancer. Eur J Nucl Med 1996;23: 312–319.
13. Wang W, Macapinlac H, Larson SM, et al.: [^{18}F]-2-Fluoro-2-deoxy-D-glucose positron emission

tomography localizes residual thyroid cancer in patients with negative diagnostic ^{131}I whole body scans and elevated serum thyroglobulin levels. J Clin Endocrinol Metab 1999;84:2291–2302.
14. Dietlein M, Scheidhauer K, Voth E, et al.: Fluorine-18 fluorodeoxyglucose positron emission tomography and iodine-131 whole body scintigraphy in the follow-up of differentiated thyroid cancer. Eur J Nucl Med 1997;24:1342–1348.
15. Altenwoerde G, Lerch H, Kuwerty T, et al.: Positron emission tomography with F-18-deoxyglucose in patients with differentiated thyroid carcinoma, elevated thyroglobulin levels, and negative iodine scans. Arch Surg 1998;383: 160–163.
16. Schluter B, Bohuslavizki KH, Beyer W, Plotkin M, Buchert R, Clausen M: Impact of FDG PET on patients with differentiated thyroid cancer who present with elevated thyroglobulin and negative ^{131}I scan. J Nucl Med 2001;42:71–76.
17. Dietlein M, Scheidhauer K, Voth E, et al.: Follow-up of differentiated thyroid cancer: What is the value of FDG and sestamibi in the diagnostic algorithm? Nuklearmedizin 1998;37:6–11.
18. Fridrich L, Messa C, Landoni C, et al.: Whole-body scintigraphy with ^{99m}Tc-MIBI, ^{18}F-FDG and ^{131}I in patents with metastatic thyroid carcinoma. Nucl Med Comm 1997;18:3–9.
19. Grünwald F, Menzel C, Bender H, et al.: Comparison of ^{18}FDG-PET with ^{131}iodine and ^{99m}Tc-sestamibi scintigraphy in differentiated thyroid cancer. Thyroid 1997;7:327–335.
20. Grunwald F, Menzel C, Bender H, et al.: Redifferentiation therapy-induced radioiodine uptake in thyroid cancer. J Nucl Med 1998;39:1903–1906.
21. Moog F, Linke R, Mentley N, et al.: Influence of thyroid-stimulating hormone levels on uptake of FDG in recurrent and metastatic differentiated thyroid carcinoma. J Nucl Med 2000;41:1989–1995.
22. Grunwald F, Biersack HJ: Invited commentary: FDG PET in thyroid cancer: Thyroxine or not? J Nucl Med 2000;41:1996–1998.
23. Gasparoni P, Rubello D, Ferlin G: Potential role of fluorine-18-deoxyglucose (FDG) positron emission tomography (PET) in the staging of primitive and recurrent medullary thyroid carcinoma. J Endocrinol Invest 1997;20(9):527–530.
24. Rigo P, Paulus P, Chasten BJ, et al.: Oncological applications of positron emission tomography with fluorine-18fluorodeoxyglucose. Eur J Nucl Med 1996;12:1641–1674.
25. Musholt TJ, Musholt PB, Dehdashti F, Moley JF: Evaluation of fluorodeoxyglucose-positron emission tomographic scanning and its association with glucose transporter expression in medullary thyroid carcinoma and pheochromocytoma: A clinical and molecular study. Surg 1997;122:1049–1061.
26. Shulkin BL, Koeppe RA, Francis IR, Deeb GM, Lloyd RV, Thompson NW: Pheochromocytomas that do not accumulate netaiodobenzylguanidine: Localization with PET and administration of FDG. Radiology 1993;186:11–15.
27. Shulkin BC, Thompson NW, Shapiro B, Francis IR, Sisson JC: Pheochromocytomas: Imaging with 2-(fluorine-(8) fluoro-s-deoxy-D-glucose PET. Radiol 1999;212:35–41.
28. Shulkin BL, Hutchinson RJ, Castle VP, Yar GA, Shapiro D, Sisson JC: Neuroblastoma: Positron emission tomography with 2-[fluorine-18]-fluoro-2-deoxy-D-glucose compared with metaiodobenzylguanidine scintigraphy. Radiology 1996;199:743–750.
29. Foidart-Willems J, Depas G, Vivegnis D, et al.: Positron emission tomography and radiolabeled octreotide scintigraphy in carcinoid tumors. Eur J Nucl Med 1995;22:635.
30. Jadvar H, Segall GM: False-negative fluorine-18-FDG-PET in metastatic carcinoid. J Nucl Med 1997;38:1382–1383.
31. Abrams HL, Spiro R, Goldstein N: Metastases in carcinoma: Analysis of 100 autopsied cases. Cancer 1950;3:74–85.
32. Korobkin M: CT characterization of adrenal masses: The time has come. Radiology 2000;217: 629–632.
33. Reinig JW, Doppman JL, Dwyer AJ, Johnson AP, Knop RH: Adrenal masses differentiated with MR imaging. Radiology 1986;158:81–84.
34. Boland GW, Goldberg MA, Lee MJ, et al.: Indeterminate adrenal mass in patients with cancer: Evaluation at PET with 2-[F-18]-fluoro-2-deoxy-D-glucose. Radiology 1995;194:131–134.
35. Erasmus JJ, Patz EF Jr, McAdams HP, et al.: Evaluation of adrenal masses in patients with broncogenic carcinoma using ^{18}F-fluorodeoxyglucose positron emission tomography. AJR 1997;168:1357–1360.
36. Griffeth LK, Dehdashti F, McGuire AH, et al.: PET evaluation of soft-tissue masses with fluorine-18 fluoro-2-deoxy-D-glucose. Radiology 1992;182:185–194.
37. Kole AC, Nieweg OE, Hoekstra HJ, et al.: Fluorine-18-fluorodeoxyglucose assessment of glucose metabolism in bone tumors. J Nucl Med 1998;39:810–815.

38. Nieweg O, Pruim J, van Ginkel RJ, et al.: Fluorine-18-fluorodeoxyglucose PET imaging of soft-tissue sarcoma. J Nucl Med 1996;37:257–261.
39. Schulte M, Brecht-Krauss D, Heymer B, et al.: Fluorodeoxyglucose positron emission tomography of soft tissue tumours: Is a non-invasive determination of biological activity possible? Eur J Nucl Med 1999;6:599–605.
40. Schulte M, Brecht-Krauss D, Werner M, et al.: Evaluation of neoadjuvant therapy response of osteogenic sarcoma using FDG PET. J Nucl Med 1999;10:1637–1643.
41. Schulte M, Brechte-Krauss D, Heymer B, et al.: Grading of tumors and tumorlike lesions of bone: Evaluation by FDG-PET. J Nucl Med 2000;41:1695–1701.
42. Messa C, Landoni C, Pozzato C, Fazio F: Is there a role for FDG PET in the diagnosis of musculoskeletal neoplasms? J Nucl Med 2000;41:1702–1703.
43. Kern KA, Brunetti A, Norton JA, et al.: Metabolic imaging of human extremity musculoskeletal tumors by PET. J Nucl Med 1988;29:181–186.
44. Adler JP, Blair HF, Williams RP, et al.: Grading liposarcomas with PET using [18F] FDG. J Comput Assist Tomogr 1990;14:960–962.
45. Eary JF, Conrad EU, Bruckner JD, et al.: Quantitative [F-18]fluorodeoxyglucose positron emission tomography in pretreatment and grading of sarcoma. Clin Cancer Res 1998;4:1215–1220.
46. Meyers PA, Heller G, Healey J, et al.: Chemotherapy for nonmetastatic osteogenic sarcoma: The Memorial Sloan-Kettering experience. J Clin Oncol 1992;10:5–15.
47. Picci P, Sangiorgi L, Rougraff BT, et al.: Relationship of chemotherapy-induced necrosis and surgical margins to local recurrence in osteosarcoma. J Clin Oncol 1994;12:2699–2705.
48. Jones DN, McCowage GB, Sostman HD, et al.: Monitoring of neoadjuvant therapy response of soft-tissue and musculoskeletal sarcoma using fluorine-18-FDG-PET. J Nucl Med 1996;37:1438–1444.
49. Van Ginkel RJ, Hoekstra HJ, Pruim J, et al.: FDG-PET to evaluate response to hyperthermic isolated limb perfusion for locally advanced soft-tissue sarcoma. J Nucl Med 1996;37:1438–1444.
50. Schulte M, Brecht-Krause D, Werner M, et al.: Evaluation of neoadjuvant therapy response of osteogenic sarcoma using FDG PET. J Nucl Med 1999;40:1637–1643.
51. Kole AC, Nieweg OE, van Ginkel RJ, et al.: Detection of local recurrence of soft-tissue sarcoma with positron emission tomography using [18F] fluorodeoxyglucose. Ann Surg Oncol 1997;4:57–63.
52. Griffeth LK, Dehdashti F, McGuire AH, et al.: PET evaluation of soft-tissue masses with fluorine-18 fluoro-2-deoxy-D-glucose. Radiology 1992;182:185–194.
53. Cook GJ, Houston S, Rubens R, Maisey MN, Fogelman I: Detection of bone metastases in breast cancer by 18FDG PET: Differing metabolic activity in osteoblastic and osteolytic lesions. J Clin Oncol 1998;10:3375–3379.
54. Cook JR, Fogelman I: The role of positron emission tomography in the management of bone metastases. Cancer 2000;88:2927–2933.
55. Dehdashti F, Siegel BA, Griffeth LK, et al.: Benign versus malignant intraosseous lesions: Discrimination by means of PET with 2-[F18] fluoro-2-deoxy-D-glucose. Radiology 1996;200:243–247.
56. Shreve PD, Grossman HB, Gross MD, Wahl RL: Metastatic prostate cancer: Initial findings of PET with 2-deoxy-2-[F18]fluoro-D-glucose. Radiology 1996;199:751–756.
57. Yeh SDJ, Imbriaco M, Garza D, et al.: Twenty percent of bony metastases of hormone resistant prostate cancer are detected by PET-FDG whole body scanning. J Nucl Med 1995;36:198.
58. Bury T, Barreto A, Daenen F, Barthelemy N, Ghaye B, Rigo P: Fluorine-18 deoxyglucose positron emission tomography for the detection of bone metastases in patients with non-small cell lung cancer. Eur J Nucl Med 1998;9:1244–1247.
59. Moog F, Bangerter M, Kotzerke J, Guhlmann A, Frickhofen N, Reske SN: 18-F-fluorodeoxyglucose-positron emission tomography as a new approach to detect lymphomatous bone marrow. J Clin Oncol 1998;2:603–609.
60. Moog F, Kotzerke J, Reske SN: FDG PET can replace bone scintigraphy in primary staging of malignant lymphoma. J Nucl Med 1999;40:1407–1413.
61. Franzius C, Sciuk J, Daldrup-Link HE, Jurgens H, Schober O: PDG-PET for the detection of osseous metastases from malignant primary bone tumours: Comparison with bone scintigraphy. Eur J Nucl Med 2000;27:1305–1311.
62. Cook JR, Maiset MN, Fogelman I, et al.: Fluorine-18-FDG-PET in Paget's disease of bone. J Nucl Med 1997;38:1495–1497.
63. Guhlmann A, Brecht-Krauss D, Suger G, et al.: Chronic osteomyelitis: Detection with FDG-PET and correlation with histopathologic findings. Radiology 1998;206:749–754.

64. Schirrmeister H, Guhlmann A, Kotzerke J, et al.: Early detection and accurate description of extent of metastatic bone disease in breast cancer with fluoride ion and positron emission tomography. J Clin Oncol 1999;8:2381–2389.
65. Schirrmeister H, Guhlmann A, Elsner K, et al.: Sensitivity in detecting osseous lesions depends on anatomic localization: Planar bone scintigraphy versus 18F PET. J Nucl Med 1999;40(10):1623–1629.
66. Cook GJC, Fogelman I: The role of positron emission tomography in skeletal disease. Semin Nucl Med 2000;31(1):50–61.

Case Presentations

Case 6.10.1

History

A 60-year-old man with a history of papillary thyroid carcinoma treated by total thyroidectomy six years prior presented with a serum thyroglobulin elevated to 87 ng/ml. On three occasions, he had been treated with high dose radioiodine therapy. The most recent posttherapy radioiodine whole-body scan revealed no evidence of cervical or distant radioiodine-avid metastases. A recent MRI of the neck and CT of the chest were reported to be negative for metastases. FDG PET imaging was requested for further assessment. Figure 6.10.1 shows coronal FDG images acquired with a dedicated PET tomograph (GE Advance) and reconstructed with iterative reconstruction and measured segmented attenuation correction.

Findings

The FDG images reveal a moderate-sized focus of markedly increased activity at the base of the left neck in the infraclavicular region or anterior mediastinum. There is a faint focus of activity in the left mid-neck. No other abnormalities are identified. The activity superior and to the right of the bladder is within the ureter.

Discussion

There are definitely one and probably two hypermetabolic foci in the left neck consistent with metastatic thyroid carcinoma. A CT of the neck with thin slices demonstrated several enlarged nodes in the left neck. A conglomerate of metastatic nodes were subsequently resected from the left neck. Four months postoperatively, serum thyroglobulin was undetectable, and a repeat CT of the neck was unrevealing.

Whole-body radioiodine scintigraphy has a sensitivity of 60 to 70% for the detection of metastases, in part dependent on the dose of radioiodine (Iodine-131) utilized. Metastases are more often seen with a 10 mCi diagnostic dose of ^{131}I than with a 2 to 5 mCi dose, and posttherapy scans obtained five to eight days after a > 100 mCi dose reveal additional lesions or clarify equivocal abnormalities seen on a diagnostic scan in as many as 35% of patients. The visualization of radioiodine-avid metastases is of utmost importance in view of the well-demonstrated efficacy of radioiodine therapy in patients with such disease. However, as these differentiated neoplasms are subjected to various therapies, they may dedifferentiate, losing the iodine symporter and thus fail to accumulate radioiodine while retaining the ability to express thyroglobulin. Other differentiated thyroid neoplasms as well as less differentiated neoplasms, including Hurthle cell, medullary, and anaplastic carcinomas, are not radioiodine-avid. These thyroid neoplasms not detected by radioiodine scintigraphy have been successfully imaged using ^{201}thallium, ^{99m}Tc-

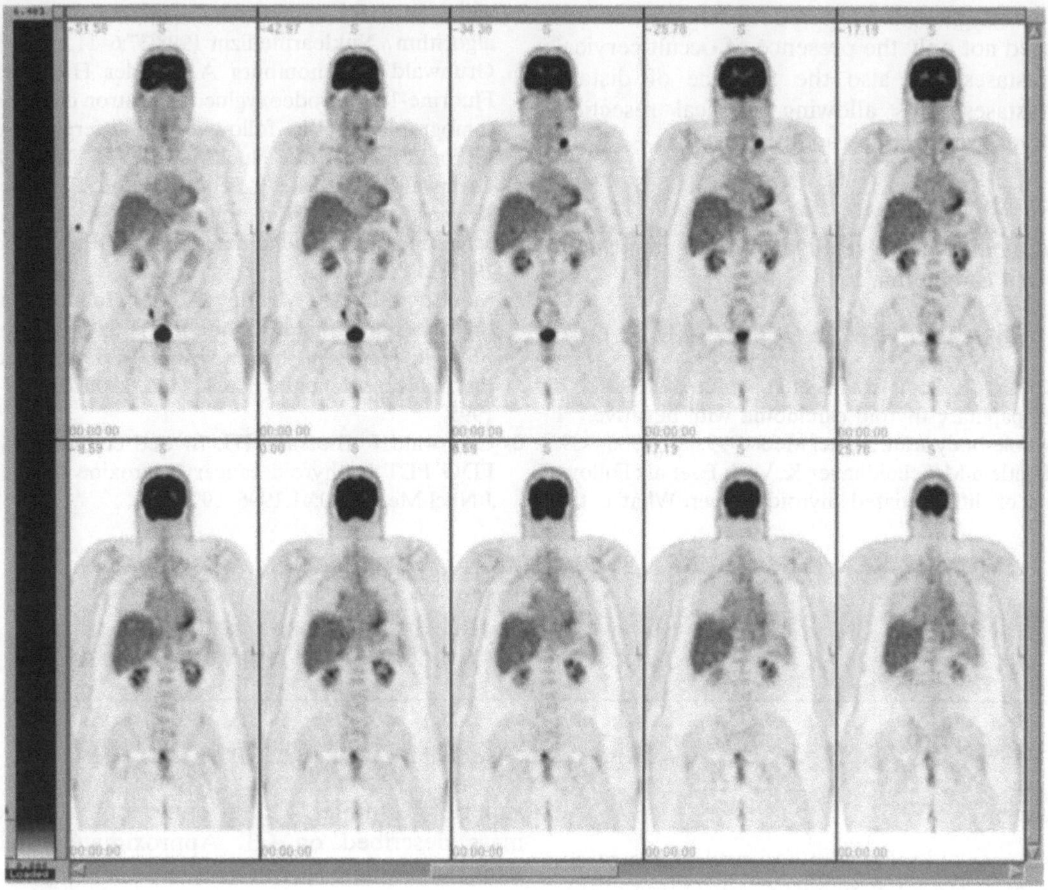

FIGURE 6.10.1.

sestamibi, and ^{99m}Tc-tetrofosmin, but FDG PET has demonstrated high sensitivity and specificity for the detection of these tumors and their metastases.[1–4]

Although FDG PET imaging may demonstrate some radioiodine-avid tumors and a heterogeneous population of radioiodine-positive/FDG-negative and radioiodine-negative/FDG-positive metastases may coexist in an individual patient, FDG PET imaging has proved most useful in the population of thyroid carcinoma patients who are suspected to harbor metastases due to elevated serum thyroglobulin levels but in whom conventional imaging and radioiodine whole-body scintigraphy are negative. PET has localized occult metastases in 50 to 82% of such patients and altered therapy in over 50%. PET has demonstrated involvement in normal-sized lymph nodes[1] but has been reported to be falsely negative in small pulmonary nodules detected by spiral CT.[2] Rare false-positive findings have been noted with inflammatory nodes, benign thymic tissue, and even benign thyroid disease. In contrast to ^{131}I whole-body scintigraphy, FDG PET imaging of thyroid cancer has typically been performed without thyroid hormone withdrawal or TSH stimulation. Preliminary data indicates that the sensitivity of FDG PET imaging for the determination of extent of disease in differentiated thyroid carcinoma may be significantly improved by thyroid hormone withdrawal or the administration of recombinant human thyrotropin (TSH) prior to FDG imaging.[5,6]

In this patient, FDG PET imaging demonstrated not only the presence of occult cervical metastases, but also the absence of distant metastases, thus allowing surgical resection with an excellent therapeutic result.

Diagnosis

Radioiodine-negative, FDG-positive metastatic thyroid carcinoma.

References

1. Chung JK, So Y, Lee JS, et al.: Value of FDG PET in papillary thyroid carcinoma with negative ^{131}I whole-body scan. J Nucl Med 1999;40(6):986–989.
2. Dietlein M, Scheidhauer K, Voth E, et al.: Follow-up of differentiated thyroid cancer: What is the value of FDG and sestamibi in the diagnostic algorithm? Nuklearmedizin 1998;37:6–11.
3. Grunwald F, Schomburg A, Bender H, et al.: Fluorine-18-fluorodeoxyglucose positron emission tomography in the follow-up of differentiated thyroid cancer. Eur J Nucl Med 1996;23:312–319.
4. Grunwald F, Kalicke T, Feine U, et al.: Fluorine-18 positron emission tomography in thyroid cancer: Results of a multicenter study. Eur J Med 1999;26:1547–1552.
5. Moog F, Linke R, Mentley N, et al.: Influence of thyroid-stimulating hormone levels on uptake of FDG in recurrent and metastatic differentiated thyroid carcinoma. J Nucl Med 2000;41:1989–1995.
6. Grunwald F, Biersack HJ: Invited commentary: FDG PET in thyroid cancer: Thyroxine or not? J Nucl Med 2000;41:1996–1998.

Case 6.10.2

History

A 42-year-old male who had undergone resection of a 14 cm left pheochromocytoma a year ago presented for FDG imaging due to the CT finding of a left para-aortic mass. A CT scan six months prior was reported to be unremarkable. At the time of the initial resection, the tumor was encapsulated, partially necrotic, and no nodal metastases were present. FDG imaging was performed to assess the presence of recurrence. Figure 6.10.2 shows coronal FDG images acquired with a dedicated PET tomograph (GE Advance) and reconstructed with iterative reconstruction and measured segmented attenuation correction.

Findings

The CT was reported to show a 7.5 by 4 cm partially necrotic mass in the left suprarenal area with no additional masses detected in the abdomen or lower thorax.

The FDG PET images demonstrate a markedly hypermetabolic mass medial and superior to the left kidney congruent with the mass described on CT. Approximately five additional small foci of increased activity are present in the surrounding area. There is a large focus of increased activity at the base of the left neck or within the anterior mediastinum, accompanied by numerous abnormal foci at the left supraclavicular and infraclavicular region and the left axilla. There is a faint focus of activity within the left hemithorax adjacent to the heart, and one additional focus is present at the sacrum.

Discussion

This constellation of findings is consistent with widespread metastatic pheochromocytoma involving abdominal, thoracic, and axillary adenopathy, probably the skeleton, and possibly the left lung. Malignant pheochromocytoma is a relatively well-differentiated tumor, and the diagnosis of malignancy can only be made in retrospect with the identification of regional or distant metastases. Although malignant pheochromocytoma typically occurs in only

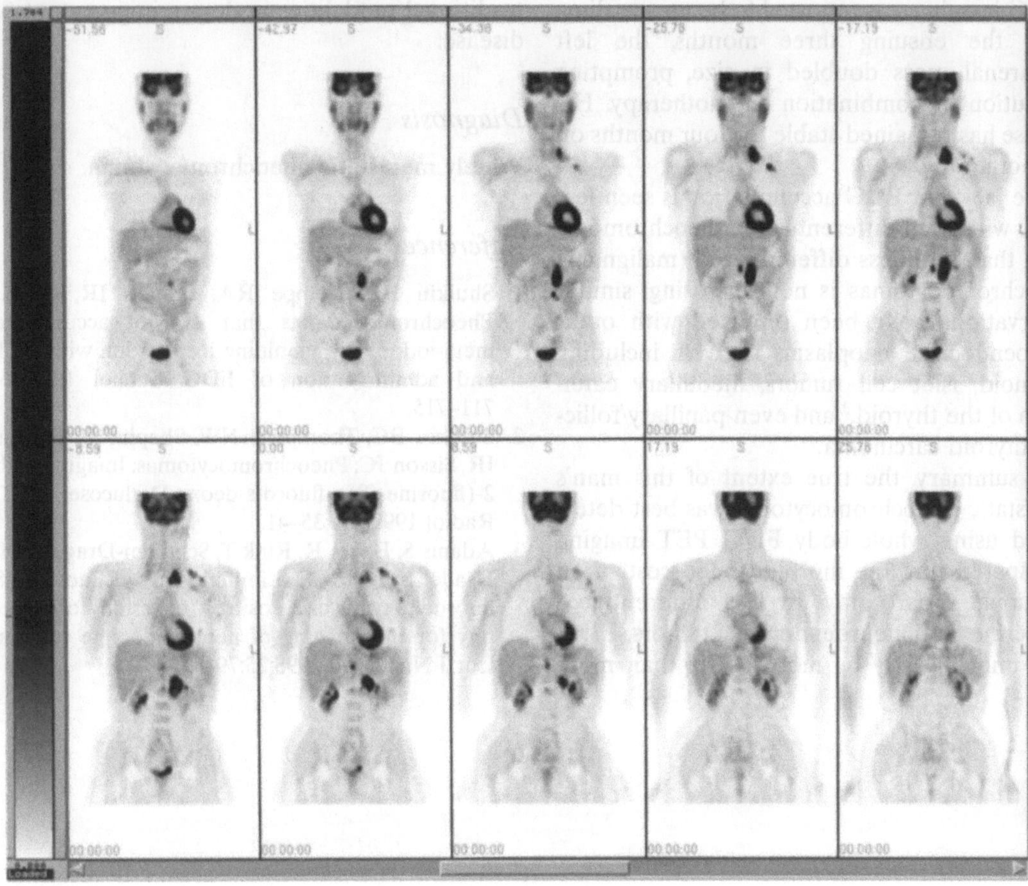

FIGURE 6.10.2.

approximately 10% of patients, the proportion of patients with metastatic malignant disease has increased to almost 50% with longer periods of follow-up. The most frequent sites of spread are bone (44%), liver and lymph nodes (37%), and lungs (27%). Extra-adrenal paragangliomas are metastatic in almost half of patients.

The sensitivity of ^{131}I-MIBG scintigraphy is 80 to 90% for the detection of pheochromocytoma and paraganglioma and their metastases with a specificity of 95%; sensitivity is even higher with ^{123}I-MIBG. An advantage of ^{131}I-MIBG scintigraphy is its ability to determine whether therapy with high activity ^{131}I-MIBG is feasible.

Similarly, the sensitivity of ^{111}In-octreotide imaging for pheochromocytoma and paraganglioma detection is approximately 90%. There is anecdotal evidence that MIBG-negative pheochromocytomas may be detected by FDG PET imaging, and in a relatively large series of pheochromocytoma patients, the same investigators have noted an 88% sensitivity for detection of malignant pheochromocytoma and its metastases with a 58% sensitivity for benign tumors using FDG PET imaging.[1] All MIBG-negative tumors in this series demonstrated intense FDG uptake.[2]

In this patient, biopsy of a left supraclavicular node was positive for metastatic pheochromocytoma; subsequent whole-body radioiodine

MIBG imaging was reported to be unrevealing. Over the ensuing three months, the left suprarenal mass doubled in size, prompting institution of combination chemotherapy. His disease has remained stable for four months on chemotherapy.

The fact that FDG accumulation is seen less often with well-differentiated pheochromocytoma than with less differentiated (malignant) pheochromocytomas is not surprising; similar observations have been reported with other neuroendocrine neoplasms as well, including carcinoid, islet cell tumors, medullary carcinoma of the thyroid,[3] and even papillary/follicular thyroid carcinoma.

In summary, the true extent of this man's metastatic pheochromocytoma was best determined using whole-body FDG PET imaging and spared him the morbidity and cost of an additional laparotomy. In less differentiated endocrine and neuroendocrine tumors, FDG PET imaging may be more useful than more traditional modalities in determining extent of disease.

Diagnosis

Widely metastatic pheochromocytoma.

References

1. Shulkin BL, Kolppe RA, Francis IR, et al.: Pheochromocytomas that do not accumulate meta-iodobenzylguanidine localization with PET and administration of FDG. Radiol 1993;86: 711–715.
2. Shulkin BC, Thompson NW, Shapiro B, Francis IR, Sisson JC: Pheochromocytomas: Imaging with 2-(fluorine-(8) fluoro-s-deoxy-D-glucose PET. Radiol 1999;212:35–41.
3. Adams S, Baum R, Rink T, Schumm-Drager PM, Usadel KH, Hor G: Limited value of fluorine-18 fluorodeoxyglucose positron emission tomography for the imaging of neuroendocrine tumors. Eur J Nucl Med 1998;25:79–83.

Case 6.10.3

History

A 50-year-old female with a history of liver metastasis from an unknown primary presented for follow-up FDG PET imaging. Three years earlier she had undergone resection of a large liver mass diagnosed as adenocarcinoma of unknown primary at that time. An extensive search for a primary lesion, including multiple CT/MR examinations and whole-body FDG PET imaging was unrevealing. Therapy was withheld. A repeat thorough workup for a primary lesion ten months later revealed no evidence of a primary neoplasm nor any metastatic lesions; this evaluation included another normal FDG PET scan. Eighteen months later, another FDG PET scan was performed and correlated with a CT scan from an outside institution (Figure 6.10.3A) performed three months prior that was interpreted as normal. Figure 6.10.3B shows transaxial FDG images acquired with a dedicated PET tomograph (GE Advance) and reconstructed with iterative reconstruction and measured segmented attenuation correction.

Findings

The FDG images demonstrate a focus of increased activity at the porta hepatis and another focus in a left para-aortic site. No other abnormalities are identified.

Discussion

The two hypermetabolic foci identified on this most recent PET scan are consistent with metastatic lymphadenopathy. A primary lesion is still not identified. At this point, three years

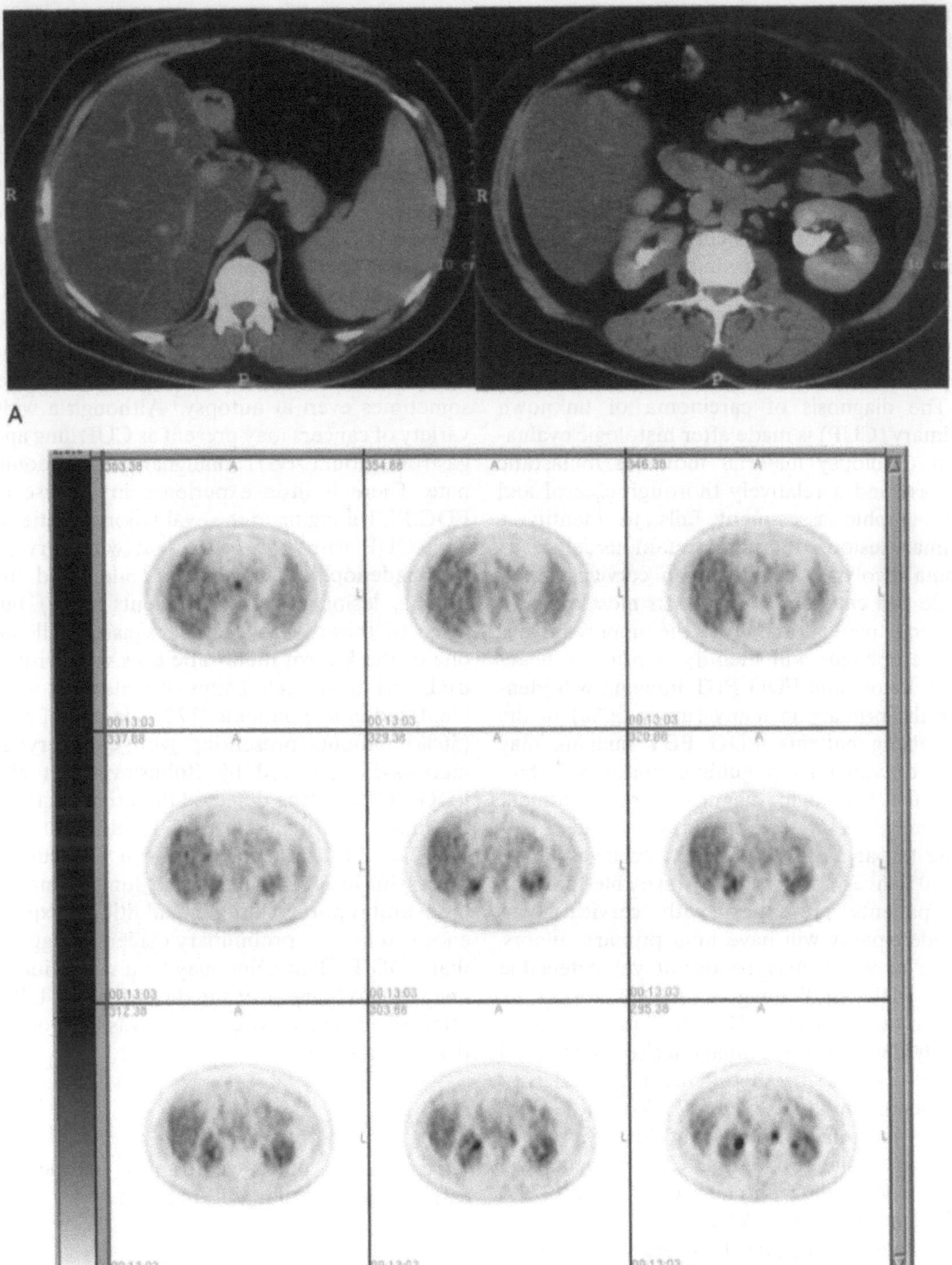

Figure 6.10.3A,B.

after a resection of a large isolated metastatic adenocarcinoma from the liver, this woman has the first identification of additional metastatic disease despite the absence of medical therapy. When the PET images were correlated with the most recent CT, the more superior lesion correlated with a 1 cm node at the hepatic hilum adjacent to the previous resection margin, and the more inferior focus correlated with a 1 cm para-aortic node seen in retrospect on the CT (Figure 6.10.3A). Repeat laparotomy confirmed the metastatic disease, and the hepatic hilar mass at histopathology was thought to represent a cholangiocarcinoma.

The diagnosis of carcinoma of unknown primary (CUP) is made after histologic evaluation of biopsy material indicates metastatic disease and a relatively thorough clinical and radiographic assessment fails to identify a primary lesion. Metastatic squamous cell carcinoma involving a mid-to-high cervical lymph node is a category by itself. In most of these patients, panendoscopy of the upper airways and esophagus will identify a primary head/neck lesion, and FDG PET imaging will identify the primary in many (up to 50%) of the remaining patients. FDG PET imaging may also be valuable in guiding endoscopic biopsy for histologic diagnosis and treatment planning.[1] Aggressive therapy of these ear-nose-throat (ENT) patients achieves a 30 to 50% five-year survival. A sizeable minority of patients presenting with cervical lymphadenopathy will have lung primary tumors, some of which may be occult yet detectable with FDG PET imaging. In the report by Bohuslavizki et al.,[2] FDG PET imaging accurately detected the primary lesion in 15 of 44 patients (34%) presenting with cervical lymphadenopathy, and seven (47%) of these were in the lung, obviously altering therapy.

Most of the rest of the CUP patients will have poorly differentiated carcinoma (27%) or adenocarcinoma (60%), representing 1 to 9% of patients with newly diagnosed cancer. In general, this is a disease with a poor prognosis with a median survival of 8 to 12 months. Except in specific circumstances, such as the finding of an occult breast carcinoma at mastectomy in women with isolated axillary adenopathy or further histopathological defining of a poorly differentiated carcinoma as compatible with a germ cell primary, neuroendocrine tumor, or undifferentiated lymphoma, the prognosis and survival are unaffected by repeated searches for a primary lesion. Although controversy surrounds the approach to these patients, most oncologists (and patients) wish to identify a primary site with the hope that survival will be impacted. The cost of such evaluations has been estimated to be approximately $18,000 (in 1995 dollars) per patient, and identification of the primary is the exception (less than 25%) rather than the rule, sometimes even at autopsy.[3] Although a wide variety of cancers may present as CUP, lung and gastrointestinal (GI) malignancies predominate. There is little experience in the use of FDG PET imaging in the evaluation of patients with CUP who do not present with cervical lymphadenopathy. Kole et al.[4] identified the primary lesion in 7 of 29 patients (24%), but three of these were head/neck cases. All but one of the known metastatic sites were visualized, and unsuspected sites of metastasis were identified in five patients (17%). In five of nine (56%) patients presenting with extracervical metastases reported by Bohuslaviski et al.,[2] FDG PET imaging detected the primary site in the lung (n = 3), colon (n = 1), and breast (n = 1). FDG PET imaging has been particularly successful in identifying occult lung primaries in several reports.[5] Although additional experience is required, preliminary evidence suggests that FDG PET imaging may be a useful initial imaging modality after the diagnosis of CUP is established and before more invasive modalities are entertained.

Diagnosis

Carcinoma of unknown primary (extracervical), probable cholangiocarcinoma.

References

1. Braams JW, Pruim J, Kole AC, et al.: Detection of unknown primary head and neck tumors by positron emission tomography. Int J Oral Maxillofac Surg 1997;26:112–115.

2. Bohuslavizki KH, Klutmann S, Kroger S, et al.: FDG PET detection of unknown primary tumors. J Nucl Med 2000;42:816–822.
3. Schapira DV, Jarrett AR: The need to consider survival, outcome, and expense when evaluating and treating patients with unknown primary carcinoma. Arch Intern Med 1995;155:2050–2054.
4. Kole AC, Nieweg OE, Pruim J, et al.: Detection of unknown occult primary tumors using positron emission tomography. Cancer 1998;82:1160–1166.
5. Lassen U, Daugaard G, Eigtved A, Damgaard K, Friberg L: 18F-FDG whole body positron emission tomography (PET) in patients with unknown primary tumours (UPT). Eur J Cancer 1999;35:1076–1082.

Case 6.10.4

History

A 33-year-old male presented with a 4 by 5 cm left axillary mass. Approximately one year earlier, he had undergone a left pneumonectomy for a partially responsive (to chemotherapy) soft tissue sarcoma involving the left hilum, pleural-based nodules, and mediastinal nodes. Bone scintigraphy (not shown) demonstrated no evidence of skeletal involvement. A chest CT (not shown) showed a 5 by 4 cm left axillary nodal mass, enlarged subcarinal and prevascular nodes, para-aortic lymphadenopathy, and a large retrosplenic soft tissue mass extending along the left chest and flank wall. These CT lesions were not present on a CT from six months prior and were less prominent on a CT from three months earlier. Figures 6.10.4A and B show coronal (Figure 6.10.4A) and transaxial (Figure 6.10.4B) FDG PET images acquired with a dedicated PET tomograph (GE Advance) and reconstructed with an iterative algorithm and measured segmented attenuation correction.

Findings

Coronal images of the thorax, abdomen, and pelvis reveal multiple abnormal foci of increased activity in the left axilla, mediastinum spanning levels T6 through T8, and left para-aortic region at T12-L1. In the left lower thorax laterally are two areas of increased activity, implying rib involvement. Also of note is volume loss of the left hemithorax with mediastinal shift to the left consistent with the patient's history of left pneumonectomy. There is no significant myocardial activity. Bilateral physiologic ureteral activity and scattered physiologic bowel activity is noted.

Discussion

These findings are consistent with widespread disease involving soft tissues, lymph nodes, and skeleton. Biopsy of the left axillary mass was consistent with recurrent follicular dendritic cell sarcoma, so the patient was started on second-line chemotherapy.

As with lymphoma, FDG PET imaging has been shown to be as useful or more useful than CT for demonstrating the extent of disease in patients with intermediate-to-high grade soft tissue sarcomas, although experience is limited. All high-grade soft tissue sarcomas and most low-grade and intermediate-grade sarcomas are FDG-avid and easily visualized, but many aggressive benign soft tissue lesions may also exhibit increased FDG accumulation. As expected, benign lesions such as lipomas and leiomyomas do not accumulate FDG, but inflammatory lesions may cause false-positive findings. The degree of FDG activity as determined by tumor-to-background (TBR) ratios of > 3 or SUVs > 2 tends to correlate with the grade (but not the histologic type) of tumor as evidenced by the finding that metastatic lesions have a mean SUV more than twice that of primary sarcomas, indicative of a more aggressive lesion.[1,2]

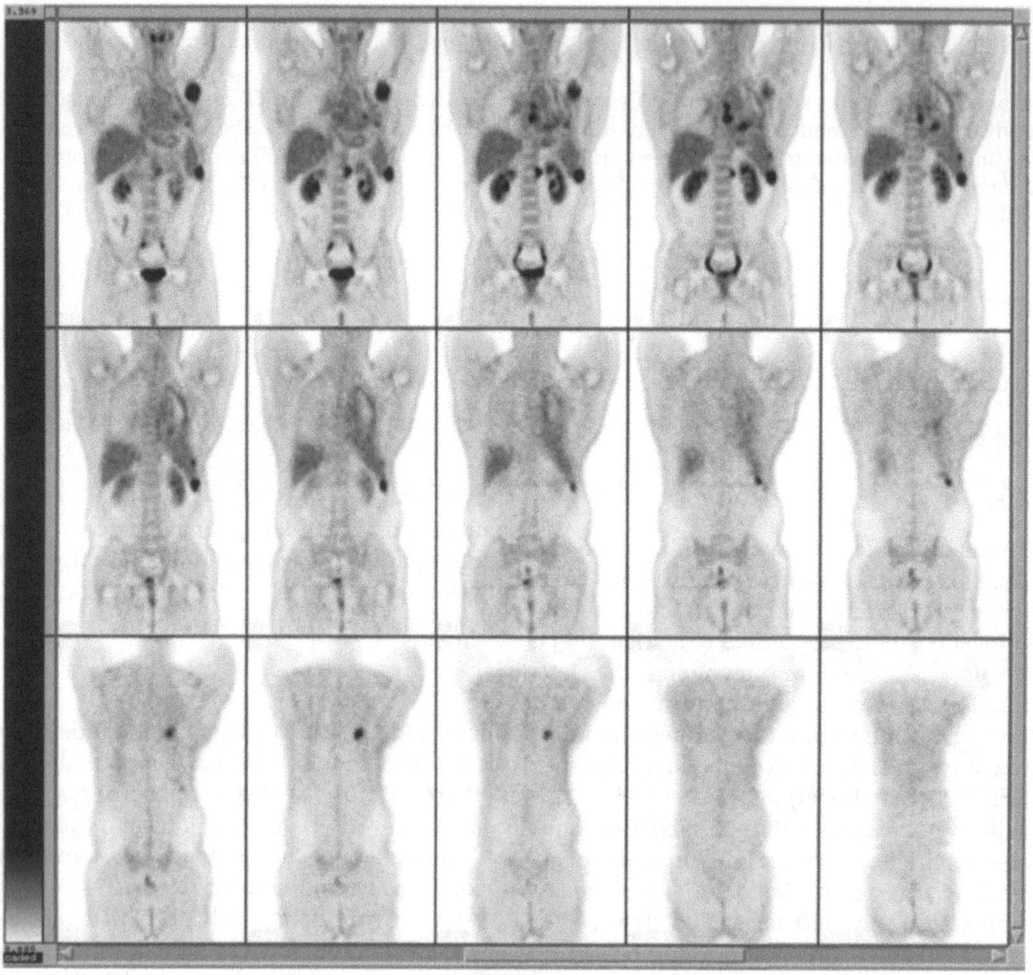

FIGURE 6.10.4A.

This patient's bone scintigraphy revealed no evidence of skeletal metastases, but the PET images are suspicious for rib involvement in the left lower thorax. In patients with osteolytic metastases, diphosphonate scintigraphy may underestimate the extent of disease in as many as 65% of patients as compared to MRI and FDG (or ^{18}F sodium fluoride) PET and may be normal in the presence of PET-demonstrated osseous metastases in as many as 18%.[3]

In view of this patient's poor response to first-line chemotherapy and widespread metastases, his prognosis is poor. He will require multiple reassessments during and after second-line and investigational therapy. Since his tumor is FDG-avid, PET may more accurately demonstrate his extent of disease, both soft tissue and skeletal, during follow-up than any other single modality.[4,5]

Diagnosis

Follicular dendritic cell sarcoma with multiple metastases.

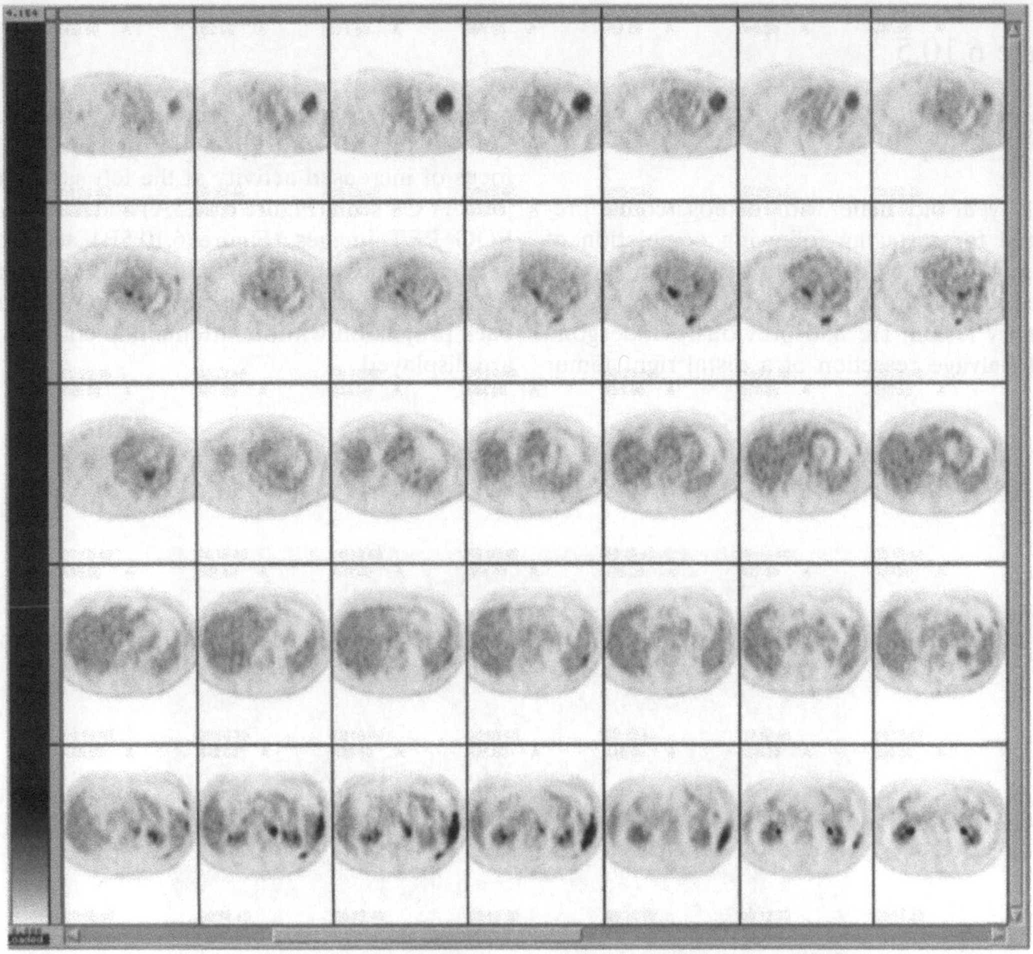

FIGURE 6.10.4B.

References

1. Schwarzbach MH, Dimitrakopoulou-Strauss A, Willeke F, et al.: Clinical value of 18-F fluorodeoxyglucose positron tomography imaging in soft tissue sarcomas. Ann Surg 2000;23:380–386.
2. Folpe AL, Lyles RH, Sprouse JT, Conrad EU, Eary JF: F-18 fluorodeoxyglucose positron emission tomography as a predictor of pathologic grade and other prognostic variables in bone and soft tissue sarcoma. Clin Cancer Res 2000;6: 1279–1287.
3. Schirrmeister H, Guhlmann CA, Kotzerke J, et al.: Early detection and accurate description of extent of metastatic bone disease in breast cancer with 18F-fluoride ion and positron emission tomography. J Clin Oncol 1999;17:2381–2389.
4. Shields AF, Mankoff DA, Link JM, et al.: Carbon-11-thymidine and FDG to measure therapy response. J Nucl Med 1998;39:1757–1762.
5. Lucas JD, O'Doherty MJ, Wong JC, et al.: Evaluation of fluorodeoxyglucose positron emission tomography in the management of soft-tissue sarcomas. J Bone Joint Surg Br 1998;80:441–447.

Case 6.10.5

History

A 17-year-old male with osteosarcoma presented for restaging following completion of chemotherapy for recurrent disease after prior resection of an isolated left metastatic pulmonary lesion. He had previously undergone limb salvage resection of a distal right femur primary osteosarcoma. Bone scintigraphy was notable for two left rib abnormalities and a focus of increased activity at the left sacroiliac joint. A CT scan (Figure 6.10.5A) and transaxial FDG PET images (Figure 6.10.5B) acquired with a dedicated PET tomograph (Siemens ECAT 933) and reconstructed using filtered back projection without attenuation correction are displayed.

A
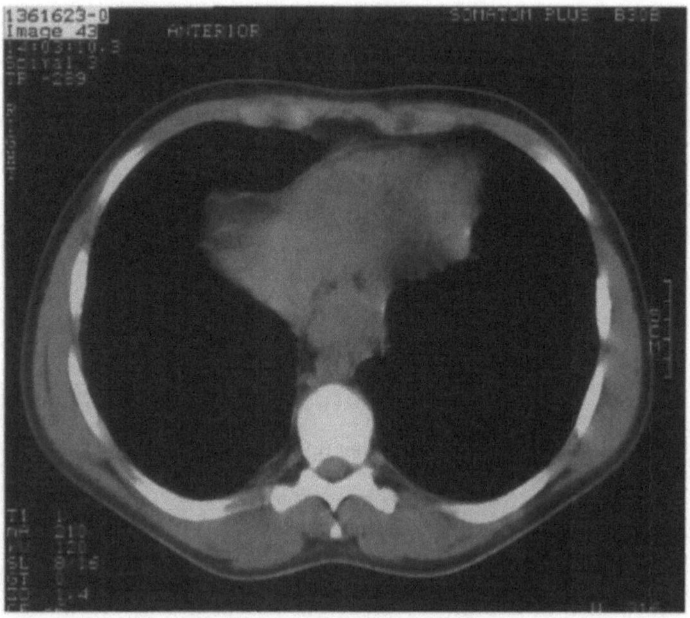

B
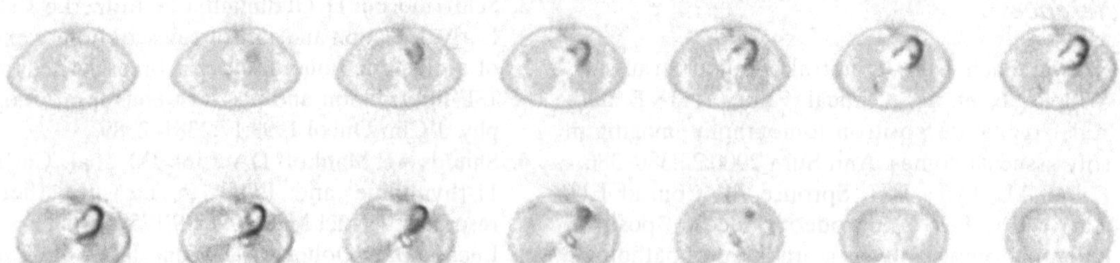

FIGURE 6.10.5A,B.

Findings

The CT images reveal a 3mm nodule in the right middle lobe, a 1cm nodule in the right lower lobe posteriorly, postthoracotomy changes in the left mid-chest (not shown), and a 4cm mass at the gastroesophageal junction (Figure 6.10.5A).

The FDG PET images demonstrate a focus of increased uptake in the right lower lobe of the lung posteriorly, corresponding to the 1cm lesion seen on CT. A faint focus of mildly increased activity is present in the right middle lobe and probably correlates with the 3mm lesion on CT (not shown). The lack of visualization of left rib uptake on PET supports a diagnosis of postthoracotomy changes rather than sarcomatous involvement. The markedly increased uptake in the posterior mediastinum corresponds to thc gastroesophageal junction mass seen on CT. The standard uptake value of 4.4 is consistent with metastasis. The photopenic center represents central necrosis.

Discussion

The FDG images are consistent with recurrent metastatic pulmonary and mediastinal disease despite several courses of chemotherapy. The small focus in the right middle lobe is suggestive of metastasis despite its relatively low apparent uptake. The spatial resolution of this older PET imaging system was approximately 8mm, so any lesion smaller than 16mm would suffer from partial volume averaging, thus underestimating the radioactivity of the lesion. Despite the findings on diphosphonate bone scintigraphy, the FDG images are not suggestive of skeletal involvement, although the sensitivity of FDG PET imaging for detection of skeletal metastases of osteosarcomas is inferior to that of bone scintigraphy.

FDG imaging has also been found to be useful in evaluating amputation stumps for recurrence, a difficult clinical problem even when CT, MRI, and diphosphonate bone scintigraphy are used. Diffuse uptake may be present postoperatively for as long as 18 months without evidence of recurrence, but a focal area of increased uptake in the absence of a clinically evident pressure sore represents recurrent disease. Most osteosarcomas and other high-grade sarcomas such as Ewing's sarcoma and chondrosarcoma accumulate FDG. Although the sensitivity of FDG PET imaging for the detection of these malignancies is over 95%, the specificity is lower due to the elevated uptake of FDG seen with aggressive benign processes such as giant cell tumors, aneursymal bone cysts, brown tumors, and Paget's disease. Inflammatory/granulomatous lesions such as osteomyelitis, eosinophilic granuloma, and sarcoidosis may cause false-positive findings, and metastatic disease cannot be differentiated from a primary tumor.[1,2] The sensitivity for the detection of recurrent disease is similarly very high, and the sensitivity for the detection of pulmonary metastases is similar to that of CT. The sensitivity of FDG PET imaging for the detection of sarcomatous skeletal involvement is controversial.

Approximately six months later, follow-up FDG PET images were obtained after completion of salvage chemotherapy (Figure 6.10.5C). The three foci of abnormal uptake in the right middle lobe, right lower lobe, and posterior mediastinum are no longer seen. A concurrent CT shows resolution of the right lower lobe nodule, no change in the tiny right middle lobe nodule, and only moderate regression of the mediastinal mass (not shown). Despite the persistence of the mediastinal mass on CT posttherapy, the absence of FDG activity is most consistent with posttherapy scarring without the presence of viable tumor.

This is similar to the situation seen with Hodgkin's lymphoma and many other malignancies, with the specificity of FDG PET imaging being significantly higher than CT posttherapy. Biopsy can be avoided, and therapy is altered on the basis of PET findings. As with many other malignancies, FDG PET imaging has been used to monitor the response of sarcomas to chemotherapy. FDG may be the best predictor of the degree of tumor necrosis occurring with neoadjuvant therapy; the differentiation of responders from nonresponders is better with FDG PET imaging than with CT/MR imaging. This can be of critical impor-

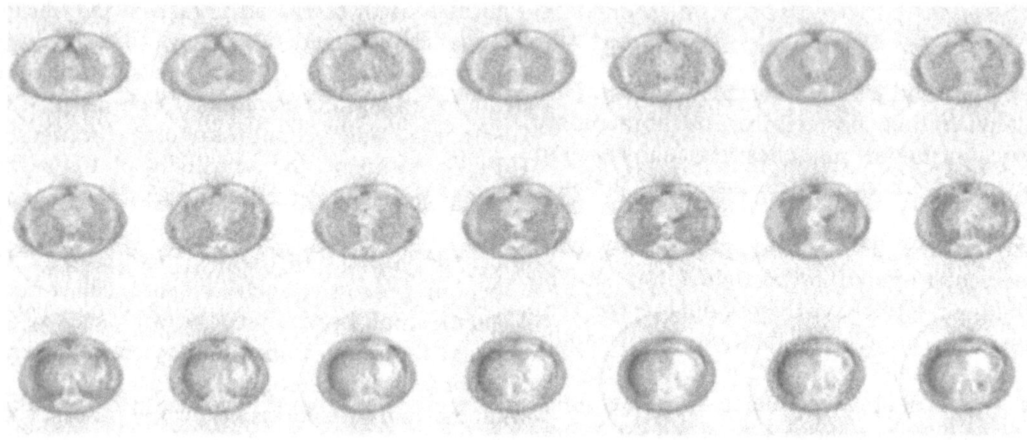

C

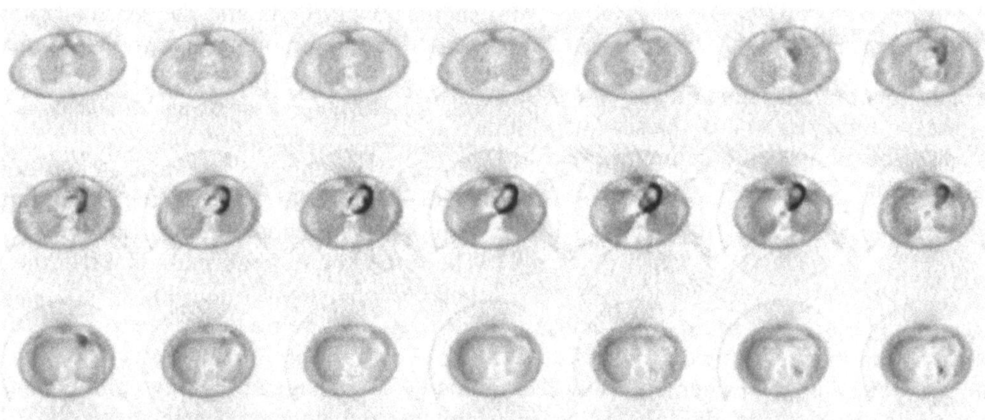

D

FIGURE 6.10.5C,D.

tance in the patient completing preoperative neoadjuvant therapy, since a limb salvage procedure cannot be advocated in a patient whose tumor has not responded well to chemotherapy.[3–5] There is insufficient experience to date to determine the utility of FDG PET imaging in the restaging of osteosarcoma following chemotherapy, but the expectation is that it will be complementary to more conventional modalities.

Five months later, a CT revealed multiple bilateral small (a few millimeters in size) lung nodules, and another FDG PET scan was performed. The lateral left upper lobe (not in the field of view) and the peripheral, posterior left lower lobe lesions can be identified on the FDG images (Figure 6.10.5D). The other nodules are not seen. The activity of lesions smaller than twice the resolution of the imaging system may be underestimated, and lesions less than the resolution of the system may go undetected, depending on the uptake within the lesion and the adjacent physiologic background activity (that is, contrast). Despite the failure to visualize all these small lesions, the detection of two of them is consistent with recurrent metastases. This patient subsequently developed brain metastases and succumbed.

Diagnosis

Recurrent metastatic osteosarcoma.

References

1. Schulte M, Brechte-Krauss D, Heymer B, et al.: Grading of tumors and tumorlike lesions of bone: Evaluation by FDG-PET. J Nucl Med 2000;41: 1695–1701.
2. Messa C, Landoni C, Pozzato C, Fazio F: Is there a role for FDG PET in the diagnosis of musculoskeletal neoplasms? J Nucl Med 2000;41:1702–1703.
3. Schulte M, Brecht-Krauss D, Werner M, et al.: Evaluation of neoadjuvant therapy response of osteogenic sarcoma using FDG PET. J Nucl Med 1999;40:1637–1643.
4. Nair N, Amjad A, Green AA, et al.: Response of osteosarcoma to chemotherapy: Evaluation with F-18 FDG-PET scans. Clin Positron Imag 2000; 3:79–83.
5. Hain SF, O'Doherty MJ, Lucas JD, Smith MA: Fluorodeoxyglucose PET in the evaluation of amputations for soft tissue sarcoma. Nucl Med Commun 1999;20:845–848.

Case 6.10.6

History

A 33-year-old male was referred for FDG PET imaging in his ongoing evaluation for suspected recurrent medullary carcinoma of the thyroid (MCT) because of a rising serum calcitonin. He was first found to have medullary thyroid carcinoma six years earlier at total thyroidectomy. Due to a rising calcitonin of > 5000 ng/ml, a thoracotomy four years later revealed metastatic mediastinal adenopathy. His calcitonin dropped to < 1,000 ng/ml postoperatively but had risen to 13,000 ng/ml at the time of his PET scan. A recent contrasted CT of the neck, thorax, and abdomen was interpreted as negative for metastases, and ^{111}In-octreotide whole-body imaging was normal (not shown). Figure 6.10.6 shows transaxial FDG PET images of the chest acquired with a dedicated PET tomograph (GE Advance) and reconstructed using an iterative algorithm and measured segmented attenuation correction.

Findings

The FDG images reveal moderate-sized foci of increased activity present in the thorax bilaterally. Small relatively faint foci of increased activity are identified at the base of the left neck, left lateral neck, and upper right posterior neck (not shown).

Discussion

The findings are consistent with multiple FDG-avid cervical and pulmonary metastases. Surgical resection of identified cervical and mediastinal metastases of medullary thyroid carcinoma has been demonstrated to normalize or decrease elevated serum levels of calcitonin and/or CEA and may favorably impact survival.[1] The presence of disease outside the cervicomediastinal region, as in this case, will generally preclude surgical therapy.

Medullary carcinoma of the thyroid is a neuroendocrine neoplasm of intermediate grade for which total thyroidectomy with regional lymphadenectomy is the only effective therapy. It accounts for only 5 to 10% of all thyroid cancers and may occur sporadically or in a familial form, either as part of the multiple endocrine neoplasia, type 2 (MEN-2) or a familial medullary thyroid carcinoma without MEN characteristics. It is bilateral in half of the sporadic cases but is bilateral and multifocal in most familial cases. MEN-2 is associated with mutations of the ret oncogene, allowing genetic screening of family members and early curative thyroidectomy in affected members. Most MCT tumors express calcitonin, CEA, and histaminase, thus providing sensitive serum tumor markers for detection of persistent or recurrent

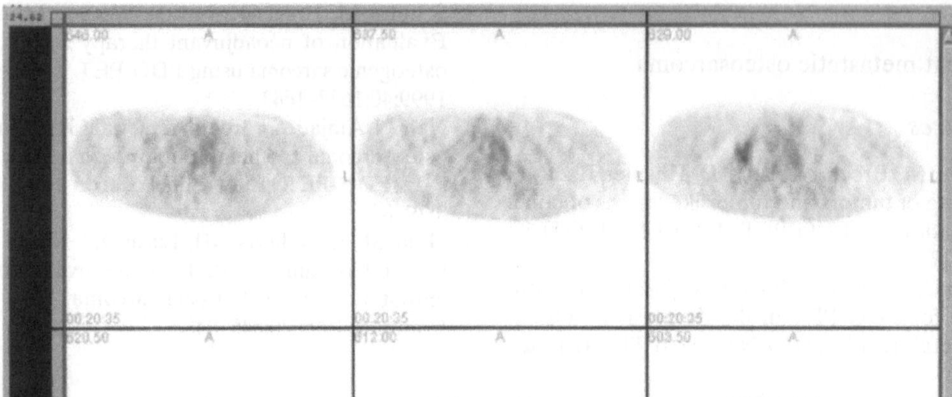

FIGURE 6.10.6.

disease. Prognosis is much better than that of anaplastic carcinoma with an 80% ten-year survival and is most influenced by early detection, absence of distant metastases, and adequate initial surgery.

In view of its poor response to external and ^{131}Iodine radiotherapy as well as chemotherapy, localization and subsequent resection of tumor deposits are the only therapeutic option for patients with medullary thyroid carcinoma. There is no single sensitive imaging modality for detection and staging of medullary thyroid carcinoma. Selective venous catheterization may be the most sensitive technique but is infrequently used. Ultrasound, CT, and MRI are insensitive for detection of small metastases outside the neck. In view of the expression of CEA by these tumors, radiolabeled anti-CEA monoclonal antibody imaging has been used to identify 40 to 86% of metastases, and similarly, somatostatin receptor imaging with ^{111}In-octreotide is able to identify approximately 50 to 70% of metastases over 1 cm in diameter. ^{201}Thallium and pentavalent ^{99m}Tc-DMSA scintigraphy have also been used with variable results. Radioiodinated MIBG scintigraphy is not useful for detection of small metastases. All of these techniques are highly dependent on the size of the metastases as well as the location of the deposits distant from regions of physiologic uptake, but in general, all have been more sensitive than ultrasound and CT. Up to 25% of patients with persistent or recurrent disease have micrometastatic disease of the liver (< 5 mm), and it is probably only in the minority of patients that disease is confined to the cervicomediastinal region.[2] For this reason, some investigators, including those at Washington University, have advocated routine laparoscopic liver examination preoperatively in addition to the use of multiple imaging modalities.[3]

In general, imaging of metastatic sites of medullary thyroid carcinoma is successful in only 60%. In preliminary studies, FDG PET imaging has a sensitivity of approximately 76% and has been especially sensitive for detection of mediastinal, pulmonary, and skeletal metastases.[4–6] Like the other modalities, very small liver metastases are difficult to detect. Although not yet proven, FDG PET imaging is likely the imaging modality of choice for the localization of metastatic medullary thyroid carcinoma.

Diagnosis

Metastatic medullary carcinoma of the thyroid.

References

1. Kebebew E, Kikuchi S, Duh QY, Clark OH: Long-term results of reoperation and localizing studies in patients with persistent or recurrent medullary thyroid cancer. Arch Surg 2000;135(8):895–901.
2. Juweid M, Sharkey RM, Swayne LC, Goldenberg DM: Improved selection of patients for reoperation for medullary thyroid cancer by imaging with radiolabeled anticarcinoembryonic antigen antibodies. Surgery 1997;122(6):1156–1165.
3. Moley JF, Debenedetti MK, Dilley WG, Tisell LE, Wells SA: Surgical management of patients with persistent or recurrent medullary thyroid cancer. J Intern Med 1998;243(6):521–526.
4. Conti PS, Durski JM, Bacqai F, Grafton ST, Singer PA: Imaging of locally recurrent and metastatic thyroid cancer with positron emission tomography. Thyroid 1999;9(8):797–804.
5. Musholt TJ, Musholt PB, Dehdashti F, Moley JF: Evaluation of fluorodeoxyglucose-positron emission tomographic scanning and its association with glucose transporter expression in medullary thyroid carcinoma and pheochromocytoma: A clinical and molecular study. Surg 1997;122:1049–1061.
6. Gasparoni P, Rubello D, Ferlin G: Potential role of fluorine-18-deoxyglucose (FDG) positron emission tomography (PET) in the staging of primitive and recurrent medullary thyroid carcinoma. J Endocrinol Invest 1997;20(9):527–530.

Case 6.10.7

History

A 65-year-old female with no history of malignancy had recently undergone craniotomy for resection of a 5 cm left posterior mass that at pathology was found to be a poorly differentiated carcinoma. CT of the thorax (Figure 6.10.7A), abdomen, and pelvis, bone scintigraphy, mammography, and colonoscopy were all unrevealing. After completion of whole brain radiation therapy, FDG PET images (Figure 6.10.7B) were acquired with a dedicated PET tomograph (GE Advance) and reconstructed with iterative reconstruction and measured segmented attenuation correction.

Findings

A small focus of markedly increased activity is present in the right lower lobe medially adjacent to the mediastinum. There is increased diffuse myocardial activity. No additional abnormalities are identified. In retrospect, a subtle abnormality is seen on CT in this region.

Discussion

The FDG PET images are compatible with a pulmonary primary carcinoma which in retrospect is visible but nonpathologic on the prior CT of two months earlier (Figure 6.10.7A).

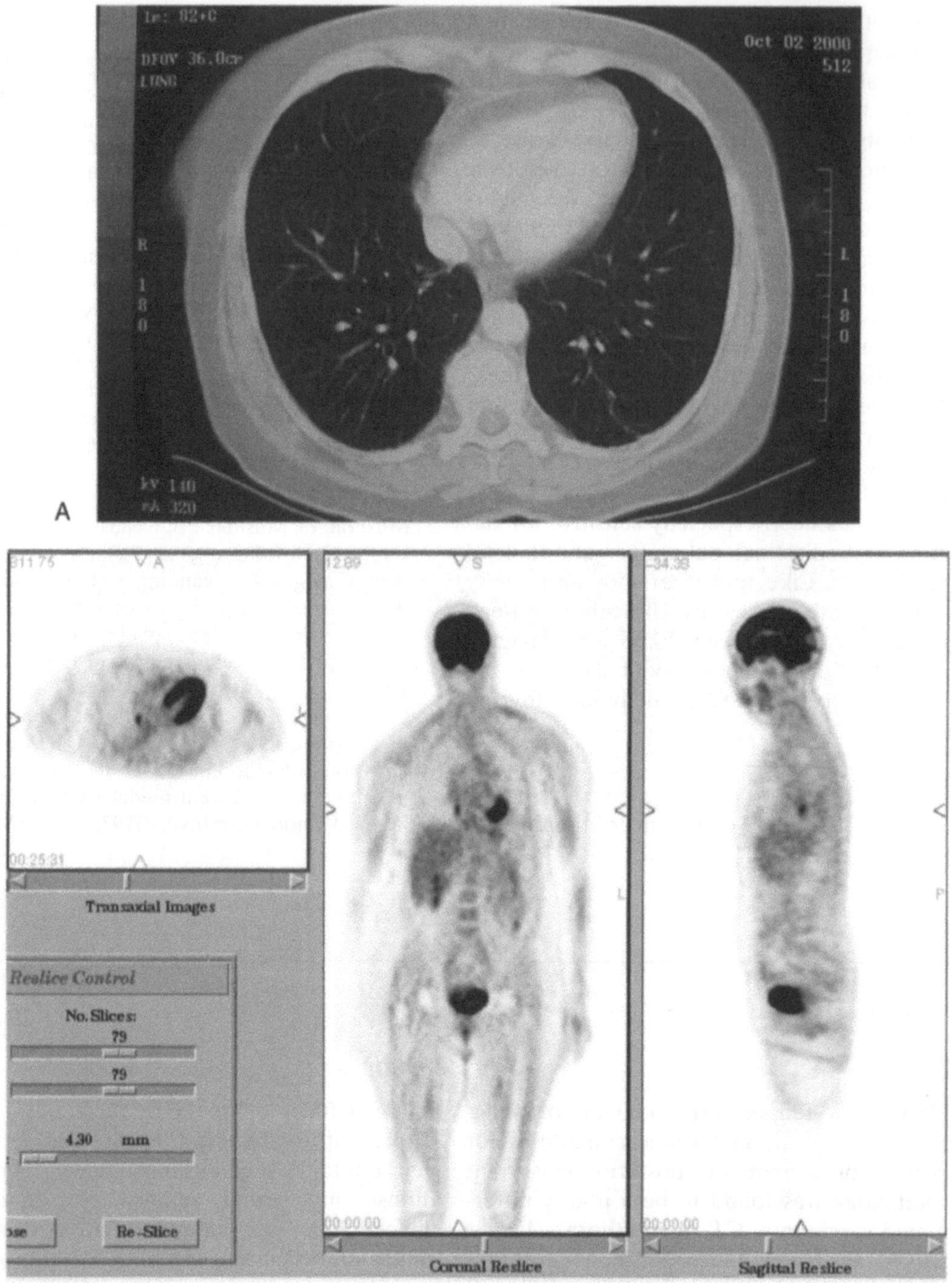

FIGURE 6.10.7A,B.

A repeat CT of the thorax with 5mm slices revealed a 1.4 by 1.6cm right lower lobe mass, congruent with the FDG PET imaging findings. This is a typical example of an occult lung cancer presenting as an isolated brain metastasis and diagnosed only by utilizing FDG PET imaging. A similar example has been reported.[1] In this particular patient, it is unlikely that this finding

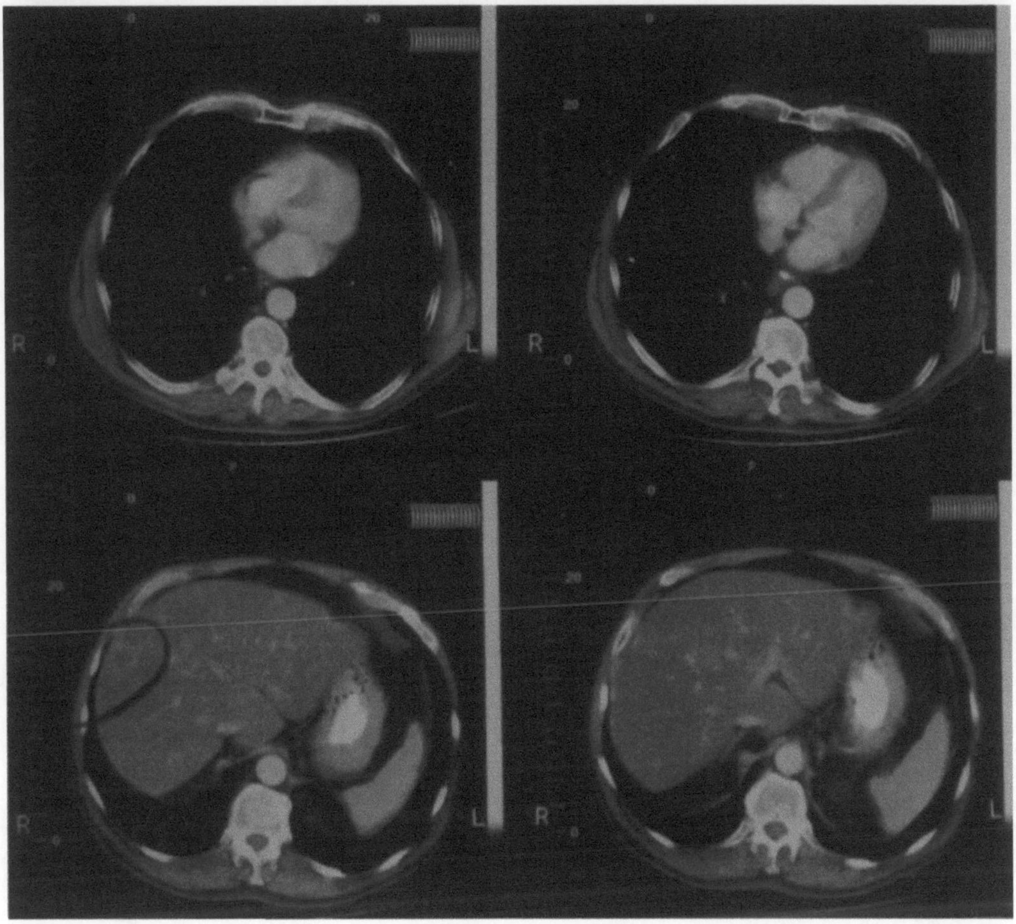

FIGURE 6.10.7C.

will significantly impact survival, but it provides important prognostic information and can be used to prescribe appropriate chemotherapy and monitor response to therapy.

A similar patient found to have poorly differentiated carcinoma metastatic to the liver but without an identifiable primary lesion despite a thorough evaluation including CT scan (Figure 6.10.7C) underwent FDG PET imaging after completion of two courses of combination chemotherapy (Figures 6.10.7D and E). The small hypermetabolic focus seen at the posteromedial right lung base is consistent with a pulmonary primary lesion. The two known hepatic metastases are barely visible, consistent with a good therapeutic response to chemotherapy. The chest CT, initially interpreted as negative for neoplasm, in retrospect shows a small soft tissue mass adjacent to the esophagus and consistent with the primary lesion (Figure 6.10.7C, upper right image).

Diagnosis

Carcinoma of unknown primary, bronchogenic primary diagnosed by FDG PET imaging.

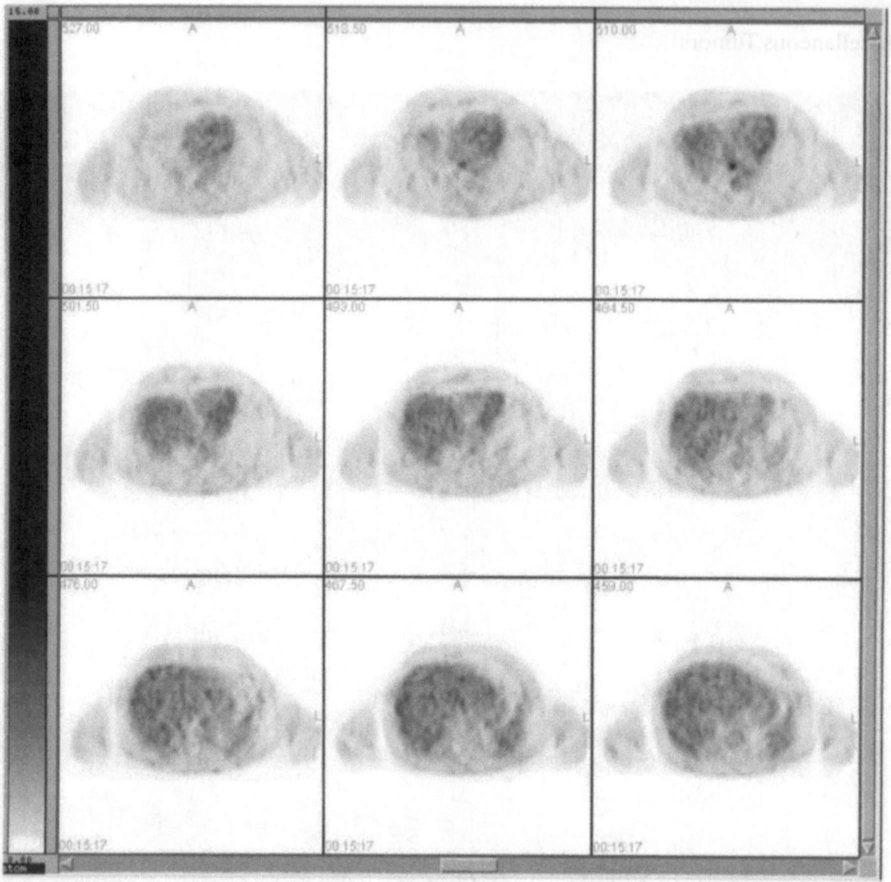

D

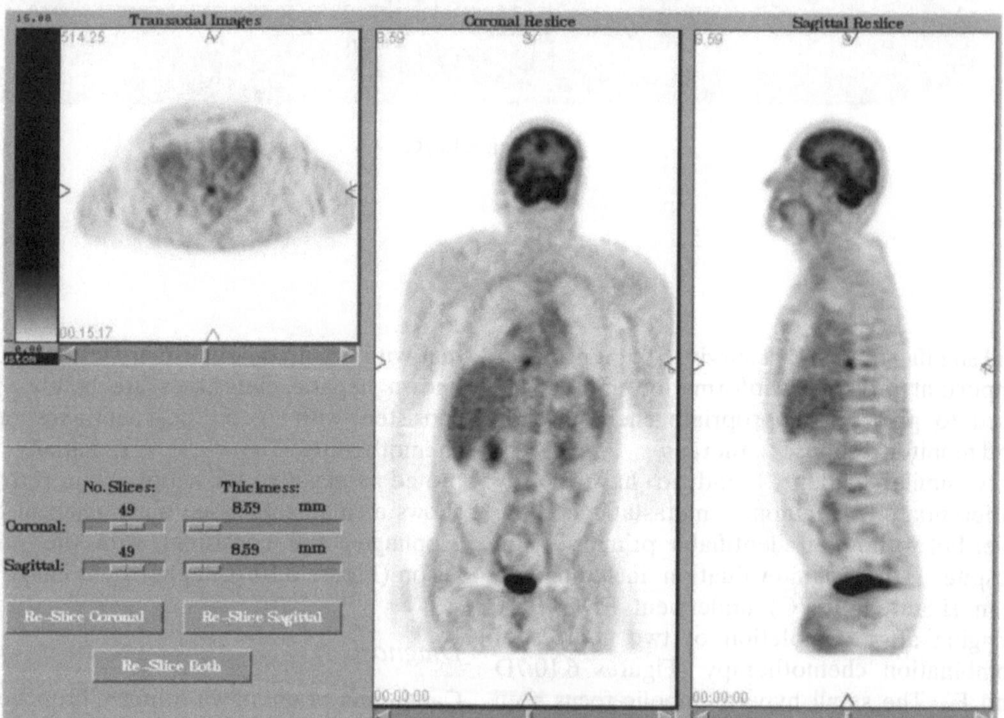

E

FIGURE 6.10.7D,E. (*Continued*)

Reference

1. Torre W, Garcia-Velloso MJ, Galbis J, Fernandez O, Richter J: FDG-PET detection of primary lung cancer in a patient with an isolated cerebral metastasis. J Cardiovasc Surg 2000;41:503–505.

Case 6.10.8

History

A 64-year-old man with hematochezia was found to have a malignant lesion at colonoscopy and was referred for staging and management. Transaxial CT images (Figure 6.10.8A) and transaxial (Figure 6.10.8B) and coronal (Figure 6.10.8C) FDG PET images acquired with a dedicated PET tomograph (Siemens ECAT 933) and reconstructed with filtered back projection without correction for attenuation are displayed. The patient moved during acquisition of the transmission images, resulting in poor quality attenuation-corrected images.

Findings

The CT images demonstrate low attenuation lesions within both lobes of the liver, two of which are approximately 5 cm in diameter in segment II and one of which is 3.5 cm in diameter in segment VI. No pathologic adenopathy is identified.

The FDG images show numerous foci of markedly increased activity within both the right and left lobes of the liver congruent with the CT lesions, as well as a large focus of markedly increased activity in the right abdomen in the region of the mid-ascending colon. Several foci of increased activity lie medial to this large abnormality.

Discussion

The hypermetabolic foci are consistent with metastatic disease to the liver in the same distribution as seen on the CT images with approximately equal sensitivity for detection.

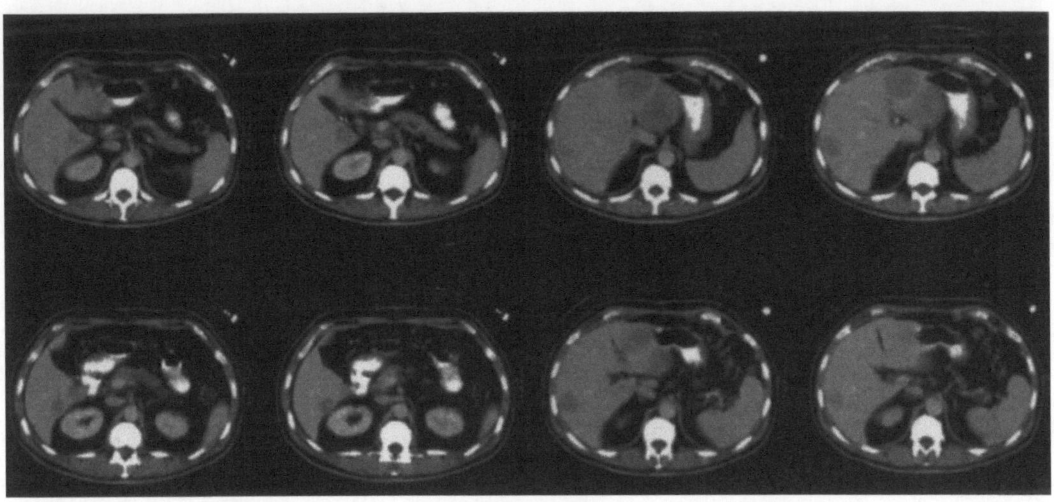

FIGURE 6.10.8A.

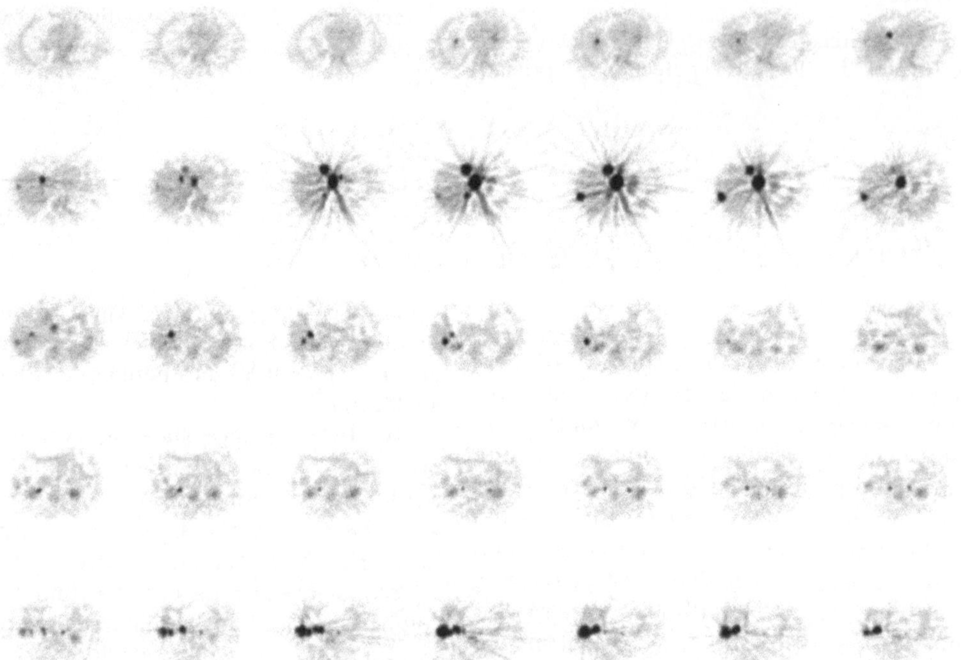

B

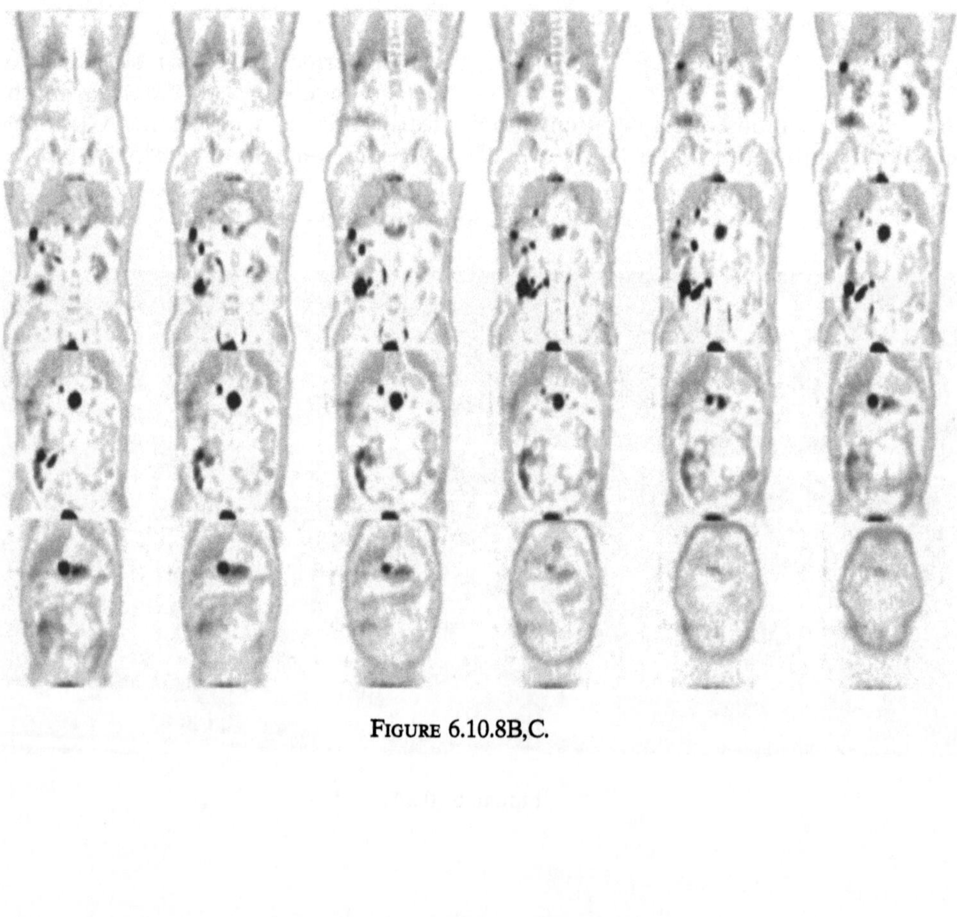

C

FIGURE 6.10.8B,C.

Although physiologic FDG activity may accumulate at the cecum and right colon related to abundant lymphoid tissue in this region, the degree of activity seen on these images is abnormal and suggestive of a primary colon malignancy with associated adjacent metastatic lymphadenopathy. At laparotomy, more than ten metastatic deposits in the liver could be palpated by the surgeon. A 4.5 cm malignant carcinoid tumor with aggressive histologic features and several adjacent metastatic nodes was resected from the mid-right colon. Therefore, the FDG images identified not only the hepatic metastases, but also the primary colonic lesion and the adjacent metastatic adenopathy. Due to the atypical histologic features, systemic cytotoxic therapy was initiated.

Most neuroendocrine tumors, including carcinoid, paraganglioma, and islet cell tumors, express somatostatin receptors (SSR) and therefore can be imaged effectively with somatostatin analogs such as ^{111}In-octreotide. This modality has been reported to be more sensitive than CT for defining the extent of metastatic disease, especially in extrahepatic and extra-abdominal sites. However, there may be significant heterogeneity in regard to SSR expression, even in the same patient in adjacent sites, probably related to dedifferentiation of the tumor. Absence of SSR positivity is reported to be a poor prognostic sign, but virtually all of these SSR-negative neuroendocrine tumors will accumulate FDG and therefore can be imaged with PET.[1,2] More differentiated SSR-positive tumors do not reliably accumulate significant FDG and therefore may be false-negative with FDG PET imaging.[3] Both techniques may detect the primary gastrointestinal or islet cell tumor in a minority of cases. FDG PET imaging is ideally suited to monitoring the success of locally directed therapy such as chemoembolization, alcohol instillation, and radiofrequency ablation.

Diagnosis

Atypical carcinoid of the colon with local and hepatic metastases.

References

1. Adams S, Baum R, Rink T, Schumm-Drager PM, Usadel KH, Hor G: Limited value of fluorine-18 fluorodeoxyglucose positron emission tomography for the imaging of neuroendocrine tumors. Eur J Nucl Med 1998;25:79–83.
2. Erasmus JJ, McAdams HP, Patz EF Jr, Coleman RE, Ahuja V, Goodman PC: Evaluation of primary pulmonary carcinoid tumors using FDG PET. AJR Am J Roentgenol 1998;170(5):1369–1373.
3. Jadvar H, Segall GM: False-negative fluorine-18-FDG PET in metastatic carcinoid. J Nucl Med 1997;38(9):1382–1383.

Case 6.10.9

History

A 52-year-old man with a history of adrenal carcinoma presented for restaging. Eighteen months earlier he had undergone a right radical adrenalectomy for Cushing's syndrome complicated by systemic nonmeningitic Cryptococcosis. Histological findings were diagnostic of a 15 by 13 cm adrenal carcinoma without vascular or capsular extension. A CT of the chest and abdomen performed six months postoperatively demonstrated no evidence of recurrence. He was referred for CT (Figure 6.10.9A) and FDG PET imaging. Figure 6.10.9B shows transaxial FDG PET images acquired with a dedicated PET tomograph (GE Advance) and reconstructed with iterative reconstruction and measured segmented attenuation correction.

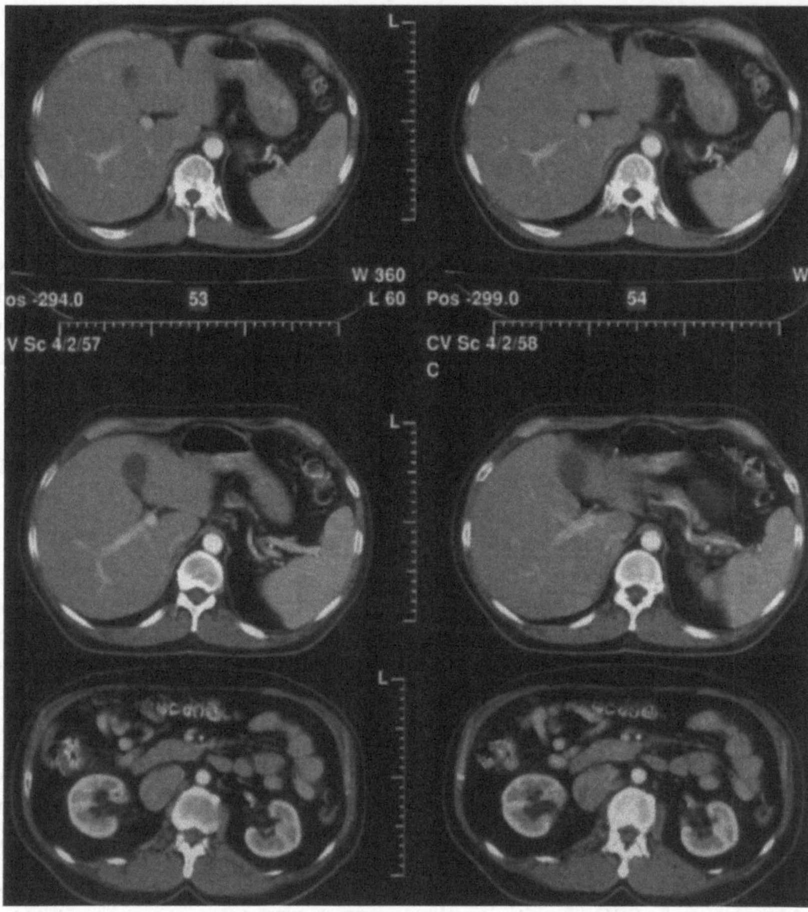

FIGURE 6.10.9A.

Findings

A new 5 cm enhancing mass is seen posterior to the inferior vena cava just below the level of the right renal vein. There is evidence of the prior right adrenalectomy. The FDG images demonstrate a large focus of intense activity anterior to the mid-polar region of the right kidney and a smaller focus of increased activity in the right adrenal bed superior to the upper pole of the right kidney.

Discussion

The CT is most consistent with a recurrence of the adrenal carcinoma inferior to the adrenal bed, but the PET images demonstrate an additional focus of recurrence in the right adrenal bed. Adrenal carcinoma is a rare entity often presenting with Cushing's syndrome and occasionally with virilism. As in this patient, the neoplasm is usually quite large, and early locoregional metastasis is the rule. Medical therapy is generally ineffective, resulting in a poor prognosis. FDG PET is able to differentiate malignant from benign adrenal masses with a high degree of accuracy, as discussed in Case 6.4.6, Case 6.5.1, and Case 6.9.3. Although the majority of malignant adrenal tumors are due to metastatic involvement, the detection of primary adrenal carcinoma by FDG PET has been reported. As seen with most other tumors, PET is superior to CT in the detection of abdominal extrahepatic metastases and differentiation of tumor recurrence from postsurgical changes, both of which are demonstrated by this case.

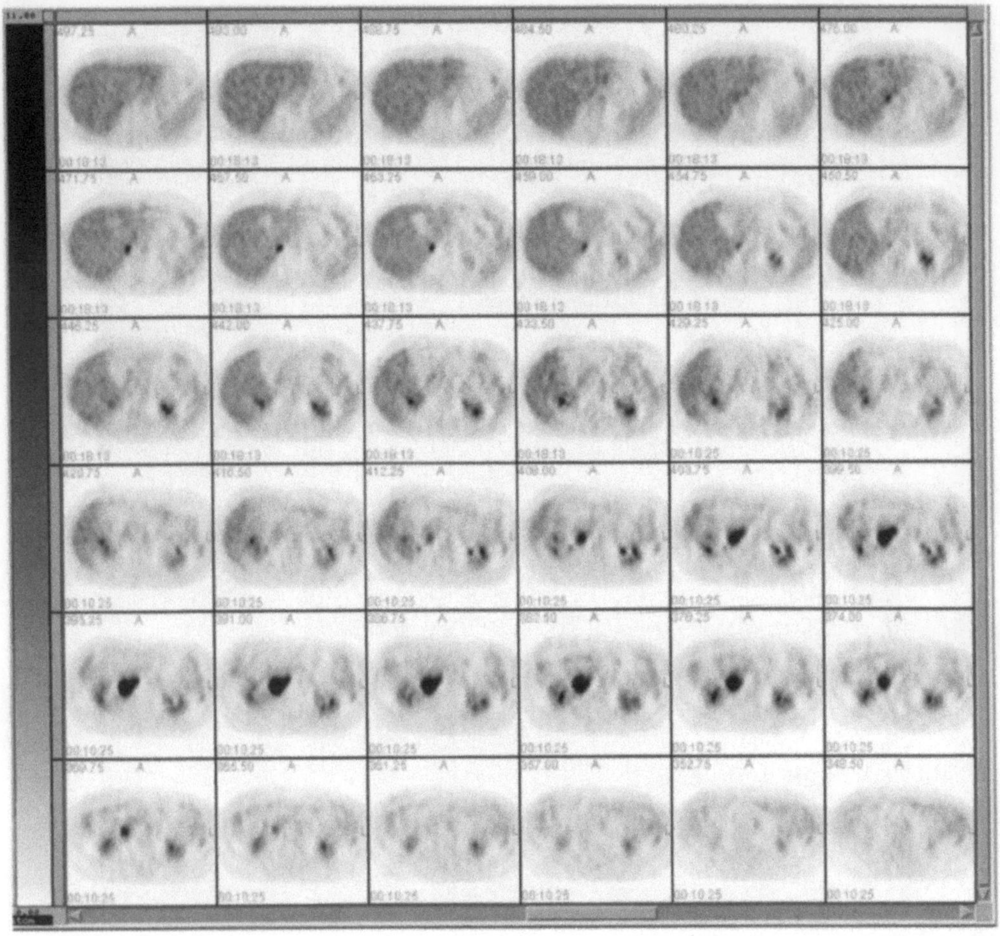

FIGURE 6.10.9B.

Diagnosis

Metastatic adrenal cortical carcinoma.

At surgical exploration, the brown recurrence was resected and the smaller metastasis was not found. Eight months later, follow-up PET and CT scan demonstrated a 3 cm metastasis in the right adrenal bed.

Index

MIX
Papier aus verantwortungsvollen Quellen
Paper from responsible sources
FSC® C105338

If you have any concerns about our products,
you can contact us on
ProductSafety@springernature.com

In case Publisher is established outside the EU,
the EU authorized representative is:
Springer Nature Customer Service Center GmbH
Europaplatz 3, 69115 Heidelberg, Germany

Printed by Libri Plureos GmbH
in Hamburg, Germany